CLINICAL GASTROENTEROLOGY

Series Editor
George Y. Wu
University of Connecticut Health Center, Farmington, CT, USA

For further volumes:
http://www.springer.com/series/7672

DIARRHEA
DIAGNOSTIC AND THERAPEUTIC ADVANCES

Edited by

STEFANO GUANDALINI, MD

The University of Chicago Celiac Disease Center, Division of Pediatric Gastroenterology, Hepatology and Nutrition, Chicago, IL

HALEH VAZIRI, MD

University of Connecticut Health Center, Division of Gastroenterology, Farmington, CT

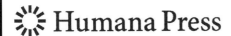

Editors
Stefano Guandalini, MD
University of Chicago
  Celiac Disease Center
Division of Pediatric Gastroenterology,
  Hepatology & Nutrition
S. Maryland Ave. 5839
60637 Chicago, IL
MC 4065
USA
sguandalini@peds.bsd.uchicago.edu

Haleh Vaziri, MD
University of Connecticut
  Health Center
Division of Gastroenterology
Farmington Ave. 263
06030-1845 Farmington, CT
USA
hvaziri@uchc.edu

ISBN 978-1-60761-182-0   e-ISBN 978-1-60761-183-7
DOI 10.1007/978-1-60761-183-7
Springer New York Dordrecht Heidelberg London

Library of Congress Control Number: 2010936275

© Springer Science+Business Media, LLC 2011
All rights reserved. This work may not be translated or copied in whole or in part without the written permission of the publisher (Humana Press, c/o Springer Science+Business Media, LLC, 233 Spring Street, New York, NY 10013, USA), except for brief excerpts in connection with reviews or scholarly analysis. Use in connection with any form of information storage and retrieval, electronic adaptation, computer software, or by similar or dissimilar methodology now known or hereafter developed is forbidden.
The use in this publication of trade names, trademarks, service marks, and similar terms, even if they are not identified as such, is not to be taken as an expression of opinion as to whether or not they are subject to proprietary rights.
While the advice and information in this book are believed to be true and accurate at the date of going to press, neither the authors nor the editors nor the publisher can accept any legal responsibility for any errors or omissions that may be made. The publisher makes no warranty, express or implied, with respect to the material contained herein.

Printed on acid-free paper

Humana Press is part of Springer Science+Business Media (www.springer.com)

PREFACE

When we were asked by the Springer Company to consider editing a new book regarding advances on diarrheal diseases, we immediately thought that this was an exciting idea. In fact, in spite of the ongoing vast interest that this wide-reaching medical problem elicits worldwide, there is an evident lack of recent books presenting updates on the numerous disorders that the clinician may be faced with when managing a patient with acute or chronic diarrhea in a concise, easy-to-read manner. Thus, we worked at building a book with the aim of providing in a conveniently accessible package a comprehensive collection of accurate and timely information on the management of diarrhea in pediatric and adult patients.

The final product has a clinically-oriented tone directed to the practicing physician in a broad range of qualifications and settings including pediatric and medicine residents' fellows pursuing a career in gastroenterology and physicians practicing in academic and non-academic medical environments.

In the 27 chapters, well-known and respected authorities from North America and Europe have joined forces in covering diverse issues, from the rarest to the most common, so as to offer the reader an exhaustive yet concise view on disorders ranging from the very benign to the life-threatening. The last two chapters, by the editors, provide a simplified empirical approach to the patient with diarrhea and an update on the emerging role of probiotics.

It is our hope and expectation that the readers will find the book enjoyable and, most importantly, helpful in their daily practice when facing patients with challenging diarrheal disorders.

Chicago, Illinois   *Stefano Guandalini*
Farmington, Connecticut   *Haleh Vaziri*

CONTENTS

Preface v

Contents vii

Contributors ix

1 *Definition, Epidemiology, Pathophysiology, Clinical Classification, and Differential Diagnosis of Diarrhea* *1*
Udayakumar Navaneethan and Ralph A. Giannella

2 *Infectious Gastroenteritis and Colitis* *33*
Jennifer M. Newton and Christina M. Surawicz

3 *Inflammatory Bowel Disease* *61*
Steven Bernick and Sunanda Kane

4 *Eosinophilic Enteritis* *81*
Charles W. DeBrosse and Li Zuo

5 *Microscopic Colitis* *93*
Darrell S. Pardi

6 *Food Allergy* *105*
Stefano Guandalini

7 *Protein-Losing Enteropathies* *117*
Jonathan Goldstein and Richard Wright

8 *Radiation Enterocolitis* *141*
Einar G. Lurix, Jorge A. Zapatier and Andrew Ukleja

9 *Congenital Disorders of Digestion and Absorption* *159*
Douglas Mogul and Eric Sibley

10 *Pancreatic Exocrine Insufficiency* *177*
Alphonso Brown and Steven D. Freedman

11 *Bacterial Overgrowth* *189*
Rosemary J. Young and Jon A. Vanderhoof

12 *Celiac Disease* *209*
Stefano Guandalini

13 *Whipple Disease* *225*
George T. Fantry

Contents

14 Surgical Conditions Presenting with Diarrhea *237*
Erica M. Carlisle and Mindy B. Statter

15 Chronic Diarrheal Disorders due to Endocrine Neoplasms . . . *265*
Tanvi Dhere, Julia Massaad and Shanthi V. Sitaraman

16 Diarrhea from Enterotoxins *281*
Gianluca Terrin and Roberto Berni Canani

17 Factitious Diarrhea *299*
Erica N. Roberson and Arnold Wald

18 Chronic Idiopathic Diarrhea *311*
Lawrence R. Schiller

19 Irritable Bowel Syndrome *325*
Arnold Wald

**20 Functional Diarrhea (Non-specific Chronic Diarrhea,
Toddler Diarrhea)** *341*
Roberto Gomez and Marc A. Benninga

21 Diarrhea Related to Non-neoplastic Endocrine Diseases *357*
Ashwani K. Singal MD, Nischita K. Reddy and Don W. Powell

22 Alcohol-Related Diarrhea *379*
Nischita K. Reddy, Ashwani Singal and Don W. Powell

23 Drug-Induced Diarrhea *393*
Bincy P. Abraham and Joseph H. Sellin

24 Runner's Diarrhea *425*
Daniel Triezenberg and Stephen M. Simons

25 Evaluation of Patients with Diarrhea and Timing of Referral . . *431*
Chami Amaratunge and Joseph H. Sellin

26 Empiric Treatment of Chronic Diarrhea *443*
Maria Soriano and Haleh Vaziri

27 Probiotics for Diarrheal Diseases *459*
Stefano Guandalini

Subject Index *475*

CONTRIBUTORS

BINCY P. ABRAHAM • *Gastroenterology and Hepatology Section, Baylor College of Medicine, Houston, TX 77030, USA*

CHAMI AMARATUNGE • *Ben Taub General Hospital, Division of Gastroenterology, Baylor College of Medicine, Houston, TX, USA*

M.A. BENNINGA • *Department of Pediatric Gastroenterology and Nutrition, Emma Children's Hospital/Academic Medical Center, Meibergdreef 9, 1105 AZ Amsterdam, the Netherlands*

STEVEN BERNICK • *Naval Hospital, San Diego, CA, USA*

ALPHONSO BROWN • *The Pancreas Center: Beth Israel Deaconess Medical, Dana 501, 330 Brookline Ave, Boston, MA 02215, USA*

ROBERTO BERNI CANANI • *Department of Pediatrics and European Laboratory for the Investigation on Food Induced Diseases University of Naples "Federico II" Via Pansini 5, 80131, Naples, Italy*

ERICA M. CARLISLE • *Department of Surgery, The University of Chicago, 5841 S. Maryland Ave., 60637, Chicago, IL, USA*

CHARLES W. DEBROSSE • *Division of Allergy and Immunology, Department of Pediatrics, Cincinnati Children's Hospital Medical Center, University of Cincinnati, College of Medicine, Cincinnati, OH, USA*

TANVI DHERE • *Department of Medicine, Division of Digestive Diseases, Emory University, 615 Michael Street, Atlanta, GA, USA*

GEORGE T. FANTRY • *Division of Gastroenterology and Hepatology, University of Maryland School of Medicine, 22 S. Greene St., Baltimore, MD 21201-1595, USA*

STEVEN D. FREEDMAN • *The Pancreas Center: Beth Israel Deaconess Medical Center, Dana 501, 330 Brookline Ave, Boston, MA 02215, USA*

RALPH A. GIANNELLA • *Division of Digestive diseases, Department of Internal Medicine, University of Cincinnati College of Medicine, 231 Albert Sabin Way ML 0595, Cincinnati, OH, USA*

JONATHAN GOLDSTEIN • *Division of Gastroenterology/Hepatology, University of Louisville School of Medicine, Louisville, KY, USA*

ROBERTO GOMEZ • *Division of Pediatric Gastroenterology, University of Alabama at Birmingham, Birmingham, AL, USA*

STEFANO GUANDALINI • *University of Chicago Comer Children's Hospital, 5841 S. Maryland Ave. MC 4065, Chicago, IL, USA*

SUNANDA KANE • *Division of Gastroenterology and Hepatology, Mayo Clinic College of Medicine, 200 First Street SW, Rochester, MN 55905, USA*

EINAR G. LURIX • *Department of Gastroenterology, Cleveland Clinic Florida, Weston, FL, USA*

JULIA MASSAAD • *Department of Medicine, Division of Digestive Diseases, Emory University, 615 Michael Street, Atlanta, GA, USA*

DOUGLAS MOGUL • *John Hopkins University School of Medicine, Baltimore, MD 21287, USA*

UDAYAKUMAR NAVANEETHAN • *Division of Digestive diseases, Department of Internal Medicine, University of Cincinnati College of Medicine, Cincinnati, OH, USA*

JENNIFER M. NEWTON • *Department of Medicine, University of Washington, Seattle, WA, USA*

DARRELL S. PARDI • *Inflammatory Bowel Disease Clinic, Division of Gastroenterology and Hepatology, Mayo Clinic College of Medicine, 200 First Street SW, Rochester, MN, USA*

DON W. POWELL • *Division of Gastroenterology and Hepatology, Department of Internal Medicine, The University of Texas Medical Branch, 301 Univ. Blvd, Galveston, TX 77555-0764, USA*

NISCHITA K. REDDY • *Division of Gastroenterology and Hepatology, Department of Internal Medicine, The University of Texas Medical Branch, Galveston, TX, USA*

ERICA N. ROBERSON • *University of Wisconsin School of Medicine and Public Health, Section of Gastroenterology and Hepatology UWHC-H6/516, 750 Highland Avenue, Madison, WI 53705-2221, USA*

LAWRENCE R. SCHILLER • *Digestive Health Associates of Texas, Baylor University Medical Center, Dallas, TX, USA, University of Texas Southwestern Medical Center, Dallas, TX, USA*

JOSEPH H. SELLIN • *Ben Taub General Hospital, Division of Gastroenterology, Baylor College of Medicine, 1709 Dryden St., Suite 800, Houston, TX, USA*

ERIC SIBLEY • *Department of Pediatrics, Division of Gastroenterology, Hepatology and Nutrition, Stanford University Medical School of Medicine, 300 Pasteur Drive G310, Stanford, CA 94305-5208, USA*

STEPHEN M. SIMONS • *611 Saint Joseph Regional Medical Center, East Douglas, Suite 137, Mishawaka, IN 46545, USA*

ASHWANI K. SINGAL • *Division of Gastroenterology and Hepatology, Department of Internal Medicine, The University of Texas Medical Branch, Galveston, TX, USA*

SHANTHI V. SITARAMAN • *Department of Medicine, Division of Digestive Diseases, Emory University, 615 Michael Street, Whitehead Research Bldg, Rm 201, Atlanta, GA 30322, USA*

MARIA SORIANO • *Division of Gastroenterology, University of Connecticut, Farmington, CT, USA*

MINDY B. STATTER • *Department of Surgery, Section of Pediatric Surgery, The University of Chicago, 5841 S. Maryland Avenue MC 4062, Chicago, IL 60637, USA*

CHRISTINA M. SURAWICZ • *Department of Medicine, Harborview Medical Center, University of Washington, Box 359773, 325 9th Ave, Seattle, WA 98104, USA*

GIANLUCA TERRIN • *Department of Pediatrics and European Laboratory for the Investigation on Food Induced Diseases University of Naples "Federico II", Naples, Italy*

DANIEL TRIEZENBERG • *Associate Director, Family Medicine Residency Saint Joseph Regional Medical Center 837 East Cedar, Suite 100 South Bend, IN 46617*

ANDREW UKLEJA • *Department of Gastroenterology, Cleveland Clinic Florida, 2950 Cleveland Clinic Boulevard, Weston, FL 33331, USA*

JON A. VANDERHOOF • *Children's Hospital, Boston, MA, USA; Harvard Medical School, Boston, MA, USA*

HALEH VAZIRI • *Department of Medicine, Division of Gastroenterology and Hepatology, 263 Farmington Avenue, University of Connecticut Health Center, Farmington, CT 06030, USA*

ARNOLD WALD • *University of Wisconsin School of Medicine and Public Health, Section of Gastroenterology and Hepatology UWHC-H6/516, 750 Highland Avenue, Madison, WI 53705-2221, USA*

RICHARD WRIGHT • *Division of Gastroenterology/Hepatology, University of Louisville School of Medicine, Louisville, KY 40292, USA*

ROSEMARY J. YOUNG • *Boys Town National Research Hospital, Boys Town, NE, USA*

JORGE A. ZAPATIER • *Department of Internal Medicine, Cleveland Clinic Florida, Weston, FL, USA*

LI ZUO • *Division of Allergy and Immunology, Department of Pediatrics, Cincinnati Children's Hospital Medical Center, University of Cincinnati, College of Medicine, Cincinnati, OH, USA*

1

Definition, Epidemiology, Pathophysiology, Clinical Classification, and Differential Diagnosis of Diarrhea

Udayakumar Navaneethan, MD and Ralph A. Giannella, MD

CONTENTS

INTRODUCTION
DEFINITION
EPIDEMIOLOGY
PATHOPHYSIOLOGY OF DIARRHEA
SECRETORY DIARRHEA
OSMOTIC DIARRHEA
INFLAMMATORY DIARRHEA
IATROGENIC-/DRUG-INDUCED DIARRHEA
FUNCTIONAL DIARRHEA
CLINICAL CLASSIFICATION
   AND DIFFERENTIAL DIAGNOSIS
REFERENCES

Summary

Diarrhea continues to be a challenge despite developments in science and remains a considerable source of morbidity and mortality. A wide variety of differential diagnoses need to be considered when evaluating patients with diarrhea. Diarrhea can be classified based

From: *Diarrhea, Clinical Gastroenterology*
Edited by: S. Guandalini, H. Vaziri, DOI 10.1007/978-1-60761-183-7_1
© Springer Science+Business Media, LLC 2011

on the duration into acute, persistent, and chronic diarrhea and this classification is important for diagnostic and treatment considerations. The epidemiological settings where diarrhea is seen help the clinician to narrow down the differential causes of diarrhea and to investigate appropriately. Acute diarrhea can happen in the setting of the community or it can be hospital acquired or acquired during travel. The etiologies and the diagnostic algorithms are different for each of these settings. The pathophysiolgy of diarrhea can be classified based on the mechanism into secretory, osmotic, inflammatory, iatrogenic/drug related, and functional/motility-related diarrhea. The differential diagnosis and the clinical classification depend on the basic pathophysiology with which diarrhea presents and can be inflammatory, watery encompassing osmotic and secretory, and fatty diarrhea. Gaining a better understanding of the pathophysiology of diarrhea will help us to initiate better preventive and treatment measures to improve the quality of life of these patients.

Key Words: Osmotic diarrhea, Secretory diarrhea, Inflammatory diarrhea, Pathophysiology, Epidemiology, Definitions, Acute diarrhea, Chronic diarrhea, Persistent diarrhea, Iatrogenic diarrhea, Drug-induced diarrhea, Functional/motility-related diarrhea

INTRODUCTION

Diarrhea is one of the most common complaints faced by internists and primary care physicians and accounts for many referrals to gastroenterologists. Acute infectious diarrhea contributes to significant morbidity and mortality worldwide with close to 70% of diarrhea being food borne [1]. The Centers for Disease Control and Prevention (CDC) estimates that 76 million food borne illnesses occur annually in the United States, resulting in 325,000 hospitalizations and 5200 deaths [2]. In a report by the American Academy of Microbiology on the global burden of gastrointestinal diseases in 2002, it was estimated that 6–60 billion cases of gastrointestinal illness occur annually throughout the world [3]. A recent World Health Organization (WHO) report estimates that 1.8 million people died, worldwide, from diarrheal diseases in 2005 [4]. Although the estimates of global mortality from diarrhea declined from approximately 4.6 million annual deaths during the mid-1980s [5] to the current estimate of 1.8 million [4], the morbidity of this syndrome remains substantial [5]. Most of the case fatalities and morbidities occur in children below the age of 5 years [5]. Also the incidence of gastrointestinal infections continues to increase [6]. A recent epidemiological study from the National Commission for

Chapter 1 / Clinical Classification and Pathophysiology of Diarrhea 3

Digestive Diseases reported that the rate of age-adjusted hospitalizations from gastrointestinal infections increased by 92.8% between 1979 (76.1 per 100,000) and 2004 (146.7 per 100,000) [6]. With the rising incidence and severity of *Clostridium difficile* infection, the morbidity and mortality is expected to increase still further [7].

Additionally, most of the morbidity estimates do not account for the malnutrition caused by persistent diarrhea and enteropathy resulting from chronic and recurring enteric infections and its attendant effect on growth and development [8]. Thus the actual morbidity may be much higher than estimated [8]. In developing countries, infectious diarrheas are frequently disabling and contribute significantly to malnutrition and mortality in children [9], while in the USA and other Western countries, they are a major cause of morbidity, physician visits/hospitalizations, and loss from work or school [10].

In contrast to acute diarrhea, chronic diarrhea is less common but often presents diagnostic challenges and can be very difficult to manage. The economic impact of chronic diarrhea has not been well studied. Available data estimate that chronic diarrhea costs more than $350,000,000 annually from work-loss alone [11]. Chronic diarrhea can also decrease quality of life. Although no studies have been done to accurately assess the effect of diarrhea on quality of life, chronic diarrhea was shown to be an independent predictor of decreased quality of life in HIV-infected patients [12].

DEFINITION

Diarrhea is generally defined as the passage of abnormally liquid or unformed stools associated with increased frequency of defecation [13]. Increased frequency is defined by three or more bowel movements a day [14]. However, most patients base their diarrhea on the consistency of the stool rather than the frequency of bowel movements [15]. Since the consistency of the stool is difficult to quantitate, diarrhea is often defined based on stool frequency or the stool weight alone. On a typical Western diet, the normal stool output varies from 100 to 200 g/day. Hence stool weight >200 g/day is considered diarrhea [13]; however, some people who consume excess fiber have stool weights of 300 g/day or more with normal consistency which does not necessarily mean diarrhea. Thus a combination of frequency, stool consistency, and stool weight should be taken into account for defining diarrhea [13].

Diarrhea may be further classified as acute if the duration is less than 2 weeks, persistent if the duration varies from 2 to 4 weeks, and chronic if it lasts more than 4 weeks in duration [13]. This distinction is important since the etiologies of each are different and the clinical approach and investigations vary.

EPIDEMIOLOGY

Acute Diarrhea

Acute diarrhea can occur in various epidemiological settings including community acquired, hospital acquired, and during travel (traveler's diarrhea). Understanding of the epidemiological settings in which diarrhea occurs directs the approach to diagnosis and treatment. Classification of acute diarrhea based on this approach is discussed in great detail in a recent article [16].

COMMUNITY-ACQUIRED DIARRHEA

In the USA and other developed nations, viral-induced diarrheas are the most common of community-acquired diarrheas and account for at least 30–40% of acute episodes of diarrhea [17]. Among the viruses, noroviruses and rotaviruses are the most common. Norovirus (old term Norwalk virus), a member of the calicivirus family, affects people of all ages. Norovirus contributes approximately to 40–60% of nonbacterial gastroenteritis affecting 23 million people annually in the USA and is the leading cause of gastroenteritis in the USA [17, 18]. Rotavirus predominantly affects children below 5 years and is also the leading cause of diarrhea-associated death in children below 5 years worldwide [19]. It is responsible for childhood diarrhea in 35% of hospitalized and 10–30% of community-based cases. Although rotavirus predominantly affects children, adults can also be affected as immunity wanes off and outbreaks tend to occur in close settings where chances of person-to-person transmission are higher such as day care centers, long-term care facilities, and schools [20].

In the USA, the most common bacterial causes of diarrhea include *Campylobacter*, nontyphoidal *Salmonella*, *Shigella*, and enterohemorrhagic *Escherichia coli* (EHEC). *Campylobacter* infection is transmitted predominantly from infected animals and their food products and most human infections (50–70%) appear to be related to consumption of improperly cooked, contaminated chicken [21]. *Campylobacter jejuni*, in fact, may be one of the most commonly encountered etiologies of acute bacterial diarrhea in the USA [22]. Nontyphoidal salmonellosis is seen worldwide and one of the most common causes of food poisoning and diarrhea in the USA. Close to 1.4 million cases of *Salmonella* food poisoning cases occur annually in the USA [2]. Transmission to humans appears to occur most commonly from infected animals and their food products. Most human infections are related to consumption of improperly cooked or contaminated poultry, although a variety of vehicles can transmit salmonellosis [21]. Shigellosis is common and accounts for 10–20% of enteric infections throughout the world. It is seen commonly in children below 5 years of age, although adults of all ages are also susceptible [21]. It can survive in acidic conditions and a very small inoculum of the organism (less than 100 organisms) is sufficient to produce disease [23]. EHEC is one of the commonest causes of bloody diarrhea in the USA [24]. The disease occurs throughout the USA but is more common in northern part of the country such as in Massachusetts, Minnesota, and the Pacific Northwest [21]. Infection usually occurs in summer between June and September and occurs primarily by ingestion of undercooked hamburgers and meat patties [25, 26]. Enteroaggregative *E. coli* (EAEC) is a recently recognized cause of community-acquired diarrhea and affects children and adults of both developing and developed countries [27]. EAEC has been shown to cause acute and/or persistent diarrhea in 10–44% of patients with HIV infection and childhood diarrheas in developing countries [28]. *Clostridium difficile* infection (CDI) is also recently reported as a cause of community-acquired diarrhea. Approximately 22–44% of patients who developed community-acquired CDI lacked the traditional risk factors like recent hospitalization, being elderly or having an underlying health condition [29, 30].

In developing countries, bacterial and protozoal infections are more common causes of acute diarrhea than in developed countries. Poor sanitation predisposes to community-acquired infection with enteric bacterial pathogens and protozoa including *Vibrio cholerae*, enterotoxigenic, enteropathogenic and enteroinvasive *E. coli* (ETEC, EPEC and EIEC, respectively), amoeba, giardia, and intestinal parasites. Worldwide, cholera is one of the most common causes of diarrhea and is seen predominantly in the Indian subcontinent, Southeast Asia, Africa, and South America. In the USA, sporadic cases have been seen along the Gulf coast [31]. Another *Vibrio* species, *Vibrio parahemolyticus* is more common in the USA occurring sporadically along the coastal USA [21]. Pathogenic *E. coli* are classified based on their pathogenic mechanisms into ETEC, EPEC, EIEC, EAEC, and EHEC. ETEC are seen in children living in developing countries. ETEC infections are not common in the USA. Some cities in the USA have reported sporadic cases [21]. It is commonly seen in travelers from USA to developing world where ETEC is prevalent. This pathogen also contributes to outbreaks of gastroenteritis on cruise ships [32]. EIEC is seen predominantly in tropical countries including Thailand [33], though occasional cases of EIEC occur in the USA. It usually presents with watery diarrhea with occasional reports of dysentery [21].

Intestinal protozoa are important causes of diarrhea in the developing world. *Entamoeba histolytica* is one of the most important causes of diarrhea/dysentery worldwide [34] with 34–50 million symptomatic (amebic colitis or abscess) infections [35] leading to 40,000–100,000 deaths annually [36]. In the USA, *Cryptosporidium* and *Giardia lamblia* are the most commonly implicated intestinal protozoa to cause diarrhea associated with 50.8 and 40.6% of waterborne outbreaks, respectively [36, 37]. *Giardia* infection is commonly seen in children in day care facilities, men who have sex with men, as well as in the normal host [37, 38]. A longitudinal study in a US day care center reported *Giardia* cysts at some time in the stool of more than 30% of children over the course of a year [39]. Worldwide, *Giardia* infects infants more commonly than adults and in highly endemic regions, recurrent infections in childhood can result in malnutrition [40, 41]. *Cryptosporidium* infection while commonly seen in HIV-infected individuals can also cause self-limited diarrhea in immunocompetent persons and severe diarrhea resulting in malnutrition in children and elderly as well [42]. It is mostly associated with outbreaks caused by contaminated water sources. The duration and severity of the infection however is directly related to the CD4 count [42]. Other protozoal and parasitic infections that are reported include *Blastocystis, microsporidia (Enterocytozoon* spp., *Encephalitozoon* spp.*), Isospora, Cyclospora, Schistosoma,* and *Strongyloides. Cyclospora* outbreaks [43, 44] are associated with Guatemalan raspberries in the USA both in HIV-infected individuals and normal hosts [45], while microsporidia are seen only in immunocompromised hosts with impaired cell-mediated immunity from AIDS or organ transplantation [46, 47]. The disease is only reported with a CD4 count of less than 200. *Isospora* is seen throughout tropical areas around the world and can affect immunocompetent children and HIV-infected individuals [48].

HOSPITAL-ACQUIRED DIARRHEA

Hospital-acquired diarrhea is defined by the onset of diarrhea 3 days after hospitalization and not incubating at the time of admission to the hospital [16]. Distinguishing community-acquired and hospital-acquired diarrhea may be difficult as the possibility of the infection incubating at the time of admission to the hospital cannot be completely excluded. Hospital-acquired diarrhea can be antibiotic associated or related to the use of nonantibiotic medications or the use of tube feeds in hospitalized patients [16]. However, CDI is the most common

Chapter 1 / Clinical Classification and Pathophysiology of Diarrhea 7

recognizable infectious cause of antibiotic-associated diarrhea in the developed world [49]. The frequency of this infection has increased dramatically and is now recognized as the most common cause of hospital-acquired infectious diarrhea in developed countries.

A recent paper reported a 23% increase in the hospitalizations attributed to CDI from 2000 to 2005 in the USA [50]. The mortality rate of CDI in the USA also increased from 5.7 per million populations in 1999 to 23.7 per million in 2004 [51]. This is attributed to a hyper-virulent form of *C. difficile* strain, BI/NAP1/027 that is associated with a more severe and complicated disease and a higher mortality [52, 53]. This hypervirulent strain is identified in at least 38 states in the USA [54, 55] and its virulence is related to increased toxin production, as well as a binary toxin and resistance to fluoroquinolones [52, 53].

Although CDI is the most common cause in developed nations, *Salmonella* has been implicated as a prominent cause of hospital-acquired diarrhea in developing countries along with other enteropathogens [56]. *Salmonella* infection occurs in a more severe form in immunocompromised patients. Similar to community-acquired infection, contaminated food, person-to-person spread, and chemotherapy predispose to *Salmonella* infection [57–59].

Although protozoa are rarely implicated in the setting of hospital-acquired diarrhea and cryptosporidial infection remains the most common cause in the USA, there are also reports of coinfection with *C. difficile* and *Cryptosporidium* [60]. Among the viruses, norovirus and rotavirus may be responsible for hospital-acquired viral diarrheas both in the developing and the developed world [61–63].

TRAVELER'S DIARRHEA

Traveler's diarrhea is defined as the passage of ≥ 3 unformed stools that occur within a 24-h period, accompanied by one other symptom or sign of enteric infection, including abdominal cramps or pain, excessive gas, nausea, fever, blood or mucous in stools, tenesmus, and vomiting [64]. The US Department of Commerce estimated that 30 million people from the USA visited developing regions with the majority traveling to Mexico [16]. Among these, it is estimated that 40–60% of US travelers to Mexico develop diarrheal illness during short periods of travel and bacterial pathogens contribute in up to 85% of cases [65].

The frequency of traveler's diarrhea varies between 4 and 40% with the highest rates (40%) seen in Latin America, Africa (except South Africa), most of the Middle East, and the Indian subcontinent [66]. The lowest rates of traveler's diarrhea (<4%) are seen in travelers to the USA, Canada, western Europe, Japan, Australia, and New Zealand, whereas intermediate rates (8–15%) are seen for travelers to China, Russia, eastern Europe, and South Africa [66, 67].

A variety of host, genetic, and environmental factors predispose to traveler's diarrhea. Genetic factors in the form of polymorphisms in the lactoferrin [68] and osteoprotegerin gene [69], young age, length of stay, immunosuppression, and low gastric acidity can predispose to traveler's diarrhea [70, 71].

Traveler's diarrhea can present either as an acute gastroenteritis with vomiting, watery diarrhea, dysenteric diarrhea, or as a persistent diarrhea and post-infectious irritable bowel syndrome [66]. The single commonest cause of traveler's diarrhea is ETEC, while EAEC and diffusely adherent *E. coli* (DAEC) are also common [66, 72]. The most common form of transmission is food borne rather than water borne [73, 74]. A majority of cases in the high-risk regions is caused by DAEC, while invasive enteropathogens, including *Campylobacter, Shigella* spp., and *Salmonella* spp. are more commonly seen in south Asia [66]. Around 20–40% of patients with traveler's diarrhea do not have an identifiable etiology even after an extensive microbiological evaluation, although they may respond to antibiotics [66]. Noroviruses are responsible for up to 15% of patients and are the most common nonbacterial cause for traveler's diarrhea [66]. Viral diarrheas are seen in people traveling in cruise ships and also among students traveling to Mexico [75, 76]. Rotavirus and astrovirus are also responsible for traveler's diarrhea in a small proportion of travelers. Travel to Asia seems to particularly predispose to *E. histolytica* as well as other parasitic causes for diarrhea [77].

Persistent Diarrhea

Persistent diarrhea is defined as diarrhea lasting from 2 to 4 weeks. Infectious etiologies predominate as a cause of persistent diarrhea similar to those of acute diarrheas [16]. The etiology varies depending on the region (developing or developed), recent travel history, and the immune function of the underlying host. Persistent diarrhea can be associated with significant morbidity due to the associated nutrient malabsorption that may often accompany the diarrhea [16]. In developing countries, EPEC and EAEC are the most commonly responsible bacterial pathogens in persistent diarrhea, whereas *Campylobacter* and *Salmonella* are rare. In developed countries, viruses including Norovirus and rotavirus can contribute to persistent diarrhea, particularly among children [78]. ETEC, EHEC, and *Shigella* are predominant causes of acute diarrhea and do not cause persistent diarrhea.

Intestinal protozoa are another common cause of persistent diarrhea. *Giardia* and *Cryptosporidium* are most often responsible followed by *Entamoeba* and *Isospora*, particularly in HIV-positive patients [79]. In the USA, protozoan infections are the most common cause of persistent diarrhea in immunocompromised patients including HIV and the elderly and *Giardia* and *Cryptosporidium* are commonly encountered [16].

Chronic Diarrhea

Chronic diarrhea is defined as diarrhea lasting more than 4 weeks. The prevalence of chronic diarrhea is variable depending on the population surveyed and the inconsistency in the definition of chronic diarrhea. However, if based on the criterion of excessive stool frequency (>3 times/day) or loose stools (more than 25% of the time), the prevalence of chronic diarrhea in the USA varies from 14 to 18% [80, 81]. A majority of these patients may have irritable bowel syndrome with co-existing abdominal pain. When patients with abdominal pain are excluded, the reported prevalence is 3% [82]. The prevalence of chronic diarrhea based on increased stool frequency alone is approximately 5% [81–83].

The etiologies of chronic diarrhea vary depending on the region and the socio-economic status. In developed countries including the USA, irritable bowel syndrome, inflammatory bowel disease, malabsorption syndrome, and chronic infections predominate [84, 85], whereas in developing countries, chronic bacterial, mycobacterial, and parasitic infections are the most common causes of chronic diarrhea [86, 87].

PATHOPHYSIOLOGY OF DIARRHEA

As diarrhea is the end result of a derangement in the normal physiology of the intestinal handling of water and electrolyte absorption and secretion, an understanding of these processes is preliminary for the understanding of the pathophysiological changes that lead to diarrhea.

Normal Physiology

Under normal physiological conditions, approximately 8 l of fluids reach the upper small bowel. This includes 2 l of ingested fluids and the remaining 6 l from salivary, gastric, biliary, and pancreatic secretions. Most of this fluid is reabsorbed before reaching the distal small bowel so that only about 1 l of fluid enters the colon [88]. The colon reabsorbs almost all of this fluid and the remaining; usually less than 200 ml is excreted in the stool. The colon has the capacity to reabsorb up to a maximum of 3–4 liters of fluid [89] and thus to salvage much of the fluid that might be lost in small intestinal malabsorptive conditions.

There is a constant bidirectional flux of water and ions across the small intestinal mucosa, i.e., absorption and secretion. Absorption occurs in villus cells and secretion largely by crypt cells [90]. Sodium and water absorption by enterocytes is mediated by an active, adenosine triphosphate (ATP)-dependent active sodium (Na) pump (Na, K-ATPase) located on the basolateral membranes of intestinal crypt and villus cells [91]. In the intestine, solute movement creates the osmotic force for fluid movement. Na absorption drives fluid reabsorption, while active Cl secretion contributes to water secretion in secretory diarrhea. Small intestinal Na absorption is mediated primarily by two mechanisms: a glucose- or amino acid-stimulated cotransport in which Na accompanies the other solute and a coupled Na–Cl mechanism. The latter is a combination of Na–H exchange and Cl–HCO$_3$ exchange. Short-chain fatty acid (SCFA)-mediated Na absorption and aldosterone-sensitive Na absorption occur in the colon [91]. Among the various mechanisms described, the coupled Na–Cl pathways are primarily regulated by cyclic adenosine monophosphate (cAMP) levels and also by cGMP and intracellular Ca levels [92]. In addition to the transporters, there are multiple extracellular factors regulating epithelial ion transport – paracrine, immunological, neural, and endocrine factors, termed together as a single regulatory system termed as PINES (paracrine–immuno-neuroendocrine system) [93].

In addition to the absorptive and secretary function of the intestine, motor functions also play a key role in facilitating digestion and absorption of fluids and nutrients. Synchronized migrating motor complexes normally occur during fasting in the stomach and small bowel with increased contractions following feeding with the total small bowel transit time of approximately 3 h for the food to reach the colon [94]. In the colon, there is further reabsorption with the ascending and transverse colon serving as reservoirs and with the sigmoid and rectum serving as volitional reservoirs [95]. Any disturbance in the coordinated flux of water and ions and motility can result in the clinical syndrome of diarrhea.

Physiological Disturbances in Diarrhea

Diarrheal syndromes result from disturbances in any of the basic pathophysiological processes including osmosis, active secretion, exudation or inflammation, and altered motility [92]. Osmotic forces contribute to diarrhea when poorly absorbable solutes remaining in the gastrointestinal lumen retain water and electrolytes resulting in

Chapter 1 / Clinical Classification and Pathophysiology of Diarrhea   11

reduced water reabsorption. Active secretion can play a vital role in the pathophysiology of diarrhea as seen in cholera [96] or in celiac disease. Other secretory stimuli include other bacterial enterotoxins [96], hormones from endocrine neoplasms, dihydroxy bile acids, hydroxylated fatty acids, and inflammatory mediators [92]. Exudation or inflammation can contribute to diarrhea when the intestinal epithelium's barrier function is compromised by loss of epithelial cells or disruption of tight junctions as occurs in invasive diarrhea due to *Shigella/Salmonella* [96] and inflammatory disease process as in ulcerative colitis (UC) or Crohn's disease (CD) [97]. Motility disturbances can result in diarrhea as occurring in thyrotoxicosis and opiate withdrawal [98]. Similarly slowing of the motor function of the small intestine as with narcotic use, scleroderma, diabetic autonomic neuropathy, and amyloidosis can result in bacterial overgrowth and hence diarrhea [98].

For understanding the pathophysiology of diarrhea, we have classified diarrheal syndromes into secretory or toxin induced, osmotic or malabsorption induced, inflammatory, iatrogenic/drug-induced, and functional diarrhea. Most etiologies will have a complex pathophysiology involving one or more of these mentioned mechanisms.

- Secretory diarrhea
- Osmotic diarrhea
- Inflammatory diarrhea
- Iatrogenic or drug-induced diarrhea
- Functional-/motility-related diarrhea

SECRETORY DIARRHEA

A number of disease processes produce secretory diarrhea. The basic pathophysiology involves either net secretion of ions (chloride or bicarbonate) or inhibition of net sodium absorption [99]. Net intestinal secretion is most often secondary to the stimulation of active chloride secretion and to the inhibition of active absorption of sodium and chloride by messengers such as cyclic AMP (see below).

The driving force for intestinal ion secretion can arise from the gut lumen as with infectious diarrhea (enterotoxins), from the subepithelial space (inflammatory mediators), or from the systemic circulation (peptide hormones produced from endocrine tumors). Most causes of secretory diarrhea alter the second messenger systems through alteration in cAMP, cGMP, or intracellular calcium-regulated ion transport pathways [91, 92]. Alterations in these mediators cause CFTR-mediated Cl secretion and inhibition of small intestinal-coupled Na–Cl transport.

Infections

The most common cause of secretory diarrhea is infection [99]. Secretory diarrheas are caused by pathogens, which usually affect the small intestine. They adhere to the mucosa disrupting the absorptive/secretary process of enterocyte producing active secretion without causing significant acute inflammation or mucosal destruction. As discussed, enterotoxins through an increase in cAMP, cGMP, or increased intracellular calcium concentration inhibit Na^+–H^+ exchange and stimulate Cl secretion in the small intestine [92, 100]. Secretory diarrhea can also be termed as noninflammatory diarrhea [96]. Thus these classically produce watery diarrhea. Microbial causes include the viruses rotavirus and norovirus, enterotoxigenic *E. coli* (ETEC), *V. cholerae*, *Giardia*, and *Cryptosporidium* infections. Some of the organisms in this group (e.g., cholera, ETEC) elaborate enterotoxins that stimulate intestinal chloride secretion along with impaired sodium absorption. Other pathogens including rotaviruses, noroviruses, and *Cryptosporidium* primarily affect the absorptive villi inhibiting sodium absorption [16].

The pathophysiology of some of the important infectious causes of secretory diarrhea is discussed in other chapters.

Noninfectious Causes of Secretory Diarrhea

Peptide hormones produced by endocrine tumors can also cause secretory diarrhea by stimulating intestinal secretion [101]. Some of these include pancreatic islet tumors which secrete vasoactive intestinal peptide, medullary carcinoma of thyroid-secreting calcitonin, carcinoid tumors which elaborate serotonin, bradykinin, substance P, and prostaglandins [101]. Diarrhea can also result from gastrin secretion from Zollinger–Ellison syndrome. Although it produces a secretory diarrhea, malabsorption also contributes due to inactivation of pancreatic lipase by the persistent acidic pH in the proximal small bowel [92]. Neurotransmitters, such as acetylcholine and serotonin, and other modulators, such as histamine in systemic mastocytosis and inflammatory cytokines, are also potent secretory stimuli [102].

Malabsorbed bile salts and fatty acids can also induce secretory diarrhea. Under normal conditions, reabsorption of conjugated bile acids occurs in the distal ileum via Na–bile acid cotransport. However with severe ileal CD or after ileal resection, some of the bile acids are not absorbed and spill into the colon and stimulate colonic secretion. This involves both intracellular Ca^{2+} (probably secondary to membrane phospholipase activation) and cAMP [92]. Similarly, following

Chapter 1 / Clinical Classification and Pathophysiology of Diarrhea   13

a large, greater than 100 cm, ileal resection, malabsorbed fatty acids enter the colon where bacteria add hydroxyl groups resulting in hydroxy fatty acids which also stimulate colonic secretion. In the inflammatory bowel diseases (IBDs), inflammatory mediators such as prostaglandins stimulate colonic secretion, contributing to diarrhea. Cytokines generated in the inflamed mucosa may also downregulate fluid-absorptive mechanisms [103, 104].

Small bowel bacterial overgrowth may also contribute to secretory diarrhea [105–107]. The small bowel is sparsely populated with bacteria. However in patients with motility disturbances (scleroderma or diabetes) or strictures in CD, overgrowth of bacteria in the small bowel can occur [106, 107]. The bacteria deconjugate bile acids and the decrease in concentration of conjugated bile salts results in fat malabsorption. Also the unabsorbed dihydroxy bile acids produce secretory diarrhea as mentioned above.

The congenital absence or alterations in the numerous transporters that maintain the constant flux of the ions and water can result in secretory diarrhea [108]. Rare congenital syndromes are caused by the absence of a specific transport molecule, such as congenital chloridorrhea, congenital sodium diarrhea, and congenital bile acid diarrhea [109–111]. In congenital chloride diarrhea, there is a defect in brush border Cl/HCO_3 exchange in the ileum and the colon and hence impaired absorption of chloride [109]. Congenital sodium diarrhea results from a defect in Na–H exchange in the small bowel, while a secretory diarrhea results from a congenital defect in Na–bile acid absorption in the colon [111].

OSMOTIC DIARRHEA

Osmotic diarrhea occurs either when nonabsorbable or poorly absorbable solutes are ingested or enterocytes or colonocytes cannot absorb them. Nonabsorbable solutes include sugar alcohols such as mannitol or sorbitol. Poorly absorbable solutes include magnesium, sulfates, and phosphates [92, 112]. The osmotic force of the unabsorbed solutes results in driving water and secondarily ions into the gut lumen resulting in diarrhea [92]. Patients with malabsorption may also have osmotic diarrhea, with the malabsorbed nutrients acting as poorly absorbed solutes [113]. Ingested disaccharides require disaccharidase digestion to their constituent monosaccharides to permit absorption, as monosaccharides are the only sugars that can be absorbed. Absence of disaccharidases as in lactase deficiency results in osmotic diarrhea.

Congenital lactase deficiency is extremely rare, while acquired deficiency of lactase may be seen with diseases of the upper small intestine causing loss of absorptive surface. Congenital sucrase–isomaltase and trehalose deficiencies are rare causes of disaccharide-induced osmotic diarrhea [114].

Both celiac disease and tropical sprue can also result in diarrhea. Although a number of mechanisms including both osmotic and secretory forces contribute to diarrhea in celiac disease, the osmotic force of unabsorbed solutes appears to play a major role [115].

INFLAMMATORY DIARRHEA

Many of the diarrheal syndromes are caused by multiple mechanisms including inflammation and exudation of the intestinal mucosa and the interaction between cytokines from immunologically reactive cells, the activity of the enteric nervous system, and the effect of secretory stimuli [108].

Inflammatory diarrhea may result from a wide variety of etiologies including infections and IBDs. Infectious pathogens causing inflammatory diarrheas primarily affect the distal small bowel or the colon [16]. They cause disease by either elaborating cytotoxins or by invading the epithelium with resultant recruitment of inflammatory cells. Cytotoxin-producing, noninvasive organisms include EAEC, EHEC, and *C. dif-ficilex*. Invasive microbes causing this syndrome include *Shigella, Campylobacter, Salmonella, Yersinia*, and *E. histolytica* [96]. Most of the pathogens causing inflammatory diarrhea do so by producing mucosal damage as well as by stimulating intestinal secretion. In some cases, the organisms elaborate enterotoxins, which stimulate intestinal secretion. In addition, the products of the inflammatory reaction and the local synthesis of inflammatory mediators including cytokines and prostaglandins contribute both to mucosal damage and to intestinal secretion. *Clostridium difficile, Shigella, Salmonella, Campylobacter*, and *Entamoeba* infections are discussed in more detail elsewhere in this book.

IBD is one of the most common and important causes of inflammatory diarrhea. Although numerous mechanisms including secretory and osmotic components lead to diarrhea, inflammation and the secondary recruitment of cytokines and eicosanoids play an important role in IBD [95, 97]. Although the initial inflammation and exudation results in diarrhea, numerous and complex mechanisms come into play once there is initial inflammation [96, 97]. The cytokines and eicosanoids initiated by inflammation downregulate the ion transporters in the colon

Chapter 1 / Clinical Classification and Pathophysiology of Diarrhea   15

and small bowel resulting in Na malabsorption [103, 104, 116, 117]. Also bacterial proteins such as flagellin further the inflammatory milieu through the activation of prochemotactic cytokines such as interleukin (IL)-8 [118]. The intestinal epithelial cells may also secrete cytokines such as IL-6 that enhance neutrophil function and hence further the inflammation [119].

Reduction in intestinal blood flow as occurs with mesenteric ischemia can also cause diarrhea [120]. However the exact mechanism is unclear. It is proposed that there may be alterations in the cytokines or neurotransmitters that produced inflammatory and secretory diarrhea. Similarly radiation enteritis can produce an inflammatory diarrhea. Radiation results in activation of intestinal transforming growth factor-β (TGF-β) which is chemotactic and pro-inflammatory, leading to neutrophil infiltration, and hyperplasia of connective tissue mast cells leading to further inflammation [121, 122].

IATROGENIC-/DRUG-INDUCED DIARRHEA

Diarrhea can also result following certain surgical procedures and usage of certain drugs. Diarrhea can follow cholecystectomy in 5–10% of patients, but the exact pathophysiology remains unclear [123]. Some respond to treatment with bile salt-binding resins. Ileal resection in CD can also result in chronic diarrhea. The pathophysiology depends on the extent of resection. With resections less than 100 cm, it is predominantly secretory with malabsorbed dihydroxy bile acids spilling into the colon and stimulating colonic secretion through increase in cyclic AMP [124, 125]. However with resections exceeding 100 cm, there is depletion of the bile acid pool resulting in chronic diarrhea due to fat malabsorption. Colonic bacteria hydroxylate malabsorbed fatty acids and such hydroxyl fatty acids then stimulate colonic secretion [124, 125].

A number of drugs can cause diarrhea. The best known of them are listed in Table 1.2. The pathophysiology of drug-induced diarrhea may involve one or more of the above-mentioned mechanisms. Antibiotic use may alter the bacterial flora in the colon resulting in impaired colonic salvage of malabsorbed carbohydrates resulting in diarrhea. Some of the drugs like lactulose may cause osmotic diarrhea, while others may cause secretory diarrhea. Theophylline may increase intracellular cAMP and fluid secretion, while erythromycin interacts with the motilin receptors increasing the motility to cause diarrhea. Similarly chemotherapeutic drugs may cause diarrhea because of decreased rate of proliferation of the enterocytes [108].

FUNCTIONAL DIARRHEA

The pathophysiology of functional diarrhea or diarrhea associated with irritable bowel syndrome (IBS) may involve multiple mechanisms. Alteration in colonic transit/motility and hypersensitivity of the rectum play a role in diarrhea [126]. In fact, a study demonstrated that up to 60% of IBS patients may have hypersensitivity [127]. This rectal hypersensitivity is more likely seen with diarrhea-predominant IBS [128]. There is also rapid and increased frequency of high-amplitude propagated contractions after food consumption in IBS [129, 130]. Disturbances in the neural control (from brain to visceral nerves) and the gut in the form of visceral nociception and abnormal motility mediated by changes in neurotransmitters like serotonin, cholecystokinin, and neurokinins are also proposed to contribute to diarrhea seen in these patients [131, 132].

In addition, mucosal inflammation is proposed as a cause of diarrhea in IBS. Increased intraepithelial lymphocytes were demonstrated in unselected IBS patients with predominant diarrhea [133]. Increased prevalence of mast cell degranulation correlating with the pain severity in IBS is also demonstrated [134]. This low-grade inflammation is suggested to represent either an abnormal reaction to the normal flora or secondary to qualitative or quantitative changes in the intrinsic flora in IBS patients [135].

In addition to the above-mentioned mechanisms, motility disorders may also cause diarrhea through both secretory and osmotic mechanisms [108]. Increased motility may decrease the time for the luminal contents to be in contact with the epithelium for absorption resulting in secretory diarrhea. This may occur in diabetes mellitus, amyloidosis, and postprandial diarrhea [108]. On the other hand, slow transit as occurring in diabetes mellitus and scleroderma may be associated with bacterial overgrowth and the ensuing bile acid deconjugation, poor micelle formation, and steatorrhea [98].

CLINICAL CLASSIFICATION AND DIFFERENTIAL DIAGNOSIS

Clinically, diarrhea can be classified into many ways, i.e. based on the time course (acute vs. persistent vs. chronic), volume (large vs. small), pathophysiology (secretory vs. osmotic vs. inflammatory vs. functional), epidemiology (community-acquired vs. hospital-acquired vs. traveler's diarrhea) or stool characteristics (watery vs. fatty vs.

Chapter 1 / Clinical Classification and Pathophysiology of Diarrhea 17

inflammatory). However, there is considerable overlap amongst these classifications. We have classified diarrhea into inflammatory, noninflammatory, fatty, and functional diarrhea. This is a simple and useful classification in which patients can usually be characterized on the basis of the history limiting the differential diagnosis and allowing rapid diagnosis with a minimum of testing.

- Inflammatory
- Noninflammatory or watery

  - Secretory
  - Osmotic

- Fatty
- Functional

The various etiologies for each type of diarrhea are summarized in Table 1.1.

The differential diagnosis of diarrhea depends on whether the diarrhea is acute or persistent or chronic. Chronic diarrheas in turn are further classified based on stool characteristics: watery, inflammatory, and fatty diarrhea.

Acute diarrhea usually lasts less than 2 weeks and infections are the usual cause. Bacteria, viruses, and protozoa all can produce acute diarrhea. Most acute diarrheas are due to viruses and generally are self-limited and usually require no workup. However, if the patient exhibits fever >101°C, has large volume diarrhea, bloody diarrhea, or severe abdominal pain, workup should be pursued. In this group, workup may reveal a treatable cause, i.e. bacterial, and treatment may abbreviate the illness and prevent complications. Sometimes infectious diarrhea can be prolonged and chronic, particularly in immunocompromised patients. The other major cause of acute diarrhea is food poisoning and drugs (see Table 1.2).

When working up patients with chronic diarrhea, one should first try to determine whether the diarrhea is an inflammatory or a non-inflammatory/watery diarrhea. This can usually be done on the basis of the history. The presence of co-existing symptoms gives a clue to the etiology. Inflammatory diarrhea is typically small volume with frequent bowel movements associated with tenesmus, abdominal cramps or pain and frequently with fever. Dehydration is uncommon because of the small-volume diarrhea [96]. Fecal leukocytes and occult blood are often seen [96]. Patients with a noninflammatory diarrhea have large volume, watery stools, and thus are susceptible to dehydration. Stools

Table 1.1
Clinical classification and differential diagnosis of diarrhea

Inflammatory diarrhea
Acute
  Intestinal infections
  – *C. difficile*
  – *C. jejuni*
  – *Salmonella*
  – *Shigella*
  – *E. coli*
  – *Yersinia*

Chronic
  Inflammatory bowel disease
  – Crohn's disease
  – Ulcerative colitis
  – Diverticulitis
  – Ulcerative jejunoileitis

  Infectious diseases
  – *C. difficile* or pseudomembranous colitis
  – Tuberculosis, yersiniosis
  – Cytomegalovirus
  – Herpes simplex
  – Amebiasis/other invasive parasites

  Other colitides
  – Radiation colitis
  – Ischemic colitis

Secretory diarrhea
Acute
  Intestinal infections
  – *Rotavirus*
  – *Norovirus*
  – *Enterotoxigenic E. coli (ETEC)*
  – *V. cholerae*
  – *Giardia*
  – *Cryptosporidium*
Chronic
  Intestinal infections
  – *Cryptosporidium*
  – *Human immunodeficiency virus*
  Inflammatory bowel diseases
  – Crohn's disease
  – Ulcerative colitis
  – Microscopic colitis
  – Diverticulitis
  – Vasculitis

Table 1.1
(continued)

Neuroendocrine tumors
- Gastrinoma
- VIPoma
- Somatostatinoma
- Mastocytosis
- Carcinoid syndrome
- Medullary carcinoma of thyroid
Drugs
Villous adenoma
Idiopathic secretory diarrhea

Osmotic diarrhea
Ingestion of poorly absorbed solutes
- Magnesium, phosphate, sulfates, magnesium-containing antacids
- Lactulose
- Sorbitol, mannitol-containing foods and drinks
Carbohydrate malabsorption
- Congenital diarrheas
- Celiac disease
- Tropical sprue
Maldigestion of food
- Lactase deficiency
- Pancreatic insufficiency

Fatty diarrhea
Malabsorption syndromes
- Mucosal diseases including celiac disease
- Short bowel syndrome
- Small bowel bacterial overgrowth
Maldigestion
- Pancreatic exocrine insufficiency
- Decreased luminal bile acid concentration

Functional/motility-related diarrhea
Irritable bowel syndrome
Disordered motility
- Postvagotomy diarrhea
- Postsympathectomy diarrhea
- Diabetic autonomic neuropathy
- Hyperthyroidism
- Addison's disease

Table 1.2
Differential diagnosis of acute diarrhea

1. Infections
   Bacterial
   – *V. cholerae*
   – *Salmonella*
   – *Shigella*
   – *Campylobacter*
   – *E. coli (enterotoxigenic, enterohemorrhagic, and enteroinvasive)*
   – *Yersinia enterocolitica*
   – *C. difficile*
   – *M. tuberculosis*
   – *Aeromonas plesoides*

   Viral
   – Norovirus
   – Rotavirus
   – Cytomegalovirus
   – Herpes simplex

   Protozoa
   – *Amebiasis*
   – *Giardiasis*
   – *Cryptosporidium*
   – *Microsporidia*
   – *Cyclospora*

2. Food poisoning
3. Food allergy
4. Medications
   – Magnesium-containing antacids
   – Anti-inflammatory agents (NSAIDs[a], 5-ASA)
   – Lactulose
   – Colchicine
   – Prostaglandin analogs (e.g., misoprostol)
   – Theophylline
   – Acid-reducing agents (e.g., histamine H2-receptor antagonists, proton pump inhibitors)
   – Antibiotics
   – Anti-retroviral agents

[a]NSAIDs, nonsteroidal anti-inflammatory drugs.

do not contain fecal leukocytes or blood. The patients may have nausea, vomiting, and occasional cramps. However, fever is not generally seen [96]. The characteristics of inflammatory vs. noninflammatory diarrhea are contrasted in Table 1.3.

Table 1.3
Characteristics of inflammatory and noninflammatory diarrhea

Characteristic	Inflammatory diarrhea	Noninflammatory diarrhea
Clinical picture	Bloody, mucoid small-volume diarrhea; tenesmus lower left quadrant abdominal cramps: may be Febrile	Large-volume, watery diarrhea; no blood, pus or tenesmus. May have nausea, vomiting, cramps, but no fever
Site of involvement	Colon	Small bowel
Fecal leukocytes	Present	Absent
Etiology	Certain Infectious diarrheas (*Shigella* spp., *Salmonella* spp., amebic colitis, *Campylobacter* spp., *Yersinia* spp., *C. difficile*), inflammatory bowel disease, radiation colitis	Certain Infectious diarrheas (norovirus, rotavirus, *V. cholerae*, *G. lamblia*, enterotoxin-producing bacteria, *Staphylococcus aureus*, *Cryptosporidium parvum*, *Clostridium perfringens*), secretory diarrhea and osmotic diarrhea

Adapted with modifications from [147].

Examination of stool can be helpful in other ways. Watery stools suggest that an osmotic or a secretory process is contributing to diarrhea, while the presence of oil suggests malabsorption such as fatty diarrhea. On the other hand, presence of blood or pus in the stools favors an inflammatory diarrhea.

In addition to gross stool appearance, simple stool tests help in distinguishing inflammatory from noninflammatory causes of diarrhea. Stool stain for polymorphonuclear leukocytes may be helpful. Positive tests point toward a possible inflammatory etiology. This test is insensitive, however. Stool tests for neutrophil products including calprotectin and lactoferrin are more sensitive and specific for the presence of neutrophils in stool and thus are a useful marker for inflammatory diarrhea [11].

Sudan stain of a random stool specimen is useful for qualitative assessment of stool fat. Fat loss is correlated with the number and size of Sudan-stained fat droplets viewed microscopically. The test is however limited by the fact that the sensitivity and specificity may vary and by interobserver variations in the interpretation of fat droplets [136]. Under certain circumstances, timed stool collections for 24 or 48 h may be helpful in the evaluation of chronic diarrhea. They allow appreciation of stool weight and thus differentiation of an osmotic from a secretory process, and ruling out the presence or the absence of steatorrhea.

Stool fat output is also measured quantitatively by chemical means of a timed (48- to 72-h) collection. In normal people without diarrhea, the upper limit of fecal fat excretion is approximately 7 g/day. However, in a study of normal subjects with induced diarrhea, 35% of the patients had increase in the fecal fat excretion above the upper limit of normal, with a maximum value of 13.6 g/day [137]. This led investigators to formulate that fecal fat excretion of 14 g/day or higher may be more specific for diseases that impair fat digestion or absorption.

Noninflammatory diarrhea (watery diarrhea) can be classified further into osmotic and secretory diarrhea. The response of stool output to fasting can be very helpful in distinguishing osmotic from secretory diarrhea. Characteristically if the diarrhea stops or is markedly reduced with fasting, it suggests an osmotic diarrhea. Persistence and continuation of diarrhea with little change during fasting is characteristic of secretory diarrhea. Stool osmotic gap is also useful for distinguishing secretory and osmotic diarrhea. The osmotic gap is calculated by subtracting twice the sum of the sodium and potassium concentrations of stool from 290 mOsm/kg. When a large osmotic gap is present (>50 mOsm/kg), much of the stool osmolality is composed of nonelectrolytes, which is characteristic of an osmotic diarrhea. On the other hand, a small (<50 mOsm/kg) osmotic gap is seen with secretory diarrhea. Some authors quote that a large osmotic gap of greater than 125 mOsm/kg is highly suggestive of osmotic diarrhea, while values between 50 and 125 mOsm/kg favor a mixed osmotic–secretory physiology [11, 138].

The presence of fatty diarrhea implies that there is malabsorption of fat and perhaps other nutrients as well. The diagnosis of fatty diarrhea can be made by macroscopic appearance of fat or oil in the commode. Malabsorption can result from diseases of the small bowel like celiac disease or Whipple's disease. Loss of absorption surface as in ileal resection or short bowel syndrome or small bowel bacterial overgrowth can also present with fatty diarrhea. Also pancreatic exocrine insufficiency produces fatty diarrhea [108].

Functional diarrhea and IBS are the most common diagnoses encountered in patients with chronic diarrhea. Patients with IBS and functional diarrhea have variable severity of diarrhea and sometimes alternate with periods of constipation [139, 140]. Patients with IBS usually present with an increased frequency of bowel movements of normal consistency, small-caliber stools, abdominal discomfort or pain relieved by having a bowel movement, bloating, mucus in the stool, and a sense of incomplete evacuation. A clustering of these symptoms may point toward the possibility of IBS. Patients with a painless variant of IBS diarrhea are classified as having functional diarrhea [108].

Patients with IBS or functional diarrhea lack alarm signs such as weight loss, anemia, fecal occult blood, and onset after the age of 50. If any of these features are present, a search for other diagnoses should be made. A minority of patients with diarrhea-predominant IBS may have celiac disease or small intestinal bacterial overgrowth; these conditions should therefore be screened for when evaluating patients with this presentation.

Other Considerations in Chronic Diarrhea

Commonly under-diagnosed entities such as celiac disease, small bowel bacterial overgrowth, microscopic colitis, drug-induced diarrhea, and giardiasis need to be excluded in cases where the diagnosis is not initially apparent.

Use of certain drugs, chemotherapeutic agents, or toxins can also be associated with watery diarrhea [141] (see Table 1.2) and should always be considered in any case of chronic diarrhea.

Microscopic colitis should be thought of as a cause of chronic watery diarrhea. A study from a tertiary care referral center highlighted that 10% of patients with chronic diarrhea had microscopic colitis [142]. A population-based epidemiologic study also highlighted that 10% of patients with chronic diarrhea had microscopic colitis and its annual incidence was similar to that of CD [143].

A major category to be considered in the differential diagnosis of chronic diarrhea is inflammatory disorders. They comprise a diverse group of infectious or idiopathic inflammatory processes. IBD (Crohn's disease, ulcerative colitis, or indeterminate colitis) is an important cause of inflammatory diarrhea [144]. Infections with protozoal and parasitic infections need to be considered. Another infection to be considered particularly in tuberculosis endemic countries is *Mycobacterium tuberculosis* [145]. In addition to infectious disorders, noninfectious disorders encompassing a wide variety of etiologies include radiation colitis, vascular disorders including ischemic bowel, and vasculitis secondary to collagen vascular disorders [146].

Specific etiologies of chronic diarrhea are discussed in detail in other chapters of this volume.

REFERENCES

1. Käfferstein FK. Food safety as a public health issue for developing countries. In: Unnevehr LJ, ed. Food safety in food security and food trade. Brief 2 of 17. Washington DC: International Food Policy Research Institute, September 2003.
2. Mead PS, Slutsker L, Dietz V, et al. Food-related illness and death in the United States. Emerg Infect Dis 1999;5:607–625.
3. http://academy.asm.org/images/stories/documents/resolvingglobalburdengidisea sebw.pdf
4. World Health Organization (WHO). Food safety and foodborne illness. Geneva, Switzerland: WHO; 2008. Available at: www.who.int/mediacentre/factsheets/fs237/en/. Accessed August 10, 2009.
5. Kosek M, Bern C, Guerrant RL. The global burden of diarrheal disease, as estimated from studies published between 1992 and 2000. Bull World Health Organ 2003;81:197–204.
6. Everhart JE, Ruhl CE. Burden of digestive diseases in the United States part II: lower gastrointestinal diseases. Gastroenterology 2009;136:741–754. Epub 2009 Jan 21.
7. Bartlett JG. Historical perspectives on studies of *Clostridium difficile* and *Clostridium difficile* infection. Clin Infec Dis 2008;46(Suppl 1).
8. Petri WA Jr, Miller M, Binder HJ, Levine MM, Dillingham R, Guerrant RL. Enteric infections, diarrhea, and their impact on function and development. J Clin Invest 2008;118:1277–1290.
9. WHO. Assainissement et diarrheé. Agir contre les Infect 2001;2:1e2.
10. Garthright WE, Archer DL, Kvenberg JE. Estimates of incidence and costs of intestinal infectious diseases in the United States. Public Health Rep 1988;103:107.
11. Fine KD, Schiller LR. AGA technical review on the evaluation and management of chronic diarrhea. Gastroenterology 1999;116:1464–1486.
12. Watson A, Samore MH, Wanke CA. Diarrhea and quality of life in ambulatory HIV-infected patients. Dig Dis Sci 1996;41:1794–1800.
13. Guerrant RL, Van Gilder T, Steiner TS, et al. Practice guidelines for the management of infectious diarrhea. Clin Infect Dis 2001;32:331–351.
14. Talley NJ, Zinsmeister AR, Van Dyke C, Melton LJ III. Epidemiology of colonic symptoms and the irritable bowel syndrome. Gastroenterology 1991;101: 927–934.
15. Talley NJ, Weaver AL, Zinsmeister AR, Melton LJ III. Self-reported diarrhea: what does it mean? Am J Gastroenterol 1994;89:1160–1164.
16. Pawlowski SW, Warren CA, Guerrant R. Diagnosis and treatment of acute or persistent diarrhea. Gastroenterology 2009;136:1874–1886. Epub 2009 May 7.
17. Musher DM, Musher BL. Contagious acute gastrointestinal infections. N Engl J Med 2004;351:2417–2428.
18. Johnston CP, Qiu H, Ticehurst JR, et al. Outbreak management and implications of a nosocomial norovirus outbreak. Clin Infect Dis 2007;45:534–540.
19. Parashar UD, Hummelman EG, Bresee JS, Miller MA, Glass RI. Global illness and deaths caused by rotavirus disease in children. Emerg Infect Dis 2003;9: 565–572.
20. Rodriguez WJ, Kim HW, Brandt CD, et al. Longitudinal study of rotavirus infection and gastroenteritis in families served by a pediatric medical practice: clinical and epidemiologic observations. Pediatr Infect Dis J 1987;6:170–176.

Chapter 1 / Clinical Classification and Pathophysiology of Diarrhea 25

21. Giannella RA. Infectious enteritis and proctocolitis and food poisoning. In: Feldman M, ed. Sleisenger & Fordtran's gastrointestinal and liver disease, 8th edn. Philadelphia: WB Saunders; 2006, pp. 2333–2391.

22. Altekruse SF, Stern NJ, Fields PI, Swerdlow DL. *Campylobacter jejuni*: an emerging food borne pathogen. Emerg Infect Dis 1999;5: 28–35.

23. Gorden J. Small PLC: acid resistance in enteric bacteria. Infect Immun 1993;61:364.

24. Slutzker LA, Ries AA, Green JG, et al. *Escherichia coli* O157:H7 diarrhea in the United States: clinical and epidemiological features. Ann Intern Med 1997;126:505.

25. Martin DL, MacDonald KL, White KE, et al. The epidemiology and clinical aspects of the hemolytic–uremic syndrome in Minnesota. N Engl J Med 1990;323:1161.

26. Bell BP, Goldoft M, Griffin PM, et al. A multistate outbreak of *Escherichia coli* O157:H7-associated bloody diarrhea and hemolytic–uremic syndrome from hamburgers: the Washington experience. JAMA 1994;272:1349.

27. Nataro JP, Mai V, Johnson J, et al. Diarrheagenic *Escherichia coli* infection in Baltimore, Maryland, and New Haven, Connecticut. Clin Infect Dis 2006;43:402–407.

28. Huang DB, Okhuysen PC, Jiang ZD, DuPont HL. Enteroaggregative *Escherichia coli*: an emerging enteric pathogen. Am J Gastroenterol 2004;99: 383–389.

29. Noren T, Akerlund T, Back E, et al. Molecular epidemiology of hospital-associated and community-acquired *Clostridium difficile* infection in a Swedish county. J Clin Microbiol 2004;42:3635–3643.

30. Price MF, Dao-Tran T, Garey KW, et al. Epidemiology and incidence of *Clostridium difficile*-associated diarrhoea diagnosed upon admission to a university hospital. J Hosp Infect 2007;65:42–46.

31. Morris JG, Black RE. Cholera and other vibrios in the United States. N Engl J Med 1985;312:343–350.

32. Daniels NA, Neimann J, Karpati A, et al. Traveler's diarrhea at sea: three outbreaks of waterborne enterotoxigenic *Escherichia coli* on cruise ships. J Infect Dis 2000;181:1491–1495.

33. Taylor DN, Echeverria P, Sethabutr O, et al. Clinical and microbiologic features of *Shigella* and enteroinvasive *Escherichia coli* infections detected by DNA hybridization. J Clin Microbiol 1988;26:1362–1366.

34. Karanis P, Kourenti C, Smith H. Waterborne transmission of protozoan parasites: a worldwide review of outbreaks and lessons learnt. J Water Health 2007;5: 1–38.

35. Haque R, Huston CD, Hughes M, Houpt E, Petri WA Jr. Amebiasis. N Engl J Med 2003 Apr 17;348(16):1565–1573.

36. Petri WA Jr, Haque R, Lyerly D, Vines RR. Estimating the impact of amebiasis on health. Parasitol Today 2000;16:320–321.

37. Kappus KD, Lundgren RG Jr, Juranek DD, et al. Intestinal parasitism in the United States: update on a continuing problem. Am J Trop Med Hyg 1994;50:705.

38. Peters CS, Sable R, Janda WM, et al. Prevalence of enteric parasites in homosexual patients attending an outpatient clinic. J Clin Microbiol 1986;24:684.

39. Pickering LK, Woodward WE, DuPont HL, Sullivan P. Occurrence of *Giardia lamblia* in children in day care centers. J Pediatr 1984;104:522.

40. Farthing MJ, Mata L, Urrutia JJ, Kronmal RA. Natural history of *Giardia* infection of infants and children in rural Guatemala and its impact on physical growth. Am J Clin Nutr 1986;43:395.
41. Fraser D, Dagan R, Naggan L, et al. Natural history of *Giardia lamblia* and *Cryptosporidium* infections in a cohort of Israeli Bedouin infants: a study of a population in transition. Am J Trop Med Hyg 1997;57:544.
42. Hoxie NJ, Davis JP, Vergeront JM, Nashold RD, Blair KA. Cryptosporidiosis-associated mortality following a massive waterborne outbreak in Milwaukee, Wisconsin. Am J Public Health 1997;87:2032–2035.
43. Ho AY, Lopez AS, Eberhart MG, et al. Outbreak of cyclosporiasis associated with imported raspberries, Philadelphia, Pennsylvania, 2000. Emerg Infect Dis 2002;8:783–788.
44. Katz D, Kumar S, Malecki J, Lowdermilk M, Koumans EH, Hopkins R. Cyclosporiasis associated with imported raspberries, Florida, 1996. Public Health Rep 1999;114:427–438.
45. Herwaldt BL, Ackers ML. An outbreak in 1996 of cyclosporiasis associated with imported raspberries. The Cyclospora Working Group. N Engl J Med 1997;336:1548–1556.
46. Bryan RT, Weber R, Schwartz DA. Microsporidiosis. In: Guerrant RL, Walker DH, Weller PF, eds. Tropical infectious diseases: principles, pathogens, and practice. Philadelphia: Churchill Livingstone; 2000, p. 840.
47. Didier ES. Microsporidiosis. Clin Infect Dis 1998; 27:1.
48. DeHovitz JA, Pape JW, Boncy M, Johnson WD. Clinical manifestations and therapy of *Isospora bella* infection in patients with the acquired immunodeficiency syndrome. N Engl J Med 1986;315:87.
49. Asha NJ, Tompkins D, Wilcox MH. Comparative analysis of prevalence, risk factors, and molecular epidemiology of antibiotic-associated diarrhea due to *Clostridium difficile*, *Clostridium perfringens*, and *Staphylococcus aureus*. J Clin Microbiol 2006;44:2785–2791.
50. Zilderberg MD, Shorr AF, Kollef MH. Increase in adult *Clostridium difficile*-related hospitalizations and case fatality rate, United States, 2000–2005. Emerg Infect Dis 2008;14:929–931.
51. Redelings MD, Sorvillo F, Mascola L. Increase in *Clostridium difficile*-related mortality rates, United States, 1999–2004. Emerg Infect Dis [serial on the Internet]. 2007 Sep [*date cited*]. Available from http://www.cdc.gov/EID/content/13/9/1417.htm
52. McDonald LC, Killgore GE, Thompson A, et al. Emergence of an epidemic, toxin gene variant strain of *Clostridium difficile* responsible for outbreaks in the United States between 2000 and 2004. N Engl J Med 2005;353:2433–2441.
53. Kazakova SV, Ware K, Baughman B, et al. A hospital outbreak of diarrhea due to an emerging epidemic strain of *Clostridium difficile*. Arch Intern Med 2006;166:2518–2524.
54. Centers for Disease Control and Prevention (CDC). Surveillance for community-associated *Clostridium difficile*--Connecticut, 2006. MMWR Morb Mortal Wkly Rep 2008;57(13):340-343.
55. CDC. Severe *Clostridium difficile*-associated disease in populations previously at low risk—four states, 2005. MMWR 2005;54:1201–1205.
56. Wall PG, Ryan MJ, Ward LR, Rowe B. Outbreaks of salmonellosis in hospitals in England and Wales: 1992–1994. J Hosp Infect 1996;33:181–190.
57. Gikas A, Kritsotakis EI, Maraki S, et al. A nosocomial, foodborne outbreak of *Salmonella enterica* serovar Enteritidis in a university hospital in Greece: the

Chapter 1 / Clinical Classification and Pathophysiology of Diarrhea   27

importance of establishing HACCP systems in hospital catering. J Hosp Infect 2007;66:194–196.

58. Alam NK, Armstrong PK, Nguyen OT, Kesson AM, Cripps TM, Corbett SJ. *Salmonella typhimurium* phage type 170 in a tertiary paediatric hospital with person-to-person transmission implicated. Commun Dis Intell 2005;29: 374–378.

59. Delaloye J, Merlani G, Petignat C, et al. Nosocomial nontyphoidal salmonellosis after antineoplastic chemotherapy: reactivation of asymptomatic colonization? Eur J Clin Microbiol Infect Dis 2004;23:751–758.

60. Neill MA, Rice SK, Ahmad NV, Flanigan TP. Cryptosporidiosis: an unrecognized cause of diarrhea in elderly hospitalized patients. Clin Infect Dis 1996;22: 168–170.

61. Kordidarian R, Kelishadi R, Arjmandfar Y. Nosocomial infection due to rotavirus in infants in Alzahra Hospital, Isfahan, Iran. J Health Popul Nutr 2007;25: 231–235.

62. Rayani A, Bode U, Habas E, et al. Rotavirus infections in paediatric oncology patients: a matched-pairs analysis. Scand J Gastroenterol 2007;42:81–87.

63. Widdowson MA, van Doornum GJ, van der Poel WH, de Boer AS, Mahdi U, Koopmans M. Emerging group-A rotavirus and a nosocomial outbreak of diarrhoea. Lancet 2000;356:1161–1162.

64. Steffen R. Epidemiology of traveler's diarrhea. Clin Infect Dis 2005;41 (Suppl 8):S536–S540.

65. Steffen R, Tornieporth N, Clemens SA, et al. Epidemiology of travelers' diarrhea: details of a global survey. J Travel Med 2004;11:231–237.

66. DuPont HL. Systematic review: the epidemiology and clinical features of travellers' diarrhoea. Aliment Pharmacol Ther 2009;30:187–196. Epub 2009 Apr 21.

67. Centers for Disease Control and Prevention. Prevention of specific infectious diseases. In: Arguin PM, Kozarsky PE, Reed C, eds. CDC health information for international travel 2008, 2008 ed. Philadelphia, PA: Elsevier; 2008. pp. 114–362.

68. Mohamed JA, DuPont HL, Jiang ZD, et al. A novel single-nucleotide polymorphism in the lactoferrin gene is associated with susceptibility to diarrhea in North American travelers to Mexico. Clin Infect Dis 2007;44:945–952.

69. Mohamed JA, Dupont HL, Jiang ZD, et al. A single-nucleotide polymorphism in the gene encoding osteoprotegerin, an anti-inflammatory protein produced in response to infection with diarrheagenic *Escherichia coli*, is associated with an increased risk of nonsecretory bacterial diarrhea in North American travelers to Mexico. J Infect Dis 2009 Jan 7.

70. Neal KR, Scott HM, Slack RC, Logan RF. Omeprazole as a risk factor for campylobacter gastroenteritis: case–control study. BMJ 1996;312:414–415.

71. Van De Winkel K, Van den Daele A, Van Gompel A, Van den Ende J. Factors influencing standard pretravel health advice—a study in Belgium. J Travel Med 2007;14:288–296.

72. Mattila L, Siitonen A, Kyronseppa H, et al. Seasonal variation in etiology of travelers' diarrhea. Finnish–Moroccan Study Group. J Infect Dis 1992;165: 385–388.

73. Adachi JA, Mathewson JJ, Jiang ZD, Ericsson CD, DuPont HL. Enteric pathogens in Mexican sauces of popular restaurants in Guadalajara, Mexico, and Houston, Texas. Ann Intern Med 2002;136:884–887.

74. DuPont HL, Ericsson CD, DuPont MW. Emporiatric enteritis: lessons learned from US students in Mexico. Trans Am Clin Climatol Assoc 1986;97:32–42.

75. Ko G, Garcia C, Jiang ZD, et al. Noroviruses as a cause of traveler's diarrhea among students from the United States visiting Mexico. J Clin Microbiol 2005;43:6126–6129.
76. Taylor DN, Houston R, Shlim DR, Bhaibulaya M, Ungar BL, Echeverria P. Etiology of diarrhea among travelers and foreign residents in Nepal. JAMA 1988;260:1245–1248.
77. Freedman DO, Weld LH, Kozarsky PE, et al. Spectrum of disease and relation to place of exposure among ill returned travelers. N Engl J Med 2006;354: 119–130.
78. Vernacchio L, Vezina RM, Mitchell AA, Lesko SM, Plaut AG, Acheson DW. Diarrhea in American infants and young children in the community setting: incidence, clinical presentation and microbiology. Pediatr Infect Dis J 2006;25: 2–7.
79. Gupta S, Narang S, Nunavath V, Singh S. Chronic diarrhoea in HIV patients: prevalence of coccidian parasites. Indian J Med Microbiol 2008;26:172–175.
80. Talley NJ, Zinsmeister AR, Van Dyke C, Melton LJ III. Epidemiology of colonic symptoms and the irritable bowel syndrome. Gastroenterology 1991;101: 927–934.
81. Talley NJ, O'Keefe EA, Zinsmeister AR, Melton LJ III. Prevalence of gastrointestinal symptoms in the elderly: a population-based study. Gastroenterology 1992;102:895–901.
82. Fine KD, Meyer RL, Lee EL. The prevalence of chronic diarrhea in patients with celiac sprue treated with a gluten-free diet. Gastroenterology 1997;112: 1830–1838.
83. Talley NJ, Weaver AL, Zinsmeister AR, Melton LJ III. Onset and disappearance of gastrointestinal symptoms and functional gastrointestinal disorders. Am J Epidemiol 1992;136:165–177.
84. Bytzer P, Stokholm M, Andersen I, Lund-Hansen B, Schaffalitzky De Muckadell OB. Aetiology, medical history, and fecal weight in adult patients referred for diarrhoea: a prospective study. Scand J Gastroenterol 1990;25:572–578.
85. Afzalpurkar RG, Schiller LR, Little KH, Santangelo WC, Fordtran JS. The self-limited nature of chronic idiopathic diarrhea. N Engl J Med 1992;327: 1849–1852.
86. Kotwal MR, Durrani HA, Shah SN. Chronic colonic diarrhoea in North-West India: a clinical study with special reference to the syndrome of irritable colon. J Indian Med Assoc 1978;70:77–80.
87. Manatsathit S, Israsena S, Kladcharoen N, Sithicharoenchai P, Roenprayoon S, Suwanakul P. Chronic diarrhoea: a prospective study in Thai patients at Chulalongkorn University Hospital, Bangkok. Southeast Asian J Trop Med Public Health 1985;16:447–452.
88. Devroede GJ, Phillips SF. Conservation of sodium, chloride, and water by the human colon. Gastroenterology 1969;56:101–109.
89. Debongnie JC, Phillips SF. Capacity of the human colon to absorb fluid. Gastroenterology 1978;74:698–703.
90. Binder, HJ, Reuben A. Nutrient digestion and absorption. In: Boron WF, Boulpaep EI, eds. Medical physiology. Philadelphia, PA: Elsevier; 2005. pp. 947–974.
91. Binder, HJ. Intestinal fluid and electrolyte movement. In: Boron WF, Boulpaep EI, eds. Medical physiology. Philadelphia, PA: Elsevier; 2005. pp. 931–946.
92. Field M. Intestinal ion transport and the pathophysiology of diarrhea. J Clin Invest 2003;111:931–943.

Chapter 1 / Clinical Classification and Pathophysiology of Diarrhea 29

93. Mourad FH, O'Donnell LJ, Dias JA, et al. Role of 5-hydroxytryptamine type 3 receptors in rat intestinal fluid and electrolyte secretion induced by cholera and *Escherichia coli* enterotoxins. Gut 1995;37:340–345.

94. Kerlin P, Zinsmeister A, Phillips S. Relationship of motility to flow of contents in the human small intestine. Gastroenterology 1982;82:701–706.

95. Proano M, Camilleri M, Phillips SF, Brown ML, Thomforde GM. Transit of solids through the human colon: regional quantification in the unprepared bowel. Am J Physiol 1990;258:G856–G862.

96. Navaneethan U, Giannella RA. Mechanisms of infectious diarrhea. Nat Clin Pract Gastroenterol Hepatol 2008;5:637–647.

97. Binder HJ. Mechanisms of diarrhea in inflammatory bowel diseases. Ann N Y Acad Sci 2009;1165:285–293.

98. Camilleri M. Chronic diarrhea: a review on pathophysiology and management for the clinical gastroenterologist. Clin Gastroenterol Hepatol 2004;2: 198–206.

99. Schiller LR. Secretory diarrhea. Curr Gastroenterol Rep 1999;1:389.

100. Janecki AJ. Why should a clinician care about the molecular biology of transport? Curr Gastroenterol Rep 2000;2:378.

101. Jensen RT. Overview of chronic diarrhea caused by functional neuroendocrine neoplasms. Semin Gastrointest Dis 1999;10:156–172.

102. Cooke HJ. Neurotransmitters in neuronal reflexes regulating intestinal secretion. Ann N Y Acad Sci 2000;915:77.

103. Rocho F, Musch MW, Lishanskiy L, et al. IFN-γ downregulates expression of Na+/H+ exchangers NHE2 and NHE3 in rat intestine and human Caco-2/bbe cells. Am J Physiol Cell Physiol 2001;280:C1224–C1232.

104. Howe K, Gauldie J, McKay DM. TGF beta effects on epithelial ion transport and barrier: reduced Cl-secretion blocked by a p38 MAPK inhibitor. Am J Physiol Cell Physiol 2002;283:C1667–C1774.

105. Riordan SM, McIver CJ, Walker BM, et al. Bacteriological method for detecting small intestinal hypomotility. Am J Gastroenterol 1996;91:2399.

106. Kaye SA, Lim SG, Taylor M, et al. Small bowel bacterial overgrowth in systemic sclerosis: detection using direct and indirect methods and treatment outcome. Br J Rheumatol 1995;34:265.

107. Virally-Monod M, Tielmans D, Kevorkian JP, et al. Chronic diarrhoea and diabetes mellitus: prevalence of small intestinal bacterial overgrowth. Diabetes Metab 1998;24:530.

108. Schiller LR, Sellin JH. Diarrhea. In: Feldman M, Friedman LS, Brandt LJ, eds. Sleisenger and Fordtran's gastrointestinal and liver disease: pathophysiology, diagnosis, management, 8th edn (Ed. Feldman M) Philadelphia: WB Saunders; 2006. pp. 159–186.

109. Kere J, Hoglund P. Inherited disorders of ion transport in the intestine. Curr Opin Genet Dev 2000;10:306.

110. Muller T, Wijmenga C, Phillips AD, et al. Congenital sodium diarrhea is an autosomal recessive disorder of sodium/proton exchange but unrelated to known candidate genes. Gastroenterology 2000;119:1506.

111. Binder HJ. Causes of chronic diarrhea. N Engl J Med 2006 20;355:236–239.

112. Hammer HF, Santa Ana CA, Schiller LR, Fordtran JS. Studies of osmotic diarrhea induced in normal subjects by ingestion of polyethylene glycol and lactulose. J Clin Invest 1989;84:1056.

113. Hammer HF, Fine KD, Santa Ana CA, et al. Carbohydrate malabsorption: its measurement and its contribution to diarrhea. J Clin Invest 1990;86:1936.

114. Naim HY. Molecular and cellular aspects and regulation of intestinal lactase–phlorizin hydrolase. Histol Histopathol 2001;16:553.
115. Vuoristo M, Miettinen TA. The role of fat and bile acid malabsorption in diarrhoea of coeliac disease. Scand J Gastroenterol 1987;22:289.
116. Amasheh S, Barmeyer C, Koch CS, et al. Cytokine-dependent transcriptional down-regulation of epithelial sodium channel in ulcerative colitis. Gastroenterology 2004;126:1711.
117. Sugi K, Musch MW, Field M, et al. Inhibition of Na+/K+-ATPase by interferon γ downregulates intestinal epithelial transport and barrier function. Gastroenterology 2001;120:1393–1403.
118. Gewirtz AT, Simon PO Jr, Schmitt CK, et al. *Salmonella typhimurium* translocates flagellin across intestinal epithelia, inducing a proinflammatory response. J Clin Invest 2001;107:99.
119. Sitaraman SV, Merlin D, Wang L, et al. Neutrophil–epithelial crosstalk at the intestinal luminal surface mediated by reciprocal secretion of adenosine and IL-6. J Clin Invest 2001;107:861.
120. Cipolla DM, Boley SJ, Luchs S, et al. Chronic mesenteric ischemia presenting as chronic diarrhea and weight loss with pneumatosis intestinalis. Gastroenterologist 1996;4:134.
121. Landberg CW, Hauer-Jensen M, Sung CC, et al. Expression of fibrogenic cytokines in rat small intestine after fractionated irradiation. Radiother Oncol 1994;32:29.
122. Richter KK, Langberg CW, Sung CC, et al. Increased transforming growth factor β (TGF-β) immunoreactivity is independently associated with chronic injury in both consequential and primary radiation enteropathy. Int J Radiat Oncol Biol Phys 1997;19:187.
123. Hearing SD, Thomas LA, Heaton KW, Hunt L. Effect of cholecystectomy on bowel function: a prospective, controlled study. Gut 1999;45:889–894.
124. Poley JR, Hofmann AF. Role of fat maldigestion in pathogenesis of steatorrhea in ileal resection: fat digestion after two sequential test meals with and without cholestyramine. Gastroenterology 1976;71:38–44.
125. Conley DR, Coyne MJ, Bonorris GG, Chung A, Schoenfield LJ. Bile acid stimulation of colonic adenylate cyclase and secretion in the rabbit. Am J Dig Dis 1976;21:453–458.
126. Drossman DA, Camilleri M, Mayer EA, Whitehead WE. AGA technical review on irritable bowel syndrome. Gastroenterology 2002;123:2108–2131.
127. Mertz H, Naliboff B, Munakata J, Niazi N, Mayer EA. Altered rectal perception is a biological marker of patients with irritable bowel syndrome. Gastroenterology 1995;109:40–52.
128. Prior A, Colgan SM, Whorwell PJ. Changes in rectal sensitivity after hypnotherapy in patients with irritable bowel syndrome. Gut 1990;31:896–898.
129. Vassallo M, Camilleri M, Phillips SF, Brown ML, Chapman NJ, Thomforde GM. Transit through the proximal colon influences stool weight in the irritable bowel syndrome. Gastroenterology 1992;102:102–108.
130. Choi MG, Camilleri M, O'Brien MD, Kammer PP, Hanson RB. A pilot study of motility and tone of the left colon in diarrhea due to functional disorders and dysautonomia. Am J Gastroenterol 1997;92:297–302.
131. Grundy D. Neuroanatomy of visceral nociception: vagal and splanchnic afferent. Gut 2002;51(Suppl 1):I2–I5.
132. Camilleri M. Serotonergic modulation of visceral sensation: lower gut. Gut 2002;51(Suppl 1):I81–I86.

Chapter 1 / Clinical Classification and Pathophysiology of Diarrhea   31

133. Chadwick VS, Chen W, Shu D, et al. Activation of the mucosal immune system in irritable bowel syndrome. Gastroenterology 2002;122:1778–1783.
134. Barbara G, Stanghellini V, De Giorgio R, et al. Activated mast cells in proximity to colonic nerves correlate with abdominal pain in irritable bowel syndrome. Gastroenterology 2004;126:693–702.
135. Quigley EM. Changing face of irritable bowel syndrome. World J Gastroenterol 2006;12:1–5.
136. Drummey GD, Benson JA, Jones CM. Microscopical examination of the stool for steatorrhea. N Engl J Med 1961;264:85–87.
137. Fine KD, Fordtran JS. The effect of diarrhea on fecal fat excretion. Gastroenterology 1992;102:1936–1939.
138. Eherer AJ, Fordtran JS. Fecal osmotic gap and pH in experimental diarrhea of various causes. Gastroenterology 1992;103:545–551.
139. Adeniji OA, Barnett CB, Di Palma JA. Durability of the diagnosis of irritable bowel syndrome based on clinical criteria. Dig Dis Sci 2004;49:572.
140. Camilleri M. Management of the irritable bowel syndrome. Gastroenterology 2001;120:652.
141. Ratnaike RN, Jones TE. Mechanisms of drug-induced diarrhoea in the elderly. Drugs Aging 1998;13:245.
142. Schiller LR, Rivera LM, Santangelo W, et al. Diagnostic value of fasting plasma peptide concentrations in patients with chronic diarrhea. Dig Dis Sci 1994;39:2216.
143. Olesen M, Eriksson S, Bohr J, et al. Microscopic colitis: a common diarrhoeal disease. An epidemiological study in Orebro, Sweden, 1993–1998. Gut 2004;53:346.
144. Su C, Lichtenstein GR. Ulcerative colitis. In: Feldman M, ed. Sleisenger and Fordtran's gastrointestinal and liver disease, 8th edn. Philadelphia: WB Saunders; 2006. pp. 2499–2538.
145. Amarapurkar DN, Patel ND, Rane PS. Diagnosis of Crohn's disease in India where tuberculosis is widely prevalent. World J Gastroenterol 2008 7;14: 741–746.
146. Sands BE. From symptom to diagnosis: clinical distinctions among various forms of intestinal inflammation. Gastroenterology 2004;126:1518–1532.
147. Park SI, Giannella RA. Approach to the adult patient with acute diarrhea. Gastroenterol Clin North Am 1993;22:483–497.

2 Infectious Gastroenteritis and Colitis

Jennifer M. Newton, MD and Christina M. Surawicz, MD, MACG

CONTENTS

INTRODUCTION
ETIOLOGY
CLINICAL PRESENTATION
SPECIFIC INFECTIONS
CLINICAL EVALUATION
DIAGNOSTIC EVALUATION
TREATMENT
CONCLUSION
REFERENCES

Summary

In this chapter, we discuss the epidemiology, etiology, presentation, diagnosis, and treatment of infectious diarrhea in immunocompetent persons. The features of small intestinal and ileocolonic disease as related to possible causative agents are presented. Additionally, there is an emphasis on specific pathogens, with a comprehensive review of viral, bacterial, and parasitic causes of diarrhea. We then discuss the intricacies of the clinical and diagnostic evaluation, as well as treatment. Specifically, we evaluate the severity of illness, historical clues to etiology, the appropriateness of diagnostic testing in various clinical situations, and which diagnostic tests are clinically relevant. Rehydration therapy is discussed along with nutrition and electrolyte

From: *Diarrhea, Clinical Gastroenterology*
Edited by: S. Guandalini, H. Vaziri, DOI 10.1007/978-1-60761-183-7_2
© Springer Science+Business Media, LLC 2011

support. The appropriate use of antidiarrheal and antimicrobial medications is reviewed, along with a brief discussion of empiric therapy and the individual and public health consequences associated with infection and treatment.

Key Words: Acute diarrhea, Infectious diarrhea, Enteritis, Colitis, Enterocolitis, Microorganisms, Virus, Bacteria, Parasites

INTRODUCTION

Infectious diarrhea is a major cause of morbidity and mortality worldwide. Children in developing countries are disproportionately affected by acute diarrhea, averaging 1–3 episodes per year. In these settings, infectious diarrhea accounts for approximately 20–25% of the mortality in children less than 5 years of age [1]. In addition, morbidity of repeated infections is manifest as malnutrition with cognitive and physical developmental delays. Around the world, there is a substantial difference in incidence of disease among children from different socioeconomic strata [1]. This difference is likely related to variability in sanitation, living quarters, and access to treated food and water. Over the last several decades, mortality from infectious diarrhea has significantly decreased, yet morbidity remains largely unchanged. The decline in mortality is believed to be the result of the widespread implementation of oral rehydration therapy as recommended by the World Health Organization (WHO) [2]. The lack of improvement in morbidity and incidence of disease is likely related to limited improvement in living conditions.

In developed nations, the mortality rate is lower, seen predominantly at the extremes of age. Morbidity still remains a major problem, with children experiencing 2–3 episodes and all persons experiencing 1–2 episodes of acute diarrhea per year [3]. In the United States alone, there are an estimated 200–300 million episodes of diarrheal illness each year, resulting in 73 million physician consultations, 1.8 million hospitalizations, and an estimated 6 billion dollars spent each year on medical costs and loss of productivity [3]. With globalization of food processing and distribution, the number of foodborne diarrheal illnesses has risen [3].

With the morbidity, mortality, and cost of infectious diarrhea, it is important to promptly determine the appropriate diagnostic evaluation and treatment.

ETIOLOGY

The major pathogens causing acute infectious diarrhea are viruses, bacteria, and parasites. Most cases are self-limited, resolve within 24–48 h,

Chapter 2 / Infectious Gastroenteritis and Colitis

and in developed nations, are likely to be viral. A pilot study in the USA identified a pathogen in approximately 70% of cases, three-quarters of which were norovirus [4]. In healthy adults, the most likely pathogens causing severe diarrheas are bacteria [5]. In developing nations and in returning travelers, enterotoxigenic *Escherichia coli* (ETEC) is the most likely pathogen. Parasites are identified less frequently as the cause of acute infectious diarrhea.

CLINICAL PRESENTATION

Diarrhea is classified as acute (duration less than 2 weeks), persistent (2–4 weeks), and chronic (greater than 4 weeks). Most infectious diarrhea are brief and self-limited, and managed by patients alone. Of those patients who do present to clinicians, their illness can generally be divided into small intestinal or ileocolonic disease (see Table 2.1).

Pathogens affecting the small intestine are usually noninvasive organisms. These patients present with high-volume watery stools and in some cases malabsorption, frequently leading to dehydration. Patients often have periumbilical pain and cramping. The most common pathogens in this category are viruses, such as norovirus and rotavirus, but also include bacteria: enterotoxigenic *E. coli*, *Vibrio cholerae*, toxin-producing *Staphylococcus aureus*, and the parasites *Giardia lamblia*, *Isospora belli*, and cryptosporidia (see Table 2.2). These enteropathogens typically cause disease via enterotoxin production, ingestion of preformed toxin, and/or bacterial adherence to epithelial cells [6].

Colonic and distal small intestinal pathogens are more likely to be invasive. They result in a syndrome of lower abdominal pain; small-volume, frequent stools which can be bloody and tenesmus (when the rectum is involved) (see Table 2.1). The most common pathogens causing this presentation are bacteria including *Campylobacter, Shigella, Salmonella* and *Shiga toxin*-producing *E. coli*, and *Clostridium difficile*.

Table 2.1
Features of small intestinal and ileocolonic disease

Features of small intestinal disease	*Features of ileocolonic disease*
Diffuse periumbilical pain	Lower abdominal pain
Large volume stools	Small-volume stools
Watery stools	Stools may be bloody
Dehydration	Tenesmus
Possible malabsorption	Dehydration

Table 2.2
Small intestinal and ileocolonic pathogens

Small intestinal pathogens	Ileocolonic pathogens
Viruses	Viruses
Caliciviruses (norovirus)	CMV
Rotavirus	Adenovirus
Enteric adenovirus	Bacteria
Bacteria	*Salmonella*
E. coli	*Shigella*
ETEC	*Campylobacter*
EPEC	STEC or EHEC
EAEC	EIEC
DAEC	*C. difficile*
V. cholera	*Yersinia*
L. monocytogenes	Non-cholera vibrios
C. perfringens	*P. shigelloides*
S. aureus	*A. hydrophila*
Parasites	Tuberculosis
G. lamblia	*K. oxytoca*
Cryptosporidium	*C. perfringens*
Microsporidium	Parasites
Cyclospora	*E. histolytica*
Isospora	*T. trichiura*
	B. coli
	B. hominis

The parasite *Entameba histolytica* has a predilection for the ileocolonic area. Fungi are rare in the immunocompetent host (see Table 2.2). The major mechanisms by which the pathogens cause ileocolonic illness are cytotoxin production and mucosal invasion leading to inflammation and ulceration [6].

Although there is some overlap between these two categories, this distinction is useful to help delineate the likely enteropathogen.

SPECIFIC INFECTIONS

Small Intestinal Pathogens

VIRUSES

Viral gastroenteritis. Viral gastroenteritis is the most common cause of self-limited, acute diarrhea worldwide, in both children and adults [7]. Viruses cause illness by diverse mechanisms. In general they infect

Chapter 2 / Infectious Gastroenteritis and Colitis

mature villous enterocytes, resulting in loss of the brush border and impaired absorption [6–8]. New evidence suggests that rotaviruses may also cause villous ischemia, produce a viral enterotoxin, and even affect the enteric nervous system [7–9]. Patients typically present with dehydrating diarrhea and vomiting, and may have associated fever. The diarrhea typically resolves within a few days, although adenovirus may cause persistent, severe disease in immunosuppressed patients [8]. Rotaviruses and noroviruses are the most common causes of diarrhea in the pediatric population [7], and noroviruses are the most common in adults. Both viruses are highly contagious as demonstrated by high rates of transmission in day cares, hospitals (rotavirus) [7], cruise ships, and banquets (noroviruses). Noroviruses can be acquired by ingestion of raw oysters from fresh water estuaries. Since viral gastroenteritis is generally self-limiting, diagnostic tests are usually unnecessary. Treatment is supportive with oral rehydration. Hand washing with soap is imperative for containment, as alcohol hand gels may not adequately kill these viruses. The American Academy of Pediatrics recommends routine immunization of infants with either of the two available rotavirus vaccines [10]. Norovirus vaccines are under development.

BACTERIA

Escherichia coli. Several groups of *E. coli* cause diarrhea. Those *E. coli* that affect the small intestine include enterotoxigenic (ETEC), enteropathogenic (EPEC), enteroaggregative (EAEC), and diffusely adherent (DAEC) *E. coli*. These bacteria all cause illness by enterotoxin production or adherence to the brush border causing effacement of cells; DAEC also has cytotoxic effects [11]. Symptoms include self-limited watery diarrhea, occurring within 2 days of ingestion and resolving within 3 days of onset. Diarrhea may occasionally be associated with nausea, vomiting, or fever. Both ETEC and EAEC are major causes of traveler's diarrhea [11, 12], and EAEC is an important cause of bacterial diarrhea in children in both the USA and developing countries [11, 13]. EAEC can also cause chronic diarrhea in persons with HIV [11]. ETEC is increasingly a cause of foodborne illness [13]. DAEC is a cause of diarrhea in children less than 2 years old [14]. EPEC is uncommon but can cause both sporadic and epidemic diarrhea, primarily in young children in developing countries. EPEC may cause severe dehydration or malnutrition, especially when infection is chronic. Historically, there have not been good diagnostic tests for these infections. However, newer techniques are allowing for identification of the different *E. coli* species when suggested by clinical history [13]. Treatment is directed at rehydration therapy. Fluoroquinolones

(FQ), trimethoprim–sulfamethoxazole (TMP–SMX), azithromycin, or rifaximin can be used in conjunction with antidiarrheals to decrease symptoms of traveler's diarrhea, when appropriate [3, 13].

Vibrio cholera. *Vibrio cholerae* causes epidemics of dehydrating diarrhea affecting all ages and may lead to high mortality rates if the public health interventions are inadequate [1]. *Vibrio cholerae* serogroups O1 (biotypes classical and El Tor) and O139 are responsible for these epidemics. Non-O1 non-O139 vibrios are pathogenic but do not cause epidemics or pandemics [15]. Studies now suggest that the majority of individuals are asymptomatic or have only mild diarrheal disease [16]. In developing countries, cholera transmission is via contaminated food and water; in the USA, it is usually associated with ingestion of undercooked seafood from the Gulf of Mexico [15]. Risk factors for infection include blood group 0, HIV [17], and low gastric acid. Cholera is rare in travelers. *Vibrio cholerae* colonizes the upper small intestine and causes diarrhea by stimulating cAMP-mediated chloride secretion, inhibiting sodium absorption, and producing platelet-activating factor with possible resultant alteration in prostaglandin synthesis. Diarrhea is abrupt in onset, resembles rice water, and is associated with vomiting. Without proper treatment, the case–fatality rate approaches 50% [15]. Treatment is initially aimed at rehydration. Antibiotics are given to shorten the duration of diarrhea. For severe cases, intravenous fluids are necessary and should be isotonic. For mild cases, oral rehydration therapy (ORT) is preferred. Recent evidence suggests that rice, wheat, or amylase-resistant starch solutions may be better than standard glucose-based solutions [18–20]. Patients should eat as soon as they can tolerate oral intake, and infants should continue to breastfeed [15, 21, 22]. Without antibiotics, patients generally recover in 4–5 days, so mild diarrhea does not require treatment. Oral vaccines are in development; the older parenteral vaccine is not recommended.

Listeria monocytogenes. Listeria was not thought to cause gastrointestinal illness until the 1990s when an outbreak of contaminated chocolate milk caused acute febrile gastroenteritis. Since then, multiple epidemics have been reported, linked to chocolate milk [23], lunch meats, and unpasteurized cheeses. Immunocompromised persons and pregnant women are at increased risk of infection and invasive disease. Watery diarrhea and fever are often accompanied by myalgias, arthralgias, headache, and fatigue or sleepiness [23–25]. Invasive infections can be fatal. The diagnosis should be considered in patients with febrile gastroenteritis when routine cultures do not identify a pathogen. Stool culture on selective media is diagnostic; blood or cerebrospinal fluid cultures may be useful in invasive disease. Since *Listeria* gastroenteritis is generally self-limited and noninvasive, treatment is not currently recommended [24]. Ampicillin or penicillin G is used for treatment of invasive disease.

Staphylococcus aureus. Enterotoxin-producing *S. aureus* has long been an important cause of food poisoning, leading to vomiting 2–7 h after ingestion of the toxin [13]. More recently, however, it has been studied as a cause of antibiotic-associated diarrhea (AAD). Studies have shown that many AAD *S. aureus* isolates can produce enterotoxins, leukotoxins, or toxic shock syndrome toxin 1 [26, 27]. *Staphylococcus aureus* can be part of normal gut flora, and colonization rises with duration of hospitalization and placement of nasogastric tubes. Among hospitalized patients with AAD, the majority of *S. aureus* isolates were methicillin-resistant *S. aureus* (MRSA). In these patients, MRSA was found in the blood, suggesting colitis as the cause of bacteremia [27]. MRSA is shed in stools. Therefore, testing for MRSA-associated AAD in *C. difficile*-negative patients should be considered to avoid dissemination of MRSA throughout the hospital. Testing may also be considered in community-acquired cases of severe *C. difficile*-negative AAD.

PARASITES

***Giardia intestinalis* (also called *Giardia lamblia*).** *Giardia* is the most commonly isolated intestinal parasite in developed countries [28]. It is prevalent throughout the world and is transmitted person-to-person or via contaminated water. Ingested cysts, which are resistant to chlorine and gastric acid, become trophozoites in the small intestine and attach to the mucosa. Genotype appears a predictor of disease severity [29, 30]. Symptoms range from asymptomatic carriage to severe cramps, bloating and gas, nausea, vomiting, and malabsorption resulting in explosive fatty diarrhea. Chronic infection can occur in immunocompetent patients as well as in those with hypogammaglobulinemia, especially IgA deficiency. Diagnosis is based on the detection of cysts in stool. Since cyst excretion is intermittent, three stools over 6 days are necessary; one stool has a yield of 50–70% and three stools have a yield of 90%. The *Giardia* stool antigen EIA is excellent, with a sensitivity of 95% and a specificity of 100%. Duodenal aspiration of trophozoites is also possible. In the USA, the principal treatment is metronidazole. Alternatives include nitazoxanide and tinidazole. Approximately 10–20% of patients will relapse and require retreatment [31].

Cryptosporidiosis. *Cryptosporidium* was recognized as a pathogen in humans in 1976 when case reports documented it to cause severe diarrhea in immunosuppressed patients. Although the organism primarily infects immunocompromised hosts, it can also infect normal hosts. Transmission is caused by fecal contamination of water and subsequent ingestion of the chlorine-resistant oocysts. Symptoms range from mild-to-severe watery diarrhea and can be chronic in patients with immunodeficiency. Patients may also have dyspepsia, weight loss, and anorexia. Diagnosis is by stool examination with acid-fast stains. In normal hosts, disease is self-limited to 2–4 weeks. While previously there was no effective antimicrobial therapy and treatment was supportive [32], recent controlled trials showed efficacy of nitazoxanide [33]. It is now FDA approved for children and immunocompetent patients.

Cyclospora cayetanensis. Cyclospora causes prolonged watery diarrhea, often lasting 4–6 weeks. The organism resembles *Cryptosporidium*, but is larger, and has blue autofluorescence when examined by UV epifluorescence microscopy, hence the older names "cyanobacter" and "blue-green algae." It is transmitted by contaminated food or water. After ingestion and excystation, trophozoites invade epithelial cells in the small intestine. Since 1990, there have been at least 11 foodborne outbreaks in the USA and Canada [34]. If untreated the diarrhea may last 10–12 weeks and follow a relapsing course. Associated symptoms include anorexia, weight loss, nausea, vomiting, abdominal pain, and myalgias. Diagnosis is made by light microscopy detecting oocysts in stool; excretion can be intermittent, so multiple stools should be examined. Treatment with TMP–SMX shortens the course of illness.

Isospora belli. Isospora belli predominantly causes disease in immunocompromised hosts; however, the organism can also cause traveler's diarrhea and outbreaks in immunocompetent individuals. Similar to cryptosporidia, *Isospora* causes self-limited watery diarrhea in normal hosts and chronic diarrhea in immunosuppressed patients. Eosinophilia may be present. Diagnosis is made by identifying oocysts in stool with a modified acid-fast stain or by small bowel biopsy. Treatment is with TMP–SMX. Metronidazole and pyrimethamine are alternatives for patients with sulfa allergies [34].

Microsporidiosis. Microsporidia are increasingly recognized as opportunistic infections. Fourteen species infect humans, two of

Chapter 2 / Infectious Gastroenteritis and Colitis 41

which cause gastrointestinal illness: *Enterocytozoon bieneusi* and *Encephalitozoon intestinalis*. These pathogens cause chronic watery diarrhea and weight loss; *E. bieneusi* can also cause acalculous cholecystitis and *E. intestinalis* can disseminate to the eye, urinary, and respiratory tracts. Diagnosis is by light microscopy, which cannot distinguish species, or electron microscopy, which is expensive and time-consuming. Treatment for *E. bieneusi* is oral fumagillin [34]. *Encephalitozoon intestinalis* and disseminated microsporidiosis are treated with albendazole [34].

Ileocolonic Pathogens

BACTERIA

Campylobacter. *Campylobacter* species are common causes of diarrheal illness worldwide. *Campylobacter jejuni* causes the overwhelming majority of illness in the USA, with *Campylobacter coli* a distant second [35]. Campylobacteriosis is primarily a foodborne illness with poultry being the leading source of infection. *Campylobacter* can also be transmitted by the fecal–oral route or by contaminated milk, eggs, or water. *Campylobacter* is an invasive organism that induces an inflammatory response which can lead to edema, mucosal bleeding, formation of microabscesses, and ulcerations [6]. Symptoms include cramping, nausea, anorexia, and watery or bloody diarrhea. Infection is self-limited and usually resolves within a week. Colitis is common and can occasionally mimic appendicitis. Complications of infection include post-infectious irritable bowel syndrome, reactive arthritis (formerly Reiter's syndrome), and is the most common cause of Guillain–Barré syndrome [13]. Diagnosis is made by stool culture. Treatment is not indicated for mild-to-moderate illness and in fact may lead to increasing antimicrobial resistance. Treatment is appropriate in patients with severe disease or symptoms lasting longer than 1 week. Macrolides are the treatment of choice [3, 13, 35]. Fluoroquinolones can still be used, but there are increasing numbers of ciprofloxacin-resistant strains [36]. Resistance to macrolides is now being reported but tends to occur more often with *C. coli* than *C. jejuni* [35].

Salmonella. *Salmonella enterica* subspecies *enterica* has multiple serotypes. The most common serotypes infecting humans are *Salmonella enteritidis*, *Salmonella heidelberg*, *Salmonella newport*, *Salmonella typhimurium*, and *Salmonella typhi*. These organisms cause two distinct clinical syndromes: enterocolitis (nontyphoidal serotypes) and typhoid fever (*S. typhi*).

Enterocolitis (gastroenteritis). Nontyphoidal *Salmonella* gastroenteritis is a major cause of bacterial diarrhea in the USA with over 1 million cases estimated yearly [37]. In North America, *S. typhimurium* and *S. enteritidis* account for over half of cases; *S. newport* and *S. heidelberg* account for approximately 20% of cases [38]. *Salmonella* enterocolitis is commonly caused by contaminated foods such as poultry, egg yolks, fresh produce, ground beef, and milk. It has also been linked to exposure to animals. It is manifest most commonly as an acute self-limited illness of the small intestine, but the colon can also be affected. Dysentery (multiple small, bloody, mucoid stools with tenesmus) is uncommon. Severe complications such as bacteremia, meningitis, and endovascular lesions may occur in 5–10% of healthy individuals [37]. Risk factors for invasive infection include corticosteroid use, extremes of age, inflammatory bowel disease, immunosuppression, and hemoglobinopathies [13]. Most nontyphoidal *Salmonella* infections are limited to uncomplicated gastroenteritis and do not require treatment. Antibiotics do not decrease duration of symptoms. Instead, they contribute to adverse public health consequences such as prolonged shedding, increased likelihood of a carrier state and emergence of resistant strains [37]. Antibiotic therapy is indicated for severe symptoms, systemic disease, and patients with severe comorbid conditions or risk factors for invasive infection [13]. Multi-drug-resistant strains have emerged and are increasing in prevalence. Several studies have shown that compared to pansusceptible strains, resistance is associated with increased risks of hospitalization, bacteremia, invasive illness, and death [37, 39–41]. Treatment of severe disease has generally been with fluoroquinolones or ceftriaxone; azithromycin may be used [13]. Ciprofloxacin-resistant strains are increasing, and ceftriaxone-resistant strains are being reported [42, 43].

Typhoid fever. Typhoid fever is caused by *S. typhi* and is common in developing countries but rare in the USA. Symptoms occur in four distinct stages each lasting about 1 week: (1) nonspecific symptoms (including fevers and chills), (2) right lower quadrant pain with diarrhea and rose spots, (3) complications of infection, and (4) resolution of illness. Diagnosis is made by blood culture early in the course of illness or stool culture late in the course. Treatment is fluoroquinolones. However, as noted above, multi-drug-resistant strains are emerging.

Shigella. *Shigella* colitis is very common worldwide and is caused by four species: *Shigella dysenteriae* (which has 13 serotypes), *Shigella flexneri*, *Shigella boydii*, and *Shigella sonnei*. *Shigella dysenteriae* serotype 1 is a major cause of dysentery worldwide, accounting for approximately 75% of all diarrhea deaths [44]. In the USA, *S. sonnei*

Chapter 2 / Infectious Gastroenteritis and Colitis

and *S. flexneri* are the most common and cause less severe illness. Transmission is fecal–oral; *S. sonnei* is transmitted by uncooked food or contaminated water. Humans are the only natural host. *Shigella* is highly contagious, requiring less than 100 organisms to cause infection. The pathogenesis of *Shigella* is via invasion of colonic epithelium and production of enterotoxins [6, 44]. Symptoms usually include a 2-day prodrome of constitutional symptoms and secretory diarrhea, followed by dysentery, fever, abdominal cramps, and tenesmus. Colitis predominantly involves the left colon and rectum, and patients may have more than 20 dysenteric stools per day [44]. Shigellosis may be complicated by intestinal perforation, toxic megacolon, dehydration, metabolic derangements, sepsis, and multiple extraintestinal manifestations including thrombotic thrombocytopenic purpura (TTP) and hemolytic uremic syndrome (HUS). *Shigella* should be suspected clinically in patients who present with watery diarrhea followed by dysentery. Diagnosis is made with stool culture; susceptibility tests should be performed on all confirmed isolates. Initial treatment is with ORT. Antibiotics are always recommended for public health reasons, although most infections would resolve within 5–7 days without treatment. Antibiotics reduce the duration of diarrhea and the period of *Shigella* excretion. TMP–SMX is the treatment for shigellosis acquired in the USA, and fluoroquinolone is recommended for disease acquired outside the USA. However, as with *Salmonella*, there are increasing numbers of fluoroquinolone-resistant isolates. Other effective antibiotics include azithromycin [3, 13, 45], second- and third-generation cephalosporins (for invasive disease), and rifaximin [46].

Escherichia coli. Two types of *E. coli* affect the colon: enteroinvasive *E. coli* (EIEC) and Shiga toxin-producing *E. coli* (STEC). STEC strains that cause hemorrhagic colitis are also called enterohemorrhagic *E. coli* (EHEC).

EIEC causes a disease similar to *S. sonnei* infection clinically and also shares some biochemical and serologic properties with the organism [44]. EIEC invades the epithelium and produces a self-limited watery diarrhea or dysentery. The symptoms are generally mild and can be treated with a fluoroquinolone or azithromycin [3, 13].

While over 470 STEC serotypes may cause human disease, only 10 serotypes are responsible for the majority of cases [47], including *E. coli* O157:H7. Both O157 and non-O157 strains cause epidemics that peak in the summer. It is estimated that non-O157 strains cause 20–40% of all STEC infections [13, 48]. Ruminants, including cattle, are a major reservoir for STEC and contribute to the contamination of beef, water, and produce, such as basil pesto and alfalfa sprouts. STEC is not invasive but produces two distinct toxins: Shiga toxin 1 (Stx1) which is identical to that of *S. dysenteriae* serotype 1 and Shiga toxin 2 (Stx2), which is responsible for the vascular endothelial injury that leads to dysentery and TTP/HUS [47]. STEC has some capacity for invasion, but the majority of systemic effects are caused by absorption of toxin from the intestine [47].

The typical presentation is nausea, vomiting, and low-grade or absent fever, followed within 2–3 days by severe abdominal pain and diarrhea, which may become bloody. The stool may lack fecal leukocytes. Symptoms generally resolve within a week unless there are complications. *Escherichia coli* O157 strains often localize to the right colon and the illness may be mistaken for ischemic colitis in the elderly and intussusception or inflammatory bowel disease in the pediatric population. The most dreaded complication is TTP/HUS, which occurs in approximately 5–10% of patients, several days after the diarrhea begins [47]. Young children and the elderly are at greatest risk. TTP/HUS may lead to permanent renal failure, seizure, and death. Thrombocytopenia is usually the first abnormality seen, followed by hemolysis and renal failure [49]. Diagnosis of STEC infection is made by stool culture, with specialized testing of lipopolysaccharides for O157 organisms, and enzyme immunoassay (EIA) for Shiga toxin. When Shiga toxin is positive and O157:H7 is negative, testing should be performed for non-O157 serotypes [13].

Treatment of both STEC and resultant TTP/HUS is supportive with hydration; there is no role for plasmapheresis since ADAMTS-13 deficiencies are not the cause of disease [50]. Antibiotics and antimotility agents should be avoided, as there is no clear reduction of symptoms, and these agents likely increase the risk of developing TTP/HUS by increasing the release of toxin by bacteriolysis and phage induction [49–52]. Recent studies show that rifaximin, azithromycin, and fosfomycin do not induce Shiga toxin production or release [13, 53] and may be future antimicrobial treatment options.

Clostridium difficile. *Clostridium difficile* infection (CDI) is an important cause of both nosocomial and community-acquired diarrhea. Epidemics have been documented in hospitals and nursing homes, and more recently, community-acquired CDI has become a serious problem. *Clostridium difficile* causes infection by production of two toxins, enterotoxin A and cytotoxin B, which cause colonic mucosal inflammation. A new strain called NAPI/B1 is responsible for recent epidemics. This strain produces a binary toxin, carries a partial gene deletion allowing increased production of toxins A and B, and has quinolone resistance [54]. These properties likely make the strain *in*

Chapter 2 / Infectious Gastroenteritis and Colitis 45

vitro more virulent and allow for selection of the strain in patients taking fluoroquinolones.

Patients with CDI may present with watery or rarely bloody diarrhea, lower abdominal cramping, fever, and leukocytosis. Signs of severe disease include severe pain, abdominal distension, hypovolemia, lactic acidosis, and marked leukocytosis (>15,000). Predictors of mortality are severe leukocytosis or leukopenia ($\geq$35,000/μL or <4,000/μL), bandemia (neutrophil bands $\geq$ 10%), age $\geq$ 70, immunosuppression, and cardiorespiratory failure (intubation or vasopressors) [55, 56]. The host immune response may play an important role in pathophysiology. For example, patients that develop IgG against toxin A are more likely to remain asymptomatic carriers [57].

CDI should be suspected in anyone who develops diarrhea during or several weeks following antibiotic therapy. Patients who develop diarrhea while hospitalized should be tested for *C. difficile*. Because of the recent epidemics, even patients with community-acquired diarrhea may need to be tested for *C. difficile*. Diagnosis may be made by detection of the toxin in the stool. Many laboratories screen stools for *C. difficile* with a glutamate dehydrogenase antigen; if negative, no further testing is done. If positive, a confirmatory test for toxin A and/or B is done, either by EIA or PCR. However, stool tests vary in sensitivity and specificity; thus if clinical suspicion is high, empiric therapy should be given.

Treatment of CDI depends on severity of disease; however, in all cases, the offending antibiotic should be discontinued if possible, and antidiarrheals should be avoided [58]. For mild-to-moderate disease, treatment with either metronidazole 250 mg QID or 500 mg TID, or vancomycin 125 mg QID for 10–14 days is recommended. The lower dose of vancomycin (compared to 250 mg QID) is sufficient for mild-to-moderate disease and is less costly [59]. Since vancomycin is more expensive and poses the public health risk of increasing vancomycin-resistant *enterococcus*, metronidazole is the recommended first-line agent [58]. If there is no improvement after 3 days of metronidazole therapy, then vancomycin should be initiated.

However, for severe colitis, vancomycin 500 mg QID for four times a day is recommended. Some patients with severe CDI develop ileus or toxic megacolon and are unable to take oral antibiotics. In these cases, intravenous metronidazole 500 mg every 6–8 h should be used. In some cases, vancomycin may be given via nasogastric tube or rectally. Colectomy may be required for severe disease [56].

Following treatment for initial CDI, approximately 15–20% of patients will develop recurrent disease, usually within 5–8 days after completing antibiotic therapy. Risk factors for recurrence include older age, intercurrent antibiotics, renal disease, and prior recurrences of CDI. There is no standard regimen for recurrent CDI. It is important to understand that recurrence is not due to resistant organisms, and therefore retreatment with the same or alternate antibiotic is recommended. Additionally, vancomycin pulses or tapers for an extended duration are often used [60]. Two weeks of rifaximin following 2 weeks of vancomycin has shown promise. The probiotic *Saccharomyces boulardii* was also found to be a beneficial adjunct to high-dose vancomycin therapy but should not be used in immunosuppressed patients. Bacteriotherapy is an area of active study: fecal enemas, colonoscopic delivery of fecal material, and delivery of colonic flora through nasogastric tubes have shown success in small studies [61, 62].

Yersinia. Two *Yersinia* species cause gastrointestinal illness: *Yersinia enterocolitica* and *Yersinia pseudotuberculosis*. *Yersinia* is not common in the USA but is common in Northern Europe and is transmitted by ingestion of contaminated milk products or pork (especially chitterlings – hog intestines). It has also rarely been associated with red blood cell transfusions [63]. These species commonly cause acute colitis with abdominal pain (often in the right lower quadrant), fever, and diarrhea which may be bloody. Symptoms may mimic appendicitis or Crohn's disease. Extraintestinal manifestations include reactive arthritis, erythema nodosum, myocarditis, pulmonary infection, nephritis, osteomyelitis, and sepsis [64]. The diagnosis can be made by stool culture on special cold-enrichment medium. Cultures from nodes, blood, and peritoneal fluid may also be diagnostic. Serology with elevated titers in a typical clinical setting may be useful. Treatment is not necessary in most cases. For severe disease including enteritis, mesenteric adenitis, erythema nodosum, and arthritis, it is probably wise to treat. Recommended antibiotics are fluoroquinolones, TMP–SMX, or doxycycline in combination with an aminoglycoside [3].

Non-cholera Vibrios. The non-O1 non-O139 vibrios are often referred to as non-cholera vibrios. These include *Vibrio vulnificus*, *Vibrio parahemolyticus*, *Vibrio fluvialis*, *Vibrio alginolyticus*, as well as other less common vibrios. These pathogens do not cause epidemics or pandemics but can cause small outbreaks, usually associated with ingestion of raw or undercooked shellfish [65]. In the USA, the Gulf states have the highest prevalence of disease, and several cases occurred following Hurricane Katrina [66]. Patients with chronic liver disease are at increased risk of infection and should not eat undercooked shellfish. The non-cholera vibrios invade the colonic mucosa causing a self-limited bloody diarrhea and fever. However, several

Chapter 2 / Infectious Gastroenteritis and Colitis 47

extraintestinal manifestations have been reported, including peritonitis, sepsis, necrotizing soft-tissue infections, septic arthritis, keratitis, and endophthalmitis [67–73]. Treatment is generally not required, but tetracycline, azithromycin, or fluoroquinolone may be used for severe illness [13].

Plesiomonas shigelloides. *Plesiomonas* is an uncommon organism that may cause an acute secretory, acute dysenteric, or persistent diarrhea. Consumption of raw seafood and international travel may be risk factors [13, 74]. Rarely, it has been associated with biliary tract disease [75–77]. Treatment is usually not necessary, but if needed, TMP–SMX, fluoroquinolones, and azithromycin may be used [3, 13]. Susceptibility testing should be performed if treatment is needed.

Aeromonas hydrophila. This organism may affect either the small bowel or the colon. Outbreaks have been associated with water, food, and day care. *Aeromonas* primarily affects children, and the reported prevalence varies significantly in studies. Symptoms include watery diarrhea that may become bloody, abdominal cramps, nausea, vomiting, and fever. Illness generally resolves in 1–2 weeks but can become persistent or chronic, requiring antibiotics. Extraintestinal manifestations include bacteremia, cellulitis, peritonitis, meningitis, and respiratory disease [76]. Susceptibility varies greatly among strains, so susceptibility testing should be performed. Possible antimicrobial agents include azithromycin, fluoroquinolones, and TMP–SMX [3, 13].

Tuberculosis. In the USA, intestinal tuberculosis is most commonly seen in immigrants from high-risk regions and in persons with HIV. It often involves the ileocecal area. Findings are nonspecific, and patients may present with chronic abdominal pain, a palpable right lower quadrant mass, or constitutional symptoms; diarrhea is uncommon. Less than half of patients will have active pulmonary tuberculosis [78]. Skin tests may be positive. Diagnosis is made with colonoscopy and biopsy. Typical colonoscopic findings are discrete ulcers, often in the cecum [79].

Klebsiella oxytoca. For decades, the role of *K. oxytoca* as a pathogen was unclear. Recent evidence suggests that certain strains produce cytotoxin and are responsible for antibiotic-associated hemorrhagic colitis (AAHC), which can be acquired in the community or nosocomially [27, 80]. AAHC typically presents with the sudden-onset bloody diarrhea 2–7 days after initiation of treatment with penicillins and some cephalosporins [27, 80]. AAHC may mimic ischemic colitis. Less commonly, the illness may be nonhemorrhagic and delayed in onset [80].

Klebsiella oxytoca leads to mucosal hemorrhage and edema, predominantly in the right colon. Diagnosis is made by stool culture or biopsy and requires selective media. Most cases studied had rapid clinical and endoscopic resolution after withdrawal of antibiotics [26].

***Clostridium perfringens* type A.** *Clostridium perfringens* is ubiquitous in the environment and has been found to be part of the residential gut flora in up to 40% of healthy persons [27]. Only about 2–5% of *C. perfringens* isolates, usually type A, produce enterotoxin and can cause food poisoning. Patients usually develop watery diarrhea without vomiting within 48 h of ingestion of contaminated poultry, vegetables, or meat [13]. New evidence suggests that these enterotoxin-producing strains may also cause *C. difficile*-negative AAC in elderly patients due to alterations in gut flora [26].

PARASITES

Entameba histolytica. Several *Entameba* species colonize humans, but most are not pathogenic. *Entameba histolytica* is a well-recognized human pathogen. The protozoa are transmitted by the ingestion of cysts in contaminated food and water or by anal–oral sexual practices. Entamebae are found worldwide, with highest incidence in developing regions with poor sanitation [34]. Therefore, travelers to and immigrants from these regions are at risk. Patients may be asymptomatic or develop invasive intestinal and/or extraintestinal amebiasis. Invasive disease is caused by adherence to and lysis of colonic epithelium. Subsequent invasion of the bloodstream and extraintestinal spread may then occur [81]. Patients may present with abdominal pain, weight loss, and watery diarrhea, sometimes with blood. In the USA, dysentery is less common, and patients may present with colicky abdominal pain and diarrhea alternating with constipation, mimicking irritable bowel syndrome [82]. Rare manifestations of disease include acute necrotizing colitis, toxic megacolon, and ameboma. Invasive extraintestinal manifestations include liver abscesses, peritonitis, pleuropulmonary abscesses, and cutaneous or genital lesions [34]. Diagnosis may be made by stool microscopy. However, this method may not differentiate *E. histolytica* from non-pathogenic *Entameba dispar*. These organisms may be distinguished by serology, stool antigen detection, or PCR [83]. Treatment for asymptomatic infection is iodoquinol or paromomycin. Oral metronidazole three times a day is the treatment for invasive disease. Parental metronidazole can be used for severe cases and should be supplemented with broad-spectrum antibiotic coverage of intestinal flora to prevent secondary sepsis. A 3-day

Chapter 2 / Infectious Gastroenteritis and Colitis 49

course of nitazoxanide is a promising new regimen. Treatment of invasive disease should be followed by treatment with a luminal amebicide: iodoquinol or paromomycin [34, 83].

Trichuriasis (whipworm). Trichuriasis is a helminthic infection caused by the nematode *Trichuris trichiura*. It is common worldwide, especially in tropical regions and in the southern USA. It is associated with poor sanitation. Transmission is by fecal–oral spread. In mild infections, the cecum and the ascending colon are primarily involved, but the entire colon can be involved with severe infection. Most infections are asymptomatic. In severe cases, patients may have symptoms of loose stools often with blood or mucus, nocturnal stools, dysentery, and rectal prolapse. Other findings can include anemia, eosinophilia, pica, finger clubbing, and impaired growth and cognition in children. Diagnosis is by stool examination for eggs. Treatment of choice is mebendazole. Albendazole is an alternative choice [34].

Blastocystis hominis. *Blastocystis hominis* has been reclassified numerous times, and most recently, was classified as a stramenopile (an assemblage of unicellular and multicellular protists). Its pathogenicity is debated. The organism occurs in both symptomatic and asymptomatic persons, suggesting that it is not pathogenic. However, others have described clinical responses to antimicrobial therapy. Reported symptoms include watery diarrhea, abdominal pain, perianal pruritus, and excessive flatulence. Diagnosis is based on finding cysts in stool. Treatment is controversial, but metronidazole, iodoquinol, and nitazoxanide have reportedly been effective [34, 84].

Balantidium coli. This protozoan parasite is a rare cause of colitis. Most cases are asymptomatic, but it can cause persistent diarrhea, occasionally dysentery, abdominal pain, and weight loss. Diagnosis is made by detecting the protozoan in stool. Treatment is tetracycline or, alternatively, metronidazole [34].

Viruses

Cytomegalovirus. CMV can affect any part of the gastrointestinal tract in immunocompromised hosts, especially those with advanced HIV. Only enteritis and colitis cause diarrhea, with colonic disease predominating. Symptoms of colitis include explosive watery diarrhea, low-grade fever, weight loss, anorexia, malaise, abdominal pain, and bleeding [85, 86]. Diffuse mucosal hemorrhage and perforation are life-threatening complications. Diagnosis is made via colonoscopy and biopsy revealing mucosal ulcerations with characteristic intranuclear and intracytoplasmic inclusions. Treatment involves IV ganciclovir or foscarnet for 3–4 weeks. Oral valganciclovir may be used if symptoms are not severe enough to cause malabsorption, or after several days of treatment with the IV medications [87]. For patients who may start anti-retroviral therapy for HIV, it is important to ensure that the patient has had an ophthalmologic exam to rule out CMV retinitis.

CLINICAL EVALUATION

The assessment of a patient with acute infectious diarrhea includes an evaluation of volume status and severity of illness, a focused epidemiologic history, and a determination of whether or not diagnostic testing is indicated.

The initial evaluation focuses on the patient's volume status. In patients with diarrhea, the physical exam finding that best predicts volume depletion is dry axillae; severe postural dizziness, supine tachycardia, and a postural pulse increment of >30 bpm are suggestive. Although not predictive alone, the combination of confusion, extremity weakness, slurred speech, dry mucous membranes, dry or furrowed tongue, and sunken eyes suggests volume depletion, with more findings making the diagnosis more likely [88]. Because it is difficult to determine volume depletion accurately with physical exam alone, additional evaluation with a serum chemistry panel, urine electrolytes, and urine output is recommended. Rehydration therapy will be discussed below.

It is useful to distinguish between ileocolonic and small intestinal disease as this can help identify the pathogen and guide diagnostic testing (see Tables 2.1 and 2.2). Epidemiologic clues include travel history, recent hospitalizations, underlying medical illnesses, sexual history, and exposures to day care, unsafe foods, untreated fresh water, animals or ill persons (see Table 2.3). Severe disease is indicated by a prolonged illness, illness that is not improving after 48 h, passage of >6 stools per day, volume depletion, bloody or dysenteric stools, fever, and severe abdominal pain in patients older than 50 years. In evaluating infectious diarrhea, physical exam helps assess volume status and disease severity (i.e., abdominal pain or wasting) (see Table 2.4).

Diagnostic testing may be indicated for individuals or public health concerns. For the individual patient, diagnostic testing is indicated if the patient has severe disease as defined above, systemic symptoms, illness lasting > 1 week, or the patient is elderly or immunocompromised. For public health reasons, diagnostic testing is also indicated

Chapter 2 / Infectious Gastroenteritis and Colitis 51

Table 2.3
Epidemiologic features

Pathogen	Epidemiologic features and risk factors
Salmonella	Poultry, livestock, milk, raw eggs, fresh produce, pet turtles, and reptiles
Shigella	Family, day-care centers
Campylobacter	Poultry, meats, dairy products
Non-cholera vibrios	Raw or undercooked seafood, liver disease, alcoholism
C. difficile	Recent or current antibiotics, hospitalizations, chemotherapy
S. aureus	Custards and cream-based foods, poultry, eggs
C. perfringens	Meat, home canned foods, poultry, gravy
Listeria	Milk, lunch meats, and unpasteurized cheeses, pregnancy
Yersinia	Pork, chitterlings (hog intestine), hemochromatosis
STEC	Undercooked ground beef, day-care centers, petting zoos, unpasteurized apple cider, raw vegetables, leaf lettuce, basil pesto, salami
Cryptosporidia	Water, day-care centers
Giardia	Untreated fresh water, anal intercourse, day-care centers
Cyclospora	Day-care centers, imported raspberries, fresh basil
Microsporidia	HIV/AIDS
Norovirus	Fresh water, food borne, cruise ships, nursing homes, raw shellfish, schools, camps
Rotavirus	Day-care centers

Adapted from Ref. [94].

Table 2.4
Historical evaluation

Important questions to ask

- Disease severity
  Duration, onset (sudden vs gradual), frequency, volume depletion
- Ileocolonic vs small intestinal disease features (see Table 2.1)
- Associated symptoms
  Nausea, vomiting, abdominal pain, fever, headache, arthralgias
- Epidemiology (see Table 2.3)

Table 2.5
Indications for diagnostic testing of stool specimens

Who should have diagnostic testing?

- Severe illness
  Prolonged illness, illness not improving after 48 h, greater than six loose
    stools per day, volume depletion, bloody stools or dysentery, fever, and
    severe abdominal pain in persons age>50 years
- Immunocompromised patients (see IDSA guidelines for
    immunocompromised patients)
- Suspected outbreak
- Persons with high risk to spread infection
  Food handlers, caregivers, healthcare workers, day-care attendees or
    workers, institutionalized persons

when an outbreak is suspected or the patient is at high risk to transmit the infection to others (see Table 2.5).

DIAGNOSTIC EVALUATION

When diagnostic evaluation is indicated, it is important to decide what type of testing is appropriate. Diagnostic testing should be selective, based on the patient's individual clinical picture [3]. When the epidemiologic history suggests a specific pathogen, individual testing for the enteropathogen can be performed. Otherwise, the following studies should be considered.

Fecal Leukocytes and the Lactoferrin Assay

The utility of fecal leukocytes and stool lactoferrin is debated. Since these tests identify inflammatory markers, they are nonspecific to infectious enterocolitis; both have high false-positive rates, and cannot distinguish infectious from inflammatory diseases. A recent meta-analysis found that these tests performed better in evaluating patients in developed countries. The sensitivity and the specificity for fecal leukocytes in developed countries were 0.73 and 0.84, respectively, although bias in favor of the test was noted [89]. The lactoferrin assay appears to be useful when negative, but not when positive [89, 90]. Also, it may miss noninvasive infections such as STEC or ETEC [3]. Until new studies put the debate to rest, it is reasonable to consider the use of fecal lactoferrin or leukocytes as a screening tool to identify colonic inflammation. However, it is important to remember that some infections may be missed.

Stool Culture

In immunocompetent patients, indications for stool culture for enteric pathogens include bloody stools, severe diarrhea, fever, severe abdominal pain, or travel to high-risk areas. If symptoms persist for more than 1 week, stool cultures may be indicated. For nosocomial diarrhea, stool should be tested for *C. difficile*. When *C. difficile* testing is negative, other etiologies such as toxin-producing *S. aureus* and *C. perfringens*, *K. oxytoca*, and non-infectious causes should be considered. Patients with persistent diarrhea should be evaluated with stool ova and parasite testing.

TREATMENT

Rehydration, Nutrition, Electrolytes

The cornerstone of treatment for diarrheal illness is rehydration. Internationally, oral rehydration therapy (ORT) is the first-line treatment, but when available, intravenous fluids may be given for severe illness. WHO and UNICEF now recommend a reduced-osmolarity oral rehydration solution (ORS) for patients with acute, non-cholera diarrhea, as this solution was found to decrease both stool output and vomiting compared to standard ORS [91]. Electrolytes should be monitored and repleted. Newer ORS with resistant starches are being studied and show promise. Adequate nutrition is also important. Adults and children should consume easily digestible foods such as soups, crackers, and mashed potatoes. Infants should continue to breastfeed or drink formula [13, 91, 92]. Zinc supplementation reduces the duration and severity of illness in children [91, 92].

ANTIDIARRHEALS

Some antidiarrheal agents (including bismuth subsalicylate and loperamide) may be given safely in patients with infectious diarrhea. In the setting of appropriate antimicrobial therapy, most antimotility agents are unlikely to be harmful [13] and have shown benefit in traveler's diarrhea [93]. However, due to the risk of precipitating toxic megacolon or systemic illness by prolonged exposure of bacteria to the intestinal mucosa, antimotility agents are to be avoided in children, as well as in adults with severe bloody diarrhea, inflammatory diarrhea, severe colitis, or *C. difficile* infection.

ANTIMICROBIALS

Since there are individual and public health risks associated with antimicrobial therapy, it is generally best to await results of diagnostic testing before treating. Some risks of antibiotics include inducing TTP/HUS with STEC infection, increasing antimicrobial resistance, and exposing patients to side effects of antibiotic therapy. However, in certain situations, the benefits of empiric therapy outweigh the risks. Empiric therapy is thus recommended for the following situations: severe illness requiring hospitalization (particularly admission to an intensive care unit), moderate-to-severe traveler's diarrhea, elderly or immunocompromised hosts, suspected *C. difficile* colitis with severe disease, suspected shigellosis, or persistent diarrhea with suspected *Giardia*. If these conditions are not present, or there is suspicion for STEC (bloody diarrhea and absence of fever) or nontyphoidal *Salmonella*, or clinical uncertainty is present, it is most appropriate to wait for culture results before treating. Once an organism is identified, then treatment should be initiated as discussed above for each pathogen. Traveler's diarrhea may be treated empirically with ciprofloxacin, azithromycin, or rifaximin. New evidence suggests that chemoprophylaxis with rifaximin or bismuth subsalicylate may decrease acquisition of traveler's diarrhea by 65–70% [13]. As new antimicrobial resistance patterns are continually emerging, it is important to check frequently updated sources for antimicrobial recommendations.

CONCLUSION

Infectious diarrhea is a major cause of morbidity and mortality worldwide and is increasing in the USA due to current food cultivation and distribution practices. Most diarrheas can be classified as small intestinal or ileocolonic, which aids in the identification of the causative agent. Viral gastroenteritis remains the most common cause of infectious diarrhea in the USA and is treated supportively. Most moderate-to-severe disease is caused by bacterial pathogens, some of which require specific treatment. Antimicrobial therapy should be avoided in suspected cases of STEC and *Salmonella*. Empiric therapy may be appropriate based on epidemiologic and historical clues, the severity of illness, or specific host factors. As resistance patterns are continuously changing, checking updated sources prior to initiating antimicrobial treatment is recommended.

ACKNOWLEDGMENTS

Special thanks to John R. Newton, MD, for his support and assistance with research.

REFERENCES

1. Bern C. Diarrhoeal diseases. In: Murray CJL, Lopez AD, Mathers CD, eds. The global epidemiology of infectious diseases. Geneva, Switzerland: World Health Organization; 2004.
2. Kosek M, Bern C, Guerrant RL. The global burden of diarrhoeal disease, as estimated from studies published between 1992 and 2000. Bulletin of the World Health Organization 2003;81(3):197–204.
3. Guerrant RL, Van Gilder T, Steiner TS, et al. Practice guidelines for the management of infectious diarrhea. Clin Infect Dis 2001;32(3):331–351.
4. Jones TF, Bulens SN, Gettner S, et al. Use of stool collection kits delivered to patients can improve confirmation of etiology in foodborne disease outbreaks. Clin Infect Dis 2004;39(10):1454–1459.
5. Dryden MS, Gabb RJ, Wright SK. Empirical treatment of severe acute community-acquired gastroenteritis with ciprofloxacin. Clin Infect Dis 1996; 22(6):1019–1025.
6. Thielman NM, Guerrant RL. Clinical practice. Acute infectious diarrhea. N Engl J Med 2004 Jan 1;350(1):38–47.
7. Wilhelmi I, Roman E, Sanchez-Fauquier A. Viruses causing gastroenteritis. Clin Microbiol Infect 2003;9(4):247–262.
8. Clark B, McKendrick M. A review of viral gastroenteritis. Curr Opin Infect Dis 2004;17(5):461–469.
9. Lorrot M, Vasseur M. How do the rotavirus NSP4 and bacterial enterotoxins lead differently to diarrhea? Virol J 2007;4:31.
10. Cortese MM, Parashar UD. Prevention of rotavirus gastroenteritis among infants and children: recommendations of the Advisory Committee on Immunization Practices (ACIP). MMWR Recomm Rep 2009;58(RR-2):1–25.
11. Flores J, Okhuysen PC. Enteroaggregative *Escherichia coli* infection. Curr Opin Gastroenterol 2009;25(1):8–11.
12. Adachi JA, Jiang ZD, Mathewson JJ, et al. Enteroaggregative *Escherichia coli* as a major etiologic agent in traveler's diarrhea in 3 regions of the world. Clin Infect Dis 2001;32(12):1706–1709.
13. DuPont HL. Clinical practice. Bacterial diarrhea. N Engl J Med 2009; 361(16):1560–1569.
14. Spano LC, Sadovsky AD, Segui PN, et al. Age-specific prevalence of diffusely adherent *Escherichia coli* in Brazilian children with acute diarrhoea. J Med Microbiol 2008;57(Pt 3):359–363.
15. Sack DA, Sack RB, Nair GB, Siddique AK. Cholera. Lancet 2004;363(9404): 223–233.
16. King AA, Ionides EL, Pascual M, Bouma MJ. Inapparent infections and cholera dynamics. Nature 2008;454(7206):877–880.
17. von Seidlein L, Wang XY, Macuamule A, et al. Is HIV infection associated with an increased risk for cholera? Findings from a case–control study in Mozambique. Trop Med Int Health 2008;13(5):683–688.
18. Gregorio GV, Gonzales ML, Dans LF, Martinez EG. Polymer-based oral rehydration solution for treating acute watery diarrhoea. Cochrane Database Syst Rev 2009(2):CD006519.
19. Raghupathy P, Ramakrishna BS, Oommen SP, et al. Amylase-resistant starch as adjunct to oral rehydration therapy in children with diarrhea. J Pediatr Gastroenterol Nutr 2006;42(4):362–368.

20. Ramakrishna BS, Subramanian V, Mohan V, et al. A randomized controlled trial of glucose versus amylase resistant starch hypo-osmolar oral rehydration solution for adult acute dehydrating diarrhea. PLoS One 2008;3(2):e1587.
21. Qureshi K, Molbak K, Sandstrom A, et al. Breast milk reduces the risk of illness in children of mothers with cholera: observations from an epidemic of cholera in Guinea-Bissau. Pediatr Infect Dis J 2006;25(12):1163–1166.
22. Coppa GV, Zampini L, Galeazzi T, et al. Human milk oligosaccharides inhibit the adhesion to Caco-2 cells of diarrheal pathogens: *Escherichia coli*, *Vibrio cholerae*, and *Salmonella fyris*. Pediatr Res 2006;59(3):377–382.
23. Dalton CB, Austin CC, Sobel J, et al. An outbreak of gastroenteritis and fever due to *Listeria monocytogenes* in milk. N Engl J Med 1997;336(2):100–105.
24. Ooi ST, Lorber B. Gastroenteritis due to *Listeria monocytogenes*. Clin Infect Dis 2005;40(9):1327–1332.
25. Aureli P, Fiorucci GC, Caroli D, et al. An outbreak of febrile gastroenteritis associated with corn contaminated by *Listeria monocytogenes*. N Engl J Med 2000;342(17):1236–1241.
26. Beaugerie L, Petit JC. Microbial–gut interactions in health and disease. Antibiotic-associated diarrhoea. Best Pract Res Clin Gastroenterol 2004;18(2):337–352.
27. Gorkiewicz G. Nosocomial and antibiotic-associated diarrhoea caused by organisms other than *Clostridium difficile*. Int J Antimicrob Agents 2009; 33(Suppl 1):S37–S41.
28. Jernigan J, Guerrant RL, Pearson RD. Parasitic infections of the small intestine. Gut 1994;35(3):289–293.
29. Haque R, Roy S, Kabir M, Stroup SE, Mondal D, Houpt ER. Giardia assemblage A infection and diarrhea in Bangladesh. J Infect Dis 2005;192(12):2171–2173.
30. Sahagun J, Clavel A, Goni P, et al. Correlation between the presence of symptoms and the *Giardia duodenalis* genotype. Eur J Clin Microbiol Infect Dis 2008;27(1):81–83.
31. Lebwohl B, Deckelbaum RJ, Green PH. Giardiasis. Gastrointest Endosc 2003;57(7):906–913.
32. Egyed Z, Sreter T, Szell Z, Varga I. Characterization of *Cryptosporidium* spp.—recent developments and future needs. Vet Parasitol 2003;111(2–3): 103–114.
33. Rossignol JF. *Cryptosporidium* and *Giardia*: treatment options and prospects for new drugs. Exp Parasitol 2009.
34. Parasites of the Intestinal Tract (Accessed Aug 20, 2009, at http://www.dpd.cdc. gov/dpdx/).
35. Alfredson DA, Korolik V. Antibiotic resistance and resistance mechanisms in *Campylobacter jejuni* and *Campylobacter coli*. FEMS Microbiol Lett 2007;277(2):123–132.
36. Nachamkin I, Ung H, Li M. Increasing fluoroquinolone resistance in *Campylobacter jejuni*, Pennsylvania, USA, 1982–2001. Emerg Infect Dis 2002; 8(12):1501–1503.
37. Su LH, Chiu CH. *Salmonella*: clinical importance and evolution of nomenclature. Chang Gung Med J 2007;30(3):210–219.
38. WHO Global Salmonella Survey, 2000–2005. WHO Press, World Health Organization, 2006 (Accessed Sept 4, 2009, at http://www.who.int/salmsurv/links/ GSSProgressReport2005.pdf).
39. Helms M, Simonsen J, Molbak K. Quinolone resistance is associated with increased risk of invasive illness or death during infection with *Salmonella serotype Typhimurium*. J Infect Dis 2004;190(9):1652–1654.

Chapter 2 / Infectious Gastroenteritis and Colitis 57

40. Molbak K. Human health consequences of antimicrobial drug-resistant *Salmonella* and other foodborne pathogens. Clin Infect Dis 2005;41(11):1613–1620.
41. Varma JK, Molbak K, Barrett TJ, et al. Antimicrobial-resistant nontyphoidal *Salmonella* is associated with excess bloodstream infections and hospitalizations. J Infect Dis 2005;191(4):554–561.
42. Su LH, Chiu CH, Chu C, Ou JT. Antimicrobial resistance in nontyphoid *Salmonella* serotypes: a global challenge. Clin Infect Dis 2004;39(4): 546–551.
43. Su LH, Wu TL, Chia JH, Chu C, Kuo AJ, Chiu CH. Increasing ceftriaxone resistance in *Salmonella* isolates from a university hospital in Taiwan. J Antimicrob Chemother 2005;55(6):846–852.
44. Niyogi SK. Shigellosis. J Microbiol 2005;43(2):133–143.
45. Khan WA, Seas C, Dhar U, Salam MA, Bennish ML. Treatment of shigellosis: V. Comparison of azithromycin and ciprofloxacin. A double-blind, randomized, controlled trial. Ann Intern Med 1997;126(9):697–703.
46. Taylor DN, McKenzie R, Durbin A, et al. Rifaximin, a nonabsorbed oral antibiotic, prevents shigellosis after experimental challenge. Clin Infect Dis 2006;42(9):1283–1288.
47. Gyles CL. Shiga toxin-producing *Escherichia coli*: an overview. J Anim Sci 2007;85(13 Suppl):E45–E62.
48. Talan D, Moran GJ, Newdow M, et al. Etiology of bloody diarrhea among patients presenting to United States emergency departments: prevalence of *Escherichia coli* O157:H7 and other enteropathogens. Clin Infect Dis 2001;32(4):573–580.
49. Tarr PI, Gordon CA, Chandler WL. Shiga-toxin-producing *Escherichia coli* and haemolytic uraemic syndrome. Lancet 2005;365(9464):1073–1086.
50. Iijima K, Kamioka I, Nozu K. Management of diarrhea-associated hemolytic uremic syndrome in children. Clin Exp Nephrol 2008;12(1):16–19.
51. Dundas S, Todd WT, Stewart AI, Murdoch PS, Chaudhuri AK, Hutchinson SJ. The central Scotland *Escherichia coli* O157:H7 outbreak: risk factors for the hemolytic uremic syndrome and death among hospitalized patients. Clin Infect Dis 2001;33(7):923–931.
52. Wong CS, Jelacic S, Habeeb RL, Watkins SL, Tarr PI. The risk of the hemolytic–uremic syndrome after antibiotic treatment of *Escherichia coli* O157:H7 infections. N Engl J Med 2000;342(26):1930–1936.
53. Ochoa TJ, Chen J, Walker CM, Gonzales E, Cleary TG. Rifaximin does not induce toxin production or phage-mediated lysis of Shiga toxin-producing *Escherichia coli*. Antimicrob Agents Chemother 2007;51(8):2837–2841.
54. McDonald LC, Killgore GE, Thompson A, et al. An epidemic, toxin gene-variant strain of *Clostridium difficile*. N Engl J Med 2005;353(23):2433–2441.
55. Sailhamer EA, Carson K, Chang Y, et al. Fulminant *Clostridium difficile* colitis: patterns of care and predictors of mortality. Arch Surg 2009;144(5):433–439; discussion 9–40.
56. Lamontagne F, Labbe AC, Haeck O, et al. Impact of emergency colectomy on survival of patients with fulminant *Clostridium difficile* colitis during an epidemic caused by a hypervirulent strain. Ann Surg 2007;245(2):267–272.
57. Kyne L, Warny M, Qamar A, Kelly CP. Asymptomatic carriage of *Clostridium difficile* and serum levels of IgG antibody against toxin A. N Engl J Med 2000;342(6):390–397.
58. Gerding DN, Johnson S, Peterson LR, Mulligan ME, Silva J Jr. *Clostridium difficile*-associated diarrhea and colitis. Infect Control Hosp Epidemiol 1995;16(8):459–477.

59. Zar FA, Bakkanagari SR, Moorthi KM, Davis MB. A comparison of vancomycin and metronidazole for the treatment of *Clostridium difficile*-associated diarrhea, stratified by disease severity. Clin Infect Dis 2007;45(3):302–307.

60. Surawicz CM. Treatment of recurrent *Clostridium difficile*-associated disease. Nat Clin Pract Gastroenterol Hepatol 2004;1(1):32–38.

61. Persky SE, Brandt LJ. Treatment of recurrent *Clostridium difficile*-associated diarrhea by administration of donated stool directly through a colonoscope. Am J Gastroenterol 2000;95(11):3283–3285.

62. Aas J, Gessert CE, Bakken JS. Recurrent *Clostridium difficile* colitis: case series involving 18 patients treated with donor stool administered via a nasogastric tube. Clin Infect Dis 2003;36(5):580–585.

63. Leclercq A, Martin L, Vergnes ML, et al. Fatal *Yersinia enterocolitica* biotype 4 serovar O:3 sepsis after red blood cell transfusion. Transfusion 2005;45(5): 814–818.

64. Zheng H, Sun Y, Lin S, Mao Z, Jiang B. *Yersinia enterocolitica* infection in diarrheal patients. Eur J Clin Microbiol Infect Dis 2008;27(8):741–752.

65. Dechet AM, Yu PA, Koram N, Painter J. Nonfoodborne *Vibrio* infections: an important cause of morbidity and mortality in the United States, 1997–2006. Clin Infect Dis 2008;46(7):970–976.

66. Centers for Disease Control and Prevention (CDC). *Vibrio* illnesses after Hurricane Katrina—multiple states, August–September 2005. MMWR Morb Mortal Wkly Rep 2005;54(37):928–931.

67. Jung EY, Kim DW, Lee DW, Cho HS, Chang SH, Park DJ. *Vibrio vulnificus* peritonitis after eating raw sea fish in a patient undergoing continuous ambulatory peritoneal dialysis (CAPD). Nephrol Dial Transplant 2007;22(5):1487.

68. Lee JY, Park JS, Oh SH, Kim HR, Lee JN, Shin JH. Acute infectious peritonitis caused by *Vibrio fluvialis*. Diagn Microbiol Infect Dis 2008;62(2):216–218.

69. You IC, Ahn M, Yoon KW, Yoon KC. A case of *Vibrio vulnificus* keratitis. Jpn J Ophthalmol 2008;52(2):131–133.

70. Tsai YH, Huang TJ, Hsu RW, et al. Necrotizing soft-tissue infections and primary sepsis caused by *Vibrio vulnificus* and *Vibrio cholerae* non-O1. J Trauma 2009;66(3):899–905.

71. Kuo CH, Dai ZK, Wu JR, Hsieh TJ, Hung CH, Hsu JH. Septic arthritis as the initial manifestation of fatal *Vibrio vulnificus* septicemia in a patient with thalassemia and iron overload. Pediatr Blood Cancer 2009;53(6):1156–1158.

72. Li XC, Xiang ZY, Xu XM, Yan WH, Ma JM. Endophthalmitis caused by *Vibrio alginolyticus*. J Clin Microbiol 2009;47(10):3379–3381.

73. Lai CH, Hwang CK, Chin C, Lin HH, Wong WW, Liu CY. Severe watery diarrhoea and bacteraemia caused by *Vibrio fluvialis*. J Infect 2006;52(3):e95–e98.

74. Kain KC, Kelly MT. Clinical features, epidemiology, and treatment of *Plesiomonas shigelloides* diarrhea. J Clin Microbiol 1989;27(5):998–1001.

75. Khan AM, Faruque AS, Hossain MS, Sattar S, Fuchs GJ, Salam MA. *Plesiomonas shigelloides*-associated diarrhoea in Bangladeshi children: a hospital-based surveillance study. J Trop Pediatr 2004;50(6):354–356.

76. Schlenker C, Surawicz CM. Emerging infections of the gastrointestinal tract. Best Pract Res Clin Gastroenterol 2009;23(1):89–99.

77. Woo PC, Lau SK, Yuen KY. Biliary tract disease as a risk factor for *Plesiomonas shigelloides* bacteraemia: a nine-year experience in a Hong Kong hospital and review of the literature. N Microbiol 2005;28(1):45–55.

78. Misra SP, Misra V, Dwivedi M, Gupta SC. Colonic tuberculosis: clinical features, endoscopic appearance and management. J Gastroenterol Hepatol 1999;14(7):723–729.

Chapter 2 / Infectious Gastroenteritis and Colitis

59

79. Kochhar R, Rajwanshi A, Goenka MK, et al. Colonoscopic fine needle aspiration cytology in the diagnosis of ileocecal tuberculosis. Am J Gastroenterol 1991;86(1):102–104.

80. Beaugerie L, Metz M, Barbut F, et al. *Klebsiella oxytoca* as an agent of antibiotic-associated hemorrhagic colitis. Clin Gastroenterol Hepatol 2003;1(5):370–376.

81. Haque R, Huston CD, Hughes M, Houpt E, Petri WA Jr. Amebiasis. N Engl J Med 2003;348(16):1565–1573.

82. Stark D, van Hal S, Marriott D, Ellis J, Harkness J. Irritable bowel syndrome: a review on the role of intestinal protozoa and the importance of their detection and diagnosis. Int J Parasitol 2007;37(1):11–20.

83. Pritt BS, Clark CG. Amebiasis. Mayo Clin Proc 2008;83(10):1154–1159; quiz 9–60.

84. Rossignol JF, Kabil SM, Said M, Samir H, Younis AM. Effect of nitazoxanide in persistent diarrhea and enteritis associated with *Blastocystis hominis*. Clin Gastroenterol Hepatol 2005;3(10):987–991.

85. Dieterich DT, Rahmin M. *Cytomegalovirus colitis* in AIDS: presentation in 44 patients and a review of the literature. J Acquir Immune Defic Syndr 1991;4 (Suppl 1):S29–S35.

86. Whitley RJ, Jacobson MA, Friedberg DN, et al. Guidelines for the treatment of cytomegalovirus diseases in patients with AIDS in the era of potent antiretroviral therapy: recommendations of an international panel. International AIDS Society—USA. Arch Intern Med 1998;158(9):957–969.

87. Kaplan JE, Benson C, Holmes KH, Brooks JT, Pau A, Masur H. Guidelines for prevention and treatment of opportunistic infections in HIV-infected adults and adolescents: recommendations from CDC, the National Institutes of Health, and the HIV Medicine Association of the Infectious Diseases Society of America. MMWR Recomm Rep 2009;58(RR-4):1–207; quiz CE1–4.

88. McGee S, Abernethy WB 3rd, Simel DL. The rational clinical examination. Is this patient hypovolemic? JAMA 1999;281(11):1022–1029.

89. Gill CJ, Lau J, Gorbach SL, Hamer DH. Diagnostic accuracy of stool assays for inflammatory bacterial gastroenteritis in developed and resource-poor countries. Clin Infect Dis 2003;37(3):365–375.

90. Silletti RP, Lee G, Ailey E. Role of stool screening tests in diagnosis of inflammatory bacterial enteritis and in selection of specimens likely to yield invasive enteric pathogens. J Clin Microbiol 1996;34(5):1161–1165.

91. WHO/UNICEF. Clinical management of acute diarrhoea. WHO/UNICEF Joint Statement 2004.

92. Gadewar S, Fasano A. Current concepts in the evaluation, diagnosis and management of acute infectious diarrhea. Curr Opin Pharmacol 2005;5(6):559–565.

93. Riddle MS, Arnold S, Tribble DR. Effect of adjunctive loperamide in combination with antibiotics on treatment outcomes in traveler's diarrhea: a systematic review and meta-analysis. Clin Infect Dis 2008;47(8):1007–1014.

94. Surawicz CM. GI infections of the small intestine and colon. In: Chang E, ed. Digestive diseases, Self Education Program (DDSEP V and 2006). Bethesda, MD: AGA, 2004.

3 Inflammatory Bowel Disease

Steven Bernick, MD and Sunanda Kane, MD, MSPH

CONTENTS

INTRODUCTION
EPIDEMIOLOGY
PATHOPHYSIOLOGY
DIFFERENTIAL DIAGNOSIS
CLINICAL PRESENTATION
EVALUATION
TREATMENT
PROGNOSIS
REFERENCES

Summary

In summary, diarrhea is a frequent complaint in patients with IBD, with a complex pathophysiologic basis. In any patient presenting with a new inflammatory diarrhea, a wide variety of etiologies must be considered, including a new diagnosis of UC or CD. In patients with pre-existing IBD, the prudent clinician must consider not only a potential exacerbation of their documented disease but also a number of other potential confounding conditions. A focused but thorough medical history, physical examination, laboratory evaluation, and imaging studies may be useful. Endoscopic examination of the upper or the lower digestive tracts may be necessary in the majority of patients. There are a number of antidiarrheal therapies that may be used for symptomatic control in these patients; however the treatment of the underlying disease is the primary goal.

From: *Diarrhea, Clinical Gastroenterology*
Edited by: S. Guandalini, H. Vaziri, DOI 10.1007/978-1-60761-183-7_3
© Springer Science+Business Media, LLC 2011

Key Words: Inflammatory bowel disease, Crohn's disease, Ulcerative colitis, CARD15, NOD2, *Clostridium difficile*, *Yersinia enterocolitica*, *Escherichia coli* 0157:H7, • TNF-α (alpha), 5-Aminosalicylate, 5-ASA, Irritable pouch syndrome, Small bowel bacterial overgrowth, Extraintestinal manifestations of IBD, Video capsule endoscopy, Endoscopy, Colonoscopy, Esophagogastroduodenoscopy, Noncaseating granulomas, Terminal ileum, Mesalamine, Sulfasalazine, Glucocorticoids, Corticosteroids, Cyclosporine, Methotrexate, Infliximab, Adalimumab, Certolizumab pegol, Natalizumab, Immunomodulators, Probiotic

INTRODUCTION

Inflammatory bowel disease (IBD) is an umbrella term that primarily incorporates both ulcerative colitis (UC) and Crohn's disease (CD), although other disorders resulting in inflammation, including microscopic (lymphocytic) colitis, collagenous colitis, and diverticulitis, also fall under this rubric. This chapter will primarily focus on UC and CD. Both diseases encompass a multisystem group of symptoms with specific clinical and pathological features, often characterized by intermittent exacerbations of symptoms and periods of disease remission that may occur spontaneously or in response to treatment.

Ulcerative colitis is a mucosal inflammatory process limited to the rectum and the colon, characterized by contiguous inflammation beginning in the rectum and progressing proximally for variable distances. Different terms are used to describe the extent of disease, with ulcerative proctitis referring to disease limited to the rectum, left-sided colitis referring to disease that extends to the splenic flexure, and pancolitis referring to inflammation that extends beyond the splenic flexure. Isolated involvement of the cecum (a cecal patch) or the terminal ileum (so-called "backwash ileitis") may also be noted.

While CD can manifest as a pure colitis, with phenotypic features that are difficult to differentiate from UC, this disorder is more notably characterized by focal, asymmetric, transmural, and occasionally granulomatous inflammation that can involve the entire gastrointestinal tract [1]. Due to the transmural nature of inflammation in CD, complications such as fistulization, intestinal strictures, obstruction, and abscesses, with the additional potential for perianal disease, may also be seen. While CD can occur anywhere in the gastrointestinal tract from the mouth to the anus, approximately 80% of patients will have some involvement of the small bowel, with one-third having disease that is exclusive to the ileum. Approximately half of all patients with CD will have ileocolitis, one-third will have perianal disease, and

10% will have rectal sparing. These differences between UC and CD are important, as they impact upon the clinical presentation of these disorders.

Diarrhea remains one of the most common symptoms reported in patients with IBD, ranging from a symptomatic nuisance to a potentially life-threatening crisis [2]. Diarrhea is the initial symptom in 50% of flares in CD and nearly 100% in UC [3]. The mechanisms of diarrhea in IBD are multifactorial and dependent in large part upon the extent and distribution of disease. It is paramount that physicians take the necessary measures to fully evaluate a patient with IBD who endorses a change in the character, frequency, or severity of their diarrhea, as differentiation between a flare of pre-existing IBD and an alternate etiology for their complaint is essential. It is important to remember that not all diarrheas in the IBD patient are the same, and the therapy must be tailored according to the presumed etiology [2].

EPIDEMIOLOGY

Despite years of investigation, the etiology of IBD has not yet been identified. Although the highest prevalence occurs in North America, the United Kingdom, and northern Europe, these diseases are increasingly being reported in other parts of the world as they become more "Westernized." In North America, prevalence rates range from 37 to 246 cases per 100,000 persons for UC and from 26 to 199 cases per 100,000 persons for CD [4]. Thus IBD is a common ailment and as such must be considered in the differential diagnosis for a patient presenting with the complaint of diarrhea.

Most cases of IBD occur in the second and third decade of life; however many studies suggest a bimodal distribution of disease, with a second peak between age 50 and 80 [5]. In addition to an increased incidence in the Ashkenazi Jewish population, patients with IBD have a 5–20% chance of having a first-degree relative with this disorder, with a positive family history noted more frequently in patients with CD than with UC [6].

PATHOPHYSIOLOGY

The pathophysiology of IBD is complex and not completely elucidated. A complete discussion is beyond the focus of this chapter. However, there is mounting evidence that IBD involves a complex interaction between four separate mechanisms, each of which may serve as specific targets for current and future therapeutic endeavors. These include a genetic predisposition that results in immune regulatory cell derangement, defects in the mucosal barrier, and a susceptibility to environmental triggers that include specific antigens as well as the patient's commensal luminal bacteria [3].

Genetic mutations in genes such as *CARD15* and *NOD2* can cause defects in important immune regulatory proteins, the consequence of which may be initiation of systemic responses that lead to uncontrolled inflammation. The presence of such mutations may also provide important prognostic information, such as preponderance for early onset disease, fistulization, and ileitis [6].

Alterations in mucosal immunity have also been demonstrated in patients with IBD, where an increase in the effect cell population (such as CD4 T-helper cells, Th1/Th2) with excessive inflammatory responses or a decreased function of regulatory-type T cells can result in mucosal inflammation. Other mediators, such as tumor necrosis factor alpha (TNF-α) and mitogen-activated protein kinases (MAPKs), are also believed to be crucial for the inflammatory process [7].

The intestinal epithelium acts as a selective barrier between the intestinal lumen and the luminal contents and mediates communication with the mucosal immune system. Derangement of this barrier results in increased permeability, with the subsequent loss of ions and water and the entry of antigens and macromolecules [7].

The role of the patient's luminal commensal bacteria has been investigated with the use of germ-free mouse models, which do not develop intestinal inflammation. From such models, we have learned that CD4 T-helper cells act as effectors, while native bacterial flora seems to drive the disease through an overly aggressive cellular response in genetically susceptible individuals [7].

Diarrhea in IBD

The mechanisms of diarrhea in IBD are complex and multifactorial, involving mucosal inflammation, malabsorption, and dysmotility. In both UC and CD, the severity and clinical manifestations are dependent upon the distribution of the disease. For example, ulcerative proctitis may result in tenesmus, urgency, and hematochezia, while small bowel CD may result in bile salt and fat malabsorption causing bloating and steatorrhea. The most important underlying mechanism for diarrhea is inflammation, which leads to stimulation of anion secretion and impaired absorption, as well as denudation of the epithelium resulting in the leakage of plasma and blood, collectively leading to secretory diarrhea [2]. When small bowel disease is present, malabsorption can result from both intestinal inflammation and surgical intervention. Compounding this is the potential for small bowel bacterial overgrowth

(SBBO) secondary to the stricturing disease and dysmotility, which may result in both fat malabsorption due to bacterial deconjugation of bile and a relative increase in the osmotic load delivered to the small bowel.

Finally, active colitis is accompanied by a relative dysmotility that decreases the absorption of water and electrolytes in the colon [2].

Diarrhea as a Side Effect of Medication

Medications available to treat IBD are available in a variety of forms, including oral tablets or capsules, foam or liquid enemas, suppositories, and subcutaneous or intravenous injections. As with many types of pharmacotherapy, the tolerance to these medications varies widely from patient to patient. It should be noted, however, that diarrhea is a well-documented side effect from all classes of medications used to treat IBD, including 5-aminosalicylate (5-ASA) compounds, antibiotics, immunomodulators, and biologics. As would be expected, the frequency of diarrhea varies among various treatment modalities. Olsalazine, a 5-ASA compound that requires colonic bacteria to cleave its azo bond, causes secretory diarrhea in up to 12.5% of patient [8]. Hypersensitivity to 5-ASA compounds can also cause worsening of diarrhea after initiation of treatment, which generally resolves after the drug is stopped. Furthermore, antibiotics, which are frequently used in the treatment of Crohn's disease, are well known for causing an osmotic form of diarrhea.

DIFFERENTIAL DIAGNOSIS

The differential diagnosis in the evaluation of diarrhea is naturally quite broad (see Table 3.1). The specific symptoms and signs that often accompany inflammatory diarrhea (abdominal pain, constitutional symptoms, hematochezia, and extraintestinal manifestations, for example) help to narrow the possible etiologies. However, a variety of causes must be considered prior to embarking upon a more extensive diagnostic evaluation and treatment for IBD. Included in this differential diagnosis are typical infectious diseases caused by organisms such as *Salmonella*, *Shigella*, and *Campylobacter*, as well as atypical infections in patients on immunosuppressive therapy, such as cytomegalovirus (CMV). Yersiniosis may mimic CD in presentation and must be considered on the list of potential pathogens. Enterohemorrhagic *Escherichia coli* (EHEC) can produce bloody diarrhea and abdominal pain, and should therefore be ruled out. Intestinal amebiasis can present with severe dysentery and should be considered in those patients with the appropriate exposure history.

Table 3.1
Differential diagnosis for diarrhea in IBD

Inflammatory diarrhea
- Infectious colitis
  - *Salmonella/Shigella/Campylobacter*
  - Yersiniosis
  - Enterohemorrhagic *E. coli* O157:H7
  - CMV colitis
  - *C. difficile* infection
  - Intestinal amebiasis
- Ischemic colitis
- Diverticulitis
- Diverticular disease-associated segmental colitis
- Inflammatory bowel disease new onset or flare of existing disease

Non-inflammatory diarrhea
- Viral enteritis
- Small bowel bacterial overgrowth (SBBO)
- Lactose intolerance or food intolerance
- Irritable pouch syndrome (IPS) or irritable bowel syndrome (IBS)
- Brisk gastrocolic reflex
- Postsurgical (bile salt diarrhea, diversion colitis, pouchitis)
- Secondary to Crohn's disease (gastrocolic fistula, intestinal stricture/ obstruction, anorectal disease)
- Fecal incontinence

Of particular consideration is *Clostridium difficile* infection (CDI), which is noted with increased incidence in patients with IBD and may present in an atypical fashion.

Patients with IBD have a four times greater mortality and higher rate of colectomy than those without underlying IBD [9]. Given the common use of immunosuppressive medications and antibiotics in this patient population, a high level of suspicion must be maintained when confronted with an IBD patient with symptoms suggestive of CDI.

Non-infectious etiologies for inflammatory diarrhea include diverticulitis, diverticular disease-associated segmental colitis, and ischemic colitis, but these can usually be discerned from IBD by history and imaging studies. Other considerations in a patient with IBD who presents with diarrhea should include bile salt-induced diarrhea, bypass of luminal contents via a fistula (such as a gastrocolic fistula), intestinal obstruction or stricture, diversion colitis, SBBO (particularly if the patient has a history of ileocolonic resection or intestinal strictures), and anorectal disease with fecal incontinence which patients may report as "diarrhea" [1].

Finally, while not inflammatory in nature, one must consider other common causes for diarrhea such as viral enteritis, medication effects, lactose intolerance (particularly in those with jejunitis or large jejunal resections, as lactase is primarily located in this segment), food intolerance, a brisk gastrocolic reflex, and irritable bowel syndrome (IBS).

CLINICAL PRESENTATION

Characteristic symptoms of IBD include chronic and often nocturnal diarrhea and abdominal pain. Constitutional symptoms (weight loss, night sweats, and fever) are frequently noted and are reflective of the underlying mucosal inflammation. Hematochezia, urgency, and tenesmus are common complaints in UC but may be absent in CD. Clinical signs include pallor, cachexia, an abdominal mass or tenderness, perianal fissures, fistulas, and abscess. In the pediatric population, growth failure or pubertal delay may be seen. Although the onset of these signs and symptoms are typically insidious, fulminant presentations with toxic megacolon and systemic toxicity can occasionally be seen.

Associated extraintestinal manifestations of IBD include spondyloarthritis (ankylosing spondylitis and sacroiliitis), peripheral arthritis (typically pauciarticular involving the large joints), cutaneous manifestations (erythema nodosum and pyoderma gangrenosum), ocular inflammation (uveitis, episcleritis, and sclera-conjunctivitis), primary sclerosing cholangitis, and hypercoagulability. Sequelae related to malabsorbtion, such as anemia, cholelithiasis, nephrolithiasis, and metabolic bone disease, may also be present. There is also an increased risk for gastrointestinal adenocarcinoma with prolonged duration of IBD [1].

There are multiple factors known to exacerbate IBD, including infections (both intra- and extracolonic), the use of nonsteroidal anti-inflammatory drugs (NSAIDS), and, in CD, cigarette smoking [10].

Although patients and practitioners believe that stress may play a role in symptomatology of IBD, this has not yet been demonstrated in a reproducible fashion [11].

EVALUATION

As with any clinical evaluation, the first step is the solicitation of a focused history. This not only can provide important diagnostic information but also may guide the clinician in identifying risk factors for the development of IBD as well as in the choice of appropriate therapeutic intervention. In addition to obtaining a complete past medical and surgical history, the patient should be queried regarding relevant travel, residence, occupation, pets, and hobbies, as these may provide important clues to an underlying infectious etiology. Family history is also important. The presence of a first-degree relative with IBD substantially increases an individual's risk, although the majority of patients with IBD lack such a genetic component to their disease. A complete accounting of current and recent medications, prescribed as well as those over the counter or administered by alternative health-care providers, should be obtained, as diarrhea is a known side effect or complication of many pharmacotherapeutic agents.

Physical Examination

Physical examination may not be useful as a diagnostic tool in evaluation of patients with possible IBD, but it helps the clinician to assess the patient's clinical status (i.e., assessment for systemic inflammatory response and hydration status). Evidence of malabsorption, such as muscle wasting or pallor, may be noted in more severe cases.

Certain clinical features may suggest either a new diagnosis of IBD or progression of documented disease. These include aphthous ulcers, cutaneous lesions consistent with erythema nodosum or pyoderma gangrenosum, ocular inflammation, anorectal fistulization, and abdominal tenderness, particularly with a palpable mass in the right lower quadrant suggestive of inflammation of the terminal ileum.

Laboratory Evaluation

Serology may be helpful in assessing disease severity, with increased white blood cell count, elevated erythrocyte sedimentation rate (ESR), and elevated C-reactive protein as indicators of inflammation. A relative anemia, low serum albumin, and variations in red blood cell indices such as the mean cell volume may serve as markers for impaired nutritional status. It should be noted, however, that normal serologic tests do not exclude the diagnosis of IBD, particularly in the pediatric population [12].

Obtaining a standard stool culture for *Campylobacter, Salmonella,* and *Shigella* should be considered as part of the initial evaluation of suspected inflammatory diarrhea. In addition, stool for *C. difficile* toxin should be obtained, even if there is no history of antibiotic use, given its current incidence in the community. Of note, there is no advantage

Chapter 3 / Inflammatory Bowel Disease

in obtaining intraluminal fluid or biopsy specimens over standard culture [13]. The evaluation of stool for ova and parasites should also be considered to rule out intestinal amebiasis. Three specimens, each separated by a 24-h period, should be analyzed to increase diagnostic yield, as parasites may be excreted intermittently.

Consideration should also be given to evaluation for other pathogens that can mimic IBD, such as *Yersinia enterocolitica* and EHEC. *Yersinia* can present with right lower quadrant abdominal pain and fevers, and thus may mimic Crohn's ileitis. To rule out yersiniosis, stool (and potentially other body fluids) should be cultured. Serologic assays have been developed and may support this diagnosis; however these are not currently widely available in the USA. The gram-negative bacteria *E. coli* O157:H7, which produces Shiga toxin, may result in a hemorrhagic colitis presenting with marked abdominal pain, similar to that of inflammatory bowel disease. Stool culture on sorbitol–MacConkey agar, or specific evaluation for Shiga toxin, should be considered as a routine test in the evaluation of inflammatory diarrhea.

Evaluation of inflammatory diarrhea traditionally has included microscopic analysis for fecal leukocytes alone, or in combination with fecal occult blood testing.

Multiple critical analyses have questioned the usefulness of this approach, given the low sensitivity and specificity of both tests. While there is about 70% agreement for both tests in predicting infection with *Shigella*, overall fecal leukocytes are a poor diagnostic test in the evaluation of inflammatory diarrhea. An alternative test is the fecal lactoferrin assay (FLA). This assay has been shown to be a more precise and technically durable marker for fecal leukocytes and hence for inflammatory diarrhea [14]. Calprotectin is another protein that is found in neutrophils and monocytes, is present in the stool samples of patients with colitis, and has also been shown to be a sensitive marker for distinguishing between inflammatory and non-inflammatory diarrhea [15].

In patients who are being treated with immunomodulators, additional consideration must be given to atypical causes of diarrhea including CMV, herpes simplex virus, *Cryptosporidium*, *Chlamydia trachomatis*, *Isospora belli*, and *Mycobacterium*.

Imaging Studies

A variety of available imaging studies offer the potential to differentiate between inflammatory and non-inflammatory ileocolitis, and provide the opportunity for disease localization as well as evaluation of both intestinal and extraintestinal complications. Contrast radiography, such as air contrast barium enema, small bowel follow-through, and enteroclysis, can be useful in the initial evaluation of either the colon or the small bowel. Transabdominal ultrasound, abdominal/pelvic computerized tomography (CT), or abdominal/pelvic magnetic resonance imaging (MRI) can define intra-abdominal complications of CD such as abscess and fistula formation, as well as perianal disease. The emergence of CT enterography and MRI enterography has largely replaced plain film imaging, where available, and in the case of MRI, without exposure to ionizing radiation. Video capsule endoscopy (VCE) has been demonstrated to be superior in its ability to detect small bowel pathology missed on standard imaging; however the risks of capsule retention in patients with CD is not insignificant and remain to be defined [16].

Endoscopy

When IBD is suspected as the cause for diarrhea, an endoscopic examination of the colon is generally considered an integral part of the initial evaluation in order to both confirm the disease and to institute appropriate medical therapy. Endoscopy provides the clinician with the opportunity to potentially differentiate UC from CD based upon gross appearance, as well as to determine the location and extent of disease. When possible, colonoscopy should be pursued over flexible sigmoidoscopy as the initial endoscopic examination, as it allows evaluation of the entire colon in addition to the terminal ileum.

Certain endoscopic findings may suggest a diagnosis of UC over that of CD. Despite its somewhat misleading name, most patients with UC develop granular or friable mucosa without deep ulcerations [17]. In addition, a sharp demarcation between inflamed and uninvolved colonic mucosa is often evident in UC. Alternatively, deep, stellate, linear, or serpiginous ulcers are more commonly found in colonic CD [18]. Furthermore, strictures and internal fistulas are suggestive of CD or underlying malignancy in patients with UC. The presence of skip areas of grossly and histologically uninvolved mucosa is more commonly found in CD; however, it should be noted that these same findings may be noted in UC patients that have received medical therapy.

Crohn's colitis can be grossly indistinguishable from UC, with continuous inflammation from the rectum to the cecum, without deep areas of ulceration. It is for this reason that intubation of the terminal ileum, along with random biopsies from this area in addition to all five major regions of the colon (ascending colon, transverse colon, descending colon, sigmoid, and rectum), are crucial. The biopsies should be obtained from both involved and uninvolved areas and

Chapter 3 / Inflammatory Bowel Disease 71

placed in separate specimen cups. Although specimens obtained during endoscopy may share similar histopathologic features, there are certain hallmarks that can be very helpful in differentiating UC from CD. Noncaseating granulomas, the key finding in CD, are noted in approximately 30% of biopsy specimens [18].

In addition to assisting in differentiation of UC and CD, colonoscopy will provide the opportunity to evaluate for other sources of inflammation, such as CMV superinfection, ischemic colitis, and CDI. The presence of inclusion bodies and cytopathic effects on colonic biopsies strongly suggests CMV superinfection. The classic appearance of ischemic bowel, particularly with an area of clear demarcation at a watershed area of vascular distribution, suggests ischemic colitis. Although the presence of pseudomembranes is not pathognomic for CDI, and its absence does not rule it out, when coupled with stool testing, the endoscopic mucosal appearance may assist the clinician in early diagnosis.

Evaluation of the upper gastrointestinal tract with esophagogastroduodenoscopy (EGD) can also be useful, particularly in patients with concomitant symptoms suggestive of upper gastrointestinal pathology such as dyspepsia, nausea, early satiety, and epigastric pain. Although inflammation of the gastric and duodenal mucosa generally suggests CD, both "focally enhanced gastritis" and duodenitis have been noted in UC patients as well [19]. The presence of duodenal strictures or fistulas would strongly favor CD. During EGD, aspiration of the luminal contents of the small bowel can be conducted to evaluate for bacterial overgrowth, further adding to the diagnostic utility of this examination in patients with IBD.

TREATMENT

The choice of medical therapy is based upon the extent and severity of the disease, with surgical options generally reserved for patients with disease refractory to standard medical therapy, fulminant disease or its complications, mucosal dysplasia, or malignancy [20]. Various indices of disease activity have been suggested, but nearly universal to all is the frequency of bowel movements and evidence of systemic toxic effects. In the absence of a "gold standard" for the measurement of disease activity, disease severity is established based on clinical parameters, systemic manifestations, and the global impact of the disease on the individual's quality of life [1]. The available pharmacologic treatment options vary between UC and CD, with a large amount of overlap between the two (see Table 3.2).

Table 3.2
Commonly used medications for the treatment of inflammatory bowel disease

Medication	Class of agent	Site of action	Average dose	Indication
Mesalamine enema	5-ASA	Rectum and left colon	1–4 g/day	Mild–moderate left-sided UC/CD
Oral mesalamine	5-ASA	Entire colon	2–4 g/day	Mild–severe distal or pancolonic UC/CD
Sulfasalazine	5-ASA bound to sulfapyridine	Entire colon	1–4 g/day	Mild–moderate distal or pancolonic UC/CD
Metronidazole, Cipro	Antibiotics	Entire colon	10–20 mg/kg/day ± Cipro 500 mg twice daily	Perianal CD
Corticosteroid enema	Corticosteroids	Rectum and left colon	Variable, up to 100 mg/day	Mild–moderate left-sided colitis
Oral/intravenous corticosteroids	Corticosteroids	Colon and small bowel	Variable, typically 40 mg/day prednisone	Mild–severe distal or pancolonic UC/CD
Cyclosporine	Immunomodulator	Colon and small bowel	4 mg/kg/day titrated to therapeutic levels	Induction for severe disease/maintenance with AZA or 6-MP in UC only

Azathioprine (AZA) and mercaptopurine (6-MP)	Immunomodulator	1.5–2.5 mg/kg/day	Mild–moderate distal or pancolonic UC/CD
Methotrexate (MTX)	Immunomodulator	25 mg weekly intramuscularly	Alternative to AZA/6-MP in CD
Infliximab (infusion)	Biologic TNF-α (alpha) antibody	5 mg/kg weeks 0, 2, 6 then every 8 weeks	Induction and maintenance of moderate–severe UC/CD
Adalimumab, certolizumab pegol	Biologic TNF-α (alpha) antibody	Variable with agent in dose and schedule	Induction and maintenance of moderate–severe CD
Natalizumab (infusion)	Biologic α-4 integrin antibody	300 mg every 4 weeks	Induction and maintenance of moderate–severe CD

5-ASA, 5-Aminosalicylic acid derivatives; UC, ulcerative colitis; CD, Crohn's disease

A complete discussion of the treatment of IBD is beyond the scope of this text; however a general review of the various modalities will be discussed in this chapter. Since these disorders are neither medially nor surgically "curable," the goals of therapy are directed toward the induction and maintenance of disease remission.

Aminosalicylates

Sulfasalazine and sulfa-free 5-ASA compounds are first-line therapy for mild to moderately active UC. The therapeutic effect of 5-ASA compounds depends on their local concentration at the inflamed mucosal surface. This may also explain their limited role in the treatment of CD, where the inflammation is transmural in nature. Various preparations with different delivery modes have been developed to prevent early absorption in the small intestine, increase local concentrations of these medications, and improve their efficacy. Overall, the 5-ASA compounds are very effective in the induction and maintenance of remission of mild to moderately active UC and should be considered first-line therapy alone or in combination with other agents, depending on the severity of the disease. Although oral mesalamine is being used in the treatment of ileal, ileocolonic, and colonic CD, new evidence suggests that this approach is minimally effective as compared with placebo and less effective than budesonide or conventional corticosteroids [1].

Antibiotics

Although antibiotics are widely used in clinical practice for the treatment of luminal CD, controlled trials have not consistently demonstrated efficacy in this setting [1]. Nonsuppurative perianal complications of CD typically respond to metronidazole alone or in combination with ciprofloxacin. Other antibiotics, such as amoxicillin/clavulanate, trimethoprim/sulfamethoxazole, levofloxacin, minocycline, and tetracycline, have also been used. Unfortunately, it appears that continuous therapy is necessary to prevent recurrence of draining fistulas. One should also know that the safety of long-term antibiotic therapy has not been established and as previously noted, antibiotic use can be associated with the development of an osmotic diarrhea, as well as increased risk for CDI.

Glucocorticoids

Glucocorticoids, or corticosteroids, are used extensively in the treatment of both UC and CD to achieve disease remission. Standard oral corticosteroid preparations, along with synthetic analogs such as budesonide, have a high affinity for the intracellular glucocorticoid receptors, leading to the inhibition of transcription of proinflammatory proteins. Intravenous corticosteroids, generally in combination with other treatment modalities, are used in the treatment of more severe or fulminant disease. Due to the adverse effects of prolonged administration of corticosteroids on nearly every organ system, the use of these drugs should be limited to short treatment courses only.

Immunomodulators

This class of medication includes the purine antimetabolite mercaptopurine and its prodrug azathioprine, as well as methotrexate (MTX). Although their exact mechanism of action is unknown, purine antimetabolites inhibit cell proliferation and induce T-lymphocyte apoptosis. Both of these drugs require several weeks to achieve therapeutic effect, and thus their usefulness in treating acute disease activity is limited. Of note is the current FDA recommendation of checking the enzyme activity level or genotype of thiopurine methyltransferase (TPMT), which converts mercaptopurine into inactive metabolites. Variations in the expression of this enzyme can lead to a higher risk for medication-induced bone marrow suppression.

Methotrexate is used primarily for the treatment of CD. Administered once weekly, either subcutaneously or intramuscularly, MTX can be effective in the induction of remission and allows steroid tapering in steroid refractory or steroid-dependent patients with CD [1]. Significant liver toxicity can occur especially in patients with concomitant liver diseases and thus monitoring of liver enzymes on a regular basis is required. Methotrexate is also a known abortifacient and absolutely contraindicated in women who are pregnant or considering pregnancy.

Cyclosporine, a calcineurin inhibitor, is another medication in this class. Unlike the purine antimetabolites, this agent achieves therapeutic levels after a few days of intravenous administration and thus can be used during acute exacerbations of ulcerative colitis or in treating pyoderma gangrenosum. Because of the need for continued measurement of cyclosporine levels and renal function, as well as adverse effects such as hypertension, renal insufficiency, seizures, and opportunistic infections, cyclosporine is used less frequently in favor of the biologic agents.

Biologic Agents

Monoclonal antibodies directed against TNF-α (TNF-α inhibitors) have been very effective in the treatment of various manifestations of IBD, including fistulizing CD. In clinical practice, these medications are generally reserved for those patients who have not responded to aminosalicylates, antibiotics, corticosteroids, and immunomodulators. However, some advocate their use early in the course of disease, with the so-called "top-down" approach to treatment. Currently there are three medications in this class: infliximab, which is delivered via intravenous infusion, adalimumab, and certolizumab pegol, which are delivered subcutaneously. At this time, infliximab is the only one of the three which has been approved by the FDA for treating UC.

Natalizumab, an antibody to α-4 integrin, is effective in the treatment of patients with moderate-to-severe CD who have not responded to standard measures, including the TNF-α inhibitors. It is delivered via intravenous infusions; however its use is currently limited due to an association with an increased risk of reactivation of human JC polyomavirus, which can lead to the development of progressive multifocal leukoencephalopathy (PML), a non-reversible infection of the central nervous system with a very high mortality rate. Prior exposure to tuberculosis should be assessed with a chest radiograph and purified protein derivative prior to the initiation of therapy with a TNF-α inhibitor, secondary to the risk for reactivation of latent tuberculosis. In addition, these patients are at increased risk for infectious complications, particularly intracellular pathogens, and should be counseled and followed appropriately. Finally, patients are at risk for medication reactions either systemically, at the time of infusion, or locally, at the site of injection. The development of antibodies with allergic reactions or loss of clinical response has also been described for each of these agents.

Surgical Management

Surgical management is generally reserved for cases refractory to medical treatment and for complications including fulminant disease. In the elective setting, the "gold standard" operation for UC is the total proctocolectomy with ileal pouch–anal anastomosis (IPAA). In older patients or those with other anal dysfunction, total proctocolectomy with end ileostomy is appropriate. These approaches can be considered "curative" in UC, although pouchitis can remain an issue. Surgical interventions in patients with CD include stricturoplasty, drainage of abscesses, ileocolectomy, and the surgical management of anorectal diseases. While not entirely curative, surgical intervention remains an important therapeutic measure in CD, and new laparoscopic techniques have helped to reduce a wide variety of post-operative complications [20].

The Role of Probiotics

The past two decades have seen a dramatic rise in the mainstream use of complementary and alternative medical approaches in the treatment of medical ailments. In parallel with this trend, there is mounting evidence that probiotic therapy may be useful in selected patients with IBD. Although trials examining the use of probiotics in CD have shown mixed results, the data for their use in UC, and more specifically in the prevention of pouchitis, have been more encouraging. Administration of probiotics such as *Lactobacillus, Bifidobacteria,* and *Saccharomyces boulardii* is reasonable in these patients; however caution must be taken when contemplating the use of these agents in patients who are severely ill, as bacterial translocation across the deranged colonic membrane and subsequent sepsis has been reported [21].

General Dietary Considerations

There are no specific dietary modifications currently recommended for patients with IBD. Given the wide spectrum of disease manifestation, dietary changes should be individually tailored. In general, minimizing fat (particularly in patients with steatorrhea) and fiber intake and eating smaller, more frequent meals may reduce intestinal gas and bloating. Other dietary factors that may contribute to the diarrhea include the consumption of fructose, non-absorbable carbohydrates such as artificial sweeteners, and stimulants such as caffeine. In addition, patients should be counseled to avoid nonsteroidal anti-inflammatory medications, as they may exacerbate colitis [2].

In addition, supplemental calcium, vitamin D, and folate are often provided, particularly in patients who have received corticosteroids and sulfasalazine, or in those with small bowel CD. Deficiencies in minerals such as iron and vitamins, such as cobalamin, should be replaced as appropriate.

Specific Antidiarrheal Treatments

In addition to the treatment measures undertaken for the underlying inflammatory process, other medications are available to treat the symptom of diarrhea, which can improve the quality of life for these patients. Loperamide, diphenoxylate, codeine sulfate, and tinctures of opium all act to retard bowel motility and thereby increase the absorption of fluids and nutrients [2]. Cholestyramine and colestipol act by binding bile salts in the ileal lumen, thus reducing diarrhea in patients with ileal involvement or resection. Anti-spasmotic medications such as dicyclomine and hyoscyamine can reduce abdominal pain, bloating, and fecal urgency. Alosetron decreases colonic motility and secretion, and is available under tight regulatory control to a selected subset of patients, having previously been withdrawn from the market because of reports of ischemic colitis and complications of severe constipation. This medication can be considered in female patients with concurrent IBS.

If bacterial overgrowth is suspected, a 7–10-day course of antibiotics such as trimethoprim/sulfamethoxazole, ciprofloxacin, metronidazole, tetracyclines, or rifaximin can be considered. Some patients may require longer therapy, combination therapy, or therapy on a rotating schedule.

It should be noted that antidiarrheal agents should be avoided in patients with evidence of obstruction, pseudo-obstruction, fever, or abdominal tenderness [22]. They should also be avoided as a primary therapy in patients with suspected invasive bacterial enterocolitis or CDI, and in severely ill patients secondary to the risk of toxic megacolon.

PROGNOSIS

The natural history of IBD depends in large part upon the extent of disease. The course of the disease typically consists of intermittent exacerbations, alternating with periods of near or complete disease remission. Crohn's disease carries an additional risk of complications related to transmural inflammation, such as stricturing disease, fistulization, abscess formation, and anorectal disease, as well as the sequelae that result from the treatment of these complications. Problems related to malabsorption, extraintestinal manifestations, iatrogenesis, and malignancy may also be seen in both disorders. While studies examining the overall effect on mortality are limited, it does not seem to be a significantly demonstrable risk.

REFERENCES

1. Lichtenstein G, Hanauer S, Sandborn W, the Practice Parameters Committee of the American College of Gastroenterology. Management of Crohn's disease in adults. Am J Gastroenterol 2009;104:465–483.
2. Shah S, Hanauer S. Treatment of diarrhea in patients with inflammatory bowel disease: concepts and cautions. Gastroenterol Disord 2007;7(Suppl 3):S3–S10.
3. Kucharzik T, Maaser, C, Lügering A, et al. Recent understanding of IBD pathogenesis: implications for future therapies. Inflamm Bowel Dis 2006;12:1068–1083.
4. Loftus EV. Clinical epidemiology of inflammatory bowel disease: incidence, prevalence, and environmental influences. Gastroenterology 2004;126(6): 1504–1517.
5. Ekbom A, Helmick C, Zack M, et al. The epidemiology of inflammatory bowel disease: a large, population-based study in Sweden. Gastroenterology 1991;100:350–358.

Chapter 3 / Inflammatory Bowel Disease 79

6. Cho J. The genetics and immunopathogenesis of inflammatory bowel disease. Nat Rev Immunol 2008;8(6):458–466.
7. Sartor R. Reviews in basic and clinical gastroenterology: microbial influences in inflammatory bowel disease. Gastroenterology 2008;134:577–594.
8. Pamukcu R, Hanauer S, Chang E. Effect of disodium azodisalicylate on electrolyte transport in rabbit ileum and colon in vitro: comparison with sulfasalazine and 5-aminosalicylic acid. Gastroenterology 1988;95:975–981.
9. Issa M, Ananthakrishnan A, Binion D. *Clostridium difficile* and inflammatory bowel disease. Inflamm Bowel Dis 2008;14:1432–1442.
10. Forrest K, Symmons D, Foster P. Systematic review: is ingestion of paracetamol or non-steroidal anti-inflammatory drugs associated with exacerbations of inflammatory bowel disease? Aliment Pharmacol Ther 2004;20:1035–1043.
11. Capril R, Gassull MA, Escer JC, et al. European evidence based consensus on the diagnosis and management of Crohn's disease: special situations. Gut 2006;55(Suppl 1):i-36–i-58.
12. Mack DR, Langton C, Markowitz J, et al. Laboratory values for children with newly diagnosed inflammatory bowel disease. Pediatrics 2007;19:1113–1119.
13. Barbut F, Beaugerie L, Delas N, et al. Comparative value of colonic biopsy and intraluminal fluid culture for diagnosis of bacterial acute colitis in immunocompetent patients. Infectious Colitis Study Group. Clin Infect Dis 1999;29:356–360.
14. Kane S, Sandborn W, Rufo P, et al. Fecal lactoferrin is a sensitive and specific marker in identifying intestinal inflammation. Am J Gastroenterol 2003;98: 1309–1314.
15. Tibble J, Teahon K, Thjodleifsson B, et al. A simple method for assessing intestinal inflammation in Crohn's disease. Gut 2000;47:506–513.
16. Eliakim R, Suissa A, Yassin K, et al. Wireless capsule video endoscopy compared to barium small bowel follow-through and computerized tomography in patients with suspected Crohn's disease—final report. Dig Liver Dis 2004;36:519–522.
17. Simpson P, Papadakis K. Endoscopic evaluation of patients with inflammatory bowel disease. Inflamm Bowel Dis 2008;14:1287–1297.
18. Lee SD, Cohen RD. Endoscopy in inflammatory bowel disease. Gastroenterol Clin North Am 2003;31:119–132.
19. Sharif F, McDermott M, Dillon M, et al. Focally enhanced gastritis in children with Crohn's disease and ulcerative colitis. Am J Gastroenterol 2002;97:1415–1420.
20. Cima R, Pemberton J. Medical and surgical management of chronic ulcerative colitis. Arch Surg 2005;140:300–310.
21. Issacs K, Herfarth H. Role of probiotic therapy in IBD. Inflamm Bowel Dis 2008;14:1597–1605.
22. Hanauer S. Drug therapy. N Engl J Med 1996;334:841–849.

4 Eosinophilic Enteritis

Charles W. DeBrosse, MD
and Li Zuo, MD

CONTENTS

INTRODUCTION
EPIDEMIOLOGY AND NATURAL HISTORY
CLINICAL PRESENTATION
  AND COMPLICATIONS
DIFFERENTIAL DIAGNOSIS
  AND DIAGNOSTIC CRITERIA
EVALUATION
TREATMENT
PATHOGENESIS AND FUTURE DIRECTIONS
SUMMARY OF KEY POINTS
REFERENCES

Summary

In summary, our knowledge of EGIDs is rapidly evolving; however, there is still much to be learned about the pathogenesis and treatment of these disorders. At the present time, it appears that eosinophilic enteritis is a chronic disorder characterized by the presence of diarrhea, abdominal pain, weight loss, and bloating. The clinical course appears to be characterized as being relapsing and remitting in nature. Successful treatment with prednisone or an elemental diet has been documented and other therapeutic interventions have been attempted with variable results. The underlying etiology for eosinophilic enteritis is unknown. The available evidence suggests a Th2-mediated process potentially driven by food antigens. The authors hope that

From: *Diarrhea, Clinical Gastroenterology*
Edited by: S. Guandalini, H. Vaziri, DOI 10.1007/978-1-60761-183-7_4
© Springer Science+Business Media, LLC 2011

they have provided a fundamental knowledge base from which the reader may be able to diagnose and treat EGIDs and hope that the readers join in the effort to further understand this fascinating group of disorders.

Key Words: Enteritis, Eosinophil-associated gastrointestinal disorders (EGIDs), Eosinophils, Esophagitis, Food allergy

INTRODUCTION

Eosinophilic enteritis can be classified as one form of the primary eosinophil-associated gastrointestinal disorders (EGIDs) and is among the common causes of chronic diarrhea. EGIDs are a heterogeneous group of disorders characterized by an inappropriate accumulation of eosinophils within the gastrointestinal (GI) tract [1–4]. Eosinophils can accumulate in any region of the GI tract from the esophagus to the colon and in different layers of the GI tract as well (mucosal, muscular, or subserosal). There appears to be an increasing incidence and recognition of eosinophilic esophagitis (EoE), the most common EGID [5]. Accordingly, there has been great research interest surrounding the treatment and pathogenesis of EoE. The number of case reports describing eosinophilic gastritis (EG), eosinophilic enteritis, and eosinophilic colitis (EC) has increased over the past decade also, suggesting that the incidence and/or the recognition of these disorders is increasing as well. However, investigations into the treatment and pathological mechanisms of EG, eosinophilic enteritis, and EC have not been as robust as EoE. This chapter highlights what is known about the clinical presentation, underlying mechanism, and treatment options for eosinophilic enteritis. Additionally, areas of uncertainty and areas for future research inquiry are addressed.

EPIDEMIOLOGY AND NATURAL HISTORY

It was originally thought that symptoms of EG and eosinophilic enteritis typically begin to manifest during the third or the fourth decade of life. It is now recognized that eosinophilic enteritis and eosinophilic gastroenteritis occur during childhood as well [6].

While there is little available data on the natural history of eosinophilic enteritis or other forms of EGIDs, these diseases appear to be chronic in nature [2]. Typically, patients with EGIDs are believed to have a waxing and waning clinical course. Clinical observations suggest that patients with eosinophilic enteritis may experience prolonged periods of disease quiescence marked by intermittent exacerbations.

A small subset of patients may develop a more severe phenotype and experience a clinical course marked by persistent symptoms and short periods of disease remission. Further studies on the natural history of eosinophilic enteritis and other forms of EGIDs are clearly needed to confirm these observations.

CLINICAL PRESENTATION AND COMPLICATIONS

Eosinophilic enteritis may present with abdominal pain, vomiting, diarrhea, weight loss, or bloating. These symptoms may result from inflammation of the mucosal layer, muscular layer, or subserosal layer of the small intestine. Classically, the symptoms of eosinophilic enteritis were thought to correspond with the area of inflammation, although this correlation is not absolute. The original literature suggests that the predominant symptom among those with mucosal layer disease is diarrhea, while patients with disease of the muscular layer present with intestinal obstruction and those with subserosal disease present with abdominal distension and eosinophilic ascites. Clinical observations have suggested that patients with eosinophilic enteritis and other EGIDs may present with diverse clinical manifestations. In a case series of 40 patients with eosinophilic gastroenteritis published by Talley and colleagues, abdominal pain was the most common presenting symptom regardless of whether the eosinophilic inflammation was present in the mucosal, muscular, or subserosal layer [7]. Nausea, vomiting, and diarrhea were also present in >50% of patients with mucosal and muscular involvement. For patients with subserosal disease, diarrhea and bloating were also commonly present (60%). Common signs and symptoms of EGIDs are summarized in Tables 4.1 and 4.2.

Table 4.1
Clinical features of
eosinophilic enteritis

Abdominal pain
Nausea
Vomiting
Diarrhea
Bloating
Eosinophilic ascites

Data recounting the common presenting symptoms of children with eosinophilic enteritis or eosinophilic gastroenteritis are limited. Anecdotally, children with eosinophilic gastroenteritis and eosinophilic

Table 4.2
Clinical features of
eosinophilic enteritis
in children

Failure to thrive
Abdominal pain
Nausea
Vomiting
Diarrhea
Bloating

enteritis present with a broad spectrum of gastrointestinal symptoms, which include abdominal pain, diarrhea, and failure to thrive.

While severe complications of EGIDs are believed to be uncommon, they can occur. There are several case reports detailing patients with eosinophilic enteritis presenting with symptoms mimicking an acute abdomen or appendicitis. Available case reports suggest that patients with eosinophilic enteritis may develop serious complications such as intestinal obstruction or perforation [8–13]. Rare complications of eosinophilic enteritis reported in the medical literature are summarized in Table 4.3.

Table 4.3
Rare complications of
eosinophilic enteritis

Stricture
Obstruction
Perforation
Intussusception
Pseudo-obstruction

DIFFERENTIAL DIAGNOSIS AND DIAGNOSTIC CRITERIA

Primary eosinophilic enteritis is likely the result of an underlying allergic etiology, mostly a food allergen-driven Th2 response. Secondary causes of eosinophilic enteritis include parasitic infection, inflammatory bowel disease, celiac disease, drug hypersensitivity, and malignancy [1–3]. Recent reports have identified that adults and children with systemic lupus erythematosus (SLE) may also present with eosinophilic inflammation of the small bowel [13–15]. Hypereosinophilic syndrome (HES) should also be considered, as patients with HES may present similarly to EGIDs with GI symptoms, eosinophilic inflammation in the GI tract, and peripheral eosinophilia. Patients with HES have sustained, markedly elevated peripheral eosinophils counts (>1500 absolute eosinophils/mm^3). Additionally, these eosinophils are activated and can lead to secondary end organ damage. Patients with HES may experience end organ damage in any organ system and HES may lead to important complications such as eosinophilic myocarditis or thrombosis. Accordingly, HES is an important diagnostic consideration when treating patients with any form of EGID. Finally, the vasculitic phase of Churg–Strauss syndrome may present with GI symptoms and eosinophilic inflammation of the GI tract. If a patient with a suspected EGID presents with additional symptoms such as recalcitrant pulmonary or sinus disease, peripheral neuropathy, purpura, or constitutional symptoms (fever, malaise, fatigue, etc.), then a diagnosis of Churg–Strauss syndrome should be entertained. The complete differential diagnosis for eosinophilic enteritis is included in Table 4.4.

Table 4.4
Differential diagnosis for eosinophilic enteritis

Crohn's disease
Ulcerative colitis
Celiac disease
Parasitic infection
Hypereosinophilic syndrome
Churg–Strauss syndrome
Connective tissue disease (SLE)
Drug hypersensitivity
Malignancy

Reprinted with permission from [16], Allen Press Publishing Services.

Because the symptoms are non-specific and the differential diagnosis is broad, the diagnosis of eosinophilic enteritis proposes several challenges to the clinician in the absence of a reliable biomarker for its diagnosis.

Table 4.5
Eosinophil levels in the GI tract of children

Gastrointestinal segment	Lamina propria		Villous lamina propria		Surface epithelium		Crypt/glandular epithelium	
	Mean	Max	Mean	Max	Mean	Max	Mean	Max
Esophagus	N/A	N/A	N/A	N/A	0.03±0.10	1	N/A	N/A
Antrum	1.9 ± 1.3	8	N/A	N/A	0.0±0.0	0	0.02±0.04	1
Fundus	2.1 ± 2.4	11	N/A	N/A	0.0±0.0	0	0.008±0.03	1
Duodenum	9.6 ± 5.3	26	2.1±1.4	9	0.06±0.09	2	0.26±0.36	6
Ileum	12.4 ± 5.4	28	4.8±2.8	15	0.47±0.25	4	0.80±0.51	4
Ascending colon	20.3 ± 8.2	50	N/A	N/A	0.29±0.25	3	1.4±1.2	11
Transverse colon	16.3 ± 5.6	42	N/A	N/A	0.22±0.39	4	0.77±0.61	4
Rectum	8.3 ± 5.9	32	N/A	N/A	0.15±0.13	2	1.2±1.1	9

The mean number of eosinophils/high-power field (±standard deviation) for each anatomical region of the gastrointestinal tract and each region of the mucosa is shown. N/A, not applicable (reprinted with permission from [16], Allen Press Publishing Services).

Currently, there are no firm diagnostic criteria for eosinophilic enteritis. Initially, a peak count of >20 eos/hpf was utilized to define eosinophilic enteritis [7]. This was based on clinical observations made in the absence of well-defined normal values. Efforts to determine the normal number of eosinophils in the small bowel have since been undertaken [16, 17]. The results of two studies suggest that eosinophil counts may be as high as 26 eos/hpf in the duodenum and 28 eos/hpf in the ileum. These studies have also identified that typically eosinophil counts in the gastrointestinal tract are lowest in the esophagus and gradually increase in number until a peak count of 50 eos/hpf is reached in the terminal ileum and the ascending colon. Peak eosinophil counts gradually descend in the transverse and sigmoid colon. A summary of the mean and peak eosinophil levels observed in healthy children is shown in Table 4.5 [16]. The peak number of eosinophils noted in the normal GI tract does vary with geographic location. This makes evaluation of GI biopsies by a pathologist familiar with normal local values critically important. In addition to elevated numbers of eosinophils, there may be evidence of cryptitis along with distorted villous architecture in biopsies consistent with eosinophilic enteritis. However, the mere presence of eosinophils in the GI tract without clinical presentation, especially in the lower part of GI tract, may not indicate a pathological process.

While approximately 50% of patients with EGIDs typically have peripheral eosinophilia, this is not a specific marker for an EGID. Likewise, elevated IgE levels, elevation of acute inflammatory markers, and the presence of other allergic disorders may coincide with eosinophilic enteritis; thus they are not sufficient for diagnosis particularly since eosinophilic enteritis may be present in their absence. Abdominal X-rays and computed topography may also demonstrate abnormalities, though they cannot provide a definitive diagnosis [18]. Primary eosinophilic enteritis is primarily a diagnosis of exclusion and is dependent upon endoscopy with biopsy, in the presence of clinical presentations as noted above.

EVALUATION

Due to the protean manifestations of EGIDs, there is no single consensus pathway for the evaluation of patients suspected of having an EGID. Once the diagnosis of an EGID is suspected, an endoscopy with biopsy is required to confirm the diagnosis. If the diagnosis is confirmed, allergy testing (skin prick testing and/or food patch testing) can be considered as part of the diagnostic evaluation. Unfortunately, there is no available data on the skin prick test or patch test results to common food allergens for patients with eosinophilic enteritis.

The most challenging aspect to the diagnosis of eosinophilic enteritis involves ruling out other causes of eosinophilic inflammation. Initially, a detailed history is required to evaluate for symptoms that may suggest the presence of a rheumatologic disorder or HES. A detailed medical history should also be taken to assess for the possibility of drug hypersensitivity. To rule out parasitic infection as a cause of eosinophilic enteritis, stool ova and parasites should be obtained. If clinical suspicion for a parasitic infection is high, titers for *Strongyloides stercoralis*, *Toxocara*, and other parasitic organisms can be considered. These titers are rarely performed locally and often need to be sent to the Center for Disease Control (CDC) for analysis.

TREATMENT

Patients with eosinophilic enteritis and other forms of EGID typically respond to treatment with prednisone [2, 6]. Reportedly, patients with the subserosal form of the disease and eosinophilic ascites respond quite well to prednisone. There are a variety of strategies that can be utilized for prednisone dosing. Starting doses of 40–60 mg once daily for 1–2 weeks followed by a slow taper over an additional 1–2 weeks are typically recommended. Elemental diets have also been used with success in patients with eosinophilic enteritis and other EGIDs [6]. Other dietary interventions such as a six-food elimination diet or antigen elimination diets based on skin prick or patch testing have been used in the treatment of EoE [19, 20]. There is currently no data on the success of these interventions among patients with eosinophilic enteritis.

While treatment with steroids or an elemental diet is highly efficacious, there are significant side effects associated with steroid treatment. Compliance with an elemental diet is likely to be low if it is required for prolonged periods.

While the data on novel therapies for eosinophilic enteritis are not robust, several other treatment options have been explored. A placebo-controlled trial investigating the effects of 10 mg of montelukast among 40 patients with duodenal eosinophilia was performed [21]. In this study, 50% of patients with duodenal eosinophilia had a reduction in clinical symptoms on montelukast. Therapy with cromolyn has also been attempted. Although the available data is limited to case reports, it suggests that oral cromolyn may provide symptomatic relief to patients with eosinophilic enteritis [22, 23]. Given that the underlying etiology of EGIDs may be allergic in nature, a clinical trial investigating the efficacy of anti-IgE therapy (omalizumab) among patients with EGIDs was performed [24]. Compared to placebo, patients taking omalizumab had a reduction in GI symptoms as well as in the expression of FcεRI on tissue basophils and dendritic cells. Unfortunately, the reduction in the number of eosinophils within the GI tract did not reach statistical significance. While many patients with EGIDs have an allergic trigger, the mechanism may not be that of a classical IgE-driven process [25]. There is some evidence to suggest that the mechanism driving eosinophilic inflammation may be a mixed process, composed of immediate and delayed allergic responses [26–28].

Perhaps the most promising new intervention for eosinophilic enteritis on the horizon is therapy with anti-IL-5. IL-5 is a cytokine responsible for eosinophil growth and differentiation [3]. Additionally, IL-5 protects eosinophils from apoptosis. As such, interventions designed to inhibit IL-5 would likely benefit patients with EGIDs. There are currently two forms of humanized anti-IL-5 being studied, mepolizumab and reslizumab. Mepolizumab has been used to successfully treat HES and has been shown to reduce the number of eosinophils in the esophagus of patients with EoE. Initial studies utilizing reslizumab for the treatment of EoE are currently ongoing.

PATHOGENESIS AND FUTURE DIRECTIONS

In addition to IL-5, other Th2-driven cytokines are likely important in the pathogenesis of EGIDs. IL-13, IL-4, and eotaxin-3 have been implicated specifically in EoE and therefore may serve as potential therapeutic targets for EoE and other forms of EGID [29]. The development of other therapeutic strategies designed to inhibit these cytokines would likely prove beneficial in treating EoE and other EGIDs. Unfortunately, investigations in the specific molecular pathways responsible for eosinophilic enteritis or eosinophilic gastroenteritis have not been performed. These studies will be critical to the development of future therapeutic treatments for these disorders. They will also help shed light on critical similarities and differences that may exist between the different forms of EGID. Finally, molecular analysis could lead to the discovery of biomarkers specific for eosinophilic enteritis. Patients with eosinophilic enteritis and other forms of EGID often undergo frequent endoscopies to assess disease severity. Noninvasive measures that could be utilized to diagnose EGID or monitor disease activity could substantially limit the number of endoscopies required for patients with EGID. In turn, this would lead to increased quality of life and decreased health-care costs for patients with EGID.

SUMMARY OF KEY POINTS

Symptoms of eosinophilic enteritis include abdominal pain, nausea, vomiting, bloating, and diarrhea.

Diagnosis is dependent upon the combination of GI symptoms and eosinophilic inflammation on biopsy.

Eosinophilic enteritis is likely due to an allergic response.

Treatment may include dietary modification, corticosteroids, or other anti-inflammatory medications.

Patients appear to experience a waxing and waning clinical course.

REFERENCES

1. DeBrosse CW, Rothenberg ME. Allergy and eosinophil-associated gastrointestinal disorders (EGID). Curr Opin Immunol 2008;20:703–708.
2. Furuta GT, Forbes D, Boey C, Dupont C, Putnam P, Roy S, Sabra A, Salvatierra A, Yamashiro Y, Husby S. Eosinophilic gastrointestinal diseases (EGIDs). J Pediatr Gastroenterol Nutr 2008;47:234–238.
3. Rothenberg ME. Eosinophilic gastrointestinal disorders (EGID). J Allergy Clin Immunol 2004;113:11–28, quiz 9.
4. Zuo L, Rothenberg ME. Eosinophil associated gastrointestinal disorders (EGID). In: Rich RR, Fleisher TA, Schroeder H, Weyand C, Frew AJ, eds. Clinical immunology, vol. **46**. Edinburgh, UK; Martin Mellor Publishing Services, Ltd, 2008, pp. 691–700.
5. Noel RJ, Putnam PE, Rothenberg ME. Eosinophilic esophagitis. N Engl J Med 2004;351:940–941.
6. Katz AJ, Twarog FJ, Zeiger RS, Falchuk ZM. Milk-sensitive and eosinophilic gastroenteropathy: similar clinical features with contrasting mechanisms and clinical course. J Allergy Clin Immunol 1984;74:72–78.
7. Talley NJ, Shorter RG, Phillips SF, Zinsmeister AR. Eosinophilic gastroenteritis: a clinicopathological study of patients with disease of the mucosa, muscle layer, and subserosal tissues. Gut 1990;31:54–58.
8. Ikenaga M, Fujimoto T, Miyake Y, Doi S, Hakata H, Naoi M. A case of eosinophilic enteritis with repeated perforation of the ileum. Nippon Shokakibyo Gakkai Zasshi 1996;93:661–665.
9. Remacha Tomey B, Velicia Llames R, del Villar A, Fernandez Orcajo P, Caro-Paton Gomez A. Eosinophilic enteritis causing intestinal obstruction. Gastroenterol Hepatol 1999;22:352–355.
10. Shin WG, Park CH, Lee YS, Kim KO, Yoo KS, Kim JH, Park CK. Eosinophilic enteritis presenting as intussusception in adult. Korean J Intern Med 2007;22: 13–17.
11. Steele RJ, Mok SD, Crofts TJ, Li AK. Two cases of eosinophilic enteritis presenting as large bowel perforation and small bowel haemorrhage. Aust N Z J Surg 1987;57:335–336.
12. Uenishi T, Sakata C, Tanaka S, Yamamoto T, Shuto T, Hirohashi K, Kubo S, Kinoshita H. Eosinophilic enteritis presenting as acute intestinal obstruction: a case report and review of the literature. Dig Surg 2003;20:326–329.
13. Yamazaki-Nakashimada MA, Rodriguez-Jurado R, Ortega-Salgado A, Gutierrez-Hernandez A, Garcia-Pavon-Osorio S, Hernandez-Bautista V. Intestinal

pseudoobstruction associated with eosinophilic enteritis as the initial presentation of systemic lupus erythematosus in children. J Pediatr Gastroenterol Nutr 2009;48:482–486.

14. Sunkureddi PR, Baethge BA. Eosinophilic gastroenteritis associated with systemic lupus erythematosus. J Clin Gastroenterol 2005;39:838–839.

15. Sunkureddi PR, Luu N, Xiao SY, Tang WW, Baethge BA. Eosinophilic enteritis with systemic lupus erythematosus. South Med J 2005;98:1049–1052.

16. DeBrosse CW, Case JW, Putnam PE, Collins MH, Rothenberg ME. Quantity and distribution of eosinophils in the gastrointestinal tract of children. Pediatr Dev Pathol 2006;9:210–218.

17. Lowichik A, Weinberg AG. A quantitative evaluation of mucosal eosinophils in the pediatric gastrointestinal tract. Mod Pathol 1996;9:110–114.

18. Zheng X, Cheng J, Pan K, Yang K, Wang H, Wu E. Eosinophilic enteritis: CT features. Abdom Imaging 2008;33:191–195.

19. Kagalwalla AF, Sentongo TA, Ritz S, Hess T, Nelson SP, Emerick KM, Melin-Aldana H, Li BU. Effect of six-food elimination diet on clinical and histologic outcomes in eosinophilic esophagitis. Clin Gastroenterol Hepatol 2006;4: 1097–1102.

20. Spergel JM, Andrews T, Brown-Whitehorn TF, Beausoleil JL, Liacouras CA. Treatment of eosinophilic esophagitis with specific food elimination diet directed by a combination of skin prick and patch tests. Ann Allergy Asthma Immunol 2005;95:336–343.

21. Friesen CA, Kearns GL, Andre L, Neustrom M, Roberts CC, Abdel-Rahman SM. Clinical efficacy and pharmacokinetics of montelukast in dyspeptic children with duodenal eosinophilia. J Pediatr Gastroenterol Nutr 2004;38:343–351.

22. Martin DM, Goldman JA, Gilliam J, Nasrallah SM. Gold-induced eosinophilic enterocolitis: response to oral cromolyn sodium. Gastroenterology 1981;80: 1567–1570.

23. Van Dellen RG, Lewis JC. Oral administration of cromolyn in a patient with protein-losing enteropathy, food allergy, and eosinophilic gastroenteritis. Mayo Clin Proc 1994;69:441–444.

24. Foroughi S, Foster B, Kim N, Bernardino LB, Scott LM, Hamilton RG, Metcalfe DD, Mannon PJ, Prussin C. Anti-IgE treatment of eosinophil-associated gastrointestinal disorders. J Allergy Clin Immunol 2007;120:594–601.

25. Spergel JM, Brown-Whitehorn T, Beausoleil JL, Shuker M, Liacouras CA. Predictive values for skin prick test and atopy patch test for eosinophilic esophagitis. J Allergy Clin Immunol 2007;119:509–511.

26. Blanchard C, Rothenberg ME. Basic pathogenesis of eosinophilic esophagitis. Gastrointest Endosc Clin N Am 2008;18:133–143, x.

27. Bullock JZ, Villanueva JM, Blanchard C, Filipovich AH, Putnam PE, Collins MH, Risma KA, Akers RM, Kirby CL, Buckmeier BK, Assa'ad AH, Hogan SP, Rothenberg ME. Interplay of adaptive th2 immunity with eotaxin-3/c-C chemokine receptor 3 in eosinophilic esophagitis. J Pediatr Gastroenterol Nutr 2007;45:22–31.

28. Vicario M, Blanchard C, Stringer KF, Collins MH, Mingler MK, Ahrens A, Putnam PE, Abonia JP, Santos J, Rothenberg ME. Local B cells and IgE production in the oesophageal mucosa in eosinophilic oesophagitis. Gut 2010; 59:12–20.

29. Blanchard C, Mingler MK, Vicario M, Abonia JP, Wu YY, Lu TX, Collins MH, Putnam PE, Wells SI, Rothenberg ME. IL-13 involvement in eosinophilic esophagitis: transcriptome analysis and reversibility with glucocorticoids. J Allergy Clin Immunol 2007;120:1292–1300.

5 Microscopic Colitis

Darrell S. Pardi, MD

CONTENTS

INTRODUCTION
BACKGROUND
EPIDEMIOLOGY
CLINICAL FEATURES
HISTOPATHOLOGY
PATHOPHYSIOLOGY
TREATMENT
CONCLUSION
REFERENCES

Summary

Microscopic colitis is a relatively common cause of chronic diarrhea. The colonic mucosa usually appears normal at endoscopy, and the diagnosis is made in the appropriate clinical setting when there is an increase in intraepithelial lymphocytes and a mixed inflammatory cell infiltrate in the lamina propria. The two main subtypes, collagenous and lymphocytic colitis, are similar clinically and histologically and are distinguished histologically by the presence or the absence of thickening of the subepithelial collagen band. The possibilities of drug-induced microscopic colitis and/or concomitant celiac sprue are important considerations when evaluating these patients. There are few controlled treatment trials to guide treatment in microscopic colitis, although a systematic approach to therapy often leads to satisfactory control of symptoms.

From: *Diarrhea, Clinical Gastroenterology*
Edited by: S. Guandalini, H. Vaziri, DOI 10.1007/978-1-60761-183-7_5
© Springer Science+Business Media, LLC 2011

Key Words: Microscopic colitis, Collagenous colitis, Lymphocytic colitis, Celiac sprue, Budesonide

INTRODUCTION

Microscopic colitis is a relatively common cause of chronic diarrhea. The colonic mucosa usually appears normal at endoscopy, and the diagnosis is made in the appropriate clinical setting when there is an increase in intraepithelial lymphocytes and a mixed inflammatory cell infiltrate in the lamina propria. The two main subtypes, collagenous and lymphocytic colitis, are similar clinically and histologically and are distinguished histologically by the presence or absence of thickening of the subepithelial collagen band. The possibility of drug-induced microscopic colitis and/or concomitant celiac sprue is an important consideration when evaluating these patients. There are few controlled treatment trials in microscopic colitis, although a systematic approach to therapy often leads to satisfactory control of symptoms.

BACKGROUND

The term "microscopic colitis" was first used to describe patients with chronic diarrhea who had normal findings on sigmoidoscopy and barium enema, but who had inflammation on colon biopsies [1]. Collagenous colitis is a related condition with similar clinical and histologic features, but with the additional finding of a thickened subepithelial collagen band [2]. It is unclear whether these two conditions are different diseases or rather are part of a spectrum. There are reports of patients in whom the diagnosis changed from one subtype to the other over time or in whom there was a "mixed" histologic picture on different biopsies from the same colonoscopy. Since the colon in collagenous colitis is grossly normal, it is also considered a form of "microscopic" colitis. Thus, the term microscopic colitis is used as an umbrella term with two subtypes: collagenous colitis, with a thickened subepithelial collagen band, and lymphocytic colitis, without collagen thickening [3].

EPIDEMIOLOGY

Microscopic colitis accounts for 4–13% of patients investigated for chronic diarrhea [4–7]. In Europe and North America, the reported incidence of collagenous colitis is 0.6–5.2/100,000 and for lymphocytic colitis, 3.7–5.5/100,000 [6–10]. In some of these studies, there was a significant increase in the incidence of microscopic colitis over time (for example, from 0.8/100,000 in 1985–1989 to 19.1/100,000 in

1998–2001 in one study from North America [7]). The reasons for this increase are not clear, but detection bias (with an increase over time in the performance of colon biopsies to evaluate patients with chronic watery diarrhea) [7] and increasing exposure to drugs that might cause microscopic colitis (see below) likely are involved.

A female predominance has been reported, particularly for collagenous colitis, with female to male ratios as high as 20:1 [6–13]. The gender difference for lymphocytic colitis is less striking than for collagenous colitis in some studies [7] but not others [10, 14]. In some recent studies, lymphocytic colitis was diagnosed more commonly than collagenous colitis [7, 14]. Microscopic colitis incidence increases significantly with age, with the diagnosis most commonly made in the sixth to seventh decade [6–14]. However, a wide age range has been reported, including pediatric cases [15, 16]. There are rare reports of familial occurrence [17, 18], including in older twin sisters (E. van Os, personal communication).

No association between microscopic colitis and colon cancer has been discovered [14, 19, 20], but long-term studies are needed to further explore this possibility. Several cases of lung cancer have been reported in patients with collagenous colitis [11, 19], perhaps related to cigarette smoking, which is more common in collagenous than lymphocytic colitis or controls [21, 22].

CLINICAL FEATURES

Microscopic colitis is characterized by chronic or intermittent watery diarrhea, ranging from mild and self-limited to severe, with dehydration and other metabolic abnormalities. Many patients will have abdominal pain or weight loss. The weight loss is typically mild but can be significant in some cases [11, 23]. Quality of life is affected in proportion to the degree of diarrhea, abdominal pain, urgency, and incontinence [24–26]. It is important to recognize that the symptoms of microscopic colitis are nonspecific. In fact, many patients with biopsy-proven microscopic colitis meet the symptom-based criteria for irritable bowel syndrome [27, 28]. Therefore, these criteria are not specific enough to distinguish microscopic colitis from IBS, which can only be done reliably with colonic mucosal biopsies. Fecal leukocytes may be present [23], but steatorrhea, fever, or hematochezia should suggest an alternate diagnosis.

Arthralgias and various autoimmune conditions (e.g., thyroid dysfunction, rheumatoid arthritis, psoriasis) are often seen in patients with microscopic colitis [11, 13, 14, 23]. In addition, an elevated erythrocyte sedimentation rate and a positive antinuclear antibody or other autoimmune markers [23, 29, 30] have been reported.

Of particular interest and clinical importance is the association between microscopic colitis and celiac sprue. In patients with celiac sprue, up to one-third have histologic changes in the colonic mucosa consistent with microscopic colitis [31, 32]. In a large cohort study of patients with celiac sprue, a clinical diagnosis of microscopic colitis was made in 4.3% of patients, which was 72 times higher than in patients without sprue [33]. Thus, microscopic colitis is relatively common in patients with celiac disease, and this diagnosis should be considered in patients who have continued or recurrent diarrhea despite a strict gluten free diet [34].

The prevalence of small bowel sprue-like changes in patients with microscopic colitis ranges from 2 to 9% in the largest series that have studied this association [11, 13, 14, 23]. However, sprue serologies are not commonly positive in patients with microscopic colitis, with anti-endomysial and anti-tissue transglutaminase antibodies found in only 0–4% and 0%, respectively [30, 35, 36], similar to rates in controls [35, 36]. Furthermore, titers of these antibodies in microscopic colitis are lower than in celiac patients [35]. Therefore, serologies may not be good diagnostic tests for celiac sprue in patients with microscopic colitis. Finally, HLA typing in microscopic colitis was similar to celiac sprue in one study [35] but not in others.

All of these data support the conclusion that celiac sprue is relatively uncommon in patients with microscopic colitis. It may not be necessary to routinely evaluate patients with microscopic colitis for celiac sprue, but this association should be considered in treatment refractory patients, those with significant weight loss or any suggestion of steatorrhea, or other clues such as unexplained iron deficiency anemia.

Endoscopic evaluation of the colon is typically normal or has mild nonspecific changes such as erythema or edema. Colonic ulceration is uncommon, and when seen is likely related to use of nonsteroidal anti-inflammatory drugs [37].

The reported natural history of microscopic colitis is variable. Symptomatic remission after many years of follow-up ranges from 60 to 93% in lymphocytic colitis [24, 38] and from 2 to 92% in collagenous colitis [11, 38–40]. One study reported remission rates of 59% in lymphocytic colitis and 34% in collagenous colitis after 6 months of follow-up, with an additional 25 and 40%, respectively, showing "significant improvement" [41]. Finally, another study reported spontaneous remission in 15% and treatment-induced remission in 48% of patients with collagenous colitis after 3.5 years of follow-up [42]. Of the remaining 37% with ongoing disease, only 60% (22% of entire cohort) required prolonged therapy. In contrast, in the clinical trials reported to date, placebo response rates after 6–8 weeks were only 12–40% [43–46], and an open-label report of patients treated with steroids indicated that 90% required some form of maintenance therapy [47].

HISTOPATHOLOGY

The hallmark histologic feature of microscopic colitis is intraepithelial lymphocytosis [41, 48]. In addition, there is a mixed infiltrate in the lamina propria, with chronic inflammatory cells most prominent [48, 49]. In collagenous colitis, the subepithelial collagen band is abnormally thickened, compared with 5–7 μm in normals [49].

Although neutrophils should not dominate the histologic picture, they are seen in microscopic colitis, and in fact, active cryptitis has been reported in 30–40% of patients with microscopic colitis [50]. These inflammatory changes are often accompanied by surface epithelial damage [48, 49], including detachment of the epithelium in some cases, despite the normal appearance of the mucosa grossly.

PATHOPHYSIOLOGY

Data on the pathophysiological mechanisms in microscopic colitis generally come from small studies and no consistent mechanism has been established [51]. Proposed mechanisms have included bile acid malabsorption, altered fluid and electrolyte absorption or secretion, infection, reaction to an unidentified luminal antigen, autoimmunity, and alteration in collagen synthesis or degradation (in collagenous colitis). Thus, it is possible that the term "microscopic colitis" encompasses different pathophysiologic mechanisms with a similar histologic phenotype.

One postulated mechanism with clinical relevance is the entity of drug-induced microscopic colitis [52, 53]. The strongest association between microscopic colitis and the use of a medication exists for nonsteroidal anti-inflammatory drugs [42, 54, 55], although not all studies have found this association to be significant [41, 56]. Patients with microscopic colitis often have arthralgias, and thus the association with NSAID use may be confounded. On the other hand, NSAIDs are known to cause colonic inflammation and may exacerbate inflammatory bowel disease [57]. Furthermore, some patients may have clinical and histologic improvement with discontinuation of NSAIDs [32, 54, 55, 58], and recurrence of collagenous colitis with NSAID rechallenge has been reported [59]. Finally, patients taking NSAIDs may be more likely to require steroid therapy [39]. Therefore, regular NSAID use should be discouraged in patients with microscopic colitis.

Several other drugs have been implicated as possible causes of microscopic colitis, including histamine-2 receptor blockers, proton pump inhibitors, selective serotonin reuptake inhibitors, carbamazepine, simvastatin, ticlopidine, and others [51–53]. In some cases, symptoms and histologic changes resolved with drug withdrawal and returned with reexposure. However, for most drugs, rechallenge is not reported, and the number of cases is small, such that a chance association cannot be excluded.

The literature on drug-induced microscopic colitis was recently analyzed to determine the strength of evidence for individual drugs or drug classes [52]. This analysis concluded that several drugs had strong or intermediate level evidence of causality, including such commonly used drugs such as aspirin, nonsteroidal anti-inflammatory drugs, proton pump inhibitors, selective serotonin reuptake inhibitors, ticlopidine, and statins. Another study showed that some drugs implicated in causing microscopic colitis are also associated with watery diarrhea, and therefore they may not actually cause colitis, but rather worsen the diarrhea and thus bring the diagnosis to attention [53].

TREATMENT

Any potential cause of drug-induced microscopic colitis and other agents that might exacerbate diarrhea (e.g., dairy products) should be discontinued if possible. Nonspecific antidiarrheal therapies, such as loperamide and diphenoxylate/atropine can be effective [11, 13, 23], and are often the first therapies prescribed in mild cases. If these agents are unsuccessful or for more moderate symptoms, bismuth subsalicylate at a dose of two or three tablets (262 mg each) three to four times per day may be beneficial [23, 60, 61]. For those who respond, long-term remission without chronic treatment has been reported [60, 61]. One study reported that most patients treated with bismuth had complete resolution of diarrhea [62]; however, others have reported that most patients have only a partial response [23].

If diarrhea does not respond to bismuth or for patients with more severe symptoms, treatment with corticosteroids, which were among the best therapies in the largest uncontrolled series [12, 14, 23], is recommended. Budesonide is the best studied treatment for microscopic colitis, having been assessed in three randomized, controlled induction studies in collagenous colitis [43–45] and two in lymphocytic colitis [46, 63]. In each of these studies, budesonide was superior to placebo for short-term treatment. In one open-label study, budesonide was as good as prednisone [47]. Thus, due to fewer side effects, budesonide should be used instead of prednisone. Unfortunately, although budesonide is effective for induction, the relapse rate is high once this medication is discontinued [13, 47, 64] and many patients become steroid dependent. Thus, before embarking on corticosteroid therapy, the diagnosis should be re-evaluated and alternative diagnoses, such as coexistent celiac sprue or infection, should be excluded, if not done already.

For steroid dependent patients, immune modifiers such as azathioprine or 6-mercaptopurine can be useful [23, 65–67]. However, many clinicians are gaining experience with long-term use of low dose (3–6 mg/day) budesonide in these patients as an alternative to immunosuppression [68]. This practice has been assessed in two randomized controlled trials, both of which showed that budesonide is superior to placebo for chronic treatment, at least through 6 months [69, 70]. With long-term budesonide therapy, patients need to be followed for steroid-related side effects [68].

Non-response to steroid therapy is uncommon [47] and when present alternate or concomitant diagnoses and non-compliance should be considered. If steroid-resistant microscopic colitis is truly present, treatment options include aminosalicylates and cholestyramine. Aminosalicylates were reported to be successful in a majority of patients in a controlled trial [71], but several large retrospective series have reported benefit in fewer than half of patients [11, 13, 23]. Cholestyramine may be more effective [11, 13, 23], although many do not tolerate the medication because of its texture.

If patients are refractory to all medical therapy, surgery can be considered, although this is rarely necessary. Reported operations include an ileostomy with or without a colectomy [23, 56, 65, 72] or an ileal pouch anal anastomosis [73, 74].

CONCLUSION

Microscopic colitis is a relatively common cause of chronic diarrhea whose incidence appears to be increasing. Colon biopsies are required to make the diagnosis and should be performed in any patient undergoing sigmoidoscopy or colonoscopy to evaluate unexplained diarrhea. The two subtypes of microscopic colitis, collagenous and lymphocytic colitis, are similar histologically and clinically and seem to respond similarly to various medical therapies. Although there are few controlled treatment trials, the approach outlined here often gives satisfactory control of diarrhea in these patients.

REFERENCES

1. Read NW, Krejs GJ, Read MG, et al. Chronic diarrhea of unknown origin. Gastroenterology 1980;76:264–271.
2. Lindstrom CG. "Collagenous colitis" with watery diarrhea – a new entity? Pathol Europa 1976;11:87–89.
3. Levison DA, Lazenby AJ, Yardley JH. Microscopic colitis cases revisited. Gastroenterology 1993;105:1594–1596.
4. Fine KD, Seidel RH, Do K. The prevalence, anatomic distrubution, and diagnosis of colonic causes of chronic diarrhea. Gastrointest Endosc 2000;51:318–326.
5. Shah RJ, Bleau B, Giannella RA. Usefulness of colonoscopy with biopsy in the evaluation of patients with chronic diarrhea. Am J Gastroenterol 2001;96: 1091–1095.
6. Fernandez-Banares F, Salas A, Forne M, et al. Incidence of collagenous and lymphocytic colitis: a 5-year population-based study. Am J Gastroenterol 1999;94:418–423.
7. Pardi DS, Loftus EV, Smyrk TC, et al. The epidemiology of microscopic colitis: a population-based study in Olmsted County, MN. Gut 2007;56:504–508.
8. Bohr J, Tysk C, Eriksson S, et al. Collagenous colitis in Orebro, Sweden, an epidemiological study 1984–1993. Gut 1995;37:394–397.
9. Agnarsdottir M, Gunnlaugsson O, Orvar KB, et al. Collagenous and lymphocytic colitis in Iceland. Dig Dis Sci 2002;47:1122–1128.
10. Williams JJ, Kaplan GG, Makhija S, et al. Microscopic colitis-defining incidence rates and risk factors: a population-based study. Clin Gastroenterol Hepatol 2008;6:35–40.
11. Bohr J, Tysk C, Eriksson S, et al. Collagenous colitis: a retrospective study of clinical presentation and treatment in 163 patients. Gut 1996;39:846–851.
12. Fernandez-Banares F, Salas A, Esteve M, et al. Collagenous colitis and lymphocytic colitis: evaluation of clinical and histological features, response to treatment and long-term follow up. Am J Gastroenterol 2003;98:340–347.
13. Olesen M, Erickson S, Bohr J, et al. Lymphocytic colitis: a retrospective study of 199 Swedish patients. Gut 2004;53:536–541.
14. Kao KT, Pedraza BA, McClune AC, et al. Microscopic colitis: a large retrospective analysis form a health maintenance organization experience. World J Gastroenterol 2009:15:3122–3127.
15. Gremse DA, Boudreaux CW, Manci EA. Collagenous colitis in children. Gastroenterology 1993;104:906–909.
16. Mahajan L, Wyllie R, Goldblum J. Lymphocytic colitis in a pediatric patient: a possible adverse reaction to carbamazepine. Am J Gastroenterol 1997;92: 2126–2127.
17. Jarnerot G, Hertervig E, Granno E, et al. Familial occurrence of microscopic colitis: a report of five families. Scand J Gastroenterol 2001;36:959–962.
18. Abdo AA, Zetler PJ, Halparin LS. Familial microscopic colitis. Can J Gastroenterol 2001;15:341–343.
19. Chan JL, Tersmette AC, Offerhaus GJA, et al. Cancer risk in collagenous colitis. Inflamm Bowel Dis 1999;5:40–43.
20. Pardi DS, Kammer PP, Loftus EV, et al. Microscopic colitis is not associated with an increased risk of colorectal cancer (abst). Am J Gastroenterol 2004;99:S115.
21. Ung KA, Kilander A, Willen R, et al. Role of bile acids in lymphocytic colitis. Hepato-gastroenterology 2002;49:432–437.

Chapter 5 / Microscopic Colitis

22. Pardi DS, Loftus EV, Kammer PP, et al. Collagenous colitis, but not lymphocytic colitis, is associated with cigarette smoking (abst). Am J Gastroenterol 2004;99:S116.

23. Pardi DS, Ramnath VR, Loftus EV, et al. Lymphocytic colitis: clinical features, treatment, and outcomes. Am J Gastroenterol 2002;97:2829–2833.

24. Mullhaupt B, Guller U, Anabitarte M, et al. Lymphocytic colitis: clinical presentation in long term course. Gut 1998;43:629–633.

25. Madisch A, Heymer P, Voss C, et al. Oral budesonide therapy improves quality of life in patients with collagenous colitis. Int J Colorectal Dis 2005;20: 312–316.

26. Hjortswang H, Tysk C, Bohr J, et al. Defining clinical criteria for clinical remission and disease activity in collagenous colitis. Inflamm Bowel Dis 2009;15: 1875–1881.

27. Limsui D, Pardi DS, Camilleri M, et al. Symptomatic overlap between irritable bowel syndrome and microscopic colitis. Inflamm Bowel Dis 2007;13: 175–181.

28. Madisch A, Bethke B, Stolte M, Miehlke S. Is there an association of microscopic colitis and irritable bowel syndrome—a subgroup analysis of placebo-controlled trials. World J Gastroenterol 2005;11:6409.

29. Giardiello FM, Bayless TM, Jessurun J, et al. Collagenous colitis: physiologic and histopathologic studies in seven patients. Ann Intern Med 1987;106:46–49.

30. Bohr J, Tysk C, Yang P, et al. Autoantibodies and immunoglobulins in collagenous colitis. Gut 1996;39:73–76.

31. Wolber R, Owen D, Freeman H. Colonic lymphocytosis in patients with celiac sprue. Hum Pathol 1990;21:1092–1096.

32. Breen EG, Coughlan G, Connolly CE, et al. Coeliac proctitis. Scand J Gastroenterol 1987;22:471–477.

33. Green PHR, Yang J, Cheng J, et al. An association between microscopic colitis and celiac disease. Clin Gastroenterol Hepatol 2009;7:1210–1216.

34. Fine KD, Meyer RL, Lee EL. The prevalence and cause of chronic diarrhea in patients with celiac sprue treated with a gluten-free diet. Gastroenterology 1997;112:1830–1838.

35. Fine KD, Do K, Schulte K, et al. High prevalence of celiac sprue-like HLA-DQ genes and enteropathy in patients with the microscopic colitis syndrome. Am J Gastroenterol 2000;95:1974–1982.

36. Ramzan NN, Shapiro MS, Pasha TM, et al. Is celiac disease associated with microscopic and collagenous colitis (abst)? Gastroenterology 2001;120:A684.

37. Kakar S, Pardi DS, Burgart LJ. Colonic ulcers accompanying collagenous colitis: implication of NSAIDs. Am J Gastroenterol 2003,98:1834–1837.

38. Bonner GF, Petras RE, Cheong DMO, et al. Short- and long-term follow-up of treatment for lymphocytic and collagenous colitis. Inflamm Bowel Dis 2000; 6:85–91.

39. Bonderup OK, Folkersen BH, Gjersoe P, et al. Collagenous colitis: a long-term follow-up study. Eur J Gastroenterol Hepatol 1999;11:493–495.

40. Madisch A, Miehlke S, Lindner M, et al. Clinical course of collagenous colitis over a period of 10 years. Z Gastroenterol 2006;44:971–974.

41. Baert F, Wouters K, D'Haens G, et al. Lymphocytic colitis: a distinct clinical entity? A clinicopathological confrontation of lymphocytic and collagenous colitis. Gut 1999;45:375–381.

42. Goff JS, Barnett JL, Pelke T, et al. Collagenous colitis: histopathology and clinical course. Am J Gastroenterol 1997;92:57–60.

43. Bonderup OK, Hansen JB, Birket-Smith L, et al. Budesonide treatment of collagenous colitis: a randomized, double-blind, placebo controlled trial with morphometric analysis. Gut 2003;52:248–251.
44. Baert F, Schmit A, D'Haens G, et al. Budesonide in collagenous colitis: a double-blind placebo-controlled trial with histologic follow-up. Gastroenterology 2002;122:20–25.
45. Miehlke S, Heymer P, Bethke B, et al. Budesonide treatment for collagenous colitis: a randomized, double-blind, placebo-controlled, multicenter trial. Gastroenterology 2002;123:978–984.
46. Miehlke S, Madish A, Karimi D, et al. A randomized double-blind, placebo-controlled study showing that budesonide is effective in treating lymphocytic colitis. Gastroenterology 2009;136:2092–2100.
47. Abdalla AA, Faubion WA, Loftus EV, et al. The natural history of microscopic colitis treated with corticosteroids. Gastroenterology 2008;134:A121.
48. Lazenby AJ, Yardley JH, Giardiello FM, et al. Lymphocytic (microscopic) colitis: a comparative histopathologic study with particular reference to collagenous colitis. Hum Pathol 1989;20:18–28.
49. Jessurun J, Yardley JH, Giardiello FM, et al. Chronic colitis with thickening of the subepithelial collagen layer (collagenous colitis). Histopathologic findings in 15 patients. Hum Pathol 1987;18:839–848.
50. Ayata G, Ithamukkala S, Sapp H, et al. Prevalence and significance of inflammatory bowel disease-like morphological features in collagenous and lymphocytic colitis. Am J Surg Pathol 2002;26:1414–1423.
51. Pardi DS. Microscopic colitis: an update. Inflamm Bowel Dis 2004;10:860–870.
52. Beaugerie L, Pardi DS. Drug-induced microscopic colitis – proposal for a scoring system and review of the literature. Aliment Pharmacol Ther 2005;22: 277–284.
53. Fernández-Bañares F, Esteve M, Espinós JC, et al. Drug consumption and the risk of microscopic colitis. Am J Gastroenterol 2007;102:324–330.
54. Riddell RH, Tanaka M, Mazzoleni G. Non-steroidal anti-inflammatory drugs as a possible cause of collagenous colitis: a case–control study. Gut 1992;33:683–686.
55. Giardiello FM, Hansen FC, Lazenby AJ, et al. Collagenous colitis in setting of nonsteroidal antiinflammatory drugs and antibiotics. Dig Dis Sci 1990;35: 257–260.
56. Veress B, Lofberg R, Bergman L. Microscopic colitis syndrome. Gut 1995;36: 880–886.
57. Bjarnason I, Hayllar J, MacPherson AJ, et al. Side effects of nonsteroidal anti-inflammatory drugs on the small and large intestine in humans. Gastroenterology 1993;104:1832–1847.
58. Yagi K, Nakamura A, Sekine A, et al. NSAID colitis with a histology of collagenous colitis. Endoscopy 2001;33:629–632.
59. al Ghamdi MY, Malatjalian DA, Veldhuyzen van Zanten S. Causation: recurrent collagenous colitis following repeated use of NSAIDs. Can J Gastroenterol 2002;16:861–862.
60. Fine KD, Lee EL. Efficacy of open-label bismuth subsalicylate for the treatment of microscopic colitis. Gastroenterology 1998;114:29–36.
61. Amaro R, Poniecka A, Rogers AI. Collagenous colitis treated successfully with bismuth subsalicylate. Dig Dis Sci 2000;45:1447–1450.
62. Fine K, Ogunji F, Lee E, et al. Randomized, double-blind, placebo-controlled trial of bismuth subsalicylate for microscopic colitis (abst). Gastroenterology 1999;116:A880.

Chapter 5 / Microscopic Colitis

63. Pardi DS, Loftus EV, Tremaine WJ, Sandborn WJ. A randomized, double-blind, placebo-controlled trial of budesonide for the treatment of active lymphocytic colitis. Gastroenterology 2009;136:A519.

64. Miehlke S, Madisch A, Voss C, et al. Long-term follow-up of collagenous colitis after induction of clinical remission with budesonide. Aliment Pharmacol Ther 2005;22:1115–1119.

65. Pardi DS, Loftus EV, Tremaine WJ, et al. Treatment of refractory microscopic colitis with azathioprine and 6-mercaptopurine. Gastroenterology 2001;120: 1483–1484.

66. Vennamaneni SR, Bonner GF. Use of azathioprine or 6-mercaptopurine for treatment of steroid-dependent lymphocytic and collagenous colitis. Am J Gastroenterol 2001;96:2798–2799.

67. Riddell J, Hillman L, Chiragakis L, Clarke A. Collagenous colitis: oral low-dose methotrexate for patients with difficult symptoms: long-term outcomes. J Gastroenterol Hepatol 2007;22:1589–1593.

68. Pardi DS. After budesonide, what next for collagenous colitis? Gut 2009;58:3–4.

69. Bonderup OK, Hansen JB, Teglbjoerg PS, et al. Long-term budesonide treatment of collagenous colitis: a randomised, double-blind, placebo-controlled trial. Gut 2009;58:68–72.

70. Miehlke S, Madish A, Bethke B, et al. Oral budesonide for maintenance treatment of collagenous colitis: a randomized, double-blind, placebo controlled trial. Gastroenterology 2008;135:1510–1516.

71. Calabrese C, Fabbri A, Areni A, et al. Mesalazine with or without cholestyramine in the treatment of microscopic colitis: randomized controlled trial. J Gastroenterol Hepatol 2007;22:809–814.

72. Jarnerot G, Tysk C, Bohr J, et al. Collagenous colitis and fecal stream diversion. Gastroenterology 1995;109:449–455.

73. Williams RA, Gelfand DV. Total proctocolectomy and ileal pouch anal anastomosis to successfully treat a patient with collagenous colitis. Am J Gastroenterol 2000;95:2147.

74. Varghese L, Galandiuk S, Tremaine WJ, et al. Lymphocytic colitis treated with proctocolectomy and ileal J-pouch anal anastomosis. Dis Colon Rect 2002; 45:123–126.

6 Food Allergy

Stefano Guandalini, MD

CONTENTS

INTRODUCTION
PATHOPHYSIOLOGY
CLINICAL PRESENTATION
REFERENCES

Summary

Adverse reactions to ingested foods are extremely common, especially in children. Different pathogenetic mechanisms underlie them, only those mediated by immune processes being defined as food allergies. Allergic reactions to food are due to several distinct immune reactions and can lead to a number of signs and symptoms, including diarrhea. Clinical presentations of the most common food allergies are illustrated, along with an outline of proper laboratory methods that are available to aid in the correct diagnostic approach. In spite of new, interesting developments, treatment of these conditions is still largely based on the elimination of the identified food allergens.

Key Words: Allergy, Food allergy, Cow's milk protein allergy, Food intolerance, Eosinophilic esophagitis, Eosinophilic gastroenteropathy

INTRODUCTION

Adverse reactions to ingested foods are extremely common. A stunning 15–20% of adults report some form of food intolerance. However, when challenged in a blinded fashion, most of the alleged intolerances cannot

From: *Diarrhea, Clinical Gastroenterology*
Edited by: S. Guandalini, H. Vaziri, DOI 10.1007/978-1-60761-183-7_6
© Springer Science+Business Media, LLC 2011

be confirmed. Still, proven food adverse reactions are very prevalent, both in children (where they are estimated to occur in about 3% of the general population, especially in the first 1–2 years) and in adults [1].

It should be noticed that not all adverse effects of food are due to allergic responses. In fact, adverse reactions to ingested foods can be classified as either nonimmune mediated (i.e., due to a variety of other conditions such as disorders of intestinal digestion/absorption, pharmacological reactions to chemicals in food, etc.) or immune mediated. Of the latter, only a few represent a true hypersensitivity reaction (i.e., have an immunoglobulin E-mediated pathogenesis). Nevertheless, the term "food allergy" is used to encompass all the specific reactions to offending food proteins that have an immunological basis, whether IgE or non-IgE mediated. Table 6.1 is a classification of adverse reactions to food.

Several food proteins, both from fluid and solid foods, can act as antigens in humans and cause an immune reaction. Cow's milk proteins are most frequently implicated as a cause of food intolerance during infancy. Soybean proteins rank second as antigens in the first months of life, particularly in infants with primary cow's milk intolerance who are switched to a soy formula. From school age on, egg protein intolerance becomes more prevalent. In childhood, there is evidence of a growing prevalence of allergy to peanuts [2, 3].

Clinical reactions to food proteins can be very heterogeneous in children as well as in adults. In children, gastrointestinal symptoms typically predominate [3, 4], with a frequency ranging from 50 to 80%, followed by skin lesions (20–40%) and respiratory symptoms (4–25%).

PATHOPHYSIOLOGY

The main proteins acting as food allergens are water-soluble glycoproteins with a molecular weight of 10,000–60,000 which are resistant to heat, low pH, and enzymatic degradation.

The uptake of intact antigens by the gastrointestinal tract is a transcellular process of endocytosis; however, some antigens can move through intercellular gaps. Under normal circumstances, the penetration of antigens through the mucosal barrier does not lead to any clinical manifestation. In fact, food antigen exposure via the gastrointestinal tract results in a local immunoglobulin A (IgA) response with activation of suppressor CD8$^+$ lymphocytes of the gut-associated lymphoid tissue, a phenomenon defined as oral tolerance.

However, in selected circumstances oral tolerance may never develop or may be lost.

In genetically susceptible individuals, oral tolerance does not develop, and different immunological and inflammatory mechanisms can be elicited by antigen entry. Local production and systemic distribution of specific reaginic IgE plays a significant role in IgE-mediated reactions to food proteins. In addition, studies have demonstrated the

Table 6.1
Adverse reactions to food

Type	Pathogenesis	Clinical entities
Non-immune mediated	Disorders of digestive–absorptive processes	Glucose–galactose malabsorption Lactase deficiency Sucrase–isomaltase deficiency Enterokinase deficiency
	Pharmacological reactions	Tyramine in aged cheeses Histamine in strawberries, caffeine, etc.
	Idiosyncratic reactions	Food additives Food colorants
	Inborn errors of metabolism	PKU (phenylketonuria) Hereditary fructose intolerance Tyrosinemia Galactosemia Lysinuric protein intolerance
Immune mediated (food allergy)	IgE mediated *(positive RAST or skin prick tests)*	Oral allergy syndrome Immediate GI hypersensitivity
	Occasionally IgE mediated	Eosinophilic esophagitis Eosinophilic gastritis Eosinophilic gastroenteritis
	Non-IgE mediated	Food protein-induced: enterocolitis (FPIES), enteropathy, proctocolitis
Autoimmune	Innate as well as adaptive immunity	Celiac disease

Table 6.2
Food proteins causing food allergies

Food	Specific protein (when identified)
Cow's milk	Caseins
	Whey proteins β-Lactoglobulin α-Lactalbumin Bovine serum albumin
Egg	Ovalbumin
Soy	2S-globulin Soy trypsin inhibitor Soy lectin
Wheat	Gluten Glutenin Globulin Albumin
Corn	50 kDa maize gamma-zein
Rice	
Fish	
Shellfish	
Beef	
Pork	
Peanuts, beans, peas	
Tree nuts and seeds, cocoa	

role of gastrointestinal T lymphocytes in the pathogenesis of gastrointestinal food allergy, so that it is now accepted that T cell-mediated or delayed hypersensitivity reactions are also responsible for food allergies.

In spite of the fact that IgG antibodies directed against food proteins can be easily detected in many individuals, the role of this immunoglobulin in the pathogenesis of clinically relevant symptoms remains unproven.

Table 6.1 lists the different clinical conditions with their corresponding underlying pathogenesis and Table 6.2 lists the most common food allergens.

CLINICAL PRESENTATION

History

Allergy to cow's milk typically develops in early infancy. The onset of symptoms is closely related to the timing of formula introduction into the diet. It is thought that the vast majority of infants with allergy to cow's milk proteins will develop clinical manifestations within 4 weeks of ingestion.

It was assumed for a long time that food allergy remits by 2 years of age, when the infant's mucosal immune system matures and the child becomes immunologically tolerant. However, it has subsequently become clear that milk protein allergy may actually persist well beyond that time or even manifest itself initially in children older than 5 years.

Occasionally patients may appear to be in remission for years, only to experience a recurrence of symptoms as teenagers or even as adults.

Signs and Symptoms

Food allergy can present with a number of different symptoms including gastrointestinal manifestations, which are the most common. Although a prominent presentation, not all food allergies are associated with diarrhea.

The following presentations describe the various entities listed in Table 6.1.

1) IgE mediated

    a. *Oral allergy syndrome*: A form of IgE-mediated contact allergy (appearing urticaria-like) that is confined almost exclusively to the oropharynx and is most commonly associated with the ingestion of various fresh fruits and vegetables [5]. Symptoms include itching, burning, and angioedema of the lips, tongue, palate, and throat.

    Immediate gastrointestinal hypersensitivity: An IgE-mediated gastrointestinal reaction that often accompanies allergic manifestations in other organs, such as the skin or lungs. The reaction usually occurs within minutes to 2 h of food ingestion. Most commonly, the involved food antigens are cow's milk or soy proteins, egg, wheat, seafood, and nuts. The patient immediately develops nausea and abdominal pain, soon followed by vomiting.

    Similar to other IgE-dependent allergic disorders, allergy to milk, egg, wheat, and soy generally resolves, whereas allergy to peanuts, tree nuts, and seafood tends to persist [3].

2) Occasionally IgE mediated: eosinophilic gastroenteropathies

A group of several disorders, all characterized by the infiltration of eosinophils into the GI mucosa and consequent various GI symptoms [6]. Peripheral eosinophilia may occur but is rarely very significant (i.e., >15–20%). Overlap exists among this group of disorders; however, it is best to consider each entity on an individual basis as described below.

a. *Eosinophilic esophagitis (EE)*: A relatively new entity occurring in both children [7] and adults [8] is characterized by heavy eosinophilic infiltration (by definition, >20 eosinophils/hpf at pathology) of the esophageal mucosa. Endoscopically, various features are described, including furrowing of the mucosa and mucosal rings.

Typically there is no concomitant involvement of the gastric or duodenal mucosa. The condition appears to be rapidly increasing in prevalence.

Affected individuals, both children and adults, may present with dysphagia, food impaction, intermittent vomiting, food refusal, epigastric or chest pain, and failure to respond to conventional antireflux medications. Of interest, EE may also be responsible for intermittent mucousy or watery, non-bloody diarrhea.

Occasionally, esophageal strictures may develop in untreated patients.

Pediatric patients have often evidence of food hypersensitivity (based on history and/or RAST test), with a response to strict elimination diets in the majority of cases [9].

Eosinophilic gastritis: Distinct from the esophagitis, and typically occurring in the absence of esophageal or duodenal involvement, this rare entity mostly presents after childhood. Its symptoms are usually typical of gastritis due to other etiologies (i.e., postprandial vomiting, abdominal pain, anorexia, and early satiety with weight loss as a consequence). Atopic features are present in about half of patients. Affected patients will often respond to an elimination diet.

b. *Eosinophilic gastroenteritis*: An ill-defined disease which is characterized by the infiltration of eosinophils into various sites of the gastrointestinal tract, extending from the stomach to the rectum.

The syndrome has been reported in children of all ages as well as in adults. The eosinophilic infiltration can be limited to the mucosa, or can extend deeper into the submucosa, muscularis, and serosa. Gastrointestinal symptoms vary according to the area of involvement and the extent of infiltration.

The most common symptoms experienced are vomiting, profuse, intermittent, non-bloody diarrhea, and weight loss. The involvement of the small and large intestine can result in anemia as well as protein-losing enteropathy, which can be severe at times.

In cases where the muscular layers are involved, gastric outlet obstruction, subacute small intestinal obstruction, and appendicitis-like symptoms have also been documented. Diagnosis requires bioptic samples showing the eosinophilic infiltration.

Unfortunately, no clear-cut line can be drawn to distinguish eosinophilic gastroenteritis from other gastrointestinal diseases and from nonpathologic, minor eosinophilic infiltrations of the lower intestine.

3) Non-IgE mediated

a. *Food protein-induced enterocolitis syndrome (FPIES)*: A symptom complex of profuse vomiting and diarrhea diagnosed in infancy involving both the small and the large intestine [10].

Food-induced enterocolitis syndrome occurs most frequently in the first few months of life. Infants younger than 3 months are especially at risk. Affected infants may develop failure to thrive quickly, if left untreated.

By far the commonest food antigens responsible for this syndrome are cow's milk and soy protein, although recently it has also been reported that solid food proteins (such as protein from rice, vegetables, and poultry) may cause it in older infants [11, 12].

Vomiting generally occurs 1–3 h after food intake, while diarrhea occurs 5–8 h after feeding.

Specific descriptions of the histologic findings are scanty because the diagnosis can be made clinically. Small bowel biopsies show mild villous injury with edema and inflammatory infiltration; while colonic specimens reveal crypt abscesses and a diffuse inflammatory infiltrate. FPIES is non-IgE mediated. Although its pathogenesis is poorly understood, it is believed to be due to a cell-mediated allergy.

b. *Food protein-induced enteropathy*: Also a cell-mediated form of food allergy involves damage to the absorptive surface of the small intestinal mucosa. Cow's milk and soy, but also rice, proteins are responsible for an uncommon syndrome appearing typically in infants 3–12 months of age. Symptoms include vomiting, pallor, chronic diarrhea, and failure to thrive or weight loss, which can be confused with celiac disease. Vomiting is present in up to two-thirds of patients. Small bowel biopsy reveals an enteropathy with variable degrees of villous atrophy. Total mucosal atrophy histologically indistinguishable from celiac disease is also a frequent finding. Intestinal protein and blood losses can aggravate the hypoalbuminemia and anemia that are frequently observed in this syndrome. In fact, protein-losing enteropathy may be a prominent feature. Overall, the frequency and severity of this syndrome has decreased over the past 20 years.

Recently described cases involve patients who tend to have patchy intestinal lesions.

c. *Food protein-induced proctocolitis*: A common cause of minor rectal bleeding in very young infants, typically 2–8 weeks of age, although recently described also in older children [13].

Again, cow's milk and soy proteins are most often responsible, but interestingly the majority of affected infants are exclusively breast-fed.

Symptoms include diarrhea with streaks of fresh blood. Affected infants typically appear healthy and have normal weight gain. The onset of bleeding is gradual and initially erratic over several days. It then progresses to streaks of blood in most stools which can elicit suspicion of an internal anal tear and is generally very alarming to the parents. Endoscopic findings include aphthae and biopsies show a mild-to-moderate eosinophilic proctitis. It should be noted, however, that endoscopy is generally not required for diagnosis in such a low-grade benign condition.

In about half of the cases, a strict maternal diet with elimination of all cow's milk and soy-based products can resolve the problem.

Diagnosis

As in every medical condition, the first step in diagnosis is to have a high level of suspicion with careful attention to history and physical exam. Family history is particularly important as it is known that the vast majority of patients with food allergy will report have a positive family history. As a general rule, once a food allergy is suspected, the incriminated foods need to be eliminated. Further diagnostic tests may or may not be necessary to confirm the diagnosis.

Oral allergy syndrome and immediate GI hypersensitivity. As these conditions are always IgE mediated, measuring food-specific IgE antibodies is helpful. This can be done either by skin prick tests or by the serum assay of food IgE antibodies through a *R*adio *A*llergo *S*orbent *T*est (RAST).

Different laboratories use different units, and it is not uncommon for the result to be reported in a "class" scheme, based on comparison with normal sera, that goes from 0 to 5. However, data should be expressed quantitatively using the parameter units/liter (U/l) in order to allow for a meaningful comparison.

Table 6.3 (from [14]) provides a guideline for the clinician, listing the probability of a clinical reaction based on levels of IgE to specific major food allergens.

It is important to notice that the positive predictive value for a test depends on the study population and the allergen being tested. In a study of 100 children in the United States, a cutoff value of 15 KU/l had a

Table 6.3
Interpretation of food-specific IgE levels (kU/l) in the diagnosis of IgE-mediated food allergy

	Egg	Milk	Peanut	Fish	Soy	Wheat	
Reactive if ≥ (no challenge necessary)	7	15	14	20	65	80	Probability of reaction
Possibly reactive (physician challenge[a])					30	26	
Unlikely reactive if < (home challenge [a])	0.35	0.35	0.35	0.35	0.35	0.35	

Reprinted with permission from [14], Elsevier.

a) In patients with a strongly suggestive history of an IgE-mediated food allergic reaction, food challenges should be performed with physician supervision, regardless of food-specific IgE value. If the food-specific IgE level is less than 0.35 kUA/L and the skin prick test response is negative, the food challenge can be performed at home unless there is a compelling history of reactivity.

positive predictive value of 95% for cow's milk [14]. A cutoff of 7 KU/l had the same positive predictive value for egg.

Eosinophilic gastroenteropathies (eosinophilic esophagitis, eosinophilic gastritis, eosinophilic gastroenteritis). Food-specific IgE antibodies should be measured, as in approximately 50% of cases these disorders may indeed be mediated by an IgE reaction. When interpreting RAST results, the same considerations that apply to IgE-mediated conditions will apply to these disorders. It is also important to note that a negative RAST does not rule out food allergy as a cause of eosinophilic gastroenteropathies.

Given the limited role of immune-allergy laboratory services and an absence of strictly defined diagnostic criteria, diagnosis relies on the clinical skills of an experienced gastroenterologist. Endoscopic procedures can help rule out conditions that have a similar presentation.

Once the diagnosis of an eosinophilic gastroenteropathy is established, an elimination diet should be implemented. The subsequent management is dictated by the response obtained during the initial trial [6]. Anti-inflammatory agents (i.e., steroids) may be necessary in some cases, especially if no food allergy is detected, which can be the case in up to 40% of patients [15].

Non-IgE mediated. Presumptive diagnoses are characteristically reached by eliminating the suspected food antigen (most commonly milk protein) and observing the clinical response.

Food protein-induced enterocolitis syndrome. A definitive diagnosis is made when there is a recurrence of symptoms upon re-challenging the patient with the offending protein. Typically no invasive diagnostic procedure is performed, as FPIES is considered a transient food allergy. Most pediatric gastroenterologists avoid the re-challenging step and simply delay the re-introduction of the suspected protein to the end of the first or early second year of life [16] . Typically no invasive diagnostic procedure is performed, as FPIES is considered a transient food allergy.

Food protein-induced enteropathy. Given the similarities with other conditions causing a malabsorption picture (and mostly celiac disease), the diagnostic workup of this condition follows that of any other malabsorptive disorder presenting in infancy and is likely to include an upper GI endoscopy with mucosal biopsies. As mentioned earlier, the pathological findings may be totally indistinguishable from those of celiac disease, including the increased number of intraepithelial lymphocytes.

Both conditions can also cause a major protein-losing enteropathy that can be detected by checking fecal α1-antitrypsin level. The diagnostic confusion in this young age group may be aggravated by the fact that the specific serology for celiac disease may be negative.

In severe cases in which both gluten and milk proteins have been eliminated from the diet of the affected infant prior to initiating the diagnostic work, repeated food challenges for a prolonged period of time may be necessary before a definitive diagnosis can be made.

Food protein-induced proctocolitis. In young breast-fed infants, the diagnostic workup is usually unnecessary as one can rely on the clinical presentation. In older children with persistent or recurrent rectal bleeding, flexible proctosigmoidoscopy should be considered. Affected children usually have mild left-sided colitis characterized by a prominent eosinophilic infiltration, focal lymphoid follicle hyperplasia, and a prompt clinical and histological response to a cow's milk free [13].

REFERENCES

1. Cochrane S, Beyer K, Clausen M, Wjst M, Hiller R, Nicoletti C, Szepfalusi Z, Savelkoul H, Breiteneder H, Manios Y, Crittenden R, Burney P. Factors influencing the incidence and prevalence of food allergy. Allergy 2009;64(9): 1246–1255.
2. Sicherer SH, Munoz-Furlong A, Sampson HA. Prevalence of seafood allergy in the United States determined by a random telephone survey. J Allergy Clin Immunol 2004;114(1):159–165.
3. Sicherer SH. Clinical aspects of gastrointestinal food allergy in childhood. Pediatrics 2003;111(6 Pt 3):1609–1616.
4. Guandalini S, Nocerino A. Food protein intolerance. In: Chris A. Liacouras M, ed. e-Medicine, 2009, http://www.emedicine.com/
5. Mari A, Ballmer-Weber BK, Vieths S. The oral allergy syndrome: improved diagnostic and treatment methods. Curr Opin Allergy Clin Immunol 2005;5(3): 267–273.
6. Rothenberg ME. Eosinophilic gastrointestinal disorders (EGID). J Allergy Clin Immunol 2004;113(1):11–28; quiz 29.
7. Liacouras CA, Ruchelli E. Eosinophilic esophagitis. Curr Opin Pediatr 2004; 16(5):560–566.
8. Sgouros SN, Bergele C, Mantides A. Eosinophilic esophagitis in adults: a systematic review. Eur J Gastroenterol Hepatol 2006;18(2):211–217.
9. Kagalwalla AF, Sentongo TA, Ritz S, Hess T, Nelson SP, Emerick KM, Melin-Aldana H, Li BU. Effect of six-food elimination diet on clinical and histologic outcomes in eosinophilic esophagitis. Clin Gastroenterol Hepatol 2006;4(9): 1097–1102.
10. Sicherer SH. Food protein-induced enterocolitis syndrome: clinical perspectives. J Pediatr Gastroenterol Nutr 2000;30 Suppl:S45–S49.
11. Nowak-Wegrzyn A, et al. Food protein-induced enterocolitis syndrome caused by solid food proteins. Pediatrics 2003;111(4 Pt 1):829–835.
12. Levy Y, Danon YL. Food protein-induced enterocolitis syndromenot only due to cow's milk and soy. Pediatr Allergy Immunol 2003;14(4):325–329.

13. Ravelli A, Villanacci V, Chiappa S, Bolognini S, Manenti S, Fuoti M. Dietary protein-induced proctocolitis in childhood. Am J Gastroenterol 2008;103(10): 2605–2612.
14. Sampson HA. Utility of food-specific IgE concentrations in predicting symptomatic food allergy. J Allergy Clin Immunol 2001;107(5):891–896.
15. Guajardo JR, et al. Eosinophil-associated gastrointestinal disorders: a world-wide-web based registry. J Pediatr 2002;141(4):576–581.
16. Hwang JB, Sohn SM, Kim AS. Prospective follow-up oral food challenge in food protein-induced enterocolitis syndrome. Arch Dis Child 2009;94(6):425–438.

7 Protein-Losing Enteropathies

*Jonathan Goldstein, MD, MPH
and Richard Wright, MD, MBA, FACP*

CONTENTS

INTRODUCTION
NORMAL PROTEIN ABSORPTION
PROTEIN MALABSORPTION AND PROTEIN
  LOSS
CLINICAL MANIFESTATIONS
DIAGNOSIS IN PROTEIN-LOSING
  GASTROENTEROPATHIES
TREATMENT
SUMMARY POINTS AND RECOMMENDATIONS
REFERENCES

Summary

Protein-losing enteropathies are a syndrome caused by mucosal disruption or increased permeability or obstruction of lymphatic drainage. Documentation of excessive intestinal protein loss is the hallmark of the diagnosis. Treatment depends on the primary disease process and is usually a combination of dietary, medical, and/or surgical therapy. Most etiologies are treatable and may be curable if the primary disease is eliminated.

Key Words: Protein losing, Enteropathy, Exudative enteropathy, Hypoalbuminemia, Hypoproteinemia

From: *Diarrhea, Clinical Gastroenterology*
Edited by: S. Guandalini, H. Vaziri, DOI 10.1007/978-1-60761-183-7_7
© Springer Science+Business Media, LLC 2011

INTRODUCTION

Protein-losing gastroenteropathy is a condition characterized by excessive loss of serum proteins into the gastrointestinal tract, which can result in systemic hypoproteinemia. This condition may be caused by a variety of underlying mucosal diseases which lead to exudation of plasma due to surface inflammation, erosion, increased permeability, or a leaky mucosa that develops for other reasons.

Maimon and colleagues first conceptualized protein-losing gastroenteropathy in 1947, by noting that fluid production from enlarged gastric folds in patients with Menetrier's disease was high in protein content. In 1949, Albright and colleagues used IV infusions of albumin to demonstrate that hypoproteinemia resulted from increased catabolism of albumin, rather than inadequate albumin synthesis. In 1956, Kimbel and colleagues observed increased gastric albumin production in chronic gastritis. Later, in 1957, Citrin and colleagues elucidated that the gastrointestinal tract was the specific site of excess protein loss in Menetrier's disease, by associating excess loss of intravenously administered radioiodinated albumin with appearance of labeled protein in the gastric secretions of these patients [1].

NORMAL PROTEIN ABSORPTION

Recommended dietary needs for protein in adults vary from 0.75 to 1 g/kg of body weight daily, although actual systemic deficiency is rare even with intake as low as 0.5 g/kg per day or less [2]. Proteins are partially broken down into large oligopeptides in the stomach by pepsins at an optimal pH of 2–3.5. Peptidases of the pancreas further hydrolyze proteins and large oligopeptides at an optimal pH of 7–8. After the combined action of gastric and pancreatic proteolytic enzymes, dietary protein is largely reduced to a combination of small oligopeptides (2–6 amino acid residues representing 75–85% of the final products of protein digestion) and free amino acids (remaining 15–25%) [2, 3].

Final digestion of the small oligopeptides to three absorbable forms (amino acids, di- and tripeptides) is catalyzed by oligopeptidases attached to the microvillous membrane.

Di- and tripeptides are absorbed more easily than amino acids [4]. Within the cytoplasm, most are quickly hydrolyzed to their constituent amino acids. A specific membrane carrier exists for the transport of the released di- and tripeptides: such transporter, designated Pept-1, is the exclusive oligopeptide transporter of the brush-border membrane of the intestinal mucosa and, in contrast to other transporters, has an

Chapter 7 / Protein-Losing Enteropathies

enormous range of substrates. Pept-1 is in fact able to transport 400 dipeptides and 8,000 tripeptides that could be produced from the digestion of dietary and body proteins [5]. In addition, a membrane carrier exists for neutral amino acids, another for basic amino acids, and a third system for proline and hydroxyproline [2]. Absorbed amino acids, particularly glutamine, are major fuels for small intestinal mucosa [2]. The absorbed amino acids and a small fraction of the dipeptides find their way to the portal venules in the lamina propria and reach the liver via the portal vein.

Approximately two thirds of protein within the lumen is dietary in origin. The remainder of protein normally leaked into the gastrointestinal lumen is from endogenous sources: 10 g/day of protein enzymes, 10 g/day of protein in exfoliated epithelial cells, and 1.4 g/day of plasma proteins [1]. Amino acids, di- and tripeptides are absorbed most efficiently in the jejunum [5]. By the time a meal enters the ileum, 80% of food protein together with the endogenous protein has been digested and absorbed. Ten percent is absorbed in the ileum. The protein content of stools equals about 10% of protein eaten, however, its source is bacteria and cellular debris [6].

PROTEIN MALABSORPTION AND PROTEIN LOSS

The most frequent causes of *protein malabsorption* are loss of normal jejunal mucosal function and loss of exocrine pancreatic secretion of peptidases. Protein malabsorption is more commonly associated with chronic generalized damage of the intestinal absorptive area such as seen in celiac disease or milk protein allergic enteropathy; in short bowel syndromes; or in conditions of severe lack of exocrine pancreatic function such as in cystic fibrosis [7].

Protein-losing enteropathy on the other hand is the consequence of a range of pathophysiologic processes that result in the loss of serum proteins into the gastrointestinal tract. Although gastrointestinal tract loss of albumin should normally account for less than 10% of the total body degradation of albumin in normal individuals, patients with protein-losing gastrointestinal disorders can increase enteric protein loss up to 60% of total systemic albumin [8, 9].

Under physiologic conditions, most endogenous proteins found in the gastrointestinal lumen are derived from sloughed enterocytes and pancreatic and biliary secretions [10]. Daily enteric loss of serum proteins accounts for less than 1–2% of the serum protein pool in healthy individuals, with enteric loss of albumin accounting for less than 10% of total albumin catabolism. The normal total albumin pool is 3.9 g/kg in women and 4.7 g/kg in men, with a rate of hepatic albumin synthesis of 0.15 g/kg/day and a half-life of 15–33 days. The rate of albumin production with albumin half-life should typically equal the rate of albumin degradation [8].

Excess proteins entering the gastrointestinal tract are digested by proteases into their constituent amino acids, which are then reabsorbed in the portal circulation [11]. Gastrointestinal losses normally are insignificant with regard to total protein metabolism, and serum protein levels thus represent a balance between protein synthesis and metabolism. However, this physiology can become severely altered in patients with protein-losing gastroenteropathy [1, 12].

Numerous disease states are associated with protein-losing gastroenteropathy, with abnormal plasma protein loss attributable to differing types of alterations in the gastrointestinal epithelial mucosa (see Table 7.1). The range of diseases causing protein-losing gastroenteropathy may be conceptualized under three descriptive mechanisms. First, mucosal injury can result in increased permeability to plasma proteins due to cell damage or loss. Second, mucosal erosions and ulcerations may cause a loss of inflammatory, protein-rich exudates. Finally, lymphatic obstruction or increased lymphatic hydrostatic pressure may allow direct leakage of lymph, which contains plasma proteins.

An important concept, with regard to the mechanisms leading to hypoproteinemia in the protein-losing gastroenteropathies, is that loss of proteins is independent of their molecular weights and is thus nonspecific. Therefore, the fraction of the intravascular pool degraded per day remains the same for various proteins, including albumin, IgG, IgA, IgM, and ceruloplasmin. A contrast, for example, is that nephrotic syndrome preferentially loses low molecular weight proteins such as albumin [13].

Although all proteins are usually lost through the gastrointestinal tract at the same rate in protein-losing gastroenteropathies, systemic deficits between various endogenous proteins may be unequal. This is due to physiological differences in the capacity to break down or synthesize specific types of proteins. For example, proteins such as insulin, clotting factors, and IgE may be relatively unaffected by gastrointestinal losses due to rapid synthetic rates. By contrast, albumin production can only be maximally increased by only 25%, and most gamma globulins (other than IgE) are limited in their ability to respond to gastrointestinal losses [14]. For this reason, abnormal protein loss from the gut can lead to an unequal systemic profile of hypoproteinemia (e.g., more commonly exhibited as hypoalbuminemia and hypoglobulinemia). Other compounding factors contributing to excessive enteric protein loss may coexist, including impaired hepatic protein

Chapter 7 / Protein-Losing Enteropathies

Table 7.1
Disease states associated with protein-losing gastroenteropathy

Primary gastrointestinal mucosal diseases (typically ulcerative/erosive)
  Erosions or ulcerations of the esophagus, stomach, or duodenum
  Regional enteritis
  Graft versus host disease
  Pseudomembranous Colitis (*Clostridium difficile*)
  Mucosal-based neoplasia
  Carcinoid syndrome
  Idiopathic ulcerative jejunoileitis
  Amyloidosis
  Kaposi sarcoma
  Protein dyscrasia
  Ulcerative colitis
  Neurofibromatosis
  Cytomegalovirus infection

Nonerosive upper gastrointestinal diseases
  Cutaneous burns
  Whipple disease
  Connective tissue disorders
  Acquired immunodeficiency syndrome (AIDS)
  Enteropathy, such as angioedema (idiopathic or hereditary) and
  Henoch-Schönlein purpura
  Celiac disease
  Tropical sprue
  Allergic gastroenteritis
  Eosinophilic gastroenteritis
  Giant hypertrophic gastritis (Menetrier disease)
  Bacterial overgrowth
  Intestinal parasites
  Microscopic colitis
  Dientamoeba fragilis

Conditions with protein loss due to increased interstitial pressure or
  lymphatic obstruction
  Tuberculosis
  Sarcoidosis
  Retroperitoneal fibrosis
  Lymphoma
  Intestinal endometriosis
  Lymphoenteric fistula
  Whipple Disease
  Cardiac disease (constrictive pericarditis or congestive heart failure)
  Intestinal lymphangiectasia

From ref. 54

synthesis and increased endogenous degradation of plasma proteins [1, 13].

Protein-losing gastroenteropathies, in addition to hypoproteinemia, can manifest in reduced concentrations of other serum components. These include lipids, iron, and trace metals. If lymphatic obstruction is the underlying mechanism, this can result in lymphocytopenia and changes in cellular immunity [1]. However, despite decreased serum gamma globulin levels, increased susceptibility to infections is uncommon [15, 16].

CLINICAL MANIFESTATIONS

Although clinical features are predominantly a manifestation of the underlying causative disease process, a low protein state with resultant edema due to reduction in oncotic pressure is the most common presenting sign. Dependent edema is a common finding; however, frank anasarca is reportedly more rare [1]. Proteins with slow catabolic turnover tend to be decreased, such as albumin and gamma globulins IgG, IgA, and IgM [17]. By contrast, rapid turnover proteins, such as pre-albumin, IgE, insulin, and retinal-binding protein are preserved [17, 18]. Intestinal lymphangiectasia may manifest as unilateral edema, upper extremity edema, facial edema, macular edema (with reversible blindness), and bilateral retinal detachments [1]. Yellow nail syndrome has been described in protein-losing enteropathy associated with primary lymphangiectasia, consisting of chronic peripheral lymphedema, yellow slow-growing nails, recurrent pleural and pericardial effusions, and chylous ascites [11, 19]. Malabsorption can be exhibited as diarrhea, such as in small bowel disorders with protein loss including celiac disease or tropical sprue. This can result decreased levels of lipids, fat-soluble vitamin malabsorption, trace metal deficiencies, anemia, and carbohydrate malabsorption [11].

Clotting factors may be lost into the gastrointestinal tract, but coagulation status typically remains unaffected [11]. Although circulating levels of proteins that bind hormones, such as cortisol and thyroid-binding proteins, may be substantially decreased, levels of circulating free hormones are not significantly altered [1].

Diseases Associated with Protein Losing Gastroenteropathy: Without Mucosal Erosions or Ulcerations

A primary example of protein-losing gastropathy without mucosal erosions includes Menetrier's disease, otherwise known as giant hypertrophic gastropathy. A pre-malignant condition, this is the most

Chapter 7 / Protein-Losing Enteropathies

common gastric disease causing severe protein loss [20]. Patients often experience dyspepsia, postprandial nausea, emesis, anorexia, edema, weight loss, and hypoproteinemia on work-up [1, 21]. Criteria for diagnosis include giant gastric folds, histological features of marked foveolar hyperplasia, atrophy of glands, and increase in mucosal thickness. Elevated TGF-α in gastric mucous cells binds to epidermal growth factor receptor. This increases gastric mucous production and cell renewal and inhibits acid secretion [22]. Hypoproteinemia occurs due to selective loss of serum proteins across the gastric mucosa. Tight junctions between cells are wider than normal, and it is thought that proteins traverse the gastric mucosa through these widened spaces [23].

A possible causal relationship appears to exist between *Helicobacter pylori* infection and Menetrier's disease with protein-losing gastroenteropathy, with a retrospective study detecting *H. pylori* in >90% of cases of Menetrier's disease [24]. Treatment of *H. pylori* has been reported to result in endoscopic and symptomatic resolution of Menetrier's disease, with normalization of hypoproteinemia [24, 25]. Of note, *H. pylori* gastritis with protein-losing gastroenteropathy from erosions may occur in the absence of Menetrier's disease. Eradication of *H. pylori* in this setting has also responded to eradication of acute infection [26].

Allergic gastroenteropathy is an additional example of a disease state without mucosal erosions or ulcerations associated with protein-losing gastroenteropathy. Although generally considered a pediatric entity, this may also be encountered in adults. Symptoms include abdominal distress, vomiting, and intermittent diarrhea. Laboratory abnormalities include hypoproteinemia, hypoalbuminemia, iron deficiency anemia, and peripheral eosinophilia. Although IgM and transferrin levels may be only moderately decreased, serum total protein, albumin, IgA, and IgG become markedly reduced [1]. Characteristic histology of the small bowel in these patients includes marked increase of eosinophils in the lamina propria and Charcot–Leyden crystals on stool examination [27].

Chehade et al. studied eight patients retrospectively, comparing controls and patients with allergic gastroenteritis and no anemia or hypoalbuminemia. Routine histological evaluation did not show any features differentiating allergic gastroenteritis from allergic gastroenteritis with protein-losing enteropathy. However, when eosinophils and mast cells were counted in intestinal biopsies, significantly more mast cells were found in biopsies of the allergic gastroenteritis with protein-losing enteropathy group despite comparable numbers of eosinophils. By contrast, eosinophils in gastric biopsies were more prominent in allergic gastroenteritis with protein-losing enteropathy, while mast cell numbers were similar in all groups [28].

Regarding treatment of this condition, Chehade et al. found that, although all patients studied had an excellent response to amino acid-based formula and tolerated gradual introduction of some foods with time, food-responsive disease persisted in all patients during 2.5–5.5 years of follow-up [28]. They thus concluded that patients with allergic gastroenteritis and protein-losing gastroenteropathy may be expected to respond well to therapy with amino acid-based formula, although food hypersensitivities may not completely resolve over up to a 5.5-year period. Also, since intestinal mast cells were significantly increased in maximally infiltrated areas of the intestine, this may be the cause of increased intestinal permeability and protein loss. Markedly elevated histamine levels have been observed in small bowel mucosal biopsy sample [29]. Histologic appearance of localized intestinal anaphylaxis correlates with mast cell migration into the intestinal lumen. Although cromolyn was an ineffective prophylaxis, it was found that sensitized animals pretreated with prostaglandin E2 or doxantrazole had inhibition of this localized anaphylactic response [30].

Another example of a disease state without mucosal erosions which may cause protein-losing gastroenteropathy is systemic lupus erythematosis. In fact, protein-losing gastroenteropathy may be the initial clinical presentation of lupus [31, 32]. The causal mechanism has been associated with mesenteric vasculitis, resulting in intestinal ischemia, edema, and intestinal capillary hyperpermeability [1]. Uniquely, although hypercholesterolemia is rare in idiopathic protein-losing gastroenteropathy due to enteric lipoprotein loss [33], this is common in lupus-associated protein-losing gastroenteropathy [34]. It is thought that leakage of cholesterol-rich lipoprotein particles in the intestinal lymph does not occur is systemic lupus, as lymphatic disruption is partial [35].

Clinically, this phenomenon may be important as outlined in YG Kim's study of 11 lupus-associated protein-losing gastroenteropathy patients. The data indicated that, if hypercholesterolemia >250 mg/dL is measured, then, corticosteroids alone were sufficient to achieve remission. Thus, the use of other immunosuppressants such as cyclophosphamide or azathioprine could be postponed in this scenario [34].

Most cases of lupus-induced protein-losing enteropathy can be treated medically with corticosteroids, plus or minus methotrexate, cyclophosphamide, or azathioprine [32]. Relapse rates of 20–30% may be expected with medical management [33]. Wang et al. published a case study in which a lupus patient with protein-losing enteropathy resistant to medical treatment was found to benefit briefly from surgical resection of the affected ascending colon segment. However, 6 months later, the patient's symptoms recurred, and Technetium

Chapter 7 / Protein-Losing Enteropathies

99m scintigraphy confirmed protein loss from the remaining colon. It was concluded that, although certain other causes of protein-losing gastroenteropathy may be effectively treated with focal resection, systemic lupus erythematosis patients are less likely to benefit, due to multi-systemic involvement [36].

Diseases Associated with Protein Losing Gastroenteropathy: with Mucosal Erosions or Ulcerations

Protein-losing gastroenteropathy secondary to mucosal erosions or ulcerations may be associated with various benign or malignant conditions. Whether the process is localized or diffuse, the mechanism of protein loss is related to inflammatory exudation secondary to erosions and ulcerations [1, 11]. The severity of protein losses depends on the degree of cellular loss, with associated inflammation and lymphatic obstruction. Diffuse ulcerations of the small intestine or colon, as seen with Crohn's disease, ulcerative colitis, and pseudomembranous colitis, can result in severe protein loss [37, 38]. Regarding causes of hypoalbuminemia in gastrointestinal tract malignancies, this may be attributable to decreased albumin synthesis as well as excessive enteric protein loss [1]. This may additionally be caused by cancer therapies, including chemotherapy, radiation-related injury, and bone marrow transplantation.

Although rare, protein-losing enteropathy can be a severe complication of Crohn's disease [37]. In fact, hypoalbuminemia can be a presenting symptom of Crohn's disease. Histology has indicated the mechanisms of intestinal leakage to include mucosal injury, increased lymphatic pressure, or dilated lymphatics [39].

The pathogenesis of nutritional disturbances in Crohn's disease is multifactorial. Hypoproteinemia in regional enteritis has correlated primarily with protein loss into the bowel, rather than with malabsorption [40]. Leakage of protein into the intestinal lumen usually does not give rise to hypoproteinemia unless this protein loss is massive. The combination of severe hypoproteinemia with lymphocytopenia may indicate intestinal loss of lymph, containing high concentrations of fat, protein, and lymphocytes [41].

Thus, whenever hypoproteinemia is accompanied by lymphocytopenia in Crohn's disease, intestinal lymphatic obstruction should be considered as a component of pathogenesis. With a sufficient rate of lymph loss into the intestinal lumen, nuclear imaging techniques can demonstrate this leakage phenomenon [41].

Nonsteroidal anti-inflammatories (NSAIDs) have been associated with protein-losing enteropathy, sometimes causing small intestinal ulcers, perforation, and strictures requiring surgery. In fact, NSAIDs produce inflammation of the small intestine in between 40 and 70% of long-term users, leading to blood loss and protein loss. In fact, a recent study utilizing capsule endoscopy in 40 healthy subjects noted macroscopic small bowel tissue damage in 68% of those ingesting slow-release diclofenac. Long-term use of NSAIDs and COX-2 inhibitors over 3 months was associated with similar rates of small bowel injury [42].

Pathogenesis of NSAID enteropathy is multi-stage, with specific biochemical and subcellular organelle damage followed by inflammatory tissue reaction. NSAID-induced injury to the intestinal epithelium results from three sources of exposure: (1) pre-absorption local effects following direct exposure after oral administration, (2) systemic effects after absorption, and (3) the recurrent local effects following enterohepatic recirculation [43]. Although the relative importance attributable to each of these mechanisms is not known, increased intestinal permeability has been suggested as the central contributing biochemical factor in small bowel NSAID-induced tissue damage [44].

Various suggested treatments for NSAID-induced enteropathy include sulphasalazine, misoprostol, and metronidazole [43]. However, the efficacy of these agents has not been adequately evaluated long term. Current strategies for prevention have been geared toward reducing intestinal permeability, since this is thought to be the most important mechanism in NSAID-induced enteropathy [44].

Diseases Associated with Protein Losing Gastroenteropathy: Altered Lymphatic Drainage

Intestinal lymphangiectasia may be primary or secondary, and is characterized by intestinal lymphatic vessel dilation and rupture of lacteals, chronic diarrhea, and loss of lymph into the gastrointestinal tract. This lymph is rich in proteins such as albumin and globulin, as well as chylomicrons and lymphocytes, resulting in chronic protein-losing enteropathy. A focal presentation is often seen in patients with acquired or secondary lymphangiectasia, in contrast to those with congenital disease who typically present with diffuse lymphangiectasia [17].

In patients with primary intestinal lymphangiectasia, tortuous, dilated mucosal and submucosal lymphatic vessels are seen. This is the most common cause of protein-losing enteropathy in children [45]. Although generally diagnosed by age 3 years, this may sometimes present up to 30 years of age [46, 47]. Signs include edema, hypoproteinemia, diarrhea, and lymphocytopenia secondary to both lymphatic leakage and rupture. Marked lymphangiectasia in the mesenteric lymph nodes and long-standing immunoglobulin deficiency favor a diagnosis of congenital lymphangiectasia [17]. Retroperitoneal processes such as adenopathy, fibrosis, and pancreatitis can also impair lymphatic drainage [1].

When central venous pressure is elevated from secondary causes, for example, congestive heart failure constrictive pericarditis, this also results in bowel wall lymphatic vessel congestion and perturbation of lymphatic drainage. An example of a secondary lymphangiectasia more predominant in the pediatric population is that induced by the Fontan procedure. This is performed for surgical correction of congenital uni-ventricular heart. It involves creation of a wide anastomosis between the right atrium and pulmonary artery and is usually completed by 18 months of age. Protein-losing gastroenteropathy has been noted in up to 15% of these patients within 10 years. Hemodynamic studies reveal increased central venous pressures. Thus, right-side pump problems may congest bowel wall lymphatic vessels, causing leakage of plasma containing lymph inside the intestinal lumen via surface epithelium [48]. Five-year survival after onset of protein-losing enteropathy is only 46–59% [49].

A more seldom observed clinical entity, Waldenstrom macroglobulinemia is characterized by lymphadenopathy, organomegaly, and a circulating monoclonal IgM paraprotein, which may lead to a hyperviscosity syndrome. Although enteric involvement is rare, this condition has been associated with protein-losing enteropathy [50]. Endoscopically this appears as edematous small intestinal mucosa, due to the dilated lymphatic channels. The most common mode of involvement is via deposition of IG light chain fragments as amyloid protein visible with Congo red staining. Small bowel biopsies may show intestinal lymphangiectasia, infiltration of the mucosa by foamy histiocytes, and intralymphatic eosinphilic acellular non-Congo staining material as IgM. The IgM produced within the lamina propria of the intestine is cleared by the lymphatic channels, but the high viscosity of the interstitial fluid may lead to lymphatic dilatation and obstruction with secondary lymphangiectasia. Infiltration of the mesenteric lymph nodes can also distort the anatomy and function of these nodes, leading to this problem, as has been observed in low-grade lymphoma [50].

DIAGNOSIS IN PROTEIN-LOSING GASTROENTEROPATHIES

The possibility of protein-losing enteropathy should be suspected in patients with hypoalbuminemia. However, hypoproteinemia with such symptoms as edema is commonly seen in multiple other disease states, including nephrotic proteinuria, liver diseases, and protein malnutrition. Thus, it is important to confirm excessive protein loss into the gastrointestinal tract in order to make the diagnosis of protein-losing gastroenteropathy [11]. Testing functional small bowel absorption, for example, with D-xylose, would be normal in cases of protein-losing gastroenteropathy due to intestinal lymphangiectasia [46], and would thus miss this diagnosis. The gold standard to confirm protein-losing enteropathy is through documenting loss of radiolabeled IV macromolecules in stool, such as with 51Cr-albumin. However, this test has such limitations as exposure to radioactive material and a 6- to 10-day collection period and is thus not usually utilized in the clinical setting [1, 51, 52].

The glycoprotein alpha 1-antitrypsin is a useful marker of intestinal protein loss, since its size is similar to that of albumin. It is also similar to albumin in that it is produced within the liver and is not actively absorbed or secreted. Alpha 1-antitrypsin is normally found in low concentrations in the stool in an intact form, since it is resistant to proteolysis in the intestinal lumen [11]. An inverse correlation is noted between enteric alpha 1-antitrypsin loss and serum albumin levels. Thus, alpha 1-antritrypsin can be used as a confirmatory measure of intestinal protein loss [32, 53]. Typically, clearance of alpha 1-antitrypsin threefold higher than the upper limits of normal (i.e., exceeding 180 mL/day) correlates with an albumin level below 3.0 g/dL [9]. However, stool alpha 1-antitrypsin concentration is a poor index of its clearance; rather, measurement of fecal concentration in conjunction with plasma levels is a more accurate indicator of intestinal protein loss [9].

A 24-h stool collection more reliable than a spot stool specimen and is thus preferred for laboratory evaluations [11]. The formula for alpha 1-antitrypsin plasma clearance (Table 7.2) can be used for both diagnosing and following response to treatment of protein-losing enteropathy [1, 54]. Interpretation of alpha 1-antitrypsin clearance should be made in the context of symptoms, with a clearance of >24 mL/day considered abnormal in patients without diarrhea and >56 mL/day as above normal limits in patients with diarrhea [1].

Table 7.2

Plasma clearance of alpha 1-antitrypsin (α-1 AT)

$$\alpha - 1 \text{ AT plasma clearance} = \frac{(\text{stool volume}) (\text{stool } \alpha - 1 \text{ AT})}{(\text{serum } \alpha - 1 \text{ AT})}$$

From ref. 54.

Chapter 7 / Protein-Losing Enteropathies

Certain pitfalls must be considered when using alpha 1-antitrypsin as a measure of protein-losing gastroenteropahty. Since alpha 1-antitrypsin is degraded by pepsin at a gastric pH < 3, this cannot be relied upon to identify protein loss from gastric sources. However, the use of a proton pump inhibitor such as lansoprazole, or H2 blockers such as cimetidine, to prevent gastric acid degradation of alpha 1-antitrypsin can allow detection of protein-losing gastropathy in such cases [55, 56]. In addition, alpha 1-antitrypsin clearance is not diagnostically useful in infants, since meconium normally contains elevated levels of this enzyme. This is due to the comparatively increased intestinal permeability found in normal neonates [57], in addition to alpha 1-antitrypsin derived from sources such as amniotic fluid [52, 58]. Finally, in patients with intestinal bleeding or occult blood loss, interpretation of alpha 1-antitrypsin clearance may be misleading, due to increased clearance rates [9].

After confirmation of excessive gastrointestinal protein loss, further evaluation should focus on identifying the responsible underlying disease. Physical and laboratory exams should be directed toward clues for further work-up, such as inflammatory states (e.g., autoantibody testing, eosinophilia, c-reactive protein levels, and sedimentation rate), hematologic work-up (e.g., protein electrophoresis, red cell indices, iron studies), endocrine work-up (e.g., thyroid studies, calcium levels), and coagulation studies. In addition, viral serological studies (e.g., for CMV or HIV) and stool studies (e.g., white blood cells, *Clostridium difficile* toxins, and examination for ova and parasites) should be included. If peripheral eosinophilia is noted, this should prompt stool analysis for Charcot–Leyden crystals [1].

Cardiac work-up may be pursued to assess for secondary lymphangiectasia as an etiology of protein loss. For instance, testing for conditions leading to right-sided heart failure, such as constrictive pericarditis, can include EKG, echocardiography, jugular venous pressure measures, or even cardiac catheterization. A simple chest radiograph may reveal cardiomegaly or granulomatous disease to direct further work-up [1, 11].

Steatorrhea may direct studies toward the upper gastrointestinal tract, such as barium gastrointestinal follow-through [1]. This may locate various mucosal abnormalities, such as ulcerations or strictures. A "stacked coin" appearance on barium x-ray with thickened, nodular small bowel folds is indicative of primary lymphagiectsia [59]. Other conditions leading to lymphatic obstruction may be diagnosed by CT scan of the abdomen and pelvis, including fibrosis, pancreatic diseases, and malignancies. In children, MRI has been successfully utilized for the diagnosis of protein-losing enteropathy secondary to intestinal lymphangiectasia [45]. A lymphangiogram may be considered in selected patients, but this test is rarely performed in most centers. Although rarely performed, lymphaniography may be pursued to further work-up lymphangiectasia if all other work-up has been negative, and exploratory laparotomy may reveal occult malignancy [1].

In addition to lab work and routine imaging, nuclear imaging can be especially helpful in the diagnosis protein-losing gastroenteropathy – especially when alpha 1-antitrypsin testing results are unclear. Such scans may utilize technetium 99m-labeled human serum albumin, 99mTc-labeled dextran *scintigraphy*, 99mTc-labeled human immunoglobulin, and indium 111-labeled transferrin. 99mTc-labeled dextran scintigraphy may be more sensitive than 99mTc-HSA. Nuclear imaging is capable of confirming and quantitating both the extent and location of the underlying disorder and thus direct evaluation toward a specific organ. These imaging studies can also be used to monitor response to therapy, however, neither test is widely available [36, 60, 61].

According to Herfarth et al., endoscopy is always recommended as verification of suspected protein-losing gastroenteropathy. Although inflammation, ulceration, or neoplastic disease may be a primary finding, endoscopy can also reveal white villi or interspersed white spots, with a milky lymph coating over the mucosa in cases of lymphangiectasia [17]. Biopsies of such mucosa can confirm the presence of lacteal exudates, dilated mucosal, submucosal, and even serosal dilation of lymphatics and polyclonal plasma cells [46].

Random endoscopic biopsies of normal-appearing mucosa can histologically exclude collagenous or lymphocytic disease states causing protein-losing enteropathy. Histologically, observation of diffuse lymphangiectasia would favor a congenital type of lymphangiectasia. By contrast, small intestinal biopsies in an acquired (secondary) form of lymphangiectasia would more classically show focal lymphangiectasia, with some villi involved and others spared [17].

Capsule endoscopy currently is considered the method of choice for evaluation of small bowel pathological processes [62], and has been observed to have a better diagnostic yield than small bowel x-rays [63]. Although also useful in the pediatric population [64], caution should be used, as up to 20% of pediatric patients experienced an adverse event associated with disposable small bowel capsule (e.g., delayed passage from the stomach or small bowel capsule retention) [62]. In addition, double balloon endoscopy has been utilized to diagnose blastomycosis, tuberculosis, and primary small bowel lymphangioma in cases of lymphangiectasia contributing to protein-losing enteropathy [65].

TREATMENT

Since protein-losing gastroenteropathy is a complex of signs and symptoms indicative of an underlying disease, rather than an actual disease in itself, treatment is generally focused correcting the underlying causative disease. For instance, antibiotics may be effective if bacterial overgrowth, *H. pylori*, or Whipple's disease is present, and autoimmune inflammatory processes, such as inflammatory bowel disease or lupus, may respond to immunosuppressive agents. Cardiovascular or other circulatory issues contributing to protein-losing enteropathy may respond to medical treatment or corrective surgery [66–68]. Nutritional status is also a primary issue that must be addressed in the treatment plan. For instance, protein loss may be offset in part by a high protein diet, and a decreased fat intake appears to have a beneficial effect on albumin metabolism, as is reviewed later in more detail.

Treatment options for Menetrier's disease may include long-term H2 receptor antagonists, proton pump inhibitors, anticholinergic agents, and octreotide [69–71]. Increased signaling of the epidermal growth factor receptor has been associated with the pathogenesis of Menetrier's disease, and medical treatment with neutralizing monoclonal antibody against this receptor has been clinically useful [72]. Patients with persistent abdominal pain, hemorrhage, or severe unrelenting protein loss may require gastrectomy. Menetrier's disease in childhood is much less common and actually appears to be an entirely different clinical entity. Although causation has not been confirmed, it has most often been associated with cytomegalovirus infection and has an excellent prognosis for spontaneous remission within approximately 5 weeks [73].

Although medical management of underlying disease is paramount in treating cases of protein-losing enteropathy associated with Crohn's disease, a retrospective analysis found that one of the most common indications for elective surgery in Crohn's disease includes protein-losing enteropathy, behind subacute intestinal obstruction and perforation-peritonitis [74]. This study noted increased postoperative morbidity after mid small bowel resection in patients who had preoperative malabsorption states, as well as anemia and immunosuppression [74]. However, examples exist in which targeted small bowel resection has alleviated protein-losing enteropathy symptoms in otherwise refractory Crohn's disease patients. For example, Ferrante, et al. reviewed a case involving a Crohn's disease patient who required resection of a severely strictured jejunal loop. After resection, the patient clinically improved without further need for albumin infusion and edema resolved [39].

In contrast to inflammatory conditions, in which treatment with steroids is often helpful in addressing resultant protein-losing enteropathies, treatment of intestinal lymphangiectasia can differ greatly. Acquired intestinal lymphangiectasia should be treated by medical or surgical correction of the underlying disease process (e.g., right-sided heart failure or pericarditis). Mechanisms for congenital enteric protein loss in primary lymphangiectasia are not well understood, although increased pressure of the lymph channels has been suggested to be a cause of protein loss [46]. Intestinal lymph flow can be reduced through fat restriction, and thus dietary fat restriction is considered to be the first choice of treatment in intestinal lymphangiectasias. Also, a diet containing medium chain triglycerides as a substitute for long-chain triglycerides is of benefit, because medium chain triglycerides are absorbed directly into the portal vein rather than the lymphatics, thus avoiding stimulation of lymph flow. Medium chain fatty acids do not require modification as would long-chain or very long-chain fatty acids and do not require energy for absorption, utilization, or storage [46, 75]. These factors may contribute to reduce the pressure within lymph channels [76].

Octreotide has been reportedly successful in treating protein-losing gastroenteropathy-associated Menetrier's disease [71], systemic lupus erythematosis [74], systemic AA amyloidosis [78], primary lymphangiectasia [79, 80], secondary lymphangiectasia and cirrhosis [81], and intestinal radiation injury [82]. Since octreotide reduces microvascular blood flow, dilation of lymphatics may be lessened through decreased local lymph formation and flow. In addition, the action of octreotide may act as an immunomodulator through its action on the somatostain receptor SST2RA, which is located on activated inflammatory cells [77, 83]. In addition, antiplasmin therapy has been used successfully to treat primary lymphangiectasia symptoms refractory to treatment with MCT's and octreotide. This halted intestinal bleeding and improved serum albumin and immunoglobulin levels [47].

Diuretics typically are not indicated because edema is due to decreased plasma oncotic pressure; however, diuretics and support hose may reduce dependent edema from hypoalbuminemia, thereby improving comfort. Exercise and adequate ambulation should be encouraged to reduce the risk of distal venous thrombosis, and attention to skin care is critical to prevent skin breakdown and cellulitis. These measures do not, in fact, affect enteric protein losses, however, they can help minimize secondary complications [1]. Although protein-losing gastroenteropathy occurs in many unrelated diseases, Bode et al.

Chapter 7 / Protein-Losing Enteropathies

used commonalities in clinical observations to identify key players in its pathogenesis. These include elevated interferon gamma (IFN-γ), the pro-inflammatory cytokine tumor necrosis factor alpha (TNF-α), venous hypertension, and the specific loss of heparin sulfate proteoglycans from the basolateral surface of intestinal epithelial cells during episodes of protein-losing enteropathy [84].

Heparin sulfate proteins have large, heavily glycosylated, heparin-like extracellular domains fixed to the plasma membrane by the protein itself (*syndecans*) or by attachment to a membrane glycolipid. Barrier function is derived from a single layer of surface epithelial cells that line the vast mucosal surface and adhere to each other to seal the space between them. For the intestine to efficiently absorb nutrient solutes, it has to separate the lamina propria from the intestinal lumen. The proteins joining the membranes between adjacent cells form the intercellular tight junctions, adherens junctions, and spot desmosomes. For most diffusible solutes, including serum proteins, the nature of these junctions defines intestinal permeability [84, 85].

Bode et al. used heparin analogues to rescue barrier function in syndecan-1-deficient mice treated with inflammatory cytokines, while Liem et al. [86] successfully used albumin infusions followed by unfractionated heparin to treat a patient with glycosylation type Ib disorder presenting with edema, diarrhea, hypoalbuminemia, and pancytopenia. A retrospective cohort study of 22 patients with single-ventricle surgical palliation who developed protein-losing enteropathy and were treated with heparin indicated that, although subcutaneous heparin was associated with symptomatic improvement in 76% of patients, this did not alter or reverse the course of disease for most patients (82%). Only three of these patients (18%) had complete remission of their disease after initiation of heparin therapy and were weaned off heparin without recurrence [49].

Lencer's analysis of Bode's heparin analogue study notes that, when examined with electron microscopy, a breakdown in the intercellular junctions was not demonstrated in syndecan-1-deficient mice unless they were also treated with the inflammatory cytokines to induce symptoms of protein-losing enteropathy. As suggested by Bode et al., it is possible that in the absence of other inciting agents, the loss of heparin sulfate proteins might cause a defect in barrier function by a mechanism separate from junction formation or maintenance. If so, then heparin sulfate proteins would have to act by affecting transcellular pathways of protein transport. Although such pathways exist, they are usually specific for certain proteins, such as the immunoglobulins [85].

SUMMARY POINTS AND RECOMMENDATIONS

Protein-losing gastroenteropathy is a syndrome, not a specific disease. Three distinct physiologic states may result in protein-losing gastroenteropathy: (1) increased mucosal permeability to proteins as a result of cell damage or cell loss, (2) mucosal erosions or ulcerations, and (3) lymphatic obstruction. Differential diagnoses other than gastroenteropathy for low protein states include nephrotic syndrome, cirrhosis, malignancy, eating disorders including bulimia and anorexia, malnutrition, and diuretic or laxative abuse. Thus, documentation of excessive protein loss into the gastrointestinal tract is required for diagnosis. Plasma clearance of alpha 1-antitrypsin is useful to both to diagnose and monitor response to therapy, and nuclear imaging may be useful for these purposes as well. Since loss of serum proteins into the gastrointestinal tract is independent of molecular weight, so proteins with limited reproductive capacity are disproportionately lower (e.g., albumin and immunoglobulins other than IgE). The goal of therapy in protein-losing gastroenteropathy is to identify the underlying disease and thus effectively directs dietary, medical, and surgical intervention, or a combination, toward it treatment. Medium chain triglycerides can help with nutrition and alleviation of lymphatic obstruction. Most etiologies of protein-losing disorders of the gastrointestinal tract are treatable once the cause is diagnosed and may be cured if the underlying disease state is successfully addressed.

REFERENCES

1. Greenwald DA. Protein-losing gastroenteropathy. In: Feldman M, Friedman LS, Sleisenger MH, eds. Sleisenger and Fordtran's gastrointestinal and liver disease, 8th ed. Philadelphia, PA: WB Saunders, 2006, pp. 557–562.
2. Farrell JJ. Digestion and absorption of nutrients and vitamins. In: Feldman M, Freidman LS, Sleisenger MH, eds. Sleisenger and Fordtran's gastrointestinal and liver disease, 8th ed. Philadelphia, PA: WB Saunders, 2006, Chapter 97.
3. Daniel H. Molecular and integrative physiology of intestinal peptide transport. Ann Rev Physiol 2004;66:361–384.
4. Silk DB, Marrs TC, Addison JM. Absorption of amino acids from an amino acid mixture simulating casein and a tryptic hydrolysate of casein in man. Clin Sci Mol Med 1973;45:715–719.
5. Adibi SA. Regulation of expression of the intestinal oligopeptide transporter (Pept-1) in health and disease. Am J Physiol Gastrointest Liver Physiol 2003; 285:G779–G788.
6. Silk DB, Grimble GK, Rees RG. Protein digestion and amino acid and peptide absorption. Proc Nutr Soc 1985;44:63–72.
7. Guandalini S, Frye RE, Tamer MA. Malabsorption syndromes. eMedicine from WebMD. Updated November 19, 2008. Available at http://www.emedicine.com/ped/topic1356.htm.

Chapter 7 / Protein-Losing Enteropathies   135

8. Waldmann TA, Wochner RD, Strober W. The role of the gastrointestinal tract in plasma protein metabolism. Studies with 51Cr Albumin. Am J Med 1969;46: 275–285.

9. Strygler B, Nicar MJ, Santangelo WC, Porter JL, Fordtran JS. Alpha 1-antitrypsin excretion in stool in normal subjects and in patients with gastrointestinal disorders. Gastroenterology 1990;99(5):1380–1387.

10. Freeman HJ, Kim YS, Sleisenger MH. Protein digestion and absorption in man. Normal mechanisms and protein–energy malnutrition. Am J Med 1979;67: 1030–1036.

11. Milovic V, Grand RJ. Protein-losing gastroenteropathy. UpToDate 17.1 Referenced October 6, 2008. Available at www.uptodate.com/patients/content/topic.do?topicKey=~zn77QAI3GZ_X6a

12. Kim KE. Protein-losing gastroenteropathy. In: Feldman M, Sleisenger MH, eds. Sleisenger and Fordtran's gastrointestinal and liver disease, 7th ed. Philadelphia, PA: WB Saunders, 2001. p. 446.

13. Landzberg BR, Pochapin MB. Protein-losing enteropathy and gastropathy. Curr Treat Options Gastroenterol 2001;4:39–49.

14. Wochner RD, Weissman SM, Waldmann TA, Houston D, Berlin NI. Direct measurement of the rates of synthesis of plasma proteins in control subjects and patients with gastrointestinal protein loss. J Clin Invest 1968;47(5):971–982.

15. Muller C, Wolf H, Gottlicher J, Zielinski CC, Eibl MM. Cellular immunodeficiency in protein-losing enteropathy. Predominant reduction of CD3+ and CD4+ lymphocytes. Dig Dis Sci 1991;36(1):116–122.

16. Strober W, Wochner RD, Carbone PP, Waldmann TA. Intestinal lymphangiectasia: a protein-losing enteropathy with hypogammaglobulinemia, lymphocytopenia and impaired homograft rejection. J Clin Invest 1967;46(10):1643–1656.

17. Herfarth H, Hofstadter F, Feuerbach S, Jurgen SH, Scholmerich J, Rogler G. A case of recurrent gastrointestinal bleeding and protein-losing gastroenteropathy. Nat Clin Pract Gastroenterol Hepatol 2007;4(5):288–293.

18. Takeda H, Ishihama K, Fukui T, Fujishima S, Orii T, Nakazawa Y, Shu HJ, Kawata S. Significance of rapid turnover proteins in protein-losing gastroenteropathy. Hepato-Gastroenterology 2003;50(54):1963–1965.

19. Malek NP, Ocran K, Tietge UJ, Maschek H, Gratz KF, Trautwein C, Wagner S, Manns MP. A case of the yellow nail syndrome associated with massive chylous ascites, pleural and pericardial effusions. Z Gastroenterol 1996;34(11):763–766.

20. Kelly DG, Miller LJ, Malagelada JR, Huizenga KA, Markowitz H. Giant hypertrophic gastropathy (Menetrier's disease): pharmacologic effects on protein leakage and mucosal ultrastructure. Gastroenterology 1982;83(3):581–589.

21. Meuwissen SG, Ridwan BU, Hasper HJ, Innemee G. Hypertrophic protein-losing gastropathy. A retrospective analysis of 40 cases in The Netherlands. The Dutch Menetrier Study Group. Scand J Gastroenterol Suppl 1992;194:1–7.

22. Warshauer DM, Thornton FJ, Nelson RC, O'Connor JB. Image of the month. Menetrier disease with premalignant transformation. Gastroenterology 2002; 123(4):968, 1419.

23. Cardenas A, Kelly C. Menetrier disease. Gut 2004;53(3):330, 338.

24. Bayerdorffer E, Ritter MM, Hatz R, Brooks W, Ruckdeschel G, Stolte M. Healing of protein losing hypertrophic gastropathy by eradication of *Helicobacter pylori* is *Helicobacter pylori* a pathogenic factor in Menetrier's disease? Gut 1994;35(5):701–704.

25. Di Vita G, Patti R, Aragona F, Leo P, Montalto G. Resolution of Menetrier's disease after *Helicobacter pylori* eradication therapy. Dig Dis 2001;19(2):179–183.

26. Yoshikawa I, Murata I, Tamura M, Kume K, Nakano S, Otsuki M. A case of protein-losing gastropathy caused by acute *Helicobacter pylori* infection. Gastrointest Endosc 1999;49(2):245–248.
27. Waldmann TA, Wochner RD, Laster L, et al. Allergic gastroenteropathy: a cause of excessive protein loss. N Engl J Med 1967;276(14):762–769.
28. Chehade M, Magid MS, Mofidi S, Nowak-Wegrzyn A, Sampson HA, Sicherer SH. Allergic eosinophilic gastroenteritis with protein-losing enteropathy: intestinal pathology, clinical course, and long-term follow-up. J Pediatr Gastroenterol Nutr 2006;42(5):516–521.
29. Raithel M, Matek M, Baenkler HW, Jorde W, Hahn EG. Mucosal histamine content and histamine secretion in Crohn's disease, ulcerative colitis and allergic enteropathy. Int Arch Allergy Immunol 1995;108(2):127–133.
30. Lake AM, Kagey-Sobotka A, Jakubowicz T, Lichtenstein LM. Histamine release in acute anaphylactic enteropathy of the rat. J Immunol 1984;133(3): 1529–1534.
31. Sultan SM, Ioannou Y, Isenberg DA. A review of gastrointestinal manifestations of systemic lupus erythematosis. Rheumatology (Oxford) 1999;38(10):917–932. Review.
32. Yaziki Y, Erkan D, Levine DM, Parker TS, Lockshin MD. Protein-losing enteropathy in systemic lupus erythematosis: report of a severe, persistent case and review of pathophysiology. Lupus 2002;11(2):119–123.
33. Perednia DA, Curosh NA. Lupus-associated protein-losing enteropathy. Arch Intern Med 1990;150(9):1806–1810.
34. Kim YG, Lee CK, Byeon JS, Myung SJ, Oh JS, Nah SS, Moon HB, Yoo B. Serum cholesterol in idiopathic and lupus-related protein-losing enteropathy. Lupus 2008;17(6):575–579.
35. Benner KG, Montanaro A. Protein-losing enteropathy in systemic lupus erythematosis. Diagnosis and monitoring immunosuppressive therapy by alpha-1-antitrypsin clearance in stool. Dig Dis Sci 1989;34:132–135.
36. Wang YF, Tseng KC, Chiu JS, Chuang MH, Chung MI, Lai NS. Outcome of surgical resection for protein-losing enteropathy in systemic lupus erythematosus. Clin Rheumatol 2008;27(10):1325–1328.
37. Acciuffi S, Ghosh S, Ferguson A. Strengths and limitations of the Crohn's disease activity index, revealed by an objective gut lavage test of gastrointestinal protein loss. Aliment Pharmacol Ther 1996;10(3):321–326.
38. Dansinger ML, Johnson S, Jansen PC, Opstad NL, Bettin KM, Gerding DN. Protein-losing enteropathy is associated with *Clostridium difficile* diarrhea but not with asymptomatic colonization: a prospective, case–control study. Clin Infect Dis 1996;22(6):932–937.
39. Ferrante M, Penninckx F, De Hertogh G, Geboes K, D'Hoore A, Noman M, Vermeire S, Rutgeerts P, Van Assche G. Protein-losing enteropathy in Crohn's disease. Acta Gastroenterol Belg 2006;69(4):384–389.
40. Steinfeld JL, Davidson JD, Gordon RS Jr, Greene FE. The mechanism of hypoproteinemia in patients with regional enteritis and ulcerative colitis. Am J Med 1960;29:405–415.
41. Baert D, Wulfrank D, Burvenich P, Lagae J. Lymph loss in the bowel and severe nutritional disturbances in Crohn's disease. J Clin Gastroenterol 1999;29(3): 277–279.
42. Maiden L. Capsule endoscopic diagnosis of nonsteroidal antiinflammatory drug-induced enteropathy. J Gastroenterol 2009;44 (Suppl 19):64–71. Epub 2009 Jan 16. Review.

Chapter 7 / Protein-Losing Enteropathies

43. Fortun PJ, Hawkey CJ. Nonsteroidal antiinflammatory drugs and the small intestine. Curr Opin Gastroenterol 2005;21(2):169–175.
44. Bjarnason I, Takeuchi K. Intestinal permeability in the pathogenesis of NSAID-induced enteropathy. J Gastroenterol 2009;44 (Suppl 19):23–29. Epub 2009 Jan 16.
45. Liu NF, Lu Q, Wang CG, Zhou JG. Magnetic resonance imaging as a new method to diagnose protein losing enteropathy. Lymphology 2008;41(3):111–115.
46. Vignes S, Bellanger J. Primary intestinal lymphangiectasia (Waldmann's disease). Orphanet J Rare Dis 2008;3:5. Review.
47. MacLean JE, Cohen E, Weinstein M. Primary intestinal and thoracic lymphangiectasia: a response to antiplasmin therapy. Pediatrics 2002;109(6): 1177–1180.
48. Nikolaidis N, Tziomalos K, Giouleme O, Gkisakis D, Kokkinomagoulou A, et al. Protein-losing enteropathy as the principal manifestation of constrictive pericarditis. J Gen Intern Med 2005;20(10):C5–C7.
49. Ryerson L, Goldberg C, Rosenthal A, Armstrong A. Usefulness of heparin therapy in protein-losing enteropathy associated with single ventricle palliation. Am J Cardiol 2008;101(2):248–251.
50. Pratz KW, Dingli D, Smyrk TC, Lust JA. Intestinal lymphangiectasia with protein-losing enteropathy in Waldenstrom macroglobulinemia. Medicine (Baltimore) 2007;86(4):210–214.
51. Karbach U, Ewe K, Bodenstein H. Alpha 1-antitrypsin, a reliable endogenous marker for intestinal protein loss and its application in patients with Crohn's disease. Gut 1983;24(8):718–723.
52. Keller KM, Knobel R, Ewe K. Fecal alpha 1-antitrypsin in newborn infants. J Pediatr Gastroenterol Nutr 1997;24(3):271–275.
53. Schmidt PN, Blirup-Jensen S, Svendsen PJ, Wandall JH. Characterization and quantification of plasma proteins excreted in faeces from healthy humans. Scand J Clin Lab Invest 1995;55(1):35–45.
54. Aslam, N. Wright R. Protein-losing enteropathy: differential diagnoses and workup. emedicine from WebMD. Updated July 11, 2008. Available at http://emedicine.medscape.com/article/182565-overview.
55. Takeda H, Nishise S, Furukawa M, Nagashima R, Shinzawa H, Takahashi T. Fecal clearance of alpha1-antitrypsin with lansoprazole can detect protein-losing gastropathy. Dig Dis Sci 1999;44(11):2313–2318.
56. Florent C, Vidon N, Flourie B, Carmantrand A, Zerbani A, et al. Gastric clearance of alpha-1-antitrypsin under cimetidine perfusion. New test to detect protein-losing gastropathy? Dig Dis Sci 1986;31(1):12–15.
57. Udall JN, Walker WA. Intestinal permeability in the newborn. In: Tanner MS, Stocks RJ, eds. Neonatal gastroenterologycontemporary issues. Newcastle Upon Tyne:. Scholium Int 1984:93–109.
58. Lisowska-Myjak B, Pachecka J, Antoniewicz B, Krawczyk A, Jozwik A. Alpha-1-antitrypsin, albumin and whole protein in meconium and stools during the first days of life in the neonate. Pediatr Pol 1995;70(10):819–826.
59. Vardy PA, Lebenthal E, Shwachman H. Intestinal lymphangiectasia: a reappraisal. Pediatrics 1975;55(6):842–851.
60. Aoki T, Noma N, Takajo I, Yamaga J, Otsuka M, Yuchi H, et al. Protein-losing gastropathy associated with autoimmune disease: successful treatment with prednisolone. J Gastroenterol 2002;37(3):204–209.
61. Seok JW, Kim S, Lee SH, et al. Protein-losing enteropathy detected on Tc-99m HSA and 99mTc-MDP scintigraphy. Clin Nucl Med 2002;27(6): 431–433.

62. Moy L. Levine J. Wireless capsule endoscopy in the pediatric age group: experience and complications. J Pediatr Gastroenterol Nutr 2007;44(4):516–520.
63. Costamagna G, Shah SK, Riccioni ME, et al. A prospective trial comparing small bowel radiographs and video capsule endoscopy for suspected small bowel disease. Gastroenterology 2002;123(4):999–1005.
64. Rivet C, Lapalus MG, Dumortier J, Le Gall C, Budin C, Bouvier R, et al. Use of capsule endoscopy in children with primary intestinal lymphangiectasia. Gastrointest Endosc 2006;64:649–650.
65. Safatle-Ribeiro AV, Iriya K, Couto DS, Kawaguti FS, Retes F, et al. Secondary lymphangiectasia of the small bowel: utility of double balloon enteroscopy for diagnosis and management. Dig Dis 26(4):383–386, 2008. Epub 2009 Jan 30.
66. Masetti PS, Marianeschi A, Capriani A, et al. Reversal of protein-losing enteropathy after ligation of systemic–pulmonary shunt. Ann Thorac Surg 1999;67: 235–236.
67. Menon S, Hagler D, Cetta F, Gloviczki P, Driscoll D. Role of caval venous manipulation in treatment of protein-losing enteropathy. Cardiol Young 2008;18(3): 275–281.
68. Jacobs ML, Rychik J, Byrum CJ, Norwood WI. Protein-losing enteropathy after Fontan operation: resolution after baffle fenestration. Ann Thorac Surg 1996;61(1):206–208.
69. Meyenberger C, Altorfer J, Munch R, Muller A, Ammann R. Long-term therapy of Menetrier disease using ranitidine and pirenzepine. Schweiz Med Worchenschr 1991;121(23):877–880.
70. Overholt BF, Jefferies GH. Hypertrophic, hypersecretory protein-losing gastropathy. Gastroenterology 1979;58:80–87.
71. Gadour MO, Salman AH, El Samman el Tel W, Tadros NM. Menetrier's disease: an excellent response to octreotide. A case report from the Middle East. Trop Gastroenterol 2005;26(3):129–131.
72. Burdick JS, Chung E, Tanner G, Sun M, et al. Treatment of Ménétrier's disease with a monoclonal antibody against the epidermal growth factor receptor. N Engl J Med 2002;343(23):1697–1701.
73. Blackstone MM, Mittal MK. The edematous toddler: a case of pediatric Menetrier disease. Pediatr Emerg Care 2008;24(10):682–684.
74. Prakash K, Varma D, Mahadevan P, Narayanan RG, Philip M. Surgical treatment for small bowel Crohn's disease: an experience of 28 cases. Indian J Gastroenterol 2008;27(1):12–15.
75. Tift WL, Lloyd JK. Intestinal lymphangiectasia. Long-term results with MCT diet. Arch Dis Child 1975;50(4):269–276.
76. Aoyagi K, Iida M, Matsumoto T, Sakisaka S. Enteral nutrition as a primary therapy for intestinal lymphangiectasia: value of elemental diet and polymeric diet compared with total parenteral nutrition. Dig Dis Sci 2005;50(8):1467–1470.
77. Ossandon A, Bombardieri M, Coari G, Graziani G, Valesini G. Protein losing enteropathy in systemic lupus erythematosus: role of diet and octreotide. Lupus 2002;11(7):465–466.
78. Fushimi T, Takahashi Y, Kashima Y, Fukushima K, Ishii W. Severe protein losing enteropathy with intractable diarrhea due to systemic AA amyloidosis, successfully treated with corticosteroid and octreotide. Amyloid 2005;12(1):48–53.
79. Kuroiwa G, Takayama T, Sato Y, Takahashi Y, Fujita T. Primary intestinal lymphangiectasia successfully treated with octreotide. J Gastroenterol 2001;36(2): 129–132.

Chapter 7 / Protein-Losing Enteropathies

80. Ballinger AB, Farthing MJ. Octreotide in the treatment of intestinal lymphangiectasia. Eur J Gastroenterol Hepatol 1998;10(8):699–702.
81. Lee HL, Han DS, Kim JB, Jeon YC, Sohn JH, et al. Successful treatment of protein-losing enteropathy induced by intestinal lymphangiectasia in a liver cirrhosis patient with octreotide: a case report. J Korean Med Sci 2004;19(3): 466–469.
82. Wang J, Zheng H, Sung CC, Hauer-Jensen M. The synthetic somatostatin analogue, octreotide, ameliorates acute and delayed intestinal radiation injury. Int J Radiat Oncol Biol Phys 1999;45(5):1289–1296.
83. Bac DJ, Van Hagen PM, Postema PT, ten Bokum AM, Zondervan PE, et al. Octreotide for protein-losing enteropathy with intestinal lymphangiectasia. Lancet 1995;345(8965):1639.
84. Bode L, Salvestrini C, Park PW, Li JP, Esko JD, et al. Heparan sulfate and syndecan-1 are essential in maintaining murine and human intestinal epithelial barrier function. J Clin Invest 2008;118(1):229–238.
85. Lencer WI. Patching a leaky intestine. N Engl J Med 2008;359(5):526–528.
86. Liem YS, Bode L, Freeze HH, Leebeek FW, Zandbergen AA,et al. Using heparin therapy to reverse protein-losing enteropathy in a patient with CDG-Ib. Nat Clin Pract Gastroenterol Hepatol 2008;5(4):220–224. Epub 2008 Feb 19.

8 Radiation Enterocolitis

Einar G. Lurix, MD,
Jorge A. Zapatier, MD,
and Andrew Ukleja, MD

CONTENTS

INTRODUCTION
CLASSIFICATION
RISK FACTORS FOR RADIATION-INDUCED
  GUT INJURY
INCIDENCE AND CLINICAL PRESENTATION
DIAGNOSTIC WORKUP
RADIOLOGIC TESTS
ENDOSCOPIC PROCEDURES
OTHER TESTS
PREVENTION
MEDICAL THERAPY
PARENTERAL NUTRITION
SURGERY
CONCLUSION
REFERENCES

Summary

This chapter is focused on review of the diagnostic tests and management of radiation enterocolitis. Radiation enterocolitis can occur after radiation therapy for urological, gynecological, and gastrointestinal cancer. Diarrhea, which is often a dominant symptom, can develop from a few weeks to many years after radiation treatment

From: *Diarrhea, Clinical Gastroenterology*
Edited by: S. Guandalini, H. Vaziri, DOI 10.1007/978-1-60761-183-7_8
© Springer Science+Business Media, LLC 2011

depending on the severity and the extent of the injury. Radiation enterocolitis can result in severe refractory diarrhea associated with progressive weight loss, abdominal pain, and malnutrition. Diagnosis of radiation enterocolitis can be a challenge. Properly selected radiographic and endoscopic studies allow for detection of subtle changes in the bowel from radiation. A history of prior radiation is a key to make the diagnosis, since other conditions can mimic radiographic, endoscopic, and histologic findings of radiation injury. Management of radiation enterocolitis is directed toward symptoms control. Surgery may be required if conservative measures fail.

Key Words: Diarrhea, Radiation enteritis, Malabsorption

INTRODUCTION

Radiation enterocolitis is defined as dysfunction of the small and/or large bowel after receiving radiation therapy for urological, gynecological, and gastrointestinal malignancies. Symptoms can develop many years after radiation treatment and depend on the severity and extent of the injury. Diarrhea is often a dominant symptom after radiation injury. Radiation enterocolitis can lead to severe refractory diarrhea associated with weight loss and malnutrition. Diagnosis of radiation enterocolitis can be difficult to establish. A history of prior radiation is a key to make the correct diagnosis. Major progress has been made in the radiographic and endoscopic evaluation of the small bowel with new diagnostic tools that can detect even subtle changes occurring secondary to radiation exposure. Endoscopic examination with biopsy of bowel mucosa may be non-diagnostic, since other conditions can mimic the endoscopic and histological findings of radiation injury. Therefore, a high index of suspicion is needed to establish a diagnosis of radiation enterocolitis. This chapter will review diagnostic tests and therapeutic options available for the management of radiation enterocolitis with focus on diarrhea.

CLASSIFICATION

The gut epithelium is at higher risk for radiation damage because of rapid cell turnover. These detrimental effects can be potentiated further when chemotherapy such as 5-fluorouracil or cisplatin is administered concurrently [1]. The terminal ileum is particularly susceptible to radiation injury because of its relatively fixed position [2]. Radiation injury can be limited to the small bowel or colon exclusively or may involve both, depending on the field of radiation. In some cases the injury may involve the rectum only presenting as radiation proctopathy. Radiation injury can range from acute to subacute or chronic condition. Acute radiation injury is typically self-limited. It can develop during radiation therapy and may last for 2 to 6 weeks after its completion. Its severity is directly related to the dose fractionation, frequency of therapy, field size, and mode of delivery (i.e., intracavital, brachytherapy, or external beam therapy) [3]. Symptoms of acute radiation injury include nausea, vomiting, abdominal pain, diarrhea, and tenesmus. Spontaneous recovery is expected to occur within weeks. Subacute bowel injury is seen between 2 and 12 months after radiation exposure. Symptoms are similar to those of acute injury. Chronic injury can overlap partially with subacute type and can develop from 6 months to 25 years following radiation. However, the majority of patients become symptomatic within 1–2 years after completion of radiation therapy. Patients who received a total dose of radiation greater than 5,000 rad or 45–50 Gy are at greatest risk of chronic radiation enteritis [3]. Chronic radiation enterocolitis is a result of obliterative endarteritis and intestinal ischemia leading to mucosal ulcerations, fibrosis, stricture, and fistula formation [1]. Radiation effects are often irreversible and permanent at this point. Chronic radiation enteritis can lead to complications including: bowel perforation, ulcerations, gastrointestinal bleeding, fistulae or strictures, and refractory diarrhea [3]. Characteristic features of radiation injury are summarized in Table 8.1.

Table 8.1
Characteristics and pathophysiology of radiation injury to the bowel

Type of injury	Timing	Histopathologic findings	Recovery
Acute	2–6 weeks	Hyperemia, edema, ulcerations inflammatory cell infiltration of the mucosa	Majority fully reversible
Subacute	2–12 months	Obliteration of submucosal arterioles, intestinal ischemia	Usually progresses to chronic
Chronic	6 months to 25 years	Obliterative endarteritis, mucosal ulceration, fibrosis, and wall thickening	Often permanent damage, symptomatic

RISK FACTORS FOR RADIATION-INDUCED GUT INJURY

There is a narrow safety margin between the desired tumoricidal dose and the maximum dose of radiation tolerated by normal gut tissue. Approximately 5,000 rad are required for sterilization of the microscopic cancer [4]. The maximum safe, tolerable dose of radiation is 4,500 rad by the small bowel and 5,500 rad for the rectum, when delivered over 4- to 6-week period. The incidence of serious gut injury increases greatly when the radiation dose exceeds 5,000 rad. In addition to the radiation dose, major risk factors for bowel injury include severe acute radiation enteritis, frequent radiation schedule, site of intestinal radiation, and the presence of intestinal adhesions that limit bowel mobility [4]. Additional risk factors include advanced age, thin body habitus, female sex, comorbidities (diabetes, hypertension, and vascular disease), tobacco abuse, prior abdominal surgery, and concurrent chemotherapy. As part of a patient's evaluation, a past record of radiation exposure should be accounted for to determine the total dose and exposure area of radiation.

INCIDENCE AND CLINICAL PRESENTATION

The exact incidence of radiation enterocolitis remains controversial. The incidence is expected to be on the rise [5]. Radiation enteritis has been reported in 2–17% of patients after abdominal or pelvic radiotherapy [6, 7]. The prevalence varies between 0.5 and 37 % and has been underestimated largely due to lack of clinical recognition [4].

Symptoms of radiation enterocolitis may include bloody or nonbloody diarrhea, intermittent colicky abdominal pain, cramping, tenesmus, abdominal distension, vomiting, and weight loss. Bowel obstruction, fistulas, bowel perforation, and massive gastrointestinal bleeding are less common but serious and life-threatening complications [8]. Massive nutrient, fluid, and electrolyte losses can be seen with fistulizing disease. Diarrhea and malnutrition may be presenting symptoms. Diarrhea is typically multifactorial in nature. (See Table 8.2) It can result from impaired bile acid absorption which can be seen in radiation ileitis or after distal ileal resection. Steatorrhea secondary to fat malabsorption can develop due to bile acid depletion from interruption of hepato-enteric circulation of bile acids following long segment resection of terminal ileum. Patients are at risk for small bowel bacterial overgrowth (SBBO) because of impaired intestinal motility, stasis due to strictures, or loss of the ileocecal valve. The incidence of SBBO in patients with radiation enteritis is unknown. Altered bowel motility is

Table 8.2
Mechanisms of diarrhea in radiation enterocolitis

	Cause	*Treatment*
Malabsorption	Jejunal/ileal resection	Nutritional supplements
	Diseased long segment of small bowel	Parenteral Nutrition (PN)
	Bile acid deficiency (ileal resection >100 cm)	
Bile acid diarrhea	Terminal ileum (TI) involvement by disease	Cholestyramine, colestid,
	Ileal resection > 50 cm	Other bile acid absorbents
Small bowel bacterial overgrowth	Small bowel stasis/ dysmotility	Antibiotics
	Strictures	Probiotics
	Resection of the terminal ileum and IC valve	
Motility disorders	Fibrosis, strictures, TI resection	Prokinetics
Fistula	Mucosal wall damage	Surgery with or without PN
	Bypass of normal bowel	
Stricture	Mucosal wall damage	Surgery with or without PN
Short gut syndrome	Massive resection of small bowel or proximal fistula	PN

seen due to strictures, diffuse wall fibrosis, or loss of the ileocecal valve (loss of inhibitory reflex). Shortened bowel following multiple bowel resections and entero-enteric fistulas can contribute to diarrhea. Large bowel involvement by radiation injury is associated with impaired water absorption and diarrhea [9]. Patients with radiation proctopathy may have diarrhea and fecal urgency. Because of limited rectal storage capacity, patients suffer from frequent, urgent small stools, or even fecal incontinence. Diarrhea can lead to dehydration, electrolyte abnormalities (sodium, potassium, and magnesium), vitamin deficiencies (B12 and fat soluble vitamins), weight loss, and malnutrition. Patients may limit their oral intake intentionally to avoid diarrhea, which leads to progressive weight loss. Iron deficiency anemia can develop secondary to malabsorption and slow gastrointestinal blood loss.

DIAGNOSTIC WORKUP

The diagnosis of radiation enterocolitis is based on clinical features combined with radiologic and/or endoscopic findings in patients who have a history of prior radiation exposure. Diagnosis can be established after the exclusion of other causes of gastrointestinal disease. Recurrence of the original tumor or development of a new tumor must be ruled out. The differential diagnosis of radiation-induced diarrhea and chronic enterocolitis includes Crohn's disease, ulcerative colitis, lymphoma, infection (tuberculosis), ischemic colitis, malabsorption syndrome, intestinal pseudo-obstruction, ulcerative jejunitis, celiac disease, and metastatic disease. Radiologic and endoscopic tests are important in confirming the diagnosis.

RADIOLOGIC TESTS

Identification of disease is more difficult in milder forms of radiation enteritis. Standard radiological tests for the evaluation of radiation enterocolitis include small bowel series, enteroclysis, barium enema, and computed tomography (CT). Newer diagnostic tools include CT enterography and magnetic resonance (MR) enteroclysis. A small bowel series is a useful initial test allowing for the detection of strictures and fistulas, but its sensitivity is low. Small bowel enteroclysis provides more detailed visualization of the small bowel mucosa and can reveal submucosal thickening, stenoses, and sinus or fistula tracts. Its sensitivity and specificity for radiation enteritis has not been well defined. Enteroclysis requires administration of contrast through a nasoenteric tube. This test is quite uncomfortable for the patient and it is available in only a few centers. It has been replaced by newer radiographic tests. CT scan can reveal thickening of bowel segments, fistulas, and strictures, but these findings are often nonspecific. CT scan is useful in distinguishing strictures from radiation enteritis and those arising from abdominal metastases or a local recurrence [10]. CT enterography is expected to be more sensitive for detection of radiation-related lesions but no data is available since this technique is relatively new. Magnetic resonance enteroclysis is the preferred radiologic method for the small bowel evaluation, but its use is limited by availability and cost [11]. It permits more detailed visualization of strictures, fistulas, or adhesions in radiated areas. Barium enema or virtual colonoscopy can be performed for colon involvement if colonic strictures are found or when colonoscopy is not feasible or incomplete. The role of virtual colonoscopy needs to be clarified in the evaluation of radiation colitis.

ENDOSCOPIC PROCEDURES

Prior to 2001, the endoscopic evaluation of the small bowel was limited to the proximal 100–120 cm. Introduction of video capsule endoscopy (VCE) and double balloon enteroscopy (DBE) began a new era in the detection of small bowel lesions including those that are radiation related [7]. Limited data is available pertaining to the diagnostic workup of radiation enteritis. Prior to VCE, small bowel series or a patency capsule should be considered to exclude strictures given the higher risk of capsule retention in the intestine. A major limitation of VCE is that it does not permit biopsies of the lesions found. DBE allows for biopsies of the small bowel lesions and helps differentiate radiation injury from that caused by malignancy, lymphoma, Crohn's disease, or tuberculosis [12, 13].

Endoscopic findings of chronic radiation exposure include an edematous, pale, hemorrhagic, friable, firm mucosa with ulcerations, erosions, telangiectasias, and neovascularization with serpiginous vessels. These findings are often nonspecific. Colonic and terminal ileum involvement can be confirmed by colonoscopy. Endoscopic findings can resemble those of inflammatory bowel disease (IBD), ischemia, or infectious colitis. Mucosal biopsies can help exclude those conditions. Special caution should be taken when performing colonoscopy in patients with radiation injury. These patients are at higher risk for colonic perforation as a friable, stiffer bowel wall develops after exposure to radiation.

Surgically obtained gross and microscopic pathology specimens can provide the most reliable information pertaining to radiation-related injury, but may still be non-diagnostic. The small bowel and colonic mucosa is flattened, atrophic with microscopic and macroscopic ulcerations. The ulcers may extend through the submucosa. Telangiectatic vessels in the submucosa, a hyalinized fibrotic lamina propria, and absence of lymphatic tissue can be seen. The serosa is typically fibrotic and thickened with obliteration of the arterioles and small arteries, consistent with an obliterating endarteritis. Occlusion of the vessel lumen by fibrin plaques and fibrosis in small arteries and elastin and fibrin thrombi in smaller vessels can be identified. Subintimal foam cells are pathognomonic for radiation enteritis [13].

OTHER TESTS

The workup of diarrhea in suspected radiation enterocolitis is shown in Fig. 8.1. Fecal leukocytes and the D-xylose absorption test are often positive in radiation enteritis. Since patients have an inflammatory type of diarrhea, leukocytes are seen in the stool. Low concentrations of

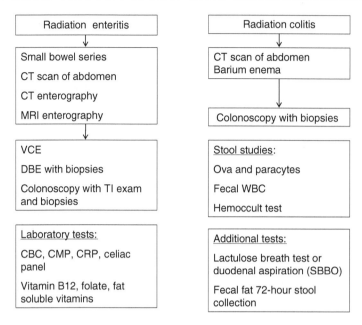

Fig. 8.1 Diagnostic tests in suspected chronic radiation enterocolitis and diarrhea.

D-xylose in blood and/or urine due to impaired absorption are found with the D-xylose absorption test. A lactulose breath test can be performed to confirm bacterial overgrowth. However, there is conflicting data about the test's sensitivity. If the breath test is not diagnostic, a sample of small bowel lumen aspirate can be obtained to determine bacterial count. Documentation of bacterial overgrowth is important before the initiation of antibiotic therapy. A 72-h stool collection for fecal fat can be performed to document steatorrhea. This test cannot, however, differentiate between fat malabsorption and maldigestion.

PREVENTION

At present, preventive measures taken during radiation therapy are the primary aim in order to reduce the risk of developing chronic radiation enteritis. Patients with severe acute injury have higher risk of progression to chronic disease months after radiation [14]. Prevention or amelioration of the initial acute phase is key. Advances in radiotherapy techniques allowed for reduction in radiation dose, field of exposure, and the amount of radiated noncancerous tissue. Brachytherapy decreases the radiation field since the radiation source

Chapter 8 / Radiation Enterocolitis

is implanted in or near the tumor. However, the combination of external beam radiotherapy (EBRT) and brachytherapy has been associated with increased morbidity and radiation toxicity when compared to brachytherapy alone [15]. Three-dimensional conformal radiotherapy (3DCRT) allows for the differentiation of the tumor from the adjacent tissues with a focused radiation beam [16]. Intensity-modulated radiation therapy (IMRT) uses a specialized CT software to increase the precision of the radiation doses by using high- and low-intensity beams within the same field and significantly reduces the incidence of acute toxicity [17].

Several drugs have been studied in the prevention and reduction of radiation injury. Amifostine, a precursor drug, is phosphorylated by alkaline phosphatase into the thiol metabolite WR-1065 and acts as a radioprotective agent by binding to free radicals. In clinical studies, amifostine has reduced the toxic effects of radiation [18].

Probiotics have been evaluated in the prevention and management of radiation damage [19]. Their mechanism of action remains unknown. *Lactobacilli* species produce exopolysaccharides, which have anti-inflammatory properties and down-regulate the severity of inflammation after radiation exposure [20]. In a double-blind placebo controlled study, a high-potency probiotic preparation, VSL#3, was given to 490 patients and significantly reduced post-radiation diarrhea [21]. The effects of probiotics on the prevention of radiation injury are controversial. Sucralfate is an aluminum–sucrose sulfate complex that binds with proteins in an acidic environment and serves as buffer, a cytoprotectant. It can also stimulate synthesis of prostaglandin E 2 [22]. In an experimental model in rats, sucralfate was associated with a reduction of radiation-induced apoptosis in colonic crypt cells and diarrhea [23]. Its use in the clinical setting is still controversial [24].

Mesalamine, 5-aminosalicylic acid (5-ASA), has anti-inflammatory properties including inhibition of leukotrienes, thromboxanes and interleukin-1, and scavenging-free radicals [25]. Prodrugs, sulfasalazine and balsalazide, have similar anti-inflammatory effects like 5-ASA, but sulfasalazine also stimulates the production of prostaglandins [26]. In the clinical setting, the use of sulfasalazine and balsalazide as prophylaxis was associated with a reduction of post-radiation diarrhea [27, 28]. No beneficial effects were seen with mesalamine compared to sulfasalazine and balsalazide, for which the reason remains unclear [29].

The use of nutritional supplementations (glutamine, vitamin E, selenium, and vitamin C), prostaglandin E2 and prostaglandin analogs, insulin-like growth factor, glucagon-like peptide, and non-steroidal anti-inflammatory drugs are novel approaches that have been supported

Table 8.3
Preventive measures in radiation enteritis

- Radiotherapy techniques (brachytherapy, 3DCRT, IMRT)[a]
- Amifostine
- Probiotics (*Lactobacillus* sp.)
- Sucralfate
- 5-ASA (sulfasalazine, balsalazide)
- Miscellaneous (nutritional supplements, biological agents, prostaglandins, non-steroidal anti-inflammatory drugs, octreotide)

[a]3DCRT, *three-dimensional conformal radiotherapy*; IMRT, *intensity-modulated radiation therapy*

by findings in experimental animal models. However, their use in human subjects has not been validated [30]. Preventive measures that can be taken are summarized in Table 8.3.

MEDICAL THERAPY

Since the hallmark of chronic radiation enteritis is irreversible bowel ischemia and fibrosis, once established, the therapeutic goals are aimed toward control of symptoms. Conservative therapy should be considered if possible. Several strategies have been recommended, but most of the evidence is limited to case reports, uncontrolled studies, or studies with a small number of subjects. The therapy should focus on improving the quality of life. Table 8.4 lists some of the available medical therapies which are being used in patients with radiation-induced diarrhea.

Table 8.4
Medical therapy in radiation-induced diarrhea

- Diet modifications (low fiber, lactose-free diet)
- Antidiarrheal drugs (loperamide)
- Cholestyramine
- Octreotide
- Hyperbaric oxygen therapy
- Pentoxifylline and tocopherol

Diet

Dietary modifications are important. However, there is no specific diet shown to alleviate the symptoms. A high fiber diet should be avoided since it may worsen the diarrhea and urgency. This diet should also be avoided in patients with obstructive symptoms as well. Instead a low fiber diet should be recommended. Some patients may develop lactose intolerance, which can be also caused by small bowel bacterial overgrowth. Lactose avoidance may help in reduction of diarrhea and bloating [31].

Caloric Supplements

Oral supplements have not been evaluated in prospective studies in patients with radiation diarrhea. Providing caloric supplements appears to be reasonable for patients with weight loss and diarrhea. If polymeric formulas (Ensure or Boost) are not tolerated, elemental formulas should be considered. The use of caloric supplements may be limited by their taste and adverse effects (bloating and diarrhea).

Antidiarrheal Drugs

Since diarrhea is often the dominant symptom experienced, antidiarrheal agents play an important therapeutic role. Loperamide has been used with success in radiation-induced diarrhea for 40 years [32]. In a crossover trial, Yeoh et al. has showed that loperamide could decrease the frequency of bowel movements significantly, slow down intestinal transit, and improve bile acid absorption in patients with post-radiation diarrhea [33]. Unfortunately abdominal bloating and nausea can limit the use of loperamide. Antidiarrheal agents should not be used in patients with suspected strictures and bowel obstruction.

Antibiotics and Probiotics

If bacterial overgrowth is suspected, a trial of antibiotics for 7–10 days may reduce symptoms including diarrhea. Establishing a diagnosis of SBBO may be important, since antibiotics can also cause diarrhea and abdominal pain. More than one antibiotic may be needed, and repeated courses of antibiotics may be required including cyclic therapy. Consideration may be given to the newer non-absorbable antibiotic, rifaximin, 200 mg three times daily for 10–14 days. However, its cost may be a limiting factor.

Efficacy of probiotic supplementation has been shown in the prevention and treatment of radiation-induced diarrhea in animal models. Probiotics have proven beneficial in a subgroup of patients with radiation-related diarrhea. However, a recent meta-analysis of four randomized controlled trials of probiotics in radiation-induced diarrhea did not show an overall benefit despite significant effects in some of the individual studies [34]. In three studies involving 632 patients prophylactic (pretreatment) use of probiotics was analyzed, while one study evaluated their role in the therapy of radiation enteritis.

Prednisone and 5-ASA Drugs

The role of prednisone in treatment of radiation diarrhea has not been well defined. A pilot study suggested a possible benefit of combination of sulfasalazine with oral prednisone [35]. No large studies with either of these drugs have been published. The results from controlled clinical trials evaluating mesalazine or sulfasalazine in the prevention of acute radiation injury have been discordant as mentioned in an earlier section [27–29].

Pentoxifylline and Tocopherol: Pentoxifylline in combination with tocopherol has been shown to reduce the severity of symptoms significantly in patients with radiation enteritis [36]. Pentoxifylline, a phosphodiesterase inhibitor, has antithrombotic and vasodilatory properties, while it also decreases blood viscosity. It also has immunomodulatory effects by reducing production of inflammatory cytokines. Severe nausea from pentoxifylline may preclude its use [37]. Tocopherol, a form of vitamin E, has antioxidant properties with scavenging of hydroxyl radicals. Based on retrospective data, patients may need more that 6 months of therapy before having symptom relief [36].

Hyperbaric Oxygen

Hyperbaric oxygen (HBO) improves tissue perfusion by induction of neoangiogenesis and inhibits bacterial growth and toxin production [30]. In an experimental model, the use of HBO resulted in less significant bowel wall fibrosis [38]. HBO therapy has been beneficial in radiation proctopathy, reduction of acute radiation injury, and closure of fistulae [39]. The limitations of HBO include the costs and its limited availability to only a few specialized centers.

Octreotide

Therapeutic properties of octreotide, somatostatin analogue, include the regulation of gastrointestinal hormones and inhibition of gastrointestinal motility [40]. In patients with radiation-induced diarrhea, octreotide has been shown to cause resolution or improvement in the diarrhea, including those patients with diarrhea refractory to loperamide [41].

Cholestyramine

Cholestyramine, a non-absorbable resin, binds bile acids and has been proposed as therapy for radiation-induced bile acid diarrhea [42]. Its beneficial effects have been limited by its side effects. Cholestyramine is not recommended as a sole therapy for radiation-induced diarrhea [43, 44].

PARENTERAL NUTRITION

In patients with severe chronic radiation enterocolitis, parenteral nutrition (PN) plays a major role when conservative therapy fails. Patients with severe malnutrition, fistulizing disease, non-correctible surgically strictures, refractory diarrhea, and short bowel from massive gut resections will require short- or long-term PN. Chronic radiation enteritis is the third most frequent indication for PN in patients with intestinal failure after ischemic bowel disease and neoplasm [45]. PN therapy for patients with radiation enteritis accounts for 14.2% of all home PN cases [45]. In a large series, the PN was initiated after a median of 20 months from radiation therapy and it was required for a median 20 months [46]. The estimated cumulative survival of patients on parenteral nutrition was 76% at 1 year and 64% at 5 years. Most early deaths resulted from cancer recurrence. PN allows to correct nutritional deficiencies, electrolyte abnormalities, and maintain weight [47]. In patients with moderate to severe malnutrition, surgery should be preferentially done after a period of nutritional rehabilitation to reduce perioperative morbidity and mortality. Therefore, preoperative PN should be considered in patients with malnutrition, serum albumin less than 3 gm/dl and absolute lymphocyte count less than 2,000 mm^3/dL [48]. PN has no role in closing radiation-induced fistulas [49].

SURGERY

Surgery for radiation enteritis can be challenging because of diffuse adhesions and fibrosis, which can make a resection difficult, the need for extensive resection resulting in short gut, and the high risk of anastomotic leak. Therefore, surgery should be avoided if possible. Unfortunately serious complications of severe radiation enteritis such as strictures, fistulas, bowel perforation, and GI bleeding often need to be managed surgically. Diarrhea is rarely the primary indication for surgery except for patients with diarrhea and short segment strictures. Approximately 30–40% of patients with chronic radiation enteritis require surgery [45]. In a large retrospective study including 14,791 patients who were treated with pelvic radiotherapy and followed for 10 years, only 48 required surgical intervention [50]. Common surgical indications were unresolving bowel obstruction, intestinal fistulas, and massive adhesions. Surgical mortality has been reported between 5 and 22 % and morbidity as high as 30–50% [51]. Surgery in patients with radiation enteritis can be technically difficult and may lead to further intra-abdominal complications including re-fistulization and intra-abdominal sepsis [49]. Many patients require more than one surgical intervention. Bowel resections are associated with a lower reoperation rate and a better 5-year survival, but a higher postoperative mortality when compared to other surgical techniques [52]. Patients with refractory radiation enteritis requiring surgical intervention are best managed by bowel resection with re-anastomosis if feasible, followed by intestinal bypass if necessary. Diversion with proximal stomas or exclusion should be attempted as a last resort [45].

CONCLUSION

In summary, radiation enterocolitis is a challenging condition to diagnose and manage. Diarrhea is a common and often a dominant symptom of chronic radiation enterocolitis. Diagnostic workup requires selected radiologic and endoscopic studies to confirm the diagnosis and exclude recurrent or new malignancy. Endoscopic and radiologic findings can overlap with other conditions including inflammatory bowel disease, lymphoma, chronic ischemic bowel making the diagnosis more difficult to establish. Standard workup for diarrhea should be performed to exclude other treatable disorders. Diarrhea can result in serious complications including dehydration, electrolyte and vitamin deficiencies, and severe malnutrition. An understanding of the mechanisms responsible for diarrhea can help with selection of appropriate therapy. In patients with refractory diarrhea and malnutrition a decision has to be made regarding long-term parenteral nutrition versus an attempt at surgical intervention. Surgery should be considered for patients with persistent bowel obstruction, enterocutaneous and entero-enteric fistulas leading to intestinal failure. Further prospective clinical studies are needed for newer regimens such as probiotics, rifaximin, and new 5-ASA products in radiation-induced diarrhea. Research on mechanisms related to fibrogenesis may help to develop effective therapeutic agents to reverse disease progression.

REFERENCES

1. Fajardo LP. Pathology of radiation injury. New York: Masson Publishers, 1982, pp. 47–76.
2. Herlinger H, Maglinte D, Birnbaum B. Clinical imaging of the small intestine. New York: Springer, 2001.
3. MacNaughton W. Review article: new insights into the pathogenesis of radiation induced intestinal dysfunction. Aliment Pharmacol Ther 2000;14:523–528.
4. Vasudeva R. Intestinal radiation injury. Emedicine 2010. Retrieved July 23, 2010 from http://emedicine.medscape.com/article/180084-print.

Chapter 8 / Radiation Enterocolitis

5. Miller AR, Martenson JA, Nelson H, et al. The incidence and clinical consequences of treatment-related bowel injury. Int J Radiat Oncol Biol Phys 1999;43:817–825.

6. Turina M, Mulhall AM, Mahid SS, et al. Frequency and surgical management of chronic complications related to pelvic radiation. Arch Surg 2008;143:46–52.

7. Kopelman Y, Groissman G, Fireman Z. Radiation enteritis diagnosed by capsule endoscopy. Gastrointest Endosc 2007;66:599.

8. Kinsella TJ, Bloomer WD. Tolerance of the intestine to radiation therapy. Surg Gynecol Obstet 1980;151:273–284.

9. Yoshimura K, Hirata I, Maemura K, et al. Radiation enteritis: a rare complication of the transverse colon in uterine cancer. Intern Med. 2000;39:1060–1063.

10. Macari M, Balthazar E. CT of bowel wall thickening: significance and pitfalls of interpretation. Am Roentgen Ray Soc 2001;176:1105–1115.

11. Lawrance IC, et al. Small bowel MRI enteroclysis or follow through: which is optimal? World J Gastroenterol 2009;15:5300–5306.

12. Yano T, Yamamoto H. Current state of double balloon endoscopy: the latest approach to small intestinal diseases. J Gastroenterol Hepatol. 2009;24: 185–192.

13. Pasha S, Harrison M, Leighton J. Obscure GI bleeding secondary to radiation enteritis diagnosed and successfully treated with retrograde double-balloon enteroscopy. Gastrointest Endosc 2007;65:552–554.

14. Weiss E, Hirnle P, Arnold-Bofinger H, et al. Therapeutic outcome and relation of acute and late side effects in the adjuvant radiotherapy of endometrial carcinoma stage I and II. Radiother Oncol 1999;53:37–44.

15. Chen AB, D'Amico AV, Neville BA, et al. Patient and treatment factors associated with complications after prostate brachytherapy. J Clin Oncol 2006;24:5298–5304.

16. Norkus D, Miller A, Kurtinaitis J, et al. A randomized trial comparing hypofractionated and conventionally fractionated three-dimensional external-beam radiotherapy for localized prostate adenocarcinoma: a report on acute toxicity. Strahlenther Onkol 2009;185:715–721.

17. Alongi F, Fiorino C, Cozzarini C, et al. IMRT significantly reduces acute toxicity of whole-pelvis irradiation in patients treated with post-operative adjuvant or salvage radiotherapy after radical prostatectomy. Radiother Oncol 2009;93: 207–212.

18. Athanassiou H, Antonadou D, Coliarakis N, et al. Protective effect of amifostine during fractionated radiotherapy in patients with pelvic carcinomas: results of a randomized trial. Int J radat Oncol Biol Phys 2003;56:1154–1160.

19. Blanarova C, Galovicova A, Petrasova D. Use of probiotics for prevention of radiation-induced diarrhea. Bratisl Lek Listy 2009;110:98–104.

20. Adler U. On control of radioenteritis by the administration of living lactobacilli in gynecological carcinoma patients. Ther Umsch 1962;19:283–285.

21. Delia P, Sansotta G, Donato V, et al. Use of probiotics for prevention of radiation-induced diarrhea. World J Gastroenterol 2007;13:912–915.

22. Burch RM, McMillan BA. Sucralfate induces proliferation of dermal fibroblasts and keratinocytes in culture and granulation tissue formation in full-thickness skin wounds. Agents Actions 1991;34:229–231.

23. Matsuu-Matsuyama M, Shichijo K, Okaichi K, et al. Sucralfate protects intestinal epithelial cells from radiation-induced apoptosis in rats. J Radiat Res 2006;47:1–8.

24. Martenson JA, Bollinger JW, Sloan JA, et al. Sucralfate in the prevention of treatment-induced diarrhea in patients receiving pelvic radiation therapy: a North Central Cancer Treatment Group phase III double-blind placebo-controlled trial. J Clin Oncol 2000;18:1239–1245.

25. Greenfield SM, Punchard NA, Teare JP, et al. Review article: the mode of action of the aminosalicylates in inflammatory bowel disease. Aliment Pharmacol Ther 1993;7:369–383.
26. Hawkey CJ, Boughton-Smith NK, Whittle BJ. Modulation of human colonic arachidonic acid metabolism by sulfasalazine. Dig Dis Sci 1985;30:1161–1165.
27. Kilic D, Egehan I, Ozenirler S, et al. Double-blinded, randomized, placebo-controlled study to evaluate the effectiveness of sulphasalazine in preventing acute gastrointestinal complications due to radiotherapy. Radiother Oncol 2000;57: 125–129.
28. Jahraus CD, Bettenhausen D, Malik U, et al. Prevention of acute radiation-induced proctosigmoiditis by balsalazide: a randomized, double-blind, placebo controlled trial in prostate cancer patients. Int J Radiat Oncol Biol Phys 2005;63: 1483–1487.
29. Resbeut M, Marteau P, Cowen D, et al. A randomized double blind placebo controlled multicenter study of mesalazine for the prevention of acute radiation enteritis. Radiother Oncol 1997;44:59–63.
30. Kountouras J, Zavos C. Recent advances in the management of radiation colitis. World J Gastroenterol 2008;14:7289–7301.
31. Sekhon S. Chronic radiation enteritis: women's food tolerances after radiation treatment for gynecologic cancer. J Am Diet Assoc 2000;100:941–943.
32. Chapaux J, Chapaux P, Royer E. Loperamide in patients with radiotherapy-induced diarrhoea. Arzneimittelforschung 1978;28:864–866.
33. Yeoh EK, Horowitz M, Russo A, et al. Gastrointestinal function in chronic radiation enteritis—effects of loperamide-N-oxide. Gut 1993;34:476–482.
34. Fuccio L, Guido A, Eusebi LH, Laterza L, et al. Effects of probiotics for the prevention and treatment of radiation-induced diarrhea. J Clin Gastroenterol 2009;43:506–513.
35. Goldstein, F, Khoury, J, Thornton, JJ. Treatment of chronic radiation enteritis and colitis with salicylazosulfapyridine and systemic corticosteroids. A pilot study. Am J Gastroenterol 1976; 65:201.
36. Hille A, Christiansen H, Pradier O, et al. Effect of pentoxifylline and tocopherol on radiation proctitis/enteritis. Strahlenther Onkol 2005;181:606–614.
37. Zimmerer T, Böcker U, Wenz F, et al. Medical prevention and treatment of acute and chronic radiation induced enteritis—is there any proven therapy? a short review. Z Gastroenterol 2008;46:441–448.
38. Feldmeier JJ, Davolt DA, Court WS, et al. Histologic morphometry confirms a prophylactic effect for hyperbaric oxygen in the prevention of delayed radiation enteropathy. Undersea Hyperb Med 1998;25:93–97.
39. Feldmeier JJ, Hampson NB. A systematic review of the literature reporting the application of hyperbaric oxygen prevention and treatment of delayed radiation injuries: an evidence based approach. Undersea Hyperb Med 2002;29:4–30.
40. Baillie-Johnson HR. Octreotide in the management of treatment-related diarrhoea. Anticancer Drugs 1996;7:11–15.
41. Topkan E, Karaoglu A. Octreotide in the management of chemoradiotherapy-induced diarrhea refractory to loperamide in patients with rectal carcinoma. Oncology 2006;71:354–360.
42. Arlow FL, Dekovich AA, Priest RJ, et al. Bile acids in radiation-induced diarrhea. South Med J 1987;80:1259–1261.
43. Chary S, Thomson DH. A clinical trial evaluating cholestyramine to prevent diarrhea in patients maintained on low-fat diets during pelvic radiation therapy. Int J Radiat Oncol Biol Phys 1984;10:1885–1890.

Chapter 8 / Radiation Enterocolitis

44. Ippoliti C. Antidiarrheal agents for the management of treatment-related diarrhea in cancer patients. Am J Health Syst Pharm 1998;55:1573–1580.
45. Vidal A, et al. Chronic radiation enteritis after ovarian cancer: from home parenteral nutrition to oral diet. Clin Nutr 2006;25:701–704.
46. Scolapio JS, Ukleja A, Burnes JU, et al. Outcome of patients with radiation enteritis treated with home parenteral nutrition. Am J Gastroenterol 2002;97:662–666.
47. Copeland EM, Souchon EA, MacFadyen BV Jr, et al. Intravenous hyperalimentation as an adjunct to radiation therapy. Cancer 1977;39:609–616.
48. Mann W. Surgical management of radiation enteropathy. Surg Clin N Am 1991;71:5.
49. Alexander-Williams J. The management of intestinal fistulae. Helv Chir Acta 1994;60:1025–1029.
50. Turina M, Mulhall AM, Mahid SS, et al. Frequency and surgical management of chronic complications related to pelvic radiation. Arch Surg 2008;143:46–52.
51. Waddell BE, Rodríguez-Bigas MA, Lee RJ, et al. Prevention of chronic radiation enteritis. J Am Coll Surg 1999;189:611–624.
52. Regimbeau JM, et al. Operative and long term results after surgery for chronic radiation enteritis. Am J Surg 2001;182:237–242.

9 Congenital Disorders of Digestion and Absorption

Douglas Mogul, MD
and Eric Sibley, MD, PhD

CONTENTS

DISORDERS OF CARBOHYDRATE
  ASSIMILATION
DISORDERS OF PROTEIN ASSIMILATION
DISORDERS OF LIPID ASSIMILATION
DISORDERS LEADING TO GENERALIZED
  MALABSORPTION
REFERENCES

Summary

Disorders of digestion and/or absorption of any of the major nutrient forms (carbohydrates, proteins, and lipids) can result in clinical symptoms of diarrhea or steatorrhea. Congenital and heritable genetic conditions associated with nutrient maldigestion and malabsorption are described below. A classification of such disorders, their genetic bases, and their clinical manifestations is presented in Table 9.1.

Key Words: Congenital diarrhea, Glucose–galactose malabsorption, Lactase deficiency, Sucrase–isomaltase deficiency, Adult-type hypolactasia, Fructose malabsorption, Fanconi–Bickel syndrome, Enterokinase deficiency, Trypsinogen deficiency, Lysinuric protein intolerance, Abetalipoproteinemia, Hypobetalipoproteinemia, Chylomicron retention disease, Primary bile acid malabsorption, Enteric anendocrinosis, Congenital zinc deficiency

From: *Diarrhea, Clinical Gastroenterology*
Edited by: S. Guandalini, H. Vaziri, DOI 10.1007/978-1-60761-183-7_9
© Springer Science+Business Media, LLC 2011

Table 9.1
Classification of main congenital digestive/absorptive disorders

Disorder	OMIM	Gene/protein	Clinical characteristics
Congenital lactase deficiency	223000	Lactase-phlorhizin hydrolase	Diarrhea, abdominal pain, distension, flatulence, failure to thrive
Adult-type hypolactasia	223100	Lactase-phlorhizin hydrolase	Diarrhea, abdominal pain, flatulence
Sucrase–isomaltase deficiency	222900	SI, sucrase–isomaltase	Diarrhea, abdominal pain, vomiting, distension, flatulence, failure to thrive
Glucose–galactose malabsorption	182380	SGLT1/SLC5A1, Na+–glucose–galactose cotransport	Severe diarrhea and dehydration, failure to thrive
Fructose malabsorption	–	GLUT5/SLC2A5, facilitative glucose/fructose cotransporter	Diarrhea, abdominal pain, flatulence
Fanconi–Bickel syndrome	227810	GLUT2, facilitative glucose transporter	Diarrhea, failure to thrive, short stature, rickets, hepatomegaly
Enterokinase deficiency	226200	PRSS7, serine protease-7	Diarrhea, failure to thrive, edema
Trypsinogen deficiency	276000	PRSS1, trypsinogen	Diarrhea, failure to thrive, edema
Lysinuric protein intolerance	222700	SLC7A7, Na$^+$-dependent system y$^+$L AA transporter	Failure to thrive, vomiting, diarrhea, abdominal pain, pancreatitis, neurodevelopmental delay, osteoporosis, immunodeficiency, hepatomegaly, anemia, thrombocytopenia, and pulmonary proteinosis and glomerulonephritis

Disorder	OMIM	Gene/protein	Clinical features
Abetalipoproteinemia	200100	MTP, microsomal transfer protein	Failure to thrive, vomiting, steatorrhea, diminished deep tendon reflexes, decreased sensation, ataxia, retinitis pigmentosa
Hypobetalipoproteinemia	107730	APOB, apolipoprotein B	Failure to thrive, vomiting, steatorrhea, diminished deep tendon reflexes, decreased sensation, ataxia, retinitis pigmentosa
Chylomicron retention disease	246700	SAR1B, Sar1b protein	Failure to thrive, vomiting, steatorrhea, diminished deep tendon reflexes, decreased sensation, ataxia, Retinitis pigmentosa
Primary bile acid malabsorption	601295	SLC10A2, ileal Na-dependent bile acid transporter	Failure to thrive, steatorrhea
Enteric anendocrinosis	610370	NEUROG3, Neurogenin-3	Failure to thrive, generalized malabsorption
Congenital zinc deficiency	201100	SLC39A4, zinc/iron-regulated transporter-like protein 4 (ZIP4)	Diarrhea, failure to thrive, bullous rash around mouth and anus

DISORDERS OF CARBOHYDRATE ASSIMILATION

The digestion of carbohydrates involves both luminal and mucosal digestion. Starch polysaccharides are initially digested within the lumen of the gastrointestinal tract via the enzymatic action of salivary and pancreatic amylase. Terminal digestion of oligosaccharides and disaccharides (lactose, sucrose, maltose, isomaltose, and trehalose) is completed by the brush-border membrane hydrolases of the intestinal cells lining the small intestinal mucosa prior to absorption of the resulting monosaccharides (glucose, fructose, galactose). In disorders of both carbohydrate digestion and absorption, non-absorbed carbohydrate molecules pass from the small intestine into the colon resulting in an osmotic diarrhea.

Congenital Lactase Deficiency

Lactose is one of the most common disaccharides in the human diet and is composed of glucose and galactose linked by a α-(1,4)-glycosidic bond. Lactose represents the principal sugar in milk, including maternal breast milk, standard infant formula, and cow's milk. Consequently, congenital lactase deficiency (OMIM #223000) presents in the immediate neonatal period as persistent diarrhea. Symptoms often present as early as 30 min after feeding, and typically include abdominal pain, distension, and increased flatulence in addition to the diarrhea.

Although relative lactose intolerance and secondary lactase deficiency from acquired inflammatory conditions are common, congenital lactase deficiency is rare. First described in the 1950s as a cause of neonatal failure to thrive and persistent diarrhea with lactose malabsorption, Levin et al. demonstrated in 1970 the histologic absence of lactase in these children [1]. Savilahti et al. reported on a large series of Finnish children with this condition, including many siblings, and currently it is believed to occur almost exclusively within Finland or amongst people of complete Finnish descent [2]. Utilizing this cohort, the gene encoding lactase-phlorhizin hydrolase (LPH) was mapped to 2q21 [3]. LPH is a 145-kDa enzyme that hydrolyzes the β-(1,4)-glycosidic bond of lactose to yield glucose and galactose and five mutations in the LCT gene encoding LPH have been discovered. An analysis of 32 patients with congenital lactase deficiency found nearly 85% are homozygous for a specific nonsense mutation in a highly conserved residue while the remaining 15% are compound heterozygotes [4].

The diagnosis of lactose intolerance, like most disorders of carbohydrate digestion, can be made on clinical grounds in the patient whose symptoms develop following the initiation of a lactose-containing

Chapter 9 / Congenital Disorders of Digestion and Absorption 163

diet and resolve when lactose is removed. Disorders of carbohydrate malabsorption can be detected by measuring stool pH and reducing substances; in the presence of nondigested sugars, colonic bacteria convert these sugars to organic acids that decrease stool pH and increase the measured reducing substances. Similarly, carbohydrate breath hydrogen testing can be used to differentiate between lactose, sucrose, glucose, and fructose malabsorption. By providing the older patient with a lactose load of 2 g/kg of bodyweight up to 25 g, malabsorbed lactose will be converted to hydrogen and an increase of greater than 20 ppm suggests lactose intolerance [5]. Genetic analyses or intestinal biopsies with immunohistochemical staining are rarely indicated, although the latter can be helpful in differentiating between isolated lactase deficiency and other malabsorptive disorders.

Treatment of congenital lactase deficiency involves cessation of all lactose-containing products from the infant's diet and using either soy-based or rice-based formulas instead. Subsequently, small amounts of lactose may be reintroduced in the presence of an oral lactase replacement.

Adult-Type Hypolactasia

While congenital lactase deficiency is rare, developmental lactase nonpersistence (adult-type hypolactasia) resulting from genetic hard-wiring occurs such that most people experience a maximal lactase production at birth that declines in childhood or adolescence. Indeed, the majority of individuals from African, Arab, and Hispanic descent and in the near totality of individuals from Asian descent experience lactase nonpersistence whereas the prevalence of lactase deficiency among Europeans is <5%. As such, lactase nonpersistence is a normal physiologic process while hereditary persistence of intestinal lactase is the result of a dominant gene mutation.

Clinically, adult-type hypolactasia is characterized by development of abdominal discomfort, flatulence, and diarrhea following lactose-containing foods. Symptoms may begin in childhood or may not be noted until adulthood. The amount of lactose tolerated varies according to the individual and in general there is not believed to be a correlation with measured lactase levels from jejunal biopsies and the degree of tolerance to a lactose challenge [6].

Diagnosis can frequently be made by clinical history and a trial of a lactose-free diet. Stool pH and reducing substances will suggest carbohydrate malabsorption but are nonspecific for lactose. Lactose challenge tests as well as a breath hydrogen test using 2 g/kg (up to 50 g) are the primary means of diagnosing lactose intolerance.

Additionally, diagnosis can be made by jejunal and duodenal biopsies that demonstrate enzyme activity of less than 0.7 U/g wet weight [7].

Treatment depends on avoidance of dairy and individuals can titrate how much lactose-containing foods they should consume based on their symptom tolerance. Alternatively, lactase-containing dairy products or supplements are readily available. Yogurt might be better tolerated since *Lactobacillus bulgaricus* and *Streptococcus thermophilus* contain lactase. Hard cheeses are lower in lactose than other cheeses and may be better tolerated than soft cheeses. Additionally, because a risk of osteoporosis is increased in individuals with adult-type hypolactasia, calcium and vitamin D supplements may be necessary as well [8].

Sucrase–Isomaltase Deficiency

Sucrose is a disaccharide composed of glucose and fructose that are linked by an α-glycosidic bond and represents an important source of carbohydrates found in fruits. Intestinal digestion depends on the enzyme sucrase–isomaltase and mutations in the allele encoding this protein lead to a condition of malabsorption and diarrhea. Sucrase–isomaltase represents the most abundant glycoprotein on the apical brush-border membrane of the epithelial cells in the small intestine [9]. The gene encoding the sucrase–isomaltase enzyme, the SI gene, has been mapped to 3q25-q26 and inheritance of two mutant alleles leads to the autosomal recessive condition. Multiple mutations have been described with a variety of phenotypic consequences including alterations in transport from the endoplasmic reticulum to the Golgi apparatus to the cell membrane, incorrect and random distribution of the enzyme on the apical and basolateral cell surface, and diminished enzyme activity.

Homozygous carriers of mutations in the SI gene have been described in 0.2% of individuals of European descent and up to 5% of indigenous people from Greenland [10, 11].

Patients with sucrase–isomaltase deficiency typically present in infancy following introduction of fruits and juices [10]. Because the sucrose molecules (like lactose) cannot be proximally digested and absorbed, these molecules provide an osmotic force that brings water into the gut lumen causing a malabsorptive diarrhea. At the same time, these sugars can be utilized by colonic bacteria providing a rich source for the fermentation of gas and the presence of reducing substances in the form of short-chain fatty acids. In addition to diarrhea and flatulence, the malabsorption can lead to failure to thrive, irritability, and

Chapter 9 / Congenital Disorders of Digestion and Absorption   165

vomiting. Older children may present with diarrhea alone or an irritable bowel picture.

Diagnosis should be suspected in the infant or toddler whose diarrhea commences with introduction of fruit juice. Stool pH less than 6.0 and the presence of reducing substances may be suggestive but these findings are not specific for sucrose malabsorption. Hydrogen breath testing can be used and rise of 20 ppm over baseline 90 and 180 min after a 2.0 g/kg load would be indicative of sucrose intolerance. Similarly, a failure to raise blood glucose at least 20 mg/ml after a 2.0 g/kg oral challenge suggests a deficiency in sucrase–isomaltase. Lastly, sucrase activity from intestinal biopsies can be measured.

Dietary sucrose restriction is a suitable and effective means of treatment; the exact amount of sucrose that is tolerated depends on the patient. Starch and glucose polymers, which depend on isomaltase activity, should also be restricted. Lyophilized baker's yeast from *Saccharomyces* cerevisae contains sucrase activity and supplementation with sacrosidase, a beta-fructofuranoside fructohydrolase produced from the yeast, has been shown to decrease symptoms [12].

Glucose–Galactose Malabsorption

Glucose, galactose, and fructose represent the principal monosaccharides in the mammalian diet and are the products of luminal and membrane-bound hydrolysis of starches and sugars in the small intestine. Glucose–Galactose malabsorption (GGM; OMIM #182380) is an extremely rare autosomal recessive disorder characterized by diarrhea, dehydration, and failure to thrive. Glucose and galactose are cotransported with sodium by SGLT1 (sodium glucose transporter 1), alternatively named SLC5A1 (solute carrier family 5, member 1), and the gene encoding this protein is localized to 22q13.1 [13, 14]. This 664 amino acid protein contains 12 transmembrane spanning domains that are localized to the apical membrane of intestinal epithelial cells. Utilizing the electrochemical gradient generated by a Na^+/K^+-ATPase on the basolateral surface of enterocytes, the low intracellular sodium levels allow for the "active" transport of glucose and galactose to be coupled to the passive transport of sodium across the apical surface. One molecule of glucose or galactose is transported for every two molecules of Na^+.

Since lactose is the primary sugar in breast milk and standard formulas, GGM usually presents in the first few days or weeks with severe diarrhea, dehydration, and acidosis which can be life threatening if untreated. Diagnosis is supported by normal intestinal biopsies, including those utilizing electron microscopy. Stool studies will be significant for an osmotic diarrhea. Stool studies are not specific for GGM, but the stool pH is typically less than 5.3 and is positive for reducing substances suggesting the presence of short-chain fatty acids produced by bacterial fermentation of unabsorbed monosaccharides. Hydrogen breath testing has also been used as well to diagnose glucose/galactose intolerance alongside fructose tolerance [15]. Genetic testing is not commercially available.

In addition to age of presentation and severity of dehydration, diagnosis would be supported if symptoms resolve after cessation of glucose and galactose, including lactose, from the diet. At the same time, these sugars are found in nearly all formulas commercially available in the United States, as well as pedialyte. The only readily available alternative for enteral nutrition in GGM is Ross Carbohydrate-Free formula, as well as modular formulas, and this intervention is diagnostic and therapeutic.

Fructose Malabsorption

Fructose (primarily derived from its sucrose derivative) is the principal monosaccharide of fruit and fruit juice. Although toddler's diarrhea from large quantities of juice is considered to be partly due to fructose intolerance, there appears to be an autosomal recessive condition of isolated fructose malabsorption. The exact mechanism of fructose absorption, however, has not been elucidated and a specific genetic defect is unknown. GLUT5 is able to transport fructose across the apical cell membrane of enterocytes [16, 17]. However, evidence exists that GLUT2 and GLUT7 may be important transporters for fructose as well [18, 19]. No relationship between toddler's diarrhea and mutations in GLUT5 have been demonstrated.

Clinically, isolated fructose malabsorption presents similarly to other forms of carbohydrate malabsorption and includes diarrhea, flatulence, and abdominal pain following a fructose load. Symptoms are dose dependent.

A fructose elimination diet is diagnostic and therapeutic. Additionally, hydrogen breath testing can be performed using fructose at 1 g/kg up to 25 g [5]. Stool pH and reducing substances will be abnormal but are nonspecific. Intestinal biopsies would reveal normal levels of other enzymes involved in carbohydrate metabolism.

Fanconi–Bickel Syndrome

Fanconi–Bickel syndrome (FBS) is a rare, autosomal recessive disorder (OMIM #227810) characterized primarily by excessive glycogen

Chapter 9 / Congenital Disorders of Digestion and Absorption 167

storage in the kidney and liver, although failure to thrive and carbohydrate malabsorption are frequently seen as well [20]. As a consequence of increased urinary losses of glucose, amino acids, protein, phosphate and calcium, patients develop hypoglycemia, poor weight gain, short stature, and rickets. Hepatomegaly is also evident but progression to renal insufficiency does not occur.

Patients with FBS are found to have mutations in GLUT2, a facilitative glucose transporter expressed in hepatocytes, beta cells of the pancreas, as well as in the intestine and lumen [21]. Although the exact pathophysiology is not well understood, it is believed that there is diminished transport and uptake of glucose into the liver and enterocytes, as well an impairment in the glucose-sensing mechanism in the pancreas. Consequently, elevated serum glucose and galactose that is observed in the fed state may be in part explained by impaired uptake of carbohydrate into the liver as well as by inappropriately low levels of insulin for the degree of hyperglycemia [22]. Likewise, hypoglycemia results from a failure to transport glucose out of hepatocytes during fasting.

In addition to genetic testing, the diagnosis can be suspected in individuals with glucosuria, aminoaciduria, phosphaturia, and calciuria with associated hypo/hyperglycemia and hepatomegaly. Diagnosis can also be supported by histologic findings of excessive glycogen stores from small bowel and liver biopsies. Treatment involves replacement of electrolyte losses as well as use of a diabetes-like diet with small frequent meals, careful monitoring of glucose, and supplemental insulin. Alternatively, the use of cornstarch or fructose may provide an alternative and stable source of carbohydrate.

DISORDERS OF PROTEIN ASSIMILATION

The digestion of dietary protein is a multi-step process beginning in the stomach with the conversion of polypeptides into smaller subunits. This initial hydrolysis is predominantly orchestrated by pepsinogen, a protease produced by chief cells in the stomach that secrete the inactive zymogen into the lumen. Subsequently, the acidic environment of the stomach allows for the cleavage of pepsinogen into its active form, pepsin. Digestion further takes place in the duodenum, where the brush border of the enterocytes is lined with enterokinase, an enzyme that is necessary for the conversion of trypsinogen to trypsin. Trypsin is subsequently responsible for activation of the endopeptidases and exopeptidades that are produced by the pancreas and that hydrolyze oligopeptides into di- and tripetides.

Enterokinase and Trypsinogen Deficiency

Although rare, cases of enterokinase deficiency have been reported in the literature (OMIM 226200). This autosomal recessive disease presents in infancy with failure to thrive and diarrhea, and most individuals are hypoproteinemic and edematous as well. Genomic analysis of three individuals with this condition identified the cause as a mutation in the serine protease-7 gene PRSS7 that encodes proenterokinase, an inactive precursor of enterokinase [23]. Treatment involves either enzyme replacement therapy or dietary modifications with a hydrolyzed formula and it has been suggested that the widespread availability and use of these formulas have led to the underdiagnosis of enterokinase deficiency.

While functional trypsinogen deficiency occurs in patients with cystic fibrosis and patients with chronic pancreatitis, congenital trypsinogen is a rare deficiency that most typically present similarly to enterokinase deficiency (OMIM 276000). At the same time, there is also emerging evidence that mutations in the gene encoding trypsinogen, PRSS1, can also lead to alterations in cleavage, activation, and stabilization of the enzyme which may ultimately lead to pancreatitis [24–26].

Lysinuric Protein Intolerance

Once polypeptides are hydrolyzed to di- and tripeptides in the intestinal lumen, they are transported into the enterocytes where they are broken down further by intracellular peptidases before being transported across the basolateral membrane. Lysinuric protein intolerance (LPI) is an autosomal recessive disorder that results from a mutation in the SLC7A7 gene that encodes the Na^+-dependent system y^+L along the basolateral surface of enterocytes, as well as along renal tubules (OMIM 222700). This transporter is responsible for exchanging dibasic amino acids – lysine, ornithine, and arginine – for sodium and neutral amino acids. As a result of impaired intestinal absorption of these amino acids as well as increased renal excretion, serum levels of these amino acids are low.

Approximately 100 cases of LPI have been reported, with the majority of individuals being of Finnish descent. Individuals with LPI present with failure to thrive, vomiting, diarrhea, abdominal pain, and pancreatitis. If undiagnosed, patients may develop hyperammonemia and mental status changes following large protein loads secondary to impairments in the urea cycle, which are dependent on ornithine and arginine. Individuals with LPI often go undiagnosed in infancy due to the relatively minimal protein load of breast

Chapter 9 / Congenital Disorders of Digestion and Absorption 169

milk and older individuals often self-impose a protein-restricted diet secondary to abdominal discomfort. Undiagnosed mental retardation can develop if prolonged hyperammonemia occurs. Long-term impairment from lysine deficiency causes osteoporosis and immunodeficiency. Hepatosplenomegaly or cirrhosis may evident on exam as well as findings related to anemia, thrombocytopenia, and pulmonary proteinosis and glomerulonephritis [27, 28].

Diagnosis of LPI is made by the presence of diminished levels of lysine, arginine, and ornithine in the blood, alongside elevated levels of lysine and orotic acid in the urine. Patients are treated with a low-protein diet of less than 1.5 g/kg/day. Supplementation of citrulline, an amino acid not dependent on the y^+L transporter, also improves function of the urea cycle and prevents hyperammonemia.

DISORDERS OF LIPID ASSIMILATION

Lipid metabolism is significantly dependent on the process of emulsification that enables an increase in the total surface area of fat as well its suspension into an aqueous phase. This process begins through mechanical means in the mouth and stomach, before utilizing bile salts that are produced in the biliary system and excreted into the duodenum. These salts are especially important in the digestion of long-chain fatty acids. Enzymatic digestion of lipids occurs alongside this emulsification and initially utilizes lingual and gastric lipase. Following exposure in the duodenum to pancreatic lipase and colipase, triglycerides are hydrolyzed to 2-triglycerol plus two fatty acids. Additionally, dietary and biliary phospholipids are broken down by phospholipase A2 and pancreatic cholesterol esterase.

After luminal metabolism is complete, fat absorption occurs in the proximal two thirds of the jejunum, with greater than 94% of fat being readily absorbed. Once inside the villi, reassembly of fatty acids to triglycerides occurs, and these triglycerides are combined with cholesterol and apoproteins to form chylomicrons. These micelles are then excreted into the bloodstream via the thoracic duct. The lipoprotein complexes excreted from the lymphatic into the bloodstream represent the principal transport mechanism for triglycerides and cholesterol and are responsible for delivering these lipids to distal tissues including adipose tissue and muscle.

Abetalipoproteinemia

Patients with abetalipoproteinemia (OMIM #200100) have significantly decreased levels of cholesterol and triglycerides and are entirely deficient in apolipoprotein B. Apolipoprotein B, including B-100 and the truncated B-48, is the only lipoprotein in chylomicrons and LDL and accounts for nearly one third of the lipoproteins in VLDL. Although initially assumed to be a mutation in the apolipoprotein B gene, the defect has been traced to the MTP gene encoding the microsomal transfer protein [29] and follows an autosomal recessive pattern of inheritance. MTP is necessary for the transport of triglycerides and cholesterol from the apical cell wall to the smooth endoplasm reticulum inside the enterocytes, as well as facilitating the formation of lipid complexes with apolipoprotein B.

Clinically, patients present with failure to thrive, vomiting, and steatorrhea. Furthermore, patients also develop neurologic manifestations secondary to, at least in part, vitamin E malabsorption. Early neurologic complications include diminished deep tendon reflexes and decreased sensation including pain and proprioception that ultimately cause ataxia and weakness. Additionally, retinitis pigmentosa progressing to retinal degeneration occurs. The constellation of ataxia and retinal disease often leads to a mistaken diagnosis of Friedrich's ataxia.

Diagnosis is made in the underweight individual who fails to gain appropriate weight when receiving adequate calories and who has low levels of triglycerides (<10 mg/dL) and total cholesterol (25–40 mg/dL) [30]. Acanthocytosis, a distinct type of spiculated pattern on red blood cells, is usually seen on peripheral smear. Imaging of the spine and head may show degeneration of the posterior column and anterior horn cells as well as the cerebellum. Finally, gross endoscopic evaluation reveals a yellowish discoloration in the small bowel while biopsies demonstrate increased fat staining within the luminal enterocytes. Treatment depends on providing a low-fat diet to avoid diarrhea as well as vitamin supplementation if serum levels are low.

Hypobetalipoproteinemia

Hypobetalipoproteinemia is an autosomal dominant disease that occurs as many as 1 in 3,000 Americans [31]. In the heterozygote state, individuals have low cholesterol and triglycerides as well as low apolipoprotein B levels. These individuals have no gastrointestinal symptoms and minimal neurologic complications. However, though significantly rarer, individuals who are homozygous for mutations in the *APOB* gene are indistinguishable from individuals with abetalipoproteinemia with regard to gastrointestinal and neurologic symptoms, laboratory values, and pathologic findings. Consequently, the treatment for homozygous hypobetalipoproteinemia and abetalipoproteinemia is the same.

Chapter 9 / Congenital Disorders of Digestion and Absorption 171

Chylomicron Retention Disease

Also known as Anderson's Disease, chylomicron retention disease (CMRD; OMIM #246700) is an additional disorder of lipid transport characterized by severe steatorrhea and neuromuscular disease. Patients typically present in infancy with growth failure and are clinically difficult to distinguish from homozygous hypobetalipoproteinemia and abetalipoproteinemia. Although not in the original description by Andersen, patients can have diminished deep tendon reflexes, mental retardation, and defects in color vision, stemming in part from vitamin E deficiency [31] and acanthocytosis has been reported as well. However, unlike defects in betalipoprotein, individuals with CMRD have normal levels of apolipoprotein B100. Treatment depends on a low-fat diet as well as supplemental vitamin E.

The defect in CMRD involves an inability to secrete chylomicrons across the enterocytes basolateral membrane and intestinal biopsies will demonstrate the accumulation of lipid droplets within the cells. These histologic findings can be explained as a consequence of the genetic defect in CMRD, the *SAR1B* gene, which encodes the Sar1b protein that plays an integral role in trafficking of chylomicrons from the endoplasmic reticulum to the Golgi apparatus [32].

Primary Bile Acid Malabsorption

Bile acids reabsorption occurs in the terminal ileum and is dependent on the ileal sodium-dependent/bile salt transporter, ISBT, on the apical membrane of the enterocytes; reabsorption of bile salts saves the liver from having to produce de novo bile salts. Mutations in this protein, encoded by the gene *SLC10A2*, lead to a primary bile acid malabsorption (PBAM, OMIM #601295), a rare, autosomal recessive disorder that was first characterized by Heubi et al. and ultimately mapped to chromosome 13q33 [33, 34].

The clinical presentation of patients with PBAM ranges from failure to thrive with diarrhea and bile acid deficiency to compensated fat malabsorption with adequate growth and normal bile acid levels. In symptomatic patients, the diarrhea is secretory and improves with use of cholestyramine as well as a low-fat diet. Diagnosis is made using the ^{75}Se-homocholic acid-taurine, a radiolabeled analogue of bile acid.

DISORDERS LEADING TO GENERALIZED MALABSORPTION

Nonspecific malabsorption of nutrients and micronutrients most often occurs in the setting of short bowel syndrome or cystic fibrosis, as well as chronic conditions that cause diffuse damage to the intestinal lumen over time such as inflammatory bowel disease. A small percentage of disorders of generalized malabsorption are due to rare, congenital disorders.

Enteric Anendocrinosis

Enteric anendocrinosis is an extremely rare form of congenital osmotic diarrhea that presents with diffuse malabsorption of all nutrients (OMIM #610370). The underlying etiology can be attributed to a relative deficiency of enteroendocrine cells from the crypts of the small bowel; patients with enteric anendocrinosis have a notable deficiency in these cells, with only one to two cells per crypt as compared to five or six in the healthy individual [35, 36]. The absence of these cells can be attributed to a mutation in *neurogenin-3*, a transcriptional factor expressed in the small bowel and pancreas, that drives stem cell fate differentiation toward enterocytes, Paneth cells, goblet cells, and enteroendocrine cells. Although these cells are extremely important in the production of enteric hormones such as CCK, secretin, and ghrelin, the direct mechanism linking an absence of these cells to the profuse diarrhea of this disease is not well understood.

Clinically, patients present shortly after birth with severe diarrhea and dehydration whose volume approximates total daily intake and which ceases when fasting. Some evidence also exists that these patients may develop diabetes in early childhood [30]. Unfortunately, singular avoidance of either carbohydrates, amino acids, or fat will not ameliorate the diarrhea. Instead, the only way to improve the diarrhea and gain weight is through total parenteral nutrition. Diagnosis is challenging because routine biopsies suggest normal crypt-villous architecture and no evidence of inflammation and no abnormalities are noted on electron microscopy as well. At the same time, staining with chromogranin A as well as with antibodies toward these hormones will reveal an absence of the enteroendocrine cells and associated hormones.

Disorders of Mixed Secretory and Osmotic Diarrhea

Congenital zinc deficiency, or primary acrodermatitis enteropathica (AE; OMIM #201100), is rare disorder characterized by severe diarrhea, failure to thrive, and a characteristic bullous rash on the hands and feet as well as perioral and perianal areas. Alopecia can be noted as well. While similar findings can be seen in nutritional zinc deficiency or as the result of severe and prolonged diarrhea, primary AE has been mapped to the gene SLC39A4, which encodes a protein from the zinc/iron-regulated transporter-like protein (ZIP) family, ZIP4

Chapter 9 / Congenital Disorders of Digestion and Absorption 173

[37]. ZIP4 can be found on the apical surface of enterocytes and is responsible for transporting zinc into the cell [38].

Diagnosis can be made by measuring serum and urine zinc levels, which are low in AE, and can be suspected in the presence of a low alkaline phosphatase, a zinc-dependent metalloenzyme. Radiolabeled zinc has also been used to assess absorptive capacity [39]. Fortunately, the reduced capacity to absorb zinc can be overcome with large doses of zinc at 1 mg elemental zinc per kilogram per day.

REFERENCES

1. Levin B, Abraham JM, Burgess EA, Wallis PG. Congenital lactose malabsorption. Arch Dis Child 1970; 45:173–177.
2. Savilahti E, Launiala K, Kuitunen P. Congenital lactase deficiency: a clinical study on 16 patients. Arch Dis Child 1983; 58:246–252.
3. Jarvela I, Enattah NS, Kokkonen J, Varilo T, Savilahti E, Peltonen L. Assignment of the locus for congenital lactase deficiency to 2q21, in the vicinity of but separate from the lactase–phlorizin hydrolase gene. Am J Hum Genet 1998; 63: 1078–1085.
4. Kuokkanen M, Kokkonen J, Enattah NS, Ylisaukko-oja T, Komu H, Varilo T, Peltonen L, Savilahti E, Jarvela I. Mutations in the translated region of the lactase gene (LCT) underlie congenital lactase deficiency. Am J Hum Genet 2006; 78:339–344.
5. Romagnuolo J, Schiller D, Bailey RJ. Using breath tests wisely in a gastroenterology practice: an evidence-based review of indications and pitfalls in interpretation. Am J Gastroenter 2002 May; 97(5):1113–1126.
6. Bedine MS, Bayless TM. Intolerance of small amounts of lactose by individuals with low lactase levels. Gastroenterology 1973 Nov; 65(5):735–743.
7. Forget P, Lombet J, Grandfils C, Dandrifosse G, Geubelle F. Lactase insufficiency revisited. J Pediatr Gastroenterol Nutr 1985 Dec; 4(6):868–872.
8. Birge SJ Jr, Keutmann HT, Cuatrecasas P, Whedon GD. Osteoporosis, intestinal lactase deficiency and low dietary calcium intake. N Engl J Med 1967 Feb 23; 276(8):445–448.
9. Naim HY, Roth J, Sterchi EE, Lentze M, Milla P, Schmitz J, Hauri HP. Sucrase–isomaltase deficiency in humans. Different mutations disrupt intracellular transport, processing, and function of an intestinal brush border enzyme. J Clin Invest 1988 Aug; 82(2):667–679.
10. Treem WR. Congenital sucrase–isomaltase deficiency. J Pediatr Gastroenterol Nutr 1995 Jul; 21(1):1–14.
11. Gudmand-Høyer E, Fenger HJ, Kern-Hansen P, Madsen PR. Sucrase deficiency in Greenland. Incidence and genetic aspects. Scand J Gastroenterol 1987 Jan; 22(1):24–28.
12. Treem WR, McAdams L, Stanford L, Kastoff G, Justinich C, Hyams J. Sacrosidase therapy for congenital sucrase–isomaltase deficiency. J Pediatr Gastroenterol Nutr 1999 Feb; 28(2):137–142.
13. Wright EM, Loo DD, Panayotova-Heiermann M, Lostao MP, Hirayama BH, Mackenzie B, Boorer K, Zampighi G. 'Active' sugar transport in eukaryotes. J Exp Biol 1994 Nov; 196:197–212.

14. Hediger MA, Budarf ML, Emanuel BS, Mohandas TK, Wright EM. Assignment of the human intestinal Na+/glucose cotransporter gene (SGLT1) to the q11.2-qter region of chromosome 22. Genomics 1989 Apr; 4(3):297–300.
15. Barnes G, McKellar W, Lawrance S. Detection of fructose malabsorption by breath hydrogen test in a child with diarrhea. J Pediatr 1983 Oct; 103(4):575–577.
16. Burant CF, Takeda J, Brot-Laroche E, Bell GI, Davidson NO. Fructose transporter in human spermatozoa and small intestine is GLUT5. J Biol Chem 1992 Jul 25; 267(21):14523–14526.
17. Davidson NO, Hausman AM, Ifkovits CA, Buse JB, Gould GW, Burant CF, Bell GI. Human intestinal glucose transporter expression and localization of GLUT5. Am J Physiol 1992 Mar; 262(3 Pt 1):C795–C800.
18. Li Q, Manolescu A, Ritzel M, Yao S, Slugoski M, Young JD, Chen XZ, Cheeseman CI. Cloning and functional characterization of the human GLUT7 isoform SLC2A7 from the small intestine. Am J Physiol Gastrointest Liver Physiol 2004 Jul; 287(1):G236–G242. Epub 2004 Mar 19.
19. Kellett GL, Brot-Laroche E. Apical GLUT2: a major pathway of intestinal sugar absorption. Diabetes 2005 Oct; 54(10):3056–3062.
20. Manz F, Bickel H, Brodehl J, Feist D, Gellissen K, Geschöll-Bauer B, Gilli G, Harms E, Helwig H, Nützenadel W, et al. Fanconi–Bickel syndrome. Pediatr Nephrol 1987 Jul; 1(3):509–518.
21. Mueckler M, Kruse M, Strube M, Riggs AC, Chiu KC, Permutt MA. A mutation in the Glut2 glucose transporter gene of a diabetic patient abolishes transport activity. J Biol Chem 1994 Jul 8; 269(27):17765–17767.
22. Santer R, Schneppenheim R, Dombrowski A, Götze H, Steinmann B, Schaub J. Mutations in GLUT2, the gene for the liver-type glucose transporter, in patients with Fanconi–Bickel syndrome. Nat Genet 1997 Nov; 17(3):324–326.
23. Holzinger A, Maier EM, Bück C, Mayerhofer PU, Kappler M, Haworth JC, Moroz SP, Hadorn HB, Sadler JE, Roscher AA. Mutations in the proenteropeptidase gene are the molecular cause of congenital enteropeptidase deficiency. Am J Hum Genet 2002 Jan; 70(1):20–25.
24. Férec C, Raguénès O, Salomon R, Roche C, Bernard JP, Guillot M, Quéré I, Faure C, Mercier B, Audrézet MP, Guillausseau PJ, Dupont C, Munnich A, Bignon JD, Le Bodic L. Mutations in the cationic trypsinogen gene and evidence for genetic heterogeneity in hereditary pancreatitis. J Med Genet 1999 Mar; 36(3):228–232.
25. Sahin-Toth M, Graf L, Toth M. Trypsinogen stabilization by mutation arg117-to-his: a unifying pathomechanism for hereditary pancreatitis? Biochem Biophys Res Commun 1999; 264:505–508.
26. Whitcomb DC, Gorry MC, Preston RA, Furey W, Sossenheimer MJ, Ulrich CD, Martin SP, Gates LK Jr, Amann ST, Toskes PP, Liddle R, McGrath K, Uomo G, Post JC., Ehrlich GD. Hereditary pancreatitis is caused by a mutation in the cationic trypsinogen gene. Nat Genet 1996; 14:141–145.
27. Parto K, Kallajoki M, Aho H, Simell O. Pulmonary alveolar proteinosis and glomerulonephritis in lysinuric protein intolerance: case reports and autopsy findings of four pediatric patients. Hum Pathol 1994; 25:400–407.
28. McManus DT, Moore R, Hill CM, Rodgers C, Carson DJ, Love AHG. Necropsy findings in lysinuric protein intolerance. J Clin Pathol 1996; 49:345–347.
29. Raabe M, Flynn LM, Zlot CH, Wong JS, Veniant MM, Hamilton RL, Young SG. Knockout of the abetalipoproteinemia gene in mice: reduced lipoprotein secretion in heterozygotes and embryonic lethality in homozygotes. Proc Natl Acad Sci 1998; 95:8686–8691.

Chapter 9 / Congenital Disorders of Digestion and Absorption 175

30. Martin MG. Congenital intestinal transport defects. In: Kleinman RE, et al., eds. Walker's pediatric gastrointestinal disease, 5th ed. Hamilton, BC Decker, pp. 289–308.

31. Roy CC, Levy E, Green PH, Sniderman A, Letarte J, Buts JP, Orquin J, Brochu P, Weber AM, Morin CL, et al. Malabsorption, hypocholesterolemia, and fat-filled enterocytes with increased intestinal apoprotein B. Chylomicron retention disease. Gastroenterology 1987 Feb; 92(2):390–399.

32. Schekman R, Orci L. Coat proteins and vesicle budding. Science 1996 Mar 15; 271(5255):1526–1533.

33. Heubi JE, Balistreri WF, Fondacaro JD, Partin JC, Schubert WK. Primary bile acid malabsorption: defective in vitro ileal active bile acid transport. Gastroenterology 1982 Oct; 83(4):804–811.

34. Wong MH, Rao PN, Pettenati MJ, Dawson PA. Localization of the ileal sodium–bile acid cotransporter gene (SLC10A2) to human chromosome 13q33. Genomics 1996 May 1; 33(3):538–540.

35. Wang J, Cortina G, Wu SV, Tran R, Cho JH, Tsai MJ, Bailey TJ, Jamrich M, Ament ME, Treem WR, Hill ID, Vargas JH, Gershman G, Farmer DG, Reyen L, Martín MG. Mutant neurogenin-3 in congenital malabsorptive diarrhea. N Engl J Med 2006 Jul 20; 355(3):270–280.

36. Cortina G, Smart CN, Farmer DG, Bhuta S, Treem WR, Hill ID, Martín MG. Enteroendocrine cell dysgenesis and malabsorption, a histopathologic and immunohistochemical characterization. Hum Pathol 2007 Apr; 38(4):570–580.

37. Küry S, Dréno B, Bézieau S, Giraudet S, Kharfi M, Kamoun R, Moisan JP. Identification of SLC39A4, a gene involved in acrodermatitis enteropathica. Nat Genet 2002 Jul; 31(3):239–240.

38. Dufner-Beattie J, Wang F, Kuo YM, Gitschier J, Eide D, Andrews GK. The acrodermatitis enteropathica gene ZIP4 encodes a tissue-specific, zinc-regulated zinc transporter in mice. J Biol Chem 2003 Aug 29; 278(35):33474–33481.

39. Van Wouwe JP. Clinical and laboratory diagnosis of acrodermatitis enteropathica. Eur J Pediatr 1989 Oct; 149(1):2–8.

10 Pancreatic Exocrine Insufficiency

*Alphonso Brown, MD, MS
and Steven D. Freedman, MD, PhD*

CONTENTS

INTRODUCTION
HOW DOES CCK STIMULATE PANCREATIC
  SECRETION?
PHYSIOLOGIC CONTROL AND
  REGULATION OF EXOCRINE
  PANCREATIC SECRETION
THE ROLE OF SECRETIN IN PANCREATIC
  DUCTAL CELL SECRETION
NON-CCK-DEPENDENT FACTORS WHICH
  AFFECT PANCREATIC SECRETION
PHYSIOLOGY AND DEFINITION OF
  PANCREATIC EXOCRINE INSUFFICIENCY
WHEN SHOULD TREATMENT BEGIN AND
  WHAT ARE THE GOALS OF ENZYME
  THERAPY?
WHICH ENZYME PREPARATION SHOULD
  BE USED?
TREATMENT GOALS AND EXPECTED
  RESPONSE TO PANCREATIC ENZYME
  THERAPY
POTENTIAL COMPLICATIONS OF THERAPY

From: *Diarrhea, Clinical Gastroenterology*
Edited by: S. Guandalini, H. Vaziri, DOI 10.1007/978-1-60761-183-7_10
© Springer Science+Business Media, LLC 2011

FUTURE RESEARCH
CONCLUSION
REFERENCES

Summary

Pancreatic enzyme replacement therapy is critical in individuals with pancreatic insufficiency. Understanding the normal physiology of pancreatic enzyme secretion and how this is deranged leading to pancreatic steatorrhea is the focus of this chapter. Several areas are detailed including how to diagnose pancreatic steatorrhea, optimal timing and use of pancreatic enzyme replacement therapy, and expected outcomes.

Key Words: Steatorrhea, Pancreatic insufficiency, Malabsorption, Pancreatic enzyme supplement, Fibrosing colonopathy

INTRODUCTION

Exocrine pancreatic insufficiency is a common complication of chronic pancreatitis which may result in several debilitating complications [1, 2]. The diagnosis and management of these patients is often challenging. This text will summarize our current understanding of the physiology of exocrine pancreatic secretion and describe the pathophysiology of exocrine pancreatic insufficiency. We will then focus on diagnostic and management strategies in the treatment of individuals with diarrhea due to pancreatic insufficiency.

HOW DOES CCK STIMULATE PANCREATIC SECRETION?

Pancreatic secretions arise from three types of cells: pancreatic acinar cells, ductal cells, and endocrine cells. The acinar cell comprises the majority of the cells involved in pancreatic secretion. The primary role of the acinar cell is to secrete a mixture of pancreatic enzymes which enable the digestion of proteins, fats, and carbohydrates [3]. The principal stimulus for the release of pancreatic enzymes is the presence of food in the proximal duodenum [4]. The pancreatic secretory response to food intake is mediated by acetylcholine from the vagus nerve and the release of the circulating hormone cholecystokinin (CCK) [5]. Acetylcholine and CCK promote the secretion of a protease-rich pancreatic fluid [6, 7]. The proteases contained in the pancreatic fluid

Chapter 10 / Pancreatic Exocrine Insufficiency

are initially secreted as pancreatic proenzymes [8]. These proenzymes become activated in the proximal duodenum. In the duodenum the enzyme enterokinase converts the pro-enzyme trypsinogen to the active enzyme trypsin. Activated trypsin then catalyzes the conversion of other proenzymes into their active forms. The pancreatic ductal cells secrete a bicarbonate-rich fluid which is produced in response to the production of the hormone secretin. Secretin is secreted by cells in the proximal duodenum [9]. The inability for pancreatic ductal cells to secrete bicarbonate in response to secretin stimulation is a sign of early chronic pancreatitis [10–13].

PHYSIOLOGIC CONTROL AND REGULATION OF EXOCRINE PANCREATIC SECRETION

Mechanism for CCK-Mediated Pancreatic Secretion in Animals

Studies performed in animals indicate that CCK not only can act directly on the acinar cell but also acts via vagal pathways to stimulate pancreatic acinar cell secretion. Studies in rats have shown that vagotomy totally abolishes the ability of physiologic doses of CCK to stimulate pancreatic secretion [14, 15]. Stimulation with supraphysiologic doses of CCK results in direct pancreatic acinar cell secretion. These studies indicate that CCK's actions on pancreatic secretion are dependent on the levels of CCK and the timing of CCK exposure. CCK stimulates pancreatic secretion via vagal high-affinity CCK-A receptors. CCK has also been shown to affect satiety and gastric motility which are mediated via vagal low-affinity CCK-A receptors [16, 17].

Mechanisms for Exocrine Pancreatic Secretion in Humans

Humans do not appear to have the same level of CCK-A receptors that are present in animals. This observation led researchers to propose that another type of receptor (s) is responsible for the activation of pancreatic enzymes. Recently it was confirmed by quantitative PCR studies that CCK-A and CCK-B receptors exist in the human pancreas. Unlike in rats it appears that there are low levels of these receptors in the human pancreas [11]. As a result, it is assumed that pancreatic enzyme release is not entirely due to the direct stimulation of CCK-A and CCK-B receptors. This hypothesis is further supported by functional studies of the human pancreas. In these studies when pancreatic acini were isolated and directly stimulated with CCK, they were not activated [18, 19]. When CCK-A receptors were transfected into these cells by adenovirus, production of pancreatic enzymes was observed when the acini were stimulated with CCK [18, 19]. These studies indicate that human pancreatic acinar cells lack large amounts of CCK-A and CCK-B receptors.

THE ROLE OF SECRETIN IN PANCREATIC DUCTAL CELL SECRETION

In humans, the main stimulator of pancreatic ductal secretion is secretin. Secretin is released from neuroendocrine cells within the mucosal layer of the proximal duodenum [20]. It is released in response to the presence of acidic chyme and via input from vagal afferent nerve fibers [9, 21]. Secretin production can also be stimulated by the presence of fatty acids in the proximal duodenum [22, 23]. Secretin stimulates pancreatic ductal secretion by increasing ductal cell cAMP levels and activation of protein kinase A (PKA) which subsequently results in the secretion of bicarbonate from these cells [24]. This leads to the stimulation of the cystic fibrosis chloride channel gene product called the cystic fibrosis transmembrane conductance regulator (CFTR) which activates a chloride–bicarbonate exchanger on the luminal plasma membrane [25] Water is thought to be transported paracellularly with the end result being a bicarbonate-rich pancreatic fluid.

NON-CCK-DEPENDENT FACTORS WHICH AFFECT PANCREATIC SECRETION

Intestinal serotonins: Studies have shown that the secretion of intestinal serotonins causes an increase in the release of pancreatic enzymes [26, 27]. It appears that serotonin release must also be accompanied by the presence of carbohydrate or hyperosmolar fluid in the duodenum [27]. Pancreatic secretion is also regulated by several different regulatory hormones. Hormones which have been shown to inhibit pancreatic enzyme secretion include somatostatin [28, 29], pancreatic peptide Y–Y [30], neuropeptide Y–Y [31–33], and calcium gene-related peptide. It can be concluded that pancreatic exocrine secretion is a complex process involving the coordinated secretion of activating and inhibitory hormones and neuropeptides in response to input from the vagus nerve as well as the contents of the intestinal lumen. The development of pancreatic insufficiency occurs when the disease process destroys the pancreatic ductal and parenchymal secretory structure and/or there is a change in the physiology of the small intestinal lumen.

PHYSIOLOGY AND DEFINITION OF PANCREATIC EXOCRINE INSUFFICIENCY

Exocrine insufficiency of the pancreas usually occurs as a result of severe destruction of the acinar and pancreatic ductal system. Due to the tremendous functional reserve of the pancreas, exocrine insufficiency becomes severely debilitating when greater than 90% of the mass of the gland is destroyed [33, 34]. The development of pancreatic exocrine insufficiency is dependent upon the degree of damage to the cells of the exocrine pancreas, the stability of the secreted pancreatic enzymes, and the small intestinal transit time. As the secretory capacity of the pancreas becomes more compromised, maximal digestion and absorption, shifts from the proximal duodenum to the distal small intestine [35, 36]. The delivery of larger, non absorbed substances to the distal small intestine has been shown to cause motor abnormalities and impaired absorption [37]. Another consequence of the destruction of pancreatic acinar cells is that pancreatic lipase secretion and activity begins to decrease which is thought to be due to a decrease in the secretion of pancreatic bicarbonate resulting in a decreased intraduodenal pH environment [38]. Small intestinal transit times have also been shown to be significantly reduced in subjects with severe pancreatic insufficiency [39], which results in less time for absorption of fats and proteins in the small intestine with subsequent increased delivery to the large intestine. The presence of undigested fats in the colon results in a net secretion of fluid into the colonic lumen which is excreted as watery liquid stools. The presence of fat and carbohydrate in these liquid stools is what leads to the classic description of steatorrhea which is foul-smelling, greasy-appearing stools that float.

WHEN SHOULD TREATMENT BEGIN AND WHAT ARE THE GOALS OF ENZYME THERAPY?

It is generally agreed upon that once the diagnosis of pancreatic steatorrhea has been established, treatment with pancreatic enzyme supplements is indicated. The diagnosis of pancreatic exocrine insufficiency can be made by performing a 72-h fecal fat test. Subjects undergoing the test should consume 100 g of fat/day. If the daily stool output exceeds 7 g/day, pancreatic exocrine insufficiency is suggested. This test is no longer routinely used due to its cumbersome nature. It also requires that subjects begin the high-fat diet at least 3 days before they begin to collect the stool samples. Many individuals are unable to complete this complex medical regimen at home resulting in inaccurate test results that are difficult to interpret. The 72-h fecal fat test has been largely replaced by the fecal elastase test. The fecal elastase test measures the presence of elastase in the stool. Low levels correlate with decreased pancreatic exocrine secretion with less than 200 μg/g of stool being abnormal and less than 100 μg/g of stool being diagnostic of pancreatic insufficiency. The fecal elastase test appears to be most sensitive and specific for detecting individuals with no pancreatic insufficiency and those with moderate-to-severe pancreatic insufficiency. Individuals with mild steatorrhea may pose a diagnostic challenge.

Once the diagnosis of exocrine pancreatic insufficiency has been established, treatment with pancreatic enzymes is indicated. In order to correct the malabsorption due to exocrine pancreatic insufficiency, it is necessary to provide approximately 5–10% of the pancreatic enzymatic output [1, 40]. Studies have shown that the quantity of enzymatic output needed to provide approximately 5–10% of pancreatic enzyme output is approximately 30,000 international units (IU) or 90,000 United States Pharmacopeia (USP) units of lipase per meal. It is important when dosing pancreatic enzymes to determine if they are in USP or IU because the number of prescribed tablets or powder will vary accordingly. The number immediately after the trade name for a pancreatic enzyme preparation is the number of lipase units per dose. For example, Creon 24 has 24,000 USP of lipase per tablet. When supplementing pancreatic enzymes, one should know that the minimum amount of lipase needed will differ among individuals, but in most cases, 90,000 USP of lipase per meal is the amount needed to abolish steatorrhea (see Table 10.1 for a list of pancreatic enzyme formulations and their lipase content per dose).

Protein malabsorption with associated diarrhea (azotorrhea) can also be seen in chronic pancreatitis. In general, protein malabsorption is easier to correct than fat malabsorption. This is due to the fact that not only are proteases much more resilient to degradation than lipases but also the proteases in the stomach and small intestine can compensate for decreased amounts of pancreatic proteases [2, 41]. Once the appropriate dose is determined, patients should then be instructed on how to take the pancreatic enzymes. Enzymes should be taken with the first bite of a meal. Depending on how rapidly a meal is consumed and the amount of food consumed, the enzyme supplements may be given entirely at the beginning of a meal or alternatively with one half of the total dose at the beginning of the meal and the other half taken in the middle of the meal. This dosing regimen ensures that there will be appropriate mixing of enzymes with food.

Chapter 10 / Pancreatic Exocrine Insufficiency

Table 10.1
Pancreatic enzyme formulations and lipase content per dose

Name	Formulation	Lipase
Cotazyme	Capsule	8,000 USP
Cotazyme-S	Enteric-coated microsphere	5,000 USP
Creon 6	Enteric-coated microsphere	6,000 USP
Creon 12	Enteric-coated microsphere	12,000 USP
Creon 24	Enteric-coated microsphere	24,000 USP
Enzym-Lefax	Tablet	2,200 PhEur
Illozyme	Tablet	11,000 USP
Ku-zyme HP	Enteric-coated microsphere	8,000 USP
Pancrease MT 4	Enteric-coated microtablets	4,000 USP
Pancrease MT 10	Enteric-coated microtablets	10,000 USP
Pancrease MT 16	Enteric-coated microtablets	16,000 USP
Pancrease MT 20	Enteric-coated microtablets	20,000 USP
Pancrease	Enteric-coated microsphere	4,500 USP
Panzytrat	Enteric-coated microtablets	10,000 PhEur
Panzytrat	Enteric-coated microtablets	25,000 PhEur
Panzytrat	Enteric-coated microtablets	40,000 PhEur
Pankreon	Tablet	10,000 PhEur
Pankreon forte	Tablet	28,000 PhEur
Ultrase MT 12	Microtablet	12,000 USP
Ultrase MT 18	Microtablet	18,000 USP
Ultrase MT 20	Microtablet	20,000 USP
Viokase	Tablet	8,000 USP
Viokase	Powder	16,800 USP

USP, United States Pharmacopeia; PhEUR, European Pharmacopeia. Tablets and powders are not enteric coated.

WHICH ENZYME PREPARATION SHOULD BE USED?

The choice of which pancreatic enzyme preparation to use is a matter of personal preference and choice. Enzyme preparations are usually enteric or non-enteric coated. The benefit of enteric-coated preparations is that the enteric coating prevents the premature degradation of pancreatic enzymes in the stomach. Non-enteric-coated enzyme preparations do not have the same protection against gastric degradation. To protect against premature gastric inactivation of non-enteric-coated pancreatic enzymes, proton-pump inhibitors are also administered. Despite being protected against gastric degradation, some enteric-coated preparations are not as effective as would be expected in treating pancreatic steatorrhea for which the reason is unclear but it may be explained by the pH gradient that exists within the duodenum. Most enteric-coated preparations are designed not to release their enzymes at low pH. There is a pH gradient that exists in the duodenum which results in a lower pH in the proximal duodenum and a higher pH in the distal duodenum. The optimal site for the activity of pancreatic enzyme preparations is believed to be the proximal duodenum. Low pH conditions in the proximal duodenum may therefore prevent the release of sufficient pancreatic enzymes in this location. The administration of proton-pump inhibitors helps to prevent the delayed release of enteric-coated preparations by raising the gastric pH and facilitating their release in the proximal duodenum.

A poor treatment response to non-enteric-coated pancreatic enzyme preparations can also be due to a delay in gastric emptying which can result in the retention of tablets in the stomach. This problem can be partially overcome by the administration of enteric-coated microspheres. These special enzyme preparations allow adequate delivery of therapeutic amounts to the proximal duodenum even when gastroparesis is present. Individuals who fail to respond to treatment with pancreatic enzymes should first be evaluated for inadequate dosing of pancreatic enzyme. If the dose is adequate, then the presence of delayed gastric emptying should be assessed. Other conditions which can mimic pancreatic insufficiency and may result in intestinal malabsorption include small-bowel bacterial overgrowth, celiac sprue, inflammatory bowel disease, giardiasis, and Whipple's disease. After ruling out these conditions in a nonresponder, gastric pH measurement should be considered and proton pump inhibitor dosing should be adjusted if gastric pH remains below 4.0. Consideration should also be given to the timing of the patient's ingestion of the pancreatic enzymes relative to the meal ingestion. In our practice, patients are recommended to take one-third of the prescribed dose at the beginning of the meal, one-third in the middle of the meal, and the final one-third at the end of the meal. If this intervention does not work, a small dose of non-enteric enzyme preparation will be added to the prescribed dose of enteric-coated pancreatic enzymes.

TREATMENT GOALS AND EXPECTED RESPONSE TO PANCREATIC ENZYME THERAPY

Studies have shown that patients with chronic pancreatitis and exocrine pancreatic insufficiency have an increased risk of cardiovascular mortality as well as overall shortened life expectancy [33, 42]. It is

Chapter 10 / Pancreatic Exocrine Insufficiency

important to treat individuals with exocrine pancreatic insufficiency in order to reduce their long-term risk of premature death. The majority of these individuals will have some decrement in their symptoms; however, total resolution of steatorrhea may be hard to achieve. Response to therapy should be based on improvement in stool output (three or less stools a day is acceptable), maintenance of weight, improvement in appetite and in the quality of life.

POTENTIAL COMPLICATIONS OF THERAPY

As with any therapeutic intervention, there are potential complications associated with pancreatic enzyme therapy. The most severe complication is the development of strictures in the colon, a condition known as fibrosing colonopathy. Several cases have been reported in children and adults after being given high doses of pancreatic enzyme supplements [43–45]. All of the children who developed strictures had cystic fibrosis but cases of affected adults without underlying cystic fibrosis have also been reported. Cystic fibrosis was the underlying etiology for pancreatic insufficiency in children who developed fibrosing colonopathy but this diagnosis was subsequently reported in some adults without CF. This complication has promoted investigators to define the maximal lipase content of pancreatic enzyme supplements in order to protect against the development of fibrosing colonopathy. Currently it is recommended that the dose of pancreatic lipase contained in pancreatic enzyme preparations should not exceed 10,000 U/kg/day [46]. In order to obtain FDA approval in the United States, the manufacturers of pancreatic enzyme preparations are required to demonstrate that the amount of lipase in their preparations does not exceed the lipase threshold recommended by the CF Foundation. Other possible side effects that may be associated with pancreatic enzyme supplementation include folic acid deficiency, constipation, hyperuricemia, and allergic reactions to the porcine components of pancreatic enzymes [47, 48].

FUTURE RESEARCH

The premature denaturation of pancreatic enzyme preparations in the stomach has led to research into the development of pancreatic enzymes that are resistant to denaturation by small intestinal proteases and gastric acid. Current research has focused on the utilization of bacterial and fungal lipases as alternatives to pancreatic enzyme preparations which have usually used porcine lipase.

The results of the studies evaluating the efficacy of these newer preparations have been mixed. Further research needs to be conducted before these enzymes replace current enzyme preparations [49].

CONCLUSION

The evaluation and management of diarrhea due to pancreatic insufficiency remains a complex process. The amount of pancreatic enzymes supplemented must be individually tailored to the clinical severity of the disease in each patient. In order to ensure the safety and efficacy of the treatment, patients must be sufficiently monitored. New FDA regulations have made it a requirement that all pancreatic enzyme preparations undergo FDA approval and manufacturers disclose the exact content of the constituent enzymes per dose. These guidelines by the FDA will help to ensure that all preparations accurately reflect the amount of pancreatic enzymes delivered per dose and will enable a more standardized approach to the treatment of pancreatic steatorrhea.

REFERENCES

1. DiMagno EP, Go VL, Summerskill WH. Relations between pancreatic enzyme outputs and malabsorption in severe pancreatic insufficiency. N Engl J Med 1973;88(16):813–815.
2. Gaskin K, et al. Improved respiratory prognosis in patients with cystic fibrosis with normal fat absorption. J Pediatr 1982;100(6):857–862.
3. Bolender RP. Stereological analysis of the guinea pig pancreas. I. Analytical model and quantitative description of nonstimulated pancreatic exocrine cells. J Cell Biol 1974;61(2):269–287.
4. Sewell WA, Young JA. Secretion of electrolytes by the pancreas of the anaesthetized rat. J Physiol 1975;252(2):379–396.
5. Konturek SJ, Tasler J, Obtulowicz W. Effect of atropine on pancreatic responses endogenous and exogenous cholecystokinin. Am J Dig Dis 1972;17(10): 911–917.
6. Grundy D, Hutson D, Scratcherd T. The response of the pancreas of the anaesthetized cat to secretin before, during and after reversible vagal blockade. J Physiol 1983;342:517–526.
7. You CH, Rominger JM, Chey WY. Potentiation effect of cholecystokinin–octapeptide on pancreatic bicarbonate secretion stimulated by a physiologic dose of secretin in humans. Gastroenterology 1983;85(1):40–45.
8. Otani T, et al. Codistribution of TAP and the granule membrane protein GRAMP-92 in rat caerulein-induced pancreatitis. Am J Physiol 1998;275(5 Pt 1): G999–G1009.
9. Chey WY, et al. Plasma secretin concentrations in fasting and postprandial state in man. Am J Dig Dis 1978;23(11):981–988.
10. Forsmark CE. The diagnosis of chronic pancreatitis. Gastrointest Endosc 2000;52(2):293–298.

Chapter 10 / Pancreatic Exocrine Insufficiency

11. Hayakawa T, et al. Relationship between pancreatic exocrine function and histological changes in chronic pancreatitis. Am J Gastroenterol 1992;87(9): 1170–1174.
12. Heij HA, et al. Relationship between functional and histological changes in chronic pancreatitis. Dig Dis Sci 1986;31(10):1009–1013.
13. Waye JD, Adler M, Dreiling DA. The pancreas: a correlation of function and structure. Am J Gastroenterol 1978;69(2):176–181.
14. Soudah HC, et al. Cholecystokinin at physiological levels evokes pancreatic enzyme secretion via a cholinergic pathway. Am J Physiol 1992;263(1 Pt 1): G102–G107.
15. Adler G, et al. Interaction of the cholinergic system and cholecystokinin in the regulation of endogenous and exogenous stimulation of pancreatic secretion in humans. Gastroenterology 1991;100(2):537–543.
16. Tang F, et al. Studies on the pleomorphism of trachoma inclusion. Wei Sheng Wu Xue Bao 1993;33(5):365–367.
17. Li Y, Zhu J, Owyang C. Electrical physiological evidence for high and low-affinity vagal CCK-A receptors. Am J Physiol 1999;277(2 Pt 1):G469–G477.
18. Ji B, et al. Human pancreatic acinar cells lack functional responses to cholecystokinin and gastrin. Gastroenterology 2001;121(6):1380–1390.
19. Miyasaka K, et al. Amylase secretion from dispersed human pancreatic acini: neither cholecystokinin a nor cholecystokinin B receptors mediate amylase secretion in vitro. Pancreas 2002;25(2):161–165.
20. Pandol SJ. Neurohumoral control of exocrine pancreatic secretion. Curr Opin Gastroenterol 2003;19(5):443–446.
21. Brooks AM, Grossman MI. Postprandial pH and neutralizing capacity of the proximal duodenum in dogs. Gastroenterology 1970;59(1):85–89.
22. Hanssen LE. Pure synthetic bile salts release immunoreactive secretin in man. Scand J Gastroenterol 1980;15(4):461–463.
23. Valnes K, et al. Plasma concentration of secretin and gastric secretion following intraduodenal calcium infusion in man. Scand J Gastroenterol 1980;15(7): 881–885.
24. Schaffalitzky de Muckadell OB, et al. Pancreatic response and plasma secretin concentration during infusion of low dose secretin in man. Scand J Gastroenterol 1978;13(3):305–311.
25. Steward MC, Ishiguro H, Case RM. Mechanisms of bicarbonate secretion in the pancreatic duct. Annu Rev Physiol 2005;67:377–409.
26. Li Y, et al. Intestinal serotonin acts as paracrine substance to mediate pancreatic secretion stimulated by luminal factors. Am J Physiol Gastrointest Liver Physiol 2001;281(4):G916–G923.
27. Zhu JX, et al. Intestinal serotonin acts as a paracrine substance to mediate vagal signal transmission evoked by luminal factors in the rat. J Physiol 2001;530 (Pt 3):431–442.
28. Li Y, Owyang C. Somatostatin inhibits pancreatic enzyme secretion at a central vagal site. Am J Physiol 1993;265(2 Pt 1):G251–G257.
29. Vinnitsky VB, Glinsky GV. Role of the binding of neuropeptides to blood plasma proteins in the control of their blood–brain barrier passage. Ann N Y Acad Sci 1987;496:278–291.
30. Jung G, Louie DS, Owyang C. Pancreatic polypeptide inhibits pancreatic enzyme secretion via a cholinergic pathway. Am J Physiol 1987;253(5 Pt 1): G706–G710.
31. Tatemoto K. Isolation and characterization of peptide YY (PYY), a candidate gut hormone that inhibits pancreatic exocrine secretion. Proc Natl Acad Sci USA 1982;79(8):2514–2518.

32. Taylor IL. Distribution and release of peptide YY in dog measured by specific radioimmunoassay. Gastroenterology 1985;88(3):731–737.
33. Layer P, et al. The different courses of early- and late-onset idiopathic and alcoholic chronic pancreatitis. Gastroenterology 1994;107(5):1481–1487.
34. Layer P, et al. Cholinergic regulation of phase II interdigestive pancreatic secretion in humans. Pancreas 1993;8(2):181–188.
35. DiMagno EP, et al. Fate of orally ingested enzymes in pancreatic insufficiency. Comparison of two dosage schedules. N Engl J Med 1977;296(23):1318–1322.
36. Keller J, Holst JJ, Layer P. Inhibition of human pancreatic and biliary output but not intestinal motility by physiological intraileal lipid loads. Am J Physiol Gastrointest Liver Physiol 2006;290(4):G704–G709.
37. Slaff J, et al. Protease-specific suppression of pancreatic exocrine secretion. Gastroenterology 1984;87(1):44–52.
38. Guarner L, et al. Fate of oral enzymes in pancreatic insufficiency. Gut 1993; 34(5):708–712.
39. Nakamura T, et al. Study of gastric emptying in patients with pancreatic diabetes (chronic pancreatitis) using acetaminophen and isotope. Acta Gastroenterol Belg 1996;59(3):173–177.
40. Regan PT, et al. Comparative effects of antacids, cimetidine and enteric coating on the therapeutic response to oral enzymes in severe pancreatic insufficiency. N Engl J Med 1977;297(16):854–858.
41. Layer P, Holtmann G. Pancreatic enzymes in chronic pancreatitis. Int J Pancreatol 1994;15(1):1–11.
42. Gullo L, et al. Cardiovascular lesions in chronic pancreatitis: a prospective study. Dig Dis Sci 1982;27(8):716–722.
43. Smyth RL, et al. Strictures of ascending colon in cystic fibrosis and high-strength pancreatic enzymes. Lancet 1994;343(8889):85–86.
44. Lebenthal E. High strength pancreatic exocrine enzyme capsules associated with colonic strictures in patients with cystic fibrosis: "more is not necessarily better". J Pediatr Gastroenterol Nutr 1994;18(4):423–425.
45. FitzSimmons SC, et al. High-dose pancreatic-enzyme supplements and fibrosing colonopathy in children with cystic fibrosis. N Engl J Med 1997;336(18): 1283–1289.
46. Lebenthal E, Rolston DD, Holsclaw DS Jr. Enzyme therapy for pancreatic insufficiency: present status and future needs. Pancreas 1994;9(1):1–12.
47. Russell RM, et al. Impairment of folic acid absorption by oral pancreatic extracts. Dig Dis Sci 1980;25(5):369–373.
48. Stapleton FB, et al. Hyperuricosuria due to high-dose pancreatic extract therapy in cystic fibrosis. N Engl J Med 1976;295(5):246–248.
49. Zentler-Munro PL, et al. Therapeutic potential and clinical efficacy of acid-resistant fungal lipase in the treatment of pancreatic steatorrhoea due to cystic fibrosis. Pancreas 1992;7(3):311–319.

11 Bacterial Overgrowth

Rosemary J. Young, APRN
and Jon A. Vanderhoof, MD

CONTENTS

INTRODUCTION
DEFINITION
MECHANISMS
SYMPTOMS
DISEASE ASSOCIATIONS
DIAGNOSIS
TREATMENT
CONCLUSION
REFERENCES

Summary

The human gastrointestinal tract typically contains 300–500 bacterial species. Most bacterial species are acquired during the birth process and although some changes to the flora may occur during later stages of life, the composition of the intestinal microflora remains relatively constant. Small bowel bacterial overgrowth (SBBO) is defined as an excessive increase in the number of bacteria in the upper gastrointestinal tract leading to the development of symptoms. Etiologic factors in the development of SBBO include anatomic abnormalities, functional abnormalities including altered intestinal motility, and multifactorial issues such as malnutrition of the host and abnormalities of the immune system. Symptoms of SBBO include abdominal cramping, bloating, diarrhea, dyspepsia, and/or weight loss. Systemic distribution of bacterial antigen–antibody complexes

From: *Diarrhea, Clinical Gastroenterology*
Edited by: S. Guandalini, H. Vaziri, DOI 10.1007/978-1-60761-183-7_11
© Springer Science+Business Media, LLC 2011

may cause rashes, arthritis, and nephritis. Colitis or ileitis may also occur due to SBBO. Although diagnosis of bacterial overgrowth is classically based upon demonstration of an increase of bacterial content by aspiration and culture of upper intestinal fluids, these methods have several limitations. For this reason, a variety of non-invasive diagnostic tests have been devised for the diagnosis of SBBO. A hydrogen breath test is the most common method used. Alternative tests include the measurement of the byproducts of luminal bacteria metabolism in urine or blood and small bowel biopsies demonstrating often inflammatory changes. Treatment of SBBO commonly involves rotating broad-spectrum oral antibiotics. When significant intestinal inflammation is present, anti-inflammatory therapy with sulfasalazine or corticosteroids may be used. Regular toileting and colonic flushing with may also be used. Surgical corrections of anatomic abnormalities, such as stricture, fistula, diverticuli, are often helpful. Segments of dilated, poorly peristaltic bowel may be corrected with lengthening operations. Probiotic therapy in SBBO may be effective in reducing the use of antibiotic therapy and controlling symptoms; however, conclusive studies are needed. Nutritional support is an essential part of the management of SBBO both as a therapeutic measure and in the prevention of malnutrition.

Key Words: Small bowel bacterial overgrowth, SIBO, Microflora, Chronic diarrhea, Breath test

INTRODUCTION

The human gastrointestinal (GI) tract is colonized with a large number of bacteria often quoted to be 10 times the number of cells in human body. Colonization of the gut begins at birth and as the infant swallows vaginal fluid during the birthing process, with the organisms rapidly proliferating throughout the intestinal tract during the next 8–24 h. Over 400 different species of microbes are present within the gut [1]. The concentration of organisms gradually increases from the proximal to the distal bowel with the usual numbers in the very proximal small intestine numbering 10^2 organisms per gram and increases to 10^{11} organisms per gram in the distal colon.

The initial establishment of the enteric flora is influenced by a variety of host and external factors [2, 3]. Gut flora tends to parallel that of the mother as most bacterial species are acquired during the birthing process [3]. Although some changes to the flora occur during the first few months of life, transient changes to the flora may occur during later stages of life and the GI flora remains remarkably constant. This feature

Chapter 11 / Bacterial Overgrowth

is largely based upon recognition and tolerance of the infant-acquired flora by the gut immune system [4] which, by sampling microbial antigens, identifies these as normal.

Mostly acid-tolerant aerobic organisms inhabit the oropharynx and upper GI tract [2, 5]. Immunoglobulins present within the salivary secretions act as a first-line defense against ingested bacteria. Gastric acidity followed by exposure to bile in the duodenum further eliminates many of the ingested microorganisms leaving, typically, aerobic and facultative anaerobes in the proximal small bowel. It has been found that in pathologic cases of bacterial overgrowth, there are excessive bacterial counts in the proximal small bowel, commonly with bacterial species including *Streptococci*, *Bacteroides*, *Escherichia*, and *Lactobacilli* [2].

In the non-resected human GI tract, bacterial counts rise and a gradual transition from aerobic to anaerobic organisms occurs in more distal segments of the gut [3, 5]. The terminal ileum represents a transition zone between the aerobic flora found in the proximal gut and the anaerobic organisms found in the colon. At the ileocecal valve, bacterial counts rise from 10^7–10^9 organisms/mL in the terminal ileum to approximately 10^{10}–10^{12} organisms/mL in the colon where predominantly fastidious anaerobic organisms such as *Bacteroides*, *Bifidobacteria*, *Clostridia*, and numerous other microbial organisms are typical residents.

Interaction of the gut bacteria with the developing immune system is imperative in regulating immune function and initiating normal immune responses [6]. The normal peristaltic activity of the gut is an important factor in keeping the number of organisms under control, and the antibacterial effects of gastric acid and bile help prevent overgrowth in the proximal small intestine. The intestinal mucosal barrier excludes most organisms from the underlying tissue and dysfunction of this barrier can have a number of adverse effects including bacteremia and inflammation.

Normal populations of bacteria in the gut vary with a number of factors. In the tropics, healthy people are colonized with higher numbers of microorganisms in the small intestine [7]. Therefore, small-bowel bacterial overgrowth in the proximal gut has been considered to be present when levels exceed that number. However, some have used lower numbers which are more consistent with values obtained from populations living in temperate zones [8]. The type of flora, such as gram-positive or gram-negative aerobic or anaerobic, may also be useful in characterizing the condition. Additionally, the presence of atypical flora in different parts of the bowel may be significant such as when colonic flora is present in the upper small bowel [9].

DEFINITION

The most common definition of small-bowel bacterial overgrowth refers to the presence of bacteria in increased concentrations in any segment of small bowel which exceeds amount and type that are typically present in a healthy, physiologic state [10]. This may or may not represent a pathogenic situation depending on a number of factors, including the specific organisms, metabolic pathways of the organisms involved, including their ability to metabolize various dietary nutrients, and whether or not the organisms have invaded or caused injury to the mucosal surface [11]. In some instances, bacteria in excessive numbers may be present but may be doing no harm or causing no symptoms so, by definition, the patient might have overgrowth but one would question whether or not it is relevant. It has even been suggested that bacterial translocation may have beneficial effects on the acquired immune system and therefore condition of bacterial overgrowth which predisposes to bacterial translocation may in fact be beneficial [12].

MECHANISMS

There are a number of factors which predispose the patient to small-bowel bacterial overgrowth. These would first include any disruption in the normal defense mechanisms which prevent overgrowth such as reduction in gastric acid secretion either through disease state or through pharmacologic therapy with proton pump inhibitors [13], impairment of normal antegrade motility either by anatomic or neuromuscular dysfunction or medication use [14], or absence of the ileocecal valve which might permit reflux of colonic flora into the small intestine [15]. Radiation injury to the small intestine is commonly associated with overgrowth [16]. Chronic infectious processes such as *Giardia* which adversely affect the ability of the mucosa to protect itself also predispose to overgrowth [17]. Likewise, achlorhydria and old age are commonly associated with small-bowel bacterial overgrowth [18]. Diabetics commonly have overgrowth which may in part be due to associated neuropathy [19]. Other disorders which affect motility including scleroderma may present with overgrowth as may disorders such as tropical sprue, celiac disease, and pancreatitis.

Spontaneous bacterial peritonitis is a potentially fatal complication of hepatic cirrhosis with high mortality and occurs with significant frequency not only in hospitalized but also in asymptomatic cirrhotic patients. The organisms involved are usually gram negative. Small-bowel bacterial overgrowth has been hypothesized as a causative factor, as overgrowth appears to be common in patients with cirrhosis [20].

Not only is the presence of increased numbers of flora important, but as noted, the specific characteristics of the bacteria down to the strain level have been shown to be increasingly relevant [21]. Broad-spectrum antibiotics may disrupt the microbiota to the extent of causing an overgrowth of a specific strain of normally present organisms and producing a pathological effect. *Clostridium difficile* is perhaps the best recognized example of this.

SYMPTOMS

Bacterial overgrowth in the small intestine can cause a variety of inflammatory changes in the mucosa and can affect mucosal permeability and micro-molecular transport [22]. Although translocation of organisms across the mucosal barrier is a normal phenomenon in healthy individuals, translocation in increased numbers, which occurs in overgrowth, predisposes the patient to septic episodes or abscess formation. Further development of immune complex deposits in the joints may result in an inflammatory arthritis [23]. Overgrowth may also result in inflammatory cytokine production and enhanced excretion of inflammatory markers into the stool [24].

Competition for nutrients commonly occurs in small-bowel bacterial overgrowth as is evidenced by the classic presentation of megaloblastic anemia due to vitamin B12 deficiency which may occur with loss of the ileum or in conditions of atrophic gastritis [25]. Steatorrhea is a relatively common occurrence, probably due to a combination of the deconjugation and the reabsorption of bile acids coupled with mucosal injury from small intestinal inflammatory changes. In such instances, these deficiencies may be accompanied by weight loss, diarrhea, bloating, and discomfort. Fat-soluble vitamin deficiencies (A, D, E, and K) may occur, although vitamin K deficiency is relatively uncommon because of endogenous production of vitamin K by luminal bacteria.

Systemic complications of overgrowth may also occur. A classic example is that of the lactic acidosis which often occurs in children with short bowel syndrome who develop overgrowth of organisms which metabolize intra-luminal carbohydrate into both D and L isomers of lactate. D-Lactate is poorly metabolized in humans despite being produced by a number of enteric organisms. Consequently, in these patients with overgrowth of predominantly D-lactate-producing organisms, neurological symptoms ranging from impaired school performance to coma may occur [25]. In such a setting, specific measurement of D-lactate in the blood is required to confirm the diagnosis, and care must be taken to make certain that the correct test is ordered. Total blood lactate may not necessarily be elevated. Yeast overgrowth may also occur, resulting in altered behavior due to elevated blood alcohol levels [26].

DISEASE ASSOCIATIONS

Short Bowel Syndrome

Of the various clinical conditions in which small-bowel bacterial overgrowth is problematic, perhaps none are more important than short bowel syndrome. In this condition the patient has acquired malabsorption as a result of resection of a major portion of the GI tract leaving behind a reduced mucosal surface area. Since these patients are already compromised, any inflammatory changes in the GI mucosa will exacerbate malabsorption. Post-operative changes resulting in anatomic abnormalities or strictures may affect antegrade propulsion of fluid through the GI tract [27]. With time, these patients often develop delayed transit and dilatation of the remaining GI tract which predisposes the patient to small-bowel bacterial overgrowth.

In many patients with short bowel syndrome, fermentation of malabsorbed carbohydrates may be an important source of energy. The products of fermentation include short-chain fatty acids, which are a good source of calories [1]. Although this happens in the colon predominantly, some of it may go on in the distal small intestine as well. Overgrowth becomes a pathologic state when the mucosal surface is damaged through inflammatory changes in the gut and it is in this group of patients that treatment is warranted, particularly in children [28].

Irritable Bowel Syndrome

One of the major controversies regarding small-bowel bacterial overgrowth is its association with irritable bowel syndrome. Irritable bowel syndrome is a condition of unknown etiology that presents with recurrent abdominal pain or discomfort along with abnormalities in stool frequency or form [29]. Visceral hypersensitivity, which has been demonstrated in both adults and children with irritable bowel syndrome, is thought to play an important role in the symptoms, and there is a possibility that inflammation associated with gut bacteria might somehow be involved in this process [30, 31]. Significant diarrhea, constipation, bloating, gas, and pain are present in patients with irritable bowel syndrome, all symptoms which may also be ascribed to small intestinal bacterial overgrowth. An abnormal glucose breath hydrogen test, lactulose breath hydrogen test, and jejunal aspirates have been observed more frequently in patients with irritable bowel syndrome than matched controls and may indicate abnormal bacterial populations

[32]. In one study, Lee and Pimentel [33] found that 84% of irritable bowel syndrome patients versus only 20% of healthy controls had abnormal lactose breath hydrogen test [33]. However, not all investigators have found similar results, and a number of negative studies also exist [34]. Specific mucosal mediators have been shown to activate human submucosal neurons in subjects with irritable bowel syndrome [35]. Likewise, the data on treatment of overgrowth associated with irritable bowel syndrome are often ineffective in both children and adults [36, 37].

Gastroesophageal Reflux

As proton pump inhibitors are commonly used in the treatment of irritable bowel syndrome, it has been hypothesized that the overgrowth found in patients with irritable bowel syndrome may simply be a result of the lack of gastric which decreases the organisms that favor acidic environments [13, 38]. Suppression of acid has been shown to contribute to small-bowel bacterial overgrowth as well as to gastrointestinal and respiratory infections in general [39]. Previous studies describing the association of overgrowth with irritable bowel syndrome have not specifically explored the confounding variable of acid suppression.

Inflammatory Bowel Disease

The role of gut flora in inflammatory bowel disease has been explored in a large number of studies. Differences in microbiota have been found in luminal samples and biopsy cultures in patients with inflammation secondary to inflammatory bowel disease [40]. Abnormal responses to bacteria and bacterial antigens have been identified in patients with Crohn's disease and overgrowth has been reported to correlate with exacerbation of disease in some patients with Crohn's disease [41]. Antibiotics have been successfully used in the treatment of Crohn's disease in a number of studies [42], and treatment with parenteral nutrition or elemental diets which significantly influence the type and numbers of bacteria in the small intestine has also been shown to be efficacious in the treatment of some forms of Crohn's disease [43]. The extent to which inflammatory bowel disease and small-bowel bacterial overgrowth are interrelated has yet to be determined.

DIAGNOSIS

The diagnosis of small-bowel bacterial overgrowth is the subject of much controversy. A number of different tests have been proposed to make the diagnosis. Analyzing breath specimens for volatile metabolites of orally administered substrates such as glucose and lactulose provides a simplified detection method for the presence of intestinal bacterial overgrowth. Probably the most commonly used substrates is glucose which is normally absorbed in the proximal small intestine, and fermentation prior to absorption in that location by GI bacteria is considered abnormal. Physiologically this occurs because when glucose interacts with bacteria, carbon dioxide and hydrogen are produced and the hydrogen is excreted into the breath, where it can be easily measured. Fasting breath hydrogen levels of more than 20 ppm are typically considered abnormal. However, glucose breath hydrogen testing depends somewhat on the specific genus and species of organisms present and will not pick up all cases of bacterial overgrowth.

In addition to glucose, lactulose has been used as a substrate for breath hydrogen testing. Lactulose consumption which results in early peaking of hydrogen production may indicate small-bowel bacterial overgrowth since lactulose is normally malabsorbed in that part of the bowel and typically is fermented in the colon. It has been suggested that lactulose breath hydrogen testing is not as reliable as it is normally malabsorbed to some degree in certain individuals [44].

Glucose and lactulose breath hydrogen testing is safe, easy to perform, and can be used in women of childbearing age and children; however, questions regarding usefulness have risen due to relatively low sensitivity and specificity [45]. Several factors may interfere with the interpretation of results, including the presence of lung disease and the potential for false-positive results following rapid delivery of the test substrate to the colon in patients who have short bowel syndrome [46]. Additionally, the hydrogen peak occurring from bacterial overgrowth in the distal small intestine may be difficult to discriminate from the normal peak seen when the test substrate reaches the colon, and false-negative results may occur in 30–40% of patients due to low anaerobic organism counts which may occur in some patients [47]. It is also possible to have no increase in hydrogen production during a lactulose breath hydrogen test if hydrogen is converted to methane or hydrogen sulfide by relatively rare, hydrogen-consuming microbes [48].

Breath testing using $[^{14}C]$-D-xylose measures the pulmonary excretion of labeled CO_2 produced from the bacterial fermentation of the labeled substrate. Xylose is a pentose sugar that is catabolized by gram-negative aerobes, which frequently are a common part of the microflora implicated in bacterial overgrowth. Breath tests are interpreted as positive for small-bowel bacterial overgrowth if significant $^{14}CO_2$ is expired before colonic H_2 and CH_4 rise or if a double H_2 and CH_4 peak occurs. Breath tests are interpreted as negative if a significant

Chapter 11 / Bacterial Overgrowth

$^{14}CO_2$ rise is detected simultaneously with the colonic H_2 and CH_4 rise [49].

The sensitivity and specificity of the [^{14}C]-D-xylose breath test approaches 90%, which is superior to other breath tests that have been used to diagnose bacterial overgrowth [49]. Disorders associated with impaired gastric emptying may lead to false-negative results, and rapid intestinal emptying may lead to false-positive results due to early presentation of the test substrate in the colon. To optimize the diagnostic performance of the [^{14}C]-D-xylose test, it is recommended that patients with severe dysmotility syndromes such as pseudo-obstruction have breath samples taken up to 3 h after ingestion of the sugar and that patients also undergo testing with the co-administration of intestinal transit markers such as barium to serve as a measure of intestinal transit time [50].

Although administration of ^{14}C is associated with trivial (10 μCi) radiation exposure, it is not recommended for children or women of childbearing age. A similar test based on ^{13}C, which does not lead to radiation exposure, is now available [51]. Because the breath tests are simple to perform, they are a reasonable choice for screening and monitoring of therapy; however, the labeled techniques are usually available only in tertiary care centers due to limited applications.

Aspirating the small bowel and culturing the intestinal fluid is usually considered the gold standard for the diagnosis of overgrowth [52]. The demonstration of more than 10^7 colony-forming units per milliliter in a jejunal aspirate is considered abnormal, although lower numbers might be considered abnormal as well if the underlying mucosa is inflamed. Unfortunately this procedure samples only the proximal small intestine and it is most common to have overgrowth only in the distal small bowel without having abnormalities in the duodenum or the jejunum [2]. Another issue concerns the contamination of the aspiration tube during procedures which may also cause false-positive results [52].

When suspicion for bacterial overgrowth is high, some clinicians use empiric treatment to make the diagnosis [11]. Although symptoms may resolve rapidly, a major drawback to this approach is possible overuse of broad-spectrum antibiotics. Additionally, antibiotics may be associated with adverse effects, some of which may mimic symptoms of bacterial overgrowth, such as diarrhea and abdominal discomfort.

Laboratory studies, including measurement of serum D-lactate and blood alcohol and qualitative urine indicans, are initial screening studies that may aid in detecting bacterial metabolites or by-products [53]. Routine electrolyte measurements may identify unexplained acidosis. Some bacteria in excess may produce high concentrations of serum folate [54]. Malabsorption due to overgrowth effects may identify low serum concentrations of fat-soluble vitamins such as vitamin A, D, and E. Although rarely performed, in patients who have vitamin B12 deficiency, bacterial overgrowth may be diagnosed during the last stage of the Schilling test if antibiotic administration normalizes the absorption of vitamin B12 [55]. Bacterial overgrowth may be suspected radiographically if an upper gastrointestinal series shows hypomotility, partial obstruction, dilatation, diverticuli, or other mechanical factors associated with delayed gastrointestinal motility as evidenced by infrequent or decreased stool output [56].

The identification of bacterial overgrowth in the small intestine by any of the previously described tests does not prove a causal relationship to the associated symptoms because some affected patients do not have clinically significant disease. In fact, in the absence of gut inflammation, bacterial overgrowth may often be asymptomatic [11]. A small-bowel biopsy can identify the inflammation associated with the negative effects of overgrowth and helps to exclude other causes of malabsorption such as celiac disease. Inflammation of the small bowel and colon due to bacterial overgrowth occurs in affected patients secondary to reactions from absorbed bacterial antigens. Successful treatment of severe bacterial overgrowth with acetylsalicylic acid preparations and corticosteroids has been reported, an observation that is consistent with the importance of intestinal inflammation in the cause of symptoms [57]. Measurement of fecal calprotectin must also be of assistance in the identification of intestinal inflammation associated with pathogenic states of bacterial overgrowth [58].

TREATMENT

Antibiotics

Treatment for small-bowel bacterial overgrowth is usually first attempted using broad-spectrum antibiotics. Several different combinations have been used by different investigators and are listed in Table 11.1 [59]. Empiric trials of therapy may also aid in the diagnostic process. The goal of antibiotic therapy should not be to eradicate the flora but to suppress the total numbers of bacteria or alter it in a way that leads to symptomatic improvement. The selection of antimicrobial agents ideally should be specific for the predominant undesirable organisms associated with bacterial overgrowth and the promotion of beneficial species such as lactobacilli and bifidobacteria.

Effective antibiotic treatment should cover both aerobic and anaerobic enteric bacteria but because of trends in microbial resistance, many

Table 11.1

Comparison of agents used for treatment of bacterial overgrowth (typical course 7–10 days, all medicines given orally!)

Medication	Pediatric dose	Adult dose	Comments	Percentage orally absorbed	Percentage renally excreted	Cisapride (Yes/No)
Amphotericin	<5 years: 100 mg bid 5–12 years: 250 mg bid	500 mg bid	Injection given orally	9	40 (2–5% active)	Yes
Augmentin	10 mg/kg/dose bid	500 mg bid		Complete (amoxicillin)	30–40%	Yes
Bactrim (TMP/SMX)	2 mg TMP/kg/dose daily	1 SS tablet daily Each tablet: sulfamethoxazole 400 mg/trimetho-prim 80 mg		Almost completely, 90–100%	Sulfamethoxazole, 10–30%; trimethoprim, 50–75%	No
Ciprofloxacin	20–40 mg/kg/day bid	500 mg bid		50–80%	30–50%	No
Clindamycin	10–30 mg/kg/day Divided tid/qid	300 mg tid		90%	10%	Yes
Colistin	<5 years: 25 mg 2–4 times/day 5-12 years: 50 mg 2–4 times/day	100 mg 2–4 times/day	Injection given orally	Insignificant	75% in 24 h	Yes
Doxycycline	Children less than 8 years: 100 mg bid	100 mg bid		100%	23%	No
Gentamicin	2 mg/kg/dose bid Others: 2.5 mg/kg/ dose tid Not to exceed 300 mg/day	2–2.5 mg/kg/dose tid Not to exceed 300 mg	Injection given orally	None	100%	Yes

Table 11.1
(continued)

Medication	Pediatric dose	Adult dose	Comments	Percentage orally absorbed	Percentage renally excreted	Cisapride (Yes/No)
Metronidazole	10 mg/kg/dose bid Others: 5—10 mg/ kg/dose bid–tid	250–500 mg tid–qid		90%	10%	No
Neomycin	50 mg/kg/day Divided every 6 h	500 mg bid 500 mg–2 g every 6–8 h	Available as tablets only	3%	0.9–1.5%	Yes
Tetracycline	Children >8 years: 25–50 mg/kg/day in divided doses every 6 h	500 mg tid		75%	60%	No
Tobramycin	<5 years: 10 mg 2–4 times/day 5–12 years: 40 mg 2–4 times/day	80 mg 2–4 times/day	Injection given orally	Poor	90–95%	Yes
Rifaximin	Not established 20–30 mg/kg/day has been used	400 mg tid	Nonformulary at Children's	<0.4%	<1%	Yes
Vancomycin	125 mg every 6 h (10 mg/kg/dose qid) Max total daily dose 2 g/day	125–500 mg every 6 h Max total daily dose 2 g/day		Poor	Oral doses primarily via feces	Yes

patients do not respond adequately to monotherapy. Adequate antimicrobial coverage can be achieved with combinations of amoxicillin–clavulanate or oral gentamicin and metronidazole [60]. A combination of cephalosporin such as cephalexin or trimethoprim–sulfamethoxazole with metronidazole has also been reported to be effective as evidenced by a decrease in overgrowth symptoms [61, 62]. More recently, trials of rifaximin, a nonabsorbable antibiotic, suggest that it has some efficacy in bacterial overgrowth [63, 64]. Probiotic therapy has been attempted in a few patients but the results are mixed [65, 66]. Probiotic therapy is not commonly recommended for the treatment of overgrowth and has the possibility of exacerbating the problem by adding additional organisms.

Antibiotics may be given during the first 5–7 days of each month, or given one out of every 2–4 weeks if needed. A single course of antibiotic therapy for 7–10 days may improve symptoms and has an effect lasting for months. They may even be given continuously until they stop working, in which case rotating to a different antibiotic protocol may be necessary. It is usually unnecessary to repeat diagnostic testing if symptoms or objective measures of malabsorption respond to treatment. Because of recurrent symptoms, some patients require repeated courses of therapy, and others need regularly scheduled treatment (such as the first 5–10 days of every month or every other week). In these patients, rotating antibiotic regimens may help to prevent the development of resistant bacterial species [67].

Dietary Support

Most small-bowel bacteria are carbohydrate fermenters and taking away the substrate for bacterial metabolism may be effective in treating some of these patients. This usually involves a high-fat, low-carbohydrate diet [68]. Fat is not significantly metabolized by the bacteria and supplies a source of energy. Decreasing the carbohydrate may lessen the development of D-lactic acidosis, the production of small-bowel gas, bloating, and discomfort. In some cases however, excess consumption of fat may be associated with the development of kidney stones and low serum calcium and magnesium levels due to the coexistence of fat malabsorption.

The type of fat administered is a subject of controversy. Substitution of medium-chain triglycerides in the diet is probably of little value because the coefficient of absorption for medium-chain triglycerides is only slightly better than for long-chain triglycerides, and their caloric density is less [69]. Furthermore, despite their water solubility, medium-chain triglycerides are at least partially absorbed via the intestinal lymphatics, which limit their usefulness. The majority of the evidence suggests that use of long-chain triglycerides significantly enhances bowel adaptation and is especially useful in early stages of rehabilitation after intestinal resection [70].

Individual nutrient support is important for all patients with bacterial overgrowth, particularly those who have significant weight loss or evidence of micronutrient deficiency as evidenced in laboratory assessments or by physical exam. Deficiencies of calcium, vitamin B12, or vitamin K are common and should be corrected. Certain nutrient changes may also alleviate symptoms. Because lactase deficiency develops in many adult patients who have bacterial overgrowth, avoidance of lactose-containing foods may be suggested.

Mechanical Methods

Periodically flushing the GI tract small intestine with polyethylene glycol solution may be needed especially in recalcitrant patients or those resistant to antibiotic therapy that may have dysmotility or dilated bowel. This technique may help to mobilize viable bacteria that are embedded in intestinal mucus [11].

Conditions associated with intestinal stasis should be corrected when possible. An example is the avoiding of the administration of drugs known to decrease intestinal motility (i.e., loperamide) or reduce gastric acidity (i.e., proton pump inhibitors). In cases of sluggish motility, which occurs naturally as a compensatory mechanism in short bowel syndrome, methods to enhance motility such as surgical bowel-tapering procedures of dilated bowel segments may be attempted [71]. The beneficial use of prokinetic drugs such as cisapride or erythromycin has not been well documented. Persistent inflammatory changes may respond to anti-inflammatory agents such as mesalamine, budesonide, or even systemic corticosteroids but are often not required.

The underlying cause of bacterial overgrowth is usually not easily reversible and may require surgery. For example, surgery may be beneficial in patients with bacterial overgrowth associated with extreme bowel dilation [71]. A variety of surgical techniques have been described, all involving intestinal tapering or lengthening. However, in many cases, surgery is not an option unless significant bowel dilatation is present [72].

CONCLUSION

Small intestinal bacterial overgrowth has been recognized for some time as a cause of malabsorption and a complication of short bowel syndrome. It has now been identified in other situations such as irritable bowel syndrome, although its contribution to pathophysiology is controversial. It is characterized by a variety of signs and symptoms resulting from an increased number and/or abnormal type of bacteria in the small intestine. The diagnosis of overgrowth is imprecise as techniques currently used have not undergone scientific validation. Treatment varies depending on the underlying cause and the presence or the absence of inflammation.

REFERENCES

1. Tappenden KA, Deutsch AS. The physiological relevance of the intestinal microbiota—contributions to human health. J Am Coll Nutr 2007 Dec;26(6):679S–683S.
2. Bouhnik Y, Alain S, Attar A, Flourie B, Raskine L, Sanson-Le Pors MJ, Rambaud JC. Bacterial populations contaminating the upper gut in patients with small intestinal bacterial overgrowth syndrome. Am J Gastroenterol 1999;94:1327–1331.
3. Mackie RI, Sghir A, Gaskins HR. Developmental microbial ecology of the neonatal gastrointestinal tract. Am J Clin Nutr 1999;69:1035S–1045S.
4. Ouwehand A, Isolauri E, Salminen S. The role of the intestinal microflora for the development of the immune system in early childhood. Eur J Nutr 2002;41 (Suppl 1):I32.
5. Berg RD. The indigenous gastrointestinal microflora. Trends Microbiol 1996;4:430–435.
6. Shi HN, Walker A. Bacterial colonization and the development of intestinal defenses. Can J Gastroenterol 2004 Aug;18(8):493–500.
7. Rana SV, Bhardwaj SB. Small Intestinal bacterial overgrowth. Scand J Gastro 2008;43(9):1030–1037.
8. Falk PG, Hooper LV, Midtvedt T, Gordon JI. Creating and maintaining the gastrointestinal ecosystem: what we know and need to know from gnotobiology. Microbiol Mol Biol Rev 1998;62:1157–1170.
9. Sullivan A, Törnblom H, Lindberg G, Hammarlund B, Palmgren AC, Einarsson C, Nord CE. The micro-flora of the small bowel in health and disease. Anaerobe 2003 Feb;9(1):11–14.
10. Wedlake L, Thomas K, McGough C, Andreyev HJ. Small bowel bacterial overgrowth and lactose intolerance during radical pelvic radiotherapy: an observational study. Eur J Cancer 2008 Oct;44(15):2212–2217.
11. DiBaise J, Young R, Vanderhoof J. Enteric microbial flora, bacterial overgrowth, and short-bowel syndrome. Clin Gastroenterol Hepatol 2006;4(1):11–20.
12. Salzedas-Netto AA, Silva RM, Martins JL, Menchaca-Diaz JL, Bugni GM, Watanabe AY, Silva FJ, Fagundes-Neto U, Morais MB, Koh IH. Can bacterial translocation be a beneficial event? Transplant Proc 2006 Jul–Aug; 38(6):1836–1837.
13. Williams C, McColl KE. Review article: proton pump inhibitors and bacterial overgrowth. Aliment Pharmacol Ther 2006 Jan 1;23(1):3–10.
14. Duval-Iflah Y, Berard H, Baumer P, Guillaume P, Raibaud P, Joulin Y, Lecomte JM. Effects of racecadotril and loperamide on bacterial proliferation and on the

central nervous system of the newborn gnotobiotic piglet. Aliment Pharmacol Ther 1999 Dec;13(Suppl 6):9–14.

15. Machado WM, Miranda JR, Morceli J, Padovani CR. The small bowel flora in individuals with cecoileal reflux. Arq Gastroenterol 2008 Jul–Sep;45(3): 212–218.

16. Wedlake L, Thomas K, McGough C, Andreyev HJ. Small bowel bacterial overgrowth and lactose intolerance during radical pelvic radiotherapy: an observational study. Eur J Cancer 2008 Oct;44(15):2212–2217.

17. Ramakrishna BS, Venkataraman S, Mukhopadhya A. Tropical malabsorption. Postgrad Med J 2006 Dec;82(974):779–787.

18. Schiffrin EJ, Parlesak A, Bode C, Bode JC, van't Hof MA, Grathwohl D, Guigoz Y. Probiotic yogurt in the elderly with intestinal bacterial overgrowth: endotoxaemia and innate immune functions. Br J Nutr 2009 Apr;101(7):961–966.

19. Cuoco L, Montalto M, Jorizzo RA, Santarelli L, Arancio F, Cammarota G, Gasbarrini G. Eradication of small intestinal bacterial overgrowth and oro-cecal transit in diabetics. Hepatogastroenterology 2002 Nov–Dec;49(48):1582–1586.

20. Bajaj JS, Zadvornova Y, Heuman DM, Hafeezullah M, Hoffmann RG, Sanyal AJ, Saeian K. Association of proton pump inhibitor therapy with spontaneous bacterial peritonitis in cirrhotic patients with ascites. Am J Gastroenterol 2009 May;104(5):1130–1134.

21. van Saene HK, Taylor N, Damjanovic V, Sarginson RE. Microbial gut overgrowth guarantees increased spontaneous mutation leading to polyclonality and antibiotic resistance in the critically ill. Curr Drug Targets 2008 May;9(5):419–421.

22. Othman M, Agüero R, Lin HC. Alterations in intestinal microbial flora and human disease. Curr Opin Gastroenterol 2008 Jan;24(1):11–16.

23. Bhangle SD, Kramer N, Rosenstein ED. Spondyloarthropathy after ampullary carcinoma resection: "post-Whipple" disease. J Clin Rheumatol 2009 Aug;15(5): 241–243.

24. Montalto M, Santoro L, Dalvai S, Curigliano V, D'Onofrio F, Scarpellini E, Cammarota G, Panunzi S, Gallo A, Gasbarrini A, Gasbarrini G. Fecal calprotectin concentrations in patients with small intestinal bacterial overgrowth. Dig Dis 2008;26(2):183–186.

25. Sentongo TA, Azzam R, Charrow J. Vitamin B12 status, methylmalonic acidemia, and bacterial overgrowth in short bowel syndrome. J Pediatr Gastroenterol Nutr 2009 Apr;48(4):495–497.

26. Spinucci G, Guidetti M, Lanzoni E, Pironi L. Endogenous ethanol production in a patient with chronic intestinal pseudo-obstruction and small intestinal bacterial overgrowth. Eur J Gastroenterol Hepatol 2006 Jul;18(7):799–802.

27. O'Keefe SJ. Bacterial overgrowth and liver complications in short bowel intestinal failure patients. Gastroenterology 2006 Feb;130(2 Suppl 1):S67–S69.

28. Kaufman SS, Loseke CA, Lupo JV, Young RJ, Murray ND, Pinch LW, Vanderhoof JA. Influence of bacterial overgrowth and intestinal inflammation on duration of parenteral nutrition in children with short bowel syndrome. J Pediatr 1997 Sep;131(3):356–361.

29. Yale SH, Musana AK, Kieke A, Hayes J, Glurich I, Chyou PH. Applying case definition criteria to irritable bowel syndrome. Clin Med Res 2008 May;6(1):9–16.

30. Collins SM, Vallance B, Barbara G, Borgaonkar M. Putative inflammatory and immunological mechanisms in functional bowel disorders. Bailliere's Best Pract Res Clin Gastroenterol 1999 Oct;13(3):429–436.

31. Lin HC. Small intestinal bacterial overgrowth: a framework for understanding irritable bowel syndrome. JAMA 2004;292:852–858.

Chapter 11 / Bacterial Overgrowth

32. Abu-Shanab A, Quigley EM. Diagnosis of small intestinal bacterial overgrowth: the challenges persist! Expert Rev Gastroenterol Hepatol 2009 Feb;3(1):77–87.
33. Lee HR, Pimentel M. Bacteria and irritable bowel syndrome: the evidence for small intestinal bacterial overgrowth. Curr Gastroenterol Rep 2006 Aug;8(4): 305–311.
34. Gilkin RJ Jr. The spectrum of irritable bowel syndrome: a clinical review. Clin Ther 2005 Nov;27(11):1696–1709.
35. Barbara G, Stanghellini V, Brandi G, Cremon C, Di Nardo G, De Giorgio R, Corinaldesi R. Interactions between commensal bacteria and gut sensorimotor function in health and disease. Am J Gastroenterol 2005 Nov;100(11):2560–2568.
36. Frissora CL, Cash BD. Review article: the role of antibiotics vs. conventional pharmacotherapy in treating symptoms of irritable bowel syndrome. Aliment Pharmacol Ther 2007 Jun 1;25(11):1271–1281.
37. Bausserman M, Michail S. The use of *Lactobacillus* GG in irritable bowel syndrome in children: a double-blind randomized control trial. J Pediatr 2005 Aug;147(2):197–201.
38. Spiegel BM, Chey WD, Chang L. Bacterial overgrowth and irritable bowel syndrome: unifying hypothesis or a spurious consequence of proton pump inhibitors? Am J Gastroenterol 2008 Dec;103(12):2972–2976.
39. Vakil N. Acid inhibition and infections outside the gastrointestinal tract. Am J Gastroenterol 2009 Mar;104(Suppl 2):S17–S20.
40. Macfarlane GT, Blackett KL, Nakayama T, Steed H, Macfarlane S. The gut microbiota in inflammatory bowel disease. Curr Pharm Des 2009;15(13):1528–1536.
41. Willing B, Halfvarson J, Dicksved J, Rosenquist M, Järnerot G, Engstrand L, Tysk C, Jansson JK. Twin studies reveal specific imbalances in the mucosaassociated microbiota of patients with ileal Crohn's disease. Inflamm Bowel Dis 2009 May;15(5):653–660.
42. Rubin DT, Kornbluth A. Role of antibiotics in the management of inflammatory bowel disease: a review. Rev Gastroenterol Disord 2005;5(Suppl 3):S10–S15.
43. Smith PA. Nutritional therapy for active Crohn's disease. World J Gastroenterol 2008 Jul 21;14(27):4420–4423.
44. Kerckhoffs AP, Visser MR, Samsom M, van der Rest ME, de Vogel J, Harmsen W, Akkermans LM. Critical evaluation of diagnosing bacterial overgrowth in the proximal small intestine. J Clin Gastroenterol 2008 Nov–Dec;42(10): 1095–1102.
45. Kerlin P, Wong L. Breath hydrogen testing in bacterial overgrowth of the small intestine. Gastroenterology 1988;95(4):982–988.
46. Corazza G, Menozzi M, Strocchi A, Rasciti L, Vaira D, Lecchini R, Avanzini P, Chezzi C, Gasbarrini G. The diagnosis of small bowel bacterial overgrowth. Reliability of jejunal culture and inadequacy of breath hydrogen testing. Gastroenterology 1990;98(2):302–309.
47. Soffer EE. Small bowel dysmotility. Curr Treat Options Gastroenterol 1998 Dec;1(1):8–14.
48. Strocchi A, Sorge M, Pranzo L. Intraindividual variability in H2 production capacity. Gastroenterol Int 1988;1:593.
49. King CE, Toskes PP, King CE, et al. Comparison of the one-gram D-$[^{14}C]$xylose breath test to the $[^{14}C]$bile acid breath test in patients with small-intestine bacterial overgrowth. Gastroenterology 1986;91:1447–1451.
50. Lewis JL, Young G, Mann M, et al. Improvement in the specificity of $[^{14}C]$D-xylose breath test for bacterial overgrowth. Dig Dis Sci 1997;42:1587–1592.
51. Klein P. 13C breath tests: visions and realities. J Nutr 2001;131:1637S–1642S.

52. Kerckhoffs AP, Visser MR, Samsom M, van der Rest ME, de Vogel J, Harmsen W, Akkermans LM Critical evaluation of diagnosing bacterial overgrowth in the proximal small intestine. J Clin Gastroenterol 2008 Nov–Dec;42(10):1095–1102.
53. Mack DR. D(–)Lactic acid-producing probiotics, D(–)lactic acidosis and infants. Can J Gastroenterol 2004;18:671–675.
54. Kirsch M. "Bacterial overgrowth". Am J Gastroenterol 1990;85(3):231–237.
55. Farivar S, Fromm H, Schindler D, Schmidt FW. Sensitivity of bile acid breath test in the diagnosis of bacterial overgrowth in the small intestine with and without the stagnant (blind) loop syndrome. Dig Dis Sci 1979 Jan;24(1):33–40.
56. Quigley E, Quera R. Small intestinal bacterial overgrowth: roles of antibiotics, prebiotics, and probiotics. Gastroenterology 2006;130(2 Suppl 1):S78–S90.
57. Vanderhoof JA, Young RJ, Murray N, Kaufman SS. Treatment strategies for small bowel bacterial overgrowth in short bowel syndrome. J Pediatr Gastroenterol Nutr 1998;27:155–160.
58. Montalto M, Santoro L, Dalvai S, Curigliano V, D'Onofrio F, Scarpellini E, Cammarota G, Panunzi S, Gallo A, Gasbarrini A, Gasbarrini G. Fecal calprotectin concentrations in patients with small intestinal bacterial overgrowth. Dig Dis 2008;26(2):183–186.
59. Personal communication. Courtesy of Kathleen Gura, PharmD. Children's Hospital Boston, 2009.
60. Vanderhoof JA, Young RJ, Thompson JS. New and emerging therapies for short bowel syndrome in children. Paediatr Drugs 2003;5(8):525–531.
61. Di Stefano M, Miceli E, Missanelli A, Mazzocchi S, Corazza GR. Absorbable vs. non-absorbable antibiotics in the treatment of small intestine bacterial overgrowth in patients with blind-loop syndrome. Aliment Pharmacol Ther 2005;21:985–992.
62. DiBaise JK, Young RJ, Vanderhoof JA. Intestinal rehabilitation and the short bowel syndrome: part 2. Am J Gastroenterol 2004;99:1823–1832.
63. Di Stefano M, Miceli E, Missanelli A, Mazzocchi S, Corazza GR. Absorbable vs. non-absorbable antibiotics in the treatment of small intestine bacterial overgrowth in patients with blind-loop syndrome. Aliment Pharmacol Ther 2005;21: 985–992.
64. Lauritano EC, Gabrielli M, Lupascu A, et al. Rifaximin dose-finding study for the treatment of small intestinal bacterial overgrowth. Aliment Pharmacol Ther 2005;22:31.
65. Sen S, Mullan MM, Parker TJ, Woolner JT, Tarry SA, Hunter JO. Effect of *Lactobacillus plantarum* 299v on colonic fermentation and symptoms of irritable bowel syndrome. Dig Dis Sci 2002;47:2615–2620.
66. Urbancsek H, Kazar T, Mezes I, Neumann K. Results of a double-blind, randomized study to evaluate the efficacy and safety of *Antibiophilus* in patients with radiation-induced diarrhoea. Eur J Gastroenterol Hepatol 2001;13:391–396.
67. Nightingale JM. The medical management of intestinal failure: methods to reduce the severity. Proc Nutr Soc 2003 Aug;62(3):703–710.
68. Bongaerts GP, Severijnen RS. Arguments for a lower carbohydrate-higher fat diet in patients with a short small bowel. Med Hypotheses 2006;67(2):280–282. Epub 2006 Apr 17.
69. Vanderhoof JA, Grandjean CJ, Kaufman SS, Burkley KT, Antonson DL. The medical management of intestinal failure: methods to reduce the severity. Proc Nutr Soc 2003 Aug;62(3):703–710.
70. Kollman KA, Lien EL, Vanderhoof JA. Dietary lipids influence intestinal adaptation after massive bowel resection. J Pediatr Gastroenterol Nutr 1999 Jan;28(1): 41–45.

71. Thompson JS. Surgical rehabilitation of intestine in short bowel syndrome. Surgery 2004;135(5):465–470.
72. Reinshagen K, Zahn K, Buch C, Zoeller M, Hagl CI, Ali M, Waag KL. The impact of longitudinal intestinal lengthening and tailoring on liver function in short bowel syndrome. Eur J Pediatr Surg 2008 Aug;18(4):249–253.

12 Celiac Disease

Stefano Guandalini, MD

CONTENTS

INTRODUCTION
EPIDEMIOLOGY
PATHOPHYSIOLOGY
CLINICAL PRESENTATION
DIAGNOSIS
TREATMENT
COMPLICATIONS
REFERENCES

Summary

Celiac disease (CD) is an autoimmune disorder occurring in genetically susceptible individuals, triggered by gluten and related prolamins, and plant storage proteins found in wheat, barley, and rye. It affects primarily the small intestine, where it progressively leads to flattening of the small intestinal mucosa and subsequent nutrient malabsorption. Its pathogenesis involves interactions among genetic, environmental, and immunological factors. Well-identified haplotypes in the HLA class II region (DQ2, DQ8) confer a large part of the genetic susceptibility to CD. Four possible presentations of CD are recognized: (1) typical, characterized mostly by gastrointestinal signs and symptoms; (2) atypical or extra-intestinal, where gastrointestinal signs/symptoms are minimal or absent and a number of extra-intestinal manifestations are present; (3) silent, where the small intestinal mucosa is damaged and CD autoimmunity can be detected by serology, but there are minimal or no symptoms; and

From: *Diarrhea, Clinical Gastroenterology*
Edited by: S. Guandalini, H. Vaziri, DOI 10.1007/978-1-60761-183-7_12
© Springer Science+Business Media, LLC 2011

finally (4) latent: these individuals, who possess genetic compatibility with CD and may also show positive autoimmune serology, have a normal mucosa morphology and may or may not be symptomatic. The diagnosis of celiac disease still rests on the demonstration of changes in the histology of the small intestinal mucosa. Currently, serological screening tests (serum levels of IgA–anti-tissue transglutaminase are generally acknowledged as the first choice) are utilized primarily to identify those individuals in need of a diagnostic endoscopic biopsy. Serology, including the newer anti-deamidated gliadin peptides, is also employed in monitoring the response to a gluten-free diet, which constitutes the only available treatment. Newer forms of treatment which will probably be available include enzymes degrading gluten to be ingested with meals; the use of substrates regulating intestinal permeability so as to prevent gluten entry across the epithelium; the development of genetically modified grains; and finally the development of different forms of immunotherapy.

Key Words: Celiac, Malabsorption, Chronic diarrhea, Autoimmunity, Diabetes, Down syndrome, Short stature, Gluten, Gliadin, Tissue transglutaminase, Anti-endomysium antibodies, Deamidated gliadin peptides, Marsh, Villous atrophy, Intraepithelial lymphocytes, Refractory sprue, EATL, Enamel hypoplasia

INTRODUCTION

Celiac disease (CD) is an autoimmune disorder which occurs in genetically susceptible individuals, is triggered by a well-identified autoantigen (gluten and related prolamins), and affects primarily the small intestine, where it progressively leads to flattening of the small intestinal mucosa. Three cereals contain gluten and are therefore toxic for celiac patients: wheat, rye, and barley [1].

The genetic susceptibility to CD is conferred by well-identified haplotypes in the HLA class II region: either DR3 (or DR5/ DR7) or HLA DR4. Such haplotypes are expressed on the antigen-presenting cells of the mucosa, with the heterodimer DQ2 being present in about 90% of all celiac disease patients and the heterodimer DQ8 occurring in 5–8% of patients. In the few remaining patients, half of the above heterodimers are found which seems to be sufficient enough to confer susceptibility to the disease. Recent studies have been able to quantify the risk conferred by different genetic assets [2].

EPIDEMIOLOGY

The availability of sensitive and specific serological tests has allowed for the detection of minimally symptomatic or even asymptomatic

Chapter 12 / Celiac Disease

cases of CD, providing a more accurate estimate of its true prevalence. This has led to an increased prevalence of CD which is thought to affect about 1% of the general population throughout Europe and North America [3]. Recent evidence suggests that the prevalence of CD continues to increase, in both Europe [4] and the USA [5].

Its prevalence in other areas of the world, however, has been less studied. Cases of CD have been reported in Latin America, North Africa, the Near and Middle East, and northwest India with an almost similar prevalence rate to those indicated above when such data are available [6]. In some ethnicities, such as in the Saharawi population, celiac disease has been found in as many as 5% of the general population [7]. Thus, it is fair to assume that celiac disease constitutes one of the most common genetically induced chronic diseases. However, it is extremely rare in people from African, Chinese, or Japanese descent, where the prevalence of the HLA haplotypes DQ2 and DQ8 is negligible.

Although gluten is the major environmental factor involved, there are other less known important risks for development of celiac disease, such as the timing of gluten introduction into the infant diet (where there is a higher risk of developing CD if gluten is introduced during the first 3 months of life [8]); the amount of gluten consumption (with an increased risk of disease with a higher intake of gluten) [9]; breast feeding at the time of gluten introduction which has been found to have a protective effect against the development of CD [10]; and lastly, there may also be a role for intestinal infections in infancy, which has been suggested by the finding that frequent rotavirus infections are more common in celiac children than in matched controls [11].

PATHOPHYSIOLOGY

Immunology

Celiac patients present with a complex immunological reaction to ingested gluten encompassing both innate and adaptive immunity and leading to progressive inflammation and severe destruction of the mucosal lining of the small bowel.

ADAPTIVE IMMUNITY

The adaptive immune response to gluten has been described with the identification of specific peptide sequences that bind to HLA-DQ2 or HLA-DQ8 molecules and stimulate gluten-specific CD4 T cells. These T cells express α/β T-cell receptor (TCR) and can be isolated from the lamina propria (LP). They have been shown to recognize specific gluten peptides presented through interaction with DQ2 or DQ8 molecules.

Gluten is a complex macromolecule containing a large amount of proline and glutamine residues which make it largely indigestible. Among the undigested peptides, one particular peptide fragment (the alpha gliadin 33-mer) contains an immunodominant peptide fragment, which after crossing the subepithelial layer is deamidated by the enzyme tissue transglutaminase 2 (TG2). Such modification creates a strong negative charge within the peptide and increases its affinity for the binding pockets of the HLA-DQ2 or HLA-DQ8 molecules on the antigen-presenting cells. This binding then leads to the induction of T-cell proliferation and a Th1 cytokine response, primarily with the release of interferon-γ.

INNATE IMMUNITY

Intraepithelial CD8+ TCRαβ T lymphocytes (IELs) play an important role in the destruction of epithelial cells. Through specific natural killer receptors, expressed on their surface, IELs recognize MHC-I molecules, induced on the enterocyte surface by stress and inflammation. This interaction activates these IELs to become lymphokine-activated killer cells, which then cause epithelial cell death [12]. This process is enhanced specifically via the cytokine IL-15, which is highly expressed in celiac mucosa.

As a result of the immunologic mechanisms, which are briefly outlined above, the following pathologic changes can be seen in celiac disease.

Pathology

The classic celiac lesion occurs in the proximal small intestine, with typical histological changes including villous atrophy, crypt hyperplasia, and increased intraepithelial lymphocytosis. Classified by Marsh ([13], see below), several distinct and progressive histological stages have been described as follows:

a. Type 0 or pre-infiltrative stage (completely normal histology);
b. Type 1 or infiltrative stage (increased intraepithelial lymphocytes);
c. Type 2 or hyperplastic stage (type 1 + crypt hyperplasia);
d. Type 3 or destructive stage (type 2 + villous atrophy with progressive severity categorized as a, b, and c).

CLINICAL PRESENTATION

While the original description of the manifestations of celiac disease was centered on its gastrointestinal and nutritional components, we have come to realize that not only can it result in a wide variety of clinical presentations, but sometimes it can exist in the complete absence of gastrointestinal symptoms. Indeed asymptomatic or minimally symptomatic cases of celiac disease are probably the most common, especially in older children and adults.

The four possible presentations of CD are described below [1] (see Table 12.1):

Table 12.1

Possible presentations of celiac disease (all subjects are positive for HLA-DQ2 and/or HLA-DQ8 *and* may also show positive celiac disease autoimmunity)

Typical	Gastrointestinal signs/symptoms predominate: • Diarrhea • Vomiting • Failure to thrive • Anorexia • Recurrent abdominal pain • Constipation
Atypical or extraintestinal	Gastrointestinal signs/symptoms are minimal or absent. Most common signs/symptoms of extraintestinal celiac disease are reported in Table 12.3
Silent	No signs/symptoms. Gluten-dependent duodenal mucosal changes confirm the diagnosis of celiac disease
Latent	No signs/symptoms. Duodenal mucosa is normal. Gluten-dependent changes with or without symptoms to appear later in time

- Typical: Gastrointestinal signs and symptoms predominate. In this category, serology for CD is almost invariably positive and bioptic findings confirm the diagnosis.
- Atypical: Gastrointestinal signs and symptoms are minimal or absent, but there are various extraintestinal manifestations present. Serology for CD is positive and bioptic findings confirm the diagnosis.
- Silent: The small intestinal mucosa is damaged (Marsh II–III) and CD autoimmunity can be detected by serology. However, these subjects do not have any overt symptoms.
- Latent (or "potential"): Asymptomatic patients, with a normal or minimally abnormal mucosa (Marsh 0–I). These individuals have a genetic susceptibility to CD and may also have positive autoimmune serology. Recent studies show that full-blown CD may ensue at a later time in at least some of these individuals [14].

"Typical" Celiac Disease: Gastrointestinal Manifestations

The so-called typical form of CD presents with gastrointestinal symptoms and is more prevalent in children than in adults, with a peak age at diagnosis between 6 and 24 months of age. A typical celiac young girl is exemplified by the patient in Fig. 12.1. Symptoms begin at variable times after the introduction of foods containing gluten.

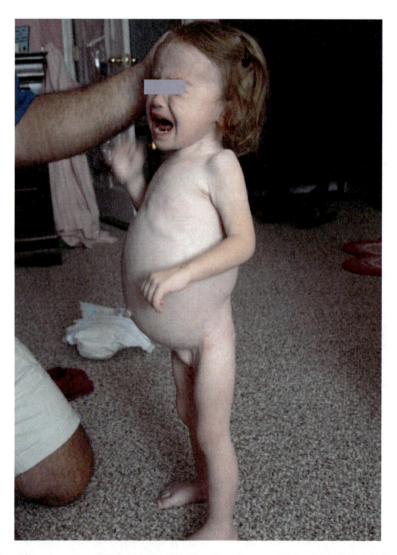

Fig. 12.1. A young child with "typical" celiac disease. This girl is 24 months old. Note the sad, irritabile expression, the emaciated extremities, and very protuberant abdomen.

Infants and young children typically present with chronic diarrhea, anorexia, abdominal distension, abdominal pain, poor weight gain or weight loss, and recurrent vomiting. The diarrhea is most commonly described as three to five bulky, foul-smelling bowel movements per day. The stools are occasionally frothy and may float in the toilet water. Undigested food particles are rarely observed, as the intraluminal digestive processes are generally intact. With delayed diagnosis severe malnutrition can occur. Behavioral changes are common and include irritability and an introverted attitude. Rarely, severely affected infants present with a "celiac crisis" characterized by explosive watery diarrhea, marked abdominal distension, dehydration, hypotension, and lethargy, often with profound electrolyte abnormalities including severe hypokalemia.

In older children and teenagers, as well as in adults, CD commonly presents with gastrointestinal manifestations consisting of intermittent, recurrent diarrhea with one to three bowel movements per day. The stools have the same appearance to those previously described for younger children, although they tend to be more watery. Other commonly associated GI and systemic symptoms commonly include abdominal bloating, discomfort, and weight loss; with the latter in part being due to a voluntary reduction in food intake secondary to a fear of feeling bloated or experiencing diarrhea upon eating. This is different from what is seen clinically in patients with irritable bowel syndrome.

"Atypical" Celiac Disease: Extraintestinal Manifestations

An increasing number of patients, especially at an older age, are being diagnosed with CD without having typical gastrointestinal manifestations [15]. It is reasonable to assume that currently more than 50% of patients with newly diagnosed CD do not present with gastrointestinal symptoms. As mentioned earlier, there appears to be a relationship between the age of onset and the type of clinical presentation with gastrointestinal symptoms and failure to thrive occurring predominantly in infants and toddlers, minor GI symptoms, inadequate weight and height gain and delayed puberty taking place in children, and anemia primarily in teenagers and young adults. In older adults and in the elderly, minor GI symptoms are more prevalent. Table 12.2 summarizes the main extraintestinal manifestations of celiac disease, which are discussed below in further detail.

- *Dermatitis herpetiformis*: A blistering skin rash which involves the elbows, knees, and buttocks and is associated with dermal granular immunoglobulin (Ig) A deposits. The rash as well as the mucosal morphology improves on a gluten-free diet (GFD). It should be emphasized

Table 12.2
"Atypical" (or "extraintestinal") celiac disease

Main presenting signs/symptoms

- Dermatitis herpetiformis
- Permanent enamel hypoplasia
- Iron deficiency anemia resistant to PO Fe
- Short stature, delayed puberty
- Chronic hepatitis with hypertransaminasemia
- Arthritis
- Osteopenia/osteoporosis
- Epilepsy with occipital calcifications
- Primary ataxia, white matter focal lesions
- Psychiatric disorders

that dermatitis herpetiformis is a rare occurrence in children and is almost exclusively described in teenagers and adults.

- *Dental enamel hypoplasia*: These enamel defects involve only the permanent dentition and may be the only presenting manifestation of celiac disease. Often, no or minimal gastrointestinal symptoms are present.
- *Iron deficiency anemia*: Iron deficiency anemia, resistant to oral iron supplementation, has been shown to be the most common extraintestinal manifestation of celiac disease in adults in several studies. In children, however, while the finding of anemia is common, iron deficiency is seldomly seen as the sole presenting sign.
- *Short stature and delayed puberty*: Short stature may be the only manifestation of celiac disease. As many as 10% of children with "idiopathic" short stature may have CD that can be detected by serologic testing. Some cases of short stature in the context of CD also have impaired growth hormone production, which can be confirmed by provocative stimulation tests. This usually normalizes with consumption of a gluten-free diet. Adolescent girls with untreated celiac disease may have delayed onset of menarche.
- *Chronic hepatitis and hypertransaminasemia*: Patients with untreated CD commonly have elevated transaminases (ALT, AST). It is estimated that as many as 9% of patients with elevated transaminase levels of unclear etiology may have silent celiac disease. Liver biopsies in these patients show nonspecific reactive hepatitis. In the majority of cases, liver enzymes normalize on a gluten-free diet.
- *Arthritis and arthralgia*: Arthritis can occur in adults with celiac disease, even while on a gluten-free diet. Up to 3% of children with juvenile chronic arthritis may have celiac disease [16].

Chapter 12 / Celiac Disease

- *Osteopenia/osteoporosis*: At the time of diagnosis approximately 50% of children and 75% of adults have a low bone mineral density, even reaching severe degrees that are consistent with osteoporosis. Bone mineral density improves in the majority of patients on a gluten-free diet and may be normalized as soon as 1 year after initiation of diet in children. However, the response to diet can be much less pronounced in adults.
- *Neurological manifestations*: A number of neurological conditions have been attributed to CD in adults and, to a lesser extent, in children. Celiac disease may cause occipital calcifications and intractable epilepsy that can be resistant to anti-seizure medications, but may benefit from a gluten-free diet if started soon after the onset of seizures [17]. An association with cerebellar ataxia is well described in adults, in which case the term "gluten-induced ataxia" has been proposed [18].
- *Psychiatric disorders*: Although in recent years a large number of behavioral disorders, such as autism, attention deficit-hyperactivity disorder, have been thought to be caused by CD, there is no evidence thus far of such a causal relationship. CD nevertheless *can* be associated with some psychiatric disorders, such as depression and anxiety. These conditions can be severe and usually will respond to a gluten-free diet.

Associated Diseases

Celiac disease is also known to be strongly associated with a number of other disorders, and specifically with certain autoimmune conditions and some genetic syndromes, the most common of which are listed in Table 12.3.

The association of CD with autoimmune conditions has been recognized for many years [19]. There is a strong positive correlation between the older age at diagnosis of CD and the presence of

Table 12.3
Main conditions associated with celiac disease

Condition	Approximate prevalence of celiac disease (%)
Insulin-dependent diabetes mellitus	8
Thyroiditis	5
Sjögren syndrome and other connective tissue diseases	4
Down syndrome	12
Williams syndrome	5
Turner syndrome	5
First-degree relatives of celiac patients	8 – 10

co-existing autoimmune disorders such as type I diabetes, thyroiditis, alopecia, which suggests that the continuous ingestion of gluten (as it occurs before the diagnosis is made) may induce the development of other autoimmune conditions [20].

- *Type 1 (insulin-dependent) diabetes*: It is estimated that approximately 10% of patients with type 1 diabetes mellitus have typical features of CD on duodenal biopsies. Many individuals with type 1 diabetes who initially test negative for CD with serologic tests will eventually test positive, which mandates the need for repeated testing. Since CD only occurs in patients with specific HLA haplotypes as indicated above, an algorithm has been developed to avoid repeated testing in **all** patients with type 1 diabetes. In this algorithm, patients should be tested for commonly associated haplotypes to determine the population at risk. Re-screening with serological tests should then be performed only in those patients who have a susceptible HLA haplotype.
- Typically, the diagnosis of diabetes precedes that of celiac disease by years, which most commonly presents with no or only mild gastrointestinal symptoms [21]. As some of these symptoms are also seen in patients with diabetes (e.g., bloating or diarrhea), the diagnosis of CD may be missed, unless screening tests are performed. Although there is no convincing evidence that a GFD has any obvious effect on the course of diabetes, the diet is still recommended, in order to prevent long-term complications of CD that can occur also in minimally symptomatic patients. Thus, the case for screening type 1 diabetic for CD seems very reasonable.
- *Down syndrome*: The best-documented and well-known association of CD with a non-autoimmune disorder is that with Down syndrome [22]. The prevalence of Down syndrome in CD, as assessed by screening methods, has been found to be between 8 and 12%. The majority of cases have some gastrointestinal symptoms, such as abdominal bloating, intermittent diarrhea, anorexia, or have failure to thrive; however, about one-third of them do not have any gastrointestinal symptoms. Similar to patients with diabetes, screening with serological markers has been suggested in genetically susceptible cases (cases with HLA-DQ2 and/or HLA-DQ8). The same approach should be applied to screen for CD in patients with Turner and Williams syndrome, where an increased incidence of CD has also been reported.

DIAGNOSIS

The diagnosis of celiac disease is made by the following:

A. Documenting the histologic changes of the duodenal mucosa, which are characterized by a progressive deterioration of the villous architecture

Chapter 12 / Celiac Disease

associated with a progressive increase in crypt length and density, while on a gluten-containing diet (see above). Biopsies are obtained by endoscopy. It is recommended that multiple biopsies be obtained (at least four), in order to avoid a false-negative result, which may occur in the occasional patients with patchy lesions. Although endoscopically visible changes have been described (scalloping or nodularity of the mucosa and sparse duodenal folds), such findings are neither sensitive nor specific and the diagnosis of CD should not depend on their presence or absence.

B. Documenting the clinical and laboratory response to a gluten-free diet particularly the disappearance of autoantibodies (anti-tissue transglutaminase or anti-endomysium antibodies) is key.

Evidence-based guidelines for the diagnosis approach of CD were introduced in 2005 by the North American Society for Pediatric Gastroenterology, Hepatology and Nutrition (NASPGHAN) [23]. These guidelines are similar to those previously proposed by the European Society for Pediatric Gastroenterology, Hepatology and Nutrition (ESPGHAN) in 1990 [24]. There is some evidence that patients may fulfill the diagnostic criteria for CD even in the presence of Marsh I or II changes only, especially when a high titer of anti-endomysium antibodies is present (see below for the role of serology in diagnosis of CD in such circumstances) [14].

The Role of Serology in the Diagnosis of Celiac Disease

In clinical practice, serologic tests are useful in identifying children who may require an intestinal biopsy in order to diagnose CD. In addition, as mentioned previously, these tests can support the diagnosis in patients with less characteristic histopathologic features of CD on small intestinal biopsy and may also have a role in monitoring the response to treatment.

There are a number of serologic tests that are commercially available. The anti-endomysial IgA antibody (EMA-IgA) and the anti-tissue transglutaminase IgA (TTG-IgA) antibody tests have both proven to be highly sensitive and specific with values approaching 95% in most studies, in both adults and children.

Elevated levels of anti-EMA, when associated with gastrointestinal symptoms, seem to have an extremely high positive predictive value. This appears to be true in both adults and children even in the presence of minimal or no enteropathy (Marsh 0–II), which may make the small bowel biopsy unnecessary in this situation. It should, however, be emphasized that this does not apply to the patients with only TTG-IgA positivity.

TREATMENT

Complete and lifelong avoidance of gluten ingestion is the only treatment currently available for celiac disease. Wheat, rye, and barley are the grains containing toxic peptides. In symptomatic patients who adhere to a gluten-free diet, the gastrointestinal symptoms resolve in a short period of time, typically within a few weeks for children, but up to a few months in adults. Normalization of hematological and biochemical parameters can be expected to follow. In children, improved rate of growth with respect to both height and weight, with an end result of normal stature, is the norm. The decrease in bone mineralization, which is seen in up to 50% of cases at the time of diagnosis, is also expected to resolve within about a year. The physical and psychological well-being of the affected child will also improve when placed on a GFD.

In some adult patients, persistence of some of the symptoms as well as of various degrees of intestinal inflammation has been recently reported [25] in spite of a reliable adherence to a gluten-free diet.

For a long time, elimination of oats from the diet had been recommended. However, a growing body of scientific evidence obtained from in vitro studies as well as from clinical investigations has demonstrated that they are safe in the vast majority of celiac patients. This is true mostly for adults but has more recently been shown to be the case in children as well [26–30]. Secondary to uncontrolled harvesting and milling procedures, as well as the possibility that lines employed in the manufacturing of wheat-based flours are also used in the preparation of oats-based foods, cross-contamination of oats with gluten is still a concern. This calls for great caution in selecting oat-containing products.

In the initial phases of dietary treatment, lactose is often eliminated too, as relative lactase deficiency is thought to accompany the flat mucosa. However, this may not be true for many of the cases that are recently being diagnosed which do not manifest with overt malabsorption. Furthermore, even in cases with obvious malabsorption, the recovery of lactase activity is typically fast, with a lactose-free diet being necessary for only a short period of time.

Although the possibility of an association between celiac disease and milk protein allergy has been repeatedly raised in past years, however, the current thought is that these two conditions may simply co-exist, which makes avoidance of "dairy products" in all patients with CD unnecessary.

The American Dietetic Association (http://www.eatright.org/) has published guidelines for the dietary treatment of CD patients. These guidelines are periodically reviewed and provide a reliable source of information for a GFD. However, given the dynamics of this field, the diet requires ongoing collaboration between patients, health-care providers, and dietitians. In this regard, a recently proposed score might prove to be useful [31].

Recently, new therapeutic possibilities are appearing at the horizon. Celiac patients appear to have a higher intestinal permeability, possibly caused by increased presence of the paracrine protein zonulin. Thus, an octapeptide (larazotide) with homology to zonulin was developed in order to block the zonulin receptor, thus increasing the tightness of the tight junctions and greatly limit the entry of gliadin peptides across them. Such preparation appeared safe in a pilot study on celiac patients in remission and controls, and it proved able to prevent the increase in intestinal permeability after a challenge with gluten [32]. Further studies are in progress with this promising strategy.

Another strategy is also actively pursued, based on the ability of some bacterial enzymes to completely digest gluten, thus potentially detoxifying it before any sizeable amounts reach the small intestinal mucosa [33]. On this basis, a commercial preparation consisting of a glutamine-specific endoprotease and a prolyl endopeptidase [34] called ALV-003 has been developed and is currently being experimented. Preliminary studies in adult patients with celiac disease with this preparation appear promising [35].

It is therefore quite likely that within the next few years celiac patients will have at their disposal some new pharmaceutical preparations to help them cope with the risk of inadvertent gluten ingestion, as they continue to follow their gluten-free diet.

COMPLICATIONS

Refractory Celiac Disease

Better known by the older terminology as "refractory sprue," refractory CD is a very severe form of celiac disease that does not respond to a gluten-free diet [36]. Refractory CD most commonly occurs in adults or elderly patients who have been suffering from malabsorptive symptoms for a long time prior to being diagnosed. This condition is further classified into type I and type II on the basis of gamma chain T-cell clonal rearrangement and aberrant T-cell phenotypes. Type II refractory celiac disease is the most aggressive form, leading to the most feared complication of celiac disease: the enteropathy-associated T-cell lymphoma (EATL). As a consequence, refractory CD results in an increased mortality rate, with a 5-year survival rate of 80–96% for patients with type I refractory CD and 44–58% for type II cases [36].

When examining the survival rate of those patients with type II refractory CD who developed EATL, then the survival rate at 5 years is a dismal 8% [37]. Of interest, epidemiological studies have shown that if EATL has not developed within 3 years of diagnosis and initiating a gluten-free diet, the risk of developing this complication diminishes significantly, to even lower than that expected in the general population [38]. Recently, in a prospective trial, treatment with an autologous stem cell transplant has been utilized with some success in these patients [39].

Increased Mortality Rate

Aside from the risks related to refractory CD, evidence is mounting that unrecognized, and hence untreated, celiac disease may carry a risk for increased mortality rate [40]. There appears to be a positive correlation between diagnostic delay and/or insufficient compliance with the diet and decreased life expectancy, which has been documented in a large retrospective study in Italy [41]. More recently, increased mortality has also been reported in undiagnosed patients (based on elevated serum TTG-IgA) in the United States [5] and in Europe [42–44].

However, a very recent population-based large study in Minnesota, USA [45], concluded that older adults with undiagnosed celiac disease, while presenting with clearly reduced bone health, had otherwise quite limited comorbidity and no increase in mortality compared to controls.

In conclusion, in spite of some uncertainties on the real long-term impact of maintaining a gluten-containing diet in asymptomatic individuals with celiac disease, it is fair to state that an aggressive strategy for early detection and treatment of patients with celiac disease, especially young ones, appears justified.

REFERENCES

1. Guandalini S. Celiac disease in essential pediatric gastroenterology. In: Guandalini S, ed. Hepatology and nutrition. New York, NY: McGraw-Hill, 2005, pp. 221–230.
2. Pietzak MM, et al. Stratifying risk for celiac disease in a large at-risk United States population by using HLA alleles. Clin Gastroenterol Hepatol 2009; 7(9):966–971.
3. Fasano A, et al. Prevalence of celiac disease in at-risk and not-at-risk groups in the United States: a large multicenter study. Arch Intern Med 2003; 163(3):286–292.
4. Lohi S, et al. Increasing prevalence of coeliac disease over time. Aliment Pharmacol Ther 2007; 26(9): 1217–1225.
5. Rubio-Tapia A, et al. Increased prevalence and mortality in undiagnosed celiac disease. Gastroenterology 2009; 137(1):88–93.
6. Cummins AG, Roberts-Thomson IC. Prevalence of celiac disease in the Asia-Pacific region. J Gastroenterol Hepatol 2009; 24(8):1347–1351.

Chapter 12 / Celiac Disease

7. Catassi C, et al. Why is coeliac disease endemic in the people of the Sahara? Lancet 1999; 354(9179):647–648.
8. Norris JM, et al. Risk of celiac disease autoimmunity and timing of gluten introduction in the diet of infants at increased risk of disease. JAMA 2005; 293(19):2343–2351.
9. Ivarsson A, et al. Breast-feeding protects against celiac disease. Am J Clin Nutr 2002 75(5):914–921.
10. Akobeng AK, et al. Effect of breast feeding on risk of coeliac disease: a systematic review and meta-analysis of observational studies. Arch Dis Child 2006; 91(1): 39–43.
11. Stene LC, et al. Rotavirus infection frequency and risk of celiac disease autoimmunity in early childhood: a longitudinal study. Am J Gastroenterol 2006: 101(10): 2333–2340.
12. Meresse B, et al. Reprogramming of CTLs into natural killer-like cells in celiac disease. J Exp Med 2006: 203(5):1343–1355.
13. Marsh MN. Gluten, major histocompatibility complex, and the small intestine. A molecular and immunobiologic approach to the spectrum of gluten sensitivity ('celiac sprue'). Gastroenterology 1992; 102(1):330–354.
14. Kurppa K, et al. Diagnosing mild enteropathy celiac disease: a randomized, controlled clinical study. Gastroenterology 2009; 136(3):816–823.
15. Bottaro G, et al. The clinical pattern of subclinical/silent celiac disease: an analysis on 1026 consecutive cases. Am J Gastroenterol 1999; 94(3):691–696.
16. Lepore L, et al. Prevalence of celiac disease in patients with juvenile chronic arthritis. J Pediatr 1996; 129(2):311–313.
17. Gobbi G. Coeliac disease, epilepsy and cerebral calcifications. Brain Dev 2005; 27(3):189–200.
18. Hadjivassiliou M, et al. Gluten ataxia. Cerebellum 2008; 7(3):494–498.
19. Barker JM, Liu E. Celiac disease: pathophysiology, clinical manifestations, and associated autoimmune conditions. Adv Pediatr 2008; 55:349–365.
20. Ventura A, Magazzu G, Greco L. Duration of exposure to gluten and risk for autoimmune disorders in patients with celiac disease. SIGEP study group for autoimmune disorders in celiac disease. Gastroenterology 1999; 117(2):297–303.
21. Holmes GK. Coeliac disease and type 1 diabetes mellitus - the case for screening. Diabet Med 2001; 18(3): 169–177.
22. Cohen WI. Current dilemmas in Down syndrome clinical care: celiac disease, thyroid disorders, and atlanto-axial instability. Am J Med Genet C Semin Med Genet 2006; 142C(3):141–148.
23. Hill ID, et al. Guideline for the diagnosis and treatment of celiac disease in children: recommendations of the North American Society for Pediatric Gastroenterology, Hepatology and Nutrition. J Pediatr Gastroenterol Nutr 2005; 40(1):1–19.
24. Walker-Smith J, et al. Revised criteria for diagnosis of coeliac disease. Report of a Working Group of ESPGAN Arch Dis Child 1990; 65:909–911.
25. Lanzini A, et al. Complete recovery of intestinal mucosa occurs very rarely in adult coeliac patients despite adherence to gluten-free diet. Aliment Pharmacol Ther 2009; 29(12):1299–1308.
26. Koskinen O, et al. Oats do not induce systemic or mucosal autoantibody response in children with coeliac disease. J Pediatr Gastroenterol Nutr 2009; 48(5): 559–565.
27. Ellis HJ, Ciclitira PJ. Should coeliac sufferers be allowed their oats? Eur J Gastroenterol Hepatol 2008; 20(6):492–493.

28. Troncone R, Auricchio R,Granata V. Issues related to gluten-free diet in coeliac disease. Curr Opin Clin Nutr Metab Care 2008; 11(3):329–333.
29. Guandalini S. The influence of gluten: weaning recommendations for healthy children and children at risk for celiac disease. Nestle Nutr Workshop Ser Pediatr Program 2007; 60:139–151; discussion 151–155.
30. Garsed K, Scott BB. Can oats be taken in a gluten-free diet? A systematic review. Scand J Gastroenterol 2007; 42(2):171–178.
31. Biagi F, et al. A gluten-free diet score to evaluate dietary compliance in patients with coeliac disease. Br J Nutr 2009; 102(6):882–887.
32. Paterson BM, et al. The safety, tolerance, pharmacokinetic and pharmacodynamic effects of single doses of AT-1001 in coeliac disease subjects: a proof of concept study. Aliment Pharmacol Ther 2007; 26(5):757–766.
33. Siegel M, et al. Rational design of combination enzyme therapy for celiac sprue. Chem Biol 2006; 13(6):649–658.
34. Gass J, et al. Combination enzyme therapy for gastric digestion of dietary gluten in patients with celiac sprue. Gastroenterology, 2007; 133(2):472–480.
35. Tye-Din JA, et al. The effects of ALV003 pre-digestion of gluten on immune response and symptoms in celiac disease in vivo. Clin Immunol 2010; 134(3): 289–295.
36. Biagi F, Corazza GR. Defining gluten refractory enteropathy. Eur J Gastroenterol Hepatol 2001; 13(5):561–565.
37. Al-Toma A, et al. Survival in refractory coeliac disease and enteropathy-associated T-cell lymphoma: retrospective evaluation of single-centre experience. Gut 2007; 56(10):1373–1378.
38. Silano M, et al. Effect of a gluten-free diet on the risk of enteropathy-associated T-cell lymphoma in celiac disease. Dig Dis Sci 2008; 53(4):972–6.
39. Al-Toma A, Verbeek WH, Mulder CJ. Update on the management of refractory coeliac disease. J Gastrointestin Liver Dis, 2007; 16(1):57–63.
40. Biagi F, Corazza GR. Mortality in celiac disease. Nat Rev Gastroenterol Hepatol 2010;7(3):158–162.
41. Corrao G, et al. Mortality in patients with coeliac disease and their relatives: a cohort study. Lancet 2001; 358(9279):356–361.
42. Lohi S, et al. Prognosis of unrecognized coeliac disease as regards mortality: a population-based cohort study. Ann Med 2009;41(7):508–515.
43. Metzger MH, et al. Mortality excess in individuals with elevated IgA anti-transglutaminase antibodies: the KORA/MONICA Augsburg cohort study 1989–1998. Eur J Epidemiol, 2006; 21(5):359–365.
44. Solaymani-Dodaran M, West J, Logan RF. Long-term mortality in people with celiac disease diagnosed in childhood compared with adulthood: a population-based cohort study. Am J Gastroenterol 2007; 102(4):864–870.
45. Godfrey JD, et al. Morbidity and mortality among older individuals with undiagnosed celiac disease. Gastroenterology 2010; doi:10.1053/j.gastro.2010.05.041.

13 Whipple Disease

George T. Fantry, MD

CONTENTS

INTRODUCTION
EPIDEMIOLOGY
ETIOLOGY AND PATHOGENESIS
PATHOLOGY
DIAGNOSIS
TREATMENT AND PROGNOSIS
REFERENCES

Summary

A rare and chronic infection occurring primarily in Caucasian males and caused by the microorganism *Tropheryma whipplei*, Whipple disease involves the small intestine, where it leads to malabsorption, but it also causes a systemic infection with extraintestinal signs and symptoms. It is currently thought that an abnormal host response may play a central role in the pathogenesis of the disease, as the monocyte/macrophage function appears impaired. The clinical manifestations vary widely: as in the majority of cases the small intestine is involved, diarrhea is a predominant symptom, often associated with various degrees of malabsorption and fatigue. Extraintestinal manifestations are less common but are well described. They include seronegative arthritis, fever or neurological symptoms. Whipple disease should be considered in the differential diagnosis of malabsorption as well as in patients with unexplained weight loss, arthritis, culture negative endocarditis and fever of unknown origin. Endoscopy with small intestinal mucosal biopsy is the diagnostic

From: *Diarrhea, Clinical Gastroenterology*
Edited by: S. Guandalini, H. Vaziri, DOI 10.1007/978-1-60761-183-7_13
© Springer Science+Business Media, LLC 2011

test of choice and is required for a definitive diagnosis. Treatment consists in a prolonged course of antibiotic therapy. Many antibiotic regimens effective against gram-positive organisms have been used successfully to treat Whipple disease. In patients who complete a course of effective antibiotic therapy, the prognosis is excellent. Extraintestinal symptoms often disappear within a few days and gastrointestinal symptoms frequently resolve within 1 month. Within a few months, most patients are asymptomatic. However, despite the initial response to antibiotic therapy, relapses are common: they can occur during treatment or even months to years after its completion.

Key Words: Whipple disease, *Tropheryma whipplei*, Diarrhea, Steatorrhea, Malabsorption, Arthritis, Fever, Weight loss, Lymphadenopathy, Hyperpigmentation, Anemia, Small intestinal Mucosal biopsy, PAS-positive macrophages, Electron microscopy, Trimethoprim–sulfamethoxazole

INTRODUCTION

Whipple disease is a rare, chronic, systemic infection caused by *Tropheryma whipplei*. The clinical manifestations vary widely. In the majority of cases, the small intestine is involved, resulting in diarrhea and malabsorption. Extraintestinal manifestations include seronegative arthritis, fever, or neurological symptoms. An important advance in our understanding of Whipple disease occurred when the uncultured bacillus of Whipple disease, *Tropheryma whippelii* [1], was identified using PCR techniques. Subsequently, the bacterium was successfully cultured in vitro, permitting antibiotic susceptibility testing [2]. These developments have led to the design of more specific diagnostic testing [3, 4].

EPIDEMIOLOGY

Whipple disease occurs primarily in Caucasians with a strong male predominance. The disease is most common between the fourth and sixth decades of life [5–10]. Although there are no clearly defined geographic or environmental risk factors, Whipple disease appears to be more common in farmers and individuals involved in farm-related trades [5].

ETIOLOGY AND PATHOGENESIS

A major advance in the understanding of the pathogenesis of Whipple disease occurred with the identification of the causal bacterium, *T. whipplei*, using PCR amplification of 16S ribosomal RNA [11]

of intestinal tissues from patients with Whipple disease [1, 12]. Subsequently, *T. whipplei* was identified in various nonintestinal sites and has been cultured from human samples, including the CSF [13–16], consistent with the systemic nature of the disease [17, 18]. Phylogenetic analysis of *T. whipplei* places it within the class of *Actinobacter* [19].

T. whipplei appears to be a ubiquitous, commensal organism whose mode of transmission remains uncertain. Although the disease has been reported in families on a few occasions [20–22] direct person-to-person transmission has not been documented. These observations are consistent with a common environmental exposure and shared genetic susceptibility.

The finding of asymptomatic carriers of *T. whipplei* [23–27] and the striking clinical features of the disease with the persistence of intracellular bacteria in macrophages of patients with Whipple disease suggests that an abnormal host response may play a central role in the pathogenesis. In addition, many studies assessing the immune response to *T. whipplei* in vitro and in patients with Whipple disease reveal findings that strongly suggest an abnormal immune response and defective host defense which leads to the inability of the host to eliminate the causal bacteria [28–37]. These data demonstrate that underlying defects of monocyte/macrophage function play an important pathophysiologic role in the development of Whipple disease. Achieving a better understanding of the process of immune evasion has important clinical implications in patients with Whipple disease. Specifically, immunomodulating therapy with interferon-γ may be beneficial [38] and immunosuppressive therapy for chronic inflammatory arthropathy may be associated with the appearance or exacerbation of gastrointestinal symptoms [39, 40].

PATHOLOGY

In Whipple disease, the lamina propria of the small intestinal mucosa is infiltrated by large foamy macrophages that grossly distort normal villus architecture resulting in a blunted, club-like appearance. The cytoplasm of these macrophages is filled with large glycoprotein granules that stain with PAS. The lymphatic channels in the mucosa and submucosa are dilated. Electron microscopy reveals the characteristic rod-shaped bacillary bodies in the lamina propria, most abundant just beneath the absorptive epithelium [41–46]. The bacilli are often seen within the PAS-positive macrophages. Most of the PAS-positive glycoprotein within the macrophages represents remnants of the cell wall of the phagocytosed bacilli. PAS-positive macrophages and the characteristic bacilli have been identified in many nonintestinal tissues [47–51] as well, consistent with the systemic nature of the disease. Treatment is associated with a marked decrease in PAS-positive macrophages in the lamina propria; however, a few PAS-positive macrophages in patchy distribution often persist at long-term follow-up [52].

Clinical Features

The clinical presentation of Whipple disease consists of multiple gastrointestinal and extraintestinal symptoms that are highly variable (Table 13.1). Due to small intestinal involvement, gastrointestinal symptoms suggestive of malabsorption, particularly steatorrhea, with associated anorexia and weight loss are common. Diarrhea is the most common presenting complaint [6] and is present in approximately three-fourths of patients at the time of diagnosis [7–9]. However, although diarrhea affects most patients with Whipple disease, it is not invariably present. When present, the diarrhea is typically characterized as multiple large, watery, or semiformed stools suggestive of steatorrhea. Weight loss is the second most common presenting complaint in patients with Whipple disease and is present in most patients [6–9]. Severe cachexia may result from anorexia and malabsorption. Other less common gastrointestinal symptoms include abdominal bloating, distention, and cramps. Occasionally, gastrointestinal bleeding can occur; however, when present it is most often occult [9]. Constitutional symptoms such as fatigue and generalized weakness are also common. If malabsorption is unrecognized and untreated, specific vitamin and nutritional deficiencies and their associated symptoms may occur. As hypoalbuminemia occurs, ascites and peripheral edema may develop.

Table 13.1
Clinical manifestations of Whipple disease

Gastrointestinal	Extraintestinal
Diarrhea	Arthritis or arthralgias
Weight loss	Fever
Anorexia	Fatigue and lethargy
Abdominal cramps	Lymphadenopathy
Abdominal bloating	Hyperpigmentation
Hepatomegaly	Heart murmurs
Splenomegaly	Cognitive deficits
	Visual changes

Occasionally patients present only with extraintestinal symptoms, such as arthritis and fever, in the absence of gastrointestinal symptoms such as diarrhea (Table 13.1). Extraintestinal symptoms may precede gastrointestinal symptoms by many years. Given the nonspecific nature of the extraintestinal symptoms, there is often a delay of months to years prior to diagnosis. Arthritis is the most common extraintestinal symptom and affects the majority of patients [6–9]. It is typically an intermittent, migratory arthritis of both large and small joints and often develops several months to years before the initial diagnosis of Whipple disease. Some patients may only have arthralgias. Fever is the second most common extraintestinal symptom and is typically low grade and intermittent [6].

Numerous additional extraintestinal symptoms affecting multiple organ systems often develop due to the systemic nature of the infection. Pulmonary involvement is frequently manifested by chronic cough or pleuritic chest pain [6, 49, 53]. Cardiac involvement is often manifested as congestive heart failure, valvular lesions, or pericarditis [6, 48, 53–57]. Endocarditis can occur in the absence of clinically evident gastrointestinal disease [58–61].

Central nervous system (CNS) involvement in Whipple disease is common; however, symptoms related to CNS involvement are present in a minority of patients [62–67]. Neurological symptoms may occur in association with gastrointestinal symptoms or as isolated symptoms [5, 50, 68, 69]. Common CNS symptoms include dementia, paralysis of gaze, and myoclonus while hypothalamic involvement may be manifested by insomnia, hyperphagia, and polydipsia [5].

On physical examination, findings vary depending on the organ systems involved (Table 13.1). Nonspecific features related to severe malabsorption, such as emaciation and muscle wasting, are often present. The most common physical findings are hyperpigmentation and peripheral lymphadenopathy [6, 8, 9]. These findings are seen in greater than 50% of patients with Whipple disease. Other potential abdominal findings include mild distention and tenderness. Hepatomegaly and splenomegaly are uncommon [6, 9]. Ascites is also uncommon but may be evident in the presence of severe hypoalbuminemia. Additional physical findings that have been described in patients with Whipple disease are related to its systemic nature. These include fever, peripheral arthritis, heart murmurs, pleural or pericardial friction rubs, and ocular abnormalities. Finally, in the setting of CNS or cranial nerve involvement, the neurological examination may reveal dementia, ataxia, muscle weakness, sensory loss, and ophthalmoplegia.

Laboratory abnormalities are very common in patients with Whipple disease. Due to malabsorption, most patients have steatorrhea with low serum carotene levels and hypoalbuminemia [6, 8, 9, 70]. Electrolyte imbalances such as hypokalemia, hypomagnesemia, and hypocalcemia may be present in patients with severe diarrhea. Normochromic-normocytic anemia suggestive of chronic disease is very common [5–9]. Occasionally, the anemia is hypochromic-microcytic due to iron deficiency. Erythrocyte sedimentation rate is often elevated and the prothrombin time is often prolonged secondary to malabsorption of vitamin K [6].

DIAGNOSIS

Although rare, Whipple disease should be considered in the differential diagnosis of malabsorption as well as in patients with unexplained weight loss, seronegative arthritis, culture negative endocarditis, and fever of unknown origin. Endoscopy with small intestinal mucosal biopsy is the diagnostic test of choice and is required for a definitive diagnosis. Although biopsy is needed for diagnosis, endoscopic mucosal lesions, including the characteristic finding of pale, shaggy, yellow mucosa in the postbulbar duodenum, have been described [71–73].

The histopathological appearance of the small bowel mucosa in Whipple disease is distinct, unique, and usually diagnostic when present. Infiltration of the lamina propria of the small intestine by PAS-positive macrophages containing gram-positive, acid-fast-negative bacilli with associated lymphatic dilation is specific and diagnostic of Whipple disease. Electron microscopy should also be performed to verify the presence of the characteristic bacillus. Electron microscopy is particularly important during the follow-up of patients treated for Whipple disease. Although PAS positivity may persist for many years [6, 41, 74], electron microscopy in successfully treated patients shows disappearance of the Whipple bacillus.

While radiologic evaluation is not diagnostic of Whipple disease, a small bowel series or abdominal CT scan obtained in the evaluation of patients with unexplained diarrhea and weight loss can provide clues. In most patients with Whipple disease, the characteristic finding of marked thickening of the mucosal folds is seen, particularly in the proximal small intestine. In addition to the small bowel thickening, abdominal CT typically reveals large paraaortic and retroperitoneal adenopathy [6, 9, 75, 76].

PCR-based diagnostic tests are useful to confirm the diagnosis of Whipple disease and to monitor the response during antibiotic treatment [1, 3, 4, 12, 17, 18, 77–79]. In addition, PCR has been shown to have clinical value in the diagnosis of extraintestinal Whipple disease

[80–83]. A PCR assay on stool specimens may provide a diagnostic tool that does not require endoscopy [84, 85].

The differential diagnosis of Whipple disease includes other malabsorptive diseases with diffuse small intestinal involvement, such as celiac disease, and infiltrative diseases of the small intestine, such as intra-abdominal lymphoma. These diseases can be readily differentiated by small intestinal mucosal biopsy. *Mycobacterium avium* complex (MAC) infection can mimic Whipple disease as it causes infiltration of the lamina propria with PAS-positive macrophages [86, 87]; however, MAC bacilli are acid-fast, whereas the Whipple bacillus is not. PAS-positive macrophages in the intestinal lamina propria can also be seen in systemic histoplasmosis and macroglobulinemia. However, in systemic histoplasmosis, large, PAS-positive, rounded, encapsulated *Histoplasma* organisms are easily seen in macrophages. In macroglobulinemia, the faintly staining, homogeneously PAS-positive macrophages are distinctly different from those found in Whipple disease.

TREATMENT AND PROGNOSIS

Whipple disease is treated with a prolonged course of antibiotic therapy. Many antibiotic regimens effective against gram-positive organisms have been used successfully to treat Whipple disease [6, 41, 47, 88, 89]. Clinical experience has been confirmed by antibiotic susceptibility testing with doxycycline, macrolides, aminoglycosides, penicillin, rifampin, chloramphenicol, and trimethoprim–sulfamethoxazole (TMP–SMX) found to be active against *T. whipplei* [90–92]. *T. whipplei* is resistant to fluoroquinolones [90]. Despite the initial response to antibiotic therapy, relapses are common. Relapses can occur during treatment or months to years after completion of treatment [5, 6, 41, 65, 88]. CNS relapses tend to occur late and respond poorly to additional antibiotic therapy.

Given the concern for CNS relapse [65, 68, 88] treating all patients initially with an antibiotic that readily crosses the blood–brain barrier, such as TMP–SMX, is usually recommended. One double-strength tablet of TMP–SMX (160 mg of TMP and 800 mg of SMX) twice daily for 1 year is the best option [88]. Starting treatment with parenteral penicillin G (1.2 million U/day) and streptomycin (1.0 g/day) for 10–14 days may be of additional benefit [6, 88], resulting in the lowest relapse rate. This should be considered in all patients with Whipple disease, since compliance with the year-long prescribed regimen can be limited. A reasonable regimen for patients who are allergic to or cannot tolerate TMP–SMX is parenteral penicillin and streptomycin for

10–14 days followed by oral ampicillin for 1 year. In addition to antibiotic treatment, if severe malabsorption and malnutrition is present, supplementation of specific nutrients, such as folic acid, vitamin B_{12}, fat-soluble vitamins, and iron, should be given as replacement or to prevent deficiency.

After 1 year of antibiotic therapy, a small intestinal mucosal biopsy should be repeated to document the absence of residual bacilli. Although PAS-positive macrophages may persist in the lamina propria for many years in patients treated for Whipple disease, the presence of bacilli on electron microscopy suggests inadequate treatment. PCR for *T. whipplei* in the intestinal mucosa, if available, may provide useful information regarding the adequacy of therapy and the likelihood of relapse [3, 4].

In patients with Whipple disease who complete a course of effective antibiotic therapy, the prognosis is excellent. Extraintestinal symptoms often disappear within a few days and gastrointestinal symptoms frequently resolve within 1 month. Within a few months, most patients are asymptomatic. Once therapy has been stopped and intestinal biopsies are negative for bacilli, patients should be carefully followed clinically for evidence of relapse. If gastrointestinal or extraintestinal symptoms recur and relapse is suspected, small intestinal biopsy should be repeated and the mucosa should be assessed for the presence of bacilli. Treatment of a relapse of Whipple disease consists of a repeat course of the initial therapy. Clinical relapses of gastrointestinal symptoms and arthritis respond favorably to further antibiotic treatment, whereas CNS relapse has a relatively poor prognosis. Combination therapy with antibiotics and interferon-γ may be beneficial in patients with refractory Whipple disease [38].

REFERENCES

1. Relman DA, Schmidt TM, MacDermott RP, Falkow S. Identification of the uncultured bacillus of Whipple's disease. N Engl J Med 1992; 327:293.
2. Raoult D, Birg ML, La Scola B, et al. Cultivation of the bacillus of Whipple's disease. N Engl J Med 2000; 342:620.
3. Von Herbay A, Ditton HJ, Maiwald M. Diagnostic application of a polymerase chain reaction assay for the Whipple's disease bacterium to intestinal biopsies. Gastroenterology 1996; 110:1735.
4. Ramzan NN, Loftus E, Burgart LJ. Diagnosis and monitoring of Whipple's disease by polymerase chain reaction. Ann Intern Med 1997; 126:520.
5. Dobbins WO III. Whipple's disease. Springfield: Charles C Thomas Publisher, 1987.
6. Fleming JL, Wiesner RH, Shorter RG. Whipple's disease: clinical, biochemical, and histopathologic features and assessment of treatment in 29 patients. Mayo Clin Proc 1988; 63:539.

Chapter 13 / Whipple Disease

7. Enzinger FM, Helwig EB. Whipple's disease: a review of the literature and report of 15 patients. Virchows Arch A Pathol Anat Histopathol 1963; 336:238.

8. Miksche LW, Blumcke S, Fritsche D, et al. Whipple's disease: etiology, pathogenesis, treatment, diagnosis and clinical course; case report and review of the world literature. Acta Hepatogastroenterol 1974; 21:307.

9. Maizel H, Ruffin JM, Dobbins WO III. Whipple's disease: a review of 19 patients from one hospital and a review of the literature since 1950. Medicine (Baltimore) 1970; 49:175.

10. Leichtentritt KG. Whipple's disease. Am J Proctol 1977; 28:59.

11. Woese CR. Bacterial evolution. Microbiol Rev 1987; 51:221.

12. Wilson KH, Blitchington R, Frothingham R, Wilson JAP. Phylogeny of the Whipple's-disease-associated bacterium. Lancet 1991; 338:474.

13. Renesto P, Crapoulet N, Ogata H, et al. Genome-based design of a cell-free culture medium for Tropheryma whipplei. Lancet 2003; 362:447.

14. Raoult D, La Scola B, Lecocq P, et al. Culture and immunological detection of Tropheryma whippelii from the duodenum of a patient with Whipple disease. JAMA 2001; 285:1039.

15. Fenollar F, Birg ML, Gauduchon V, Raoult D. Culture of Tropheryma whipplei from human samples: a 3-year experience (1999-2002). J Clin Microbiol 2003; 41:3816.

16. Maiwald M, von Herbay A, Fredricks DN, et al. Cultivation of Tropheryma whipplei from cerebrospinal fluid. J Infect Dis 2003; 188:801.

17. Muller C, Stain C, Burghuber O. *Tropheryma whippelii* in peripheral blood mononuclear cells and cells of pleural effusion. Lancet 1993; 341:701.

18. Lowsky R, Archer GL, Fyles G, et al. Diagnosis of Whipple's disease by molecular analysis of peripheral blood. N Engl J Med 1994; 331:1343.

19. Maiwald M, Lepp PW, Relman DA. Analysis of conserved non-rRNA genes of Tropheryma whipplei. Syst Appl Microbiol 2003; 26:3.

20. Gross JB, Wollaeger EE, Sauer WG, et al. Whipple's disease: a report of four cases, including two in brothers, with observations on pathologic physiology, diagnosis, and treatment. Gastroenterology 1959; 36:65.

21. Puite RH, Tesluk H. Whipple's disease. Am J Med 1955; 19:383.

22. Dykman DD, Cuccherini BA, Fuss IJ, et al. Whipple's disease in a father-daughter pair. Dig Dis Sci 1999; 44:2542.

23. Ehrbar HU, Bauerfeind P, Dutly F, et al. PCR-positive tests for *Tropheryma whippelii* in patients without Whipple's disease. Lancet 1999; 353:2214.

24. Street S, Donoghue HD, Neild GH. *Tropheryma whippelii* DNA in saliva of healthy people. Lancet 1999; 354:1178.

25. Dutly F, Hinrikson HP, Seidel T, et al. *Tropheryma whippelii* DNA in saliva of patients without Whipple's disease. Infection 2000; 28:219.

26. Amsler L, Bauernfeind P, Nigg C, et al. Prevalence of Tropheryma whipplei DNA in patients with various gastrointestinal diseases and in healthy controls. Infection 2003; 31:81.

27. Fenollar F, Trani M, Davoust B, et al. Prevalence of asymptomatic Tropheryma whipplei carriage among humans and nonhuman primates. J Infect Dis 2008; 197:880.

28. Dobbins WO III. Is there an immune deficit in Whipple's disease? Dig Dis Sci 1981; 26:247.

29. Marth T, Feurle GE. Cutaneous anergy to streptococcal antigens in Whipple's disease. Am J Gastroenterol 1996; 91:2254.

30. Marth T, Roux M, Von Herbay A, et al. Persistent reduction of complement receptor 3 alpha-chain expressing mononuclear blood cells and transient inhibitory serum factors in Whipple's disease. Clin Immunol Immunopathol 1994; 72:217.
31. Marth T, Neurath M, Cuccherini BA, Strober W. Defects of monocyte interleukin 12 production and humoral immunity in Whipple's disease. Gastroenterology 1997; 113:442.
32. Marth T, Kleen N, Stallmach A, et al. Dysregulated peripheral and mucosal Th1/Th2 response in Whipple's disease. Gastroenterology 2002; 123:1468.
33. Ring S, Schneider T, Marth T. Mucosal immune response to Tropheryma whipplei. Int J Med Microbiol 2003; 293:69.
34. Kalt A, Schneider T, Ring S, et al. Decreased levels of interleukin-12p40 in the serum of patients with Whipple's disease. Int J Colorectal Dis 2006; 21:114–120.
35. Desnues B, Lepidi H, Raoult D, Mege JL. Whipple disease: Intestinal infiltrating cells exhibit a transcriptional pattern of m2/alternatively activated macrophages. J Infect Dis 2005; 192:1642.
36. Desnues B, Raoult D, Mege JL. IL-16 is critical for Tropheryma whipplei replication in Whipple's disease. J Immunol 2005; 175:4575.
37. Moos V, Schmidt C, Geelhaar A, et al. Impaired immune functions of monocytes and macrophages in Whipple's disease. Gastroenterology 2010; 138:210.
38. Schneider T, Stallmach A, Von Herbay A, et al. Treatment of refractory Whipple disease with interferon-γ. Ann Intern Med 1998; 129:875.
39. Kneitz C, Suerbaum S, Beer M, et al. Exacerbation of Whipple's disease associated with infliximab treatment. Scand J Rheumatol 2005; 34:148.
40. Mahnel R, Kalt A, Ring S, et al. Immunosuppressive therapy in Whipple's disease is associated with the appearance of gastrointestinal manifestations. Am J Gastroenterol 2005; 100:1167.
41. Trier JS, Phelps PC, Eidelman S, Rubin CE. Whipple's disease: light and electron microscope correlation of jejunal mucosal histology with antibiotic treatment and clinical status. Gastroenterology 1965; 48:684.
42. Yardley JH, Hendrix TR. Combined electron and light microscopy in Whipple's disease: demonstration of "bacillary bodies" in the intestine. Bull Johns Hopkins Hosp 1961; 109:80.
43. Chears WC, Ashworth CT. Electron microscopic study of the intestinal mucosa in Whipple's disease: demonstration of encapsulated bacilliform bodies in the lesion. Gastroenterology 1961; 41:129.
44. Rubin CE, Dobbins WO III. Peroral biopsy of the small intestine: a review of its diagnostic usefulness. Gastroenterology 1965; 49:676.
45. Dobbins WO III, Ruffin JM. A light- and electron microscopic study of bacterial invasion in Whipple's disease. Am J Pathol 1967; 51:225.
46. Dobbins WO III, Kawanishi H. Bacillary characteristics in Whipple's disease: an electron microscopic study. Gastroenterology 1981; 80:1468.
47. Viteri AL, Stinson JC, Barnes MC, Dyck WP. Rod-shaped organism in the liver of a patient with Whipple's disease. Dig Dis Sci 1979; 24:560.
48. Lie JT, David JS. Pancarditis in Whipple's disease: electron microscopic demonstration of intracardiac bacillary bodies. Am J Clin Pathol 1976; 66:22.
49. Winberg CD, Rose ME, Rappaport H. Whipple's disease of the lung. Am J Med 1978; 65:873.
50. Johnson L, Diamond I. Cerebral Whipple's disease: diagnosis by brain biopsy. Am J Clin Pathol 1980; 74:486.
51. Silvestry FE, Kim B, Pollack BJ, et al. Cardiac Whipple disease: identification of Whipple bacillus by electron microscopy in the myocardium of a patient before death. Ann Intern Med 1997; 126:214.

Chapter 13 / Whipple Disease

52. Von Herbay A, Maiwald M, Ditton HJ, Otto HF. Histology of intestinal Whipple's disease revisited. A study of 48 patients. Virchows Arch 1996; 429:335.
53. Pastor BM, Geerken RG. Whipple's disease presenting as pleuropericarditis. Am J Med 1973; 55:827.
54. Rose AG. Mitral stenosis in Whipple's disease. Thorax 1978; 33:500.
55. Wright CB, Hiratzka LF, Crossland S, et al. Aortic insufficiency requiring valve replacement in Whipple's disease. Ann Thorac Surg 1978; 25:466.
56. McAllister HA, Fenoglio JJ. Cardiac involvement in Whipple's disease. Circulation 1975; 52:152.
57. Vliestra RE, Lie JT, Kuhl WE, et al. Whipple's disease involving the pericardium: pathological confirmation during life. Aust N Z J Med 1978; 8:649.
58. Gubler JGH, Kuster M, Dutly F, et al. Whipple endocarditis without overt gastrointestinal disease: report of 4 cases. Ann Intern Med 1999; 131:112.
59. Smith M. Whipple endocarditis without gastrointestinal disease. Ann Intern Med 2000; 132:595.
60. Horton JM, Sing RF, Jenkin SJ. Polymerase chain reaction analysis for diagnosis of *Tropheryma whippelii* infective endocarditis in two patients with no previous evidence of Whipple's disease. Clin Infect Dis 1999; 29:1348.
61. Elkins C, Shuman TA, Pirolo JS. Cardiac Whipple's disease without digestive symptoms. Ann Thorac Surg 1999; 67:250.
62. Schmitt BP, Richardson H, Smith E, Kaplan R. Encephalopathy complicating Whipple's disease: failure to respond to antibiotics. Ann Intern Med 1981; 94:51.
63. Badenoch J, Richards WCD, Oppenheimer DR. Encephalopathy in a case of Whipple's disease. J Neurol Neurosurg Psychiatry 1963; 26:203.
64. Koudouris SD, Stern TN, Utterback RA. Involvement of central nervous system in Whipple's disease. Neurology (Minneap) 1963; 13:397.
65. Knox DL, Bayless TM, Pittman FE. Neurologic disease in patients with treated Whipple's disease. Medicine (Baltimore) 1976; 55:467.
66. Lampert P, Tom MI, Cumings JN. Encephalopathy in Whipple's disease: a histochemical study. Neurology 1962; 12:65.
67. Romanul FCA, Radvany J, Rosales RK. Whipple's disease confined to the brain: a case studied clinically and pathologically. J Neurol Neurosurg Psychiatry 1977; 40:901.
68. Feurle GE, Volk B, Waldherr R. Cerebral Whipple's disease with negative jejunal histology. N Engl J Med 1979; 300:907.
69. Grossman RI, Davis KR, Halperin J. Cranial computed tomography in Whipple's disease. J Comput Assist Tomogr 1981; 5:246.
70. Laster L, Waldmann TA, Fenster LF, Singleton JW. Albumin metabolism in patients with Whipple's disease. J Clin Invest 1966; 45:637.
71. Crane S, Schlippert W. Duodenoscopic findings in Whipple's disease. Gastrointest Endosc 1978; 24:248.
72. Geboes K, Ectors N, Heidbuchel H, et al. Whipple's disease. Endoscopic aspects before and after therapy. Gastrointest Endosc 1990; 36:247.
73. Fritscher-Ravens A, Swain CP, von Herbay A. Refractory Whipple's disease with anaemia: first lessons from capsule endoscopy. Endoscopy 2004; 36:659.
74. Hargrove MD, Verner JV, Smith AG, et al. Whipple's disease: report of two cases with intestinal biopsy before and after treatment. Gastroenterology 1960; 39:619.
75. Philips RL, Carlson HC. The roentgenographic and clinical findings in Whipple's disease: a review of 8 patients. Am J Roentgenol 1975; 123:268.
76. Li DK, Rennie CS. Abdominal computed tomography in Whipple's disease. J Comput Assist Tomogr 1981; 5:249.

77. Muller C, Petermann D, Stain C, et al. Whipple's disease: comparison of histology with diagnosis based on polymerase chain reaction in four consecutive cases. Gut 1997; 40:425.
78. Pron B, Poyart C, Abachin C, et al. Diagnosis and follow-up of Whipple's disease by amplification of the 16S rRNA gene of *Tropheryma whippelii*. World J Clin Microbiol Infect Dis 1999; 18:62.
79. Petrides PE, Muller-Hocker J, Fredricks DN, Relman DA. PCR analysis of *T whippelii* DNA in a case of Whipple's disease: effect of antibiotics and correlation with histology. Am J Gastroenterol 1998; 93:1579.
80. Tasken K, Schulz T, Elgjo K, et al. Diagnostic utility of the polymerase chain reaction in 2 cases of suspected Whipple disease. Arch Intern Med 1998; 158:801.
81. Lynch T, Odel J, Fredericks DN, et al. Polymerase chain reaction-based detection of *Tropheryma whippelii* in central nervous system Whipple's disease. Ann Neurol 1997; 42:120.
82. Gras E, Matius-Guiu X, Garcia A, et al. PCR analysis in the pathological diagnosis of Whipple's disease: emphasis on extraintestinal involvement or atypical morphological features. J Pathol 1999; 188:318.
83. Von Herbay A, Ditton HJ, Schuhmacher F, Maiwald M. Whipple's disease: staging and monitoring by cytology and polymerase chain reaction analysis of cerebrospinal fluid. Gastroenterology 1997; 113:434.
84. Maibach RC, Dutly F, Altwegg M. Detection of Tropheryma whipplei DNA in feces by PCR using a target capture method. J Clin Microbiol 2002; 40:2466.
85. Fenollar F, Laouira S, Lepidi H, et al. Value of Tropheryma whipplei quantitative polymerase chain reaction assay for the diagnosis of Whipple disease: usefulness of saliva and stool specimens for first-line screening. Clin Infect Dis 2008; 47:659.
86. Gillen JS, Urmacher C, West R, Shike M. Disseminated *Mycobacterium avium-intracellulare* infection in acquired immunodeficiency syndrome mimicking Whipple's disease. Gastroenterology 1983; 85:1187.
87. Roth RI, Owen RL, Keren DF, Valberding PA. Intestinal infection with *Mycobacterium avium-intracellulare* infection in acquired immunodeficiency syndrome (AIDS). Histological and clinical comparison with Whipple's disease. Dig Dis Sci 1985; 30:497.
88. Keinath RD, Merrell DE, Vlietstra R, Dobbins WO III. Antibiotic treatment and relapse in Whipple's disease. Long-term follow-up of 88 patients. Gastroenterology 1985; 88:1867.
89. Ryser RJ, Locksley RM, Eng SC, et al. Reversal of dementia associated with Whipple's disease by trimethoprim-sulfamethoxazole, drugs that penetrate the blood-brain barrier. Gastroenterology 1984; 86:745.
90. Boulos A, Rolain JM, Raoult D. Antibiotic susceptibility of Tropheryma whipplei in MRC5 cells. Antimicrob Agents Chemother 2004; 48:747.
91. Boulos A, Rolain JM, Mallet MN, Raoult D. Molecular evaluation of antibiotic susceptibility of Tropheryma whipplei in axenic medium. J Antimicrob Chemother 2005; 55:178.
92. Masselot F, Boulos A, Maurin M, et al. Molecular evaluation of antibiotic susceptibility: Tropheryma whipplei paradigm. Antimicrob Agents Chemother 2003; 47:1658.

14 Surgical Conditions Presenting with Diarrhea

Erica M. Carlisle, MD
and Mindy B. Statter, MD

CONTENTS

INTRODUCTION
PEDIATRIC SURGICAL DISORDERS
  PRESENTING WITH DIARRHEA
CHRONIC DIARRHEAL DISORDERS
  IN PEDIATRICS
SURGICAL DISORDERS PRESENTING
  WITH DIARRHEA IN ADULTS
CHRONIC DIARRHEAL DISORDERS
  IN ADULTS
REFERENCES

Summary

This chapter will focus on those surgical conditions that present with diarrhea in the child and the adult. The diarrheal disorders will be classified as acute or chronic, typed as bloody or non-bloody, with suggested management for children and adults, respectively.

Key Words: NEC, Intussusception, Malrotation, Volvulus, Appendicitis, Short gut, Hemolytic-uremic syndrome, Colo-cutaneous fistula, IBD, Tumors, PTLD, Polyposis, Intestinal ischemia, Chronic mesenteric ischemia, Mesenteric venous thrombosis (MVT), Colitis, Carcinoid, Zollinger–Ellison, Chronic pancreatitis

From: *Diarrhea, Clinical Gastroenterology*
Edited by: S. Guandalini, H. Vaziri, DOI 10.1007/978-1-60761-183-7_14
© Springer Science+Business Media, LLC 2011

INTRODUCTION

Diarrhea, as defined in Chapter 1 can be the result of numerous causes. Although infectious agents are the most common causes of acute and persistent diarrhea, a wide range of causes, both congenital and acquired, can be responsible for chronic diarrheal disorders. In this chapter, we will focus on those diarrheal conditions occurring both in children and in adults that recognize a surgically treatable one. We will distinguish them based on their duration: acute or chronic diarrheal disorders (see Chapter 1 for definitions), examining them separately as they occur in children and in adults, with the understanding that some conditions (e.g., inflammatory bowel disease or *Clostridium difficile* colitis) may well occur in both age groups.

PEDIATRIC SURGICAL DISORDERS PRESENTING WITH DIARRHEA

Necrotizing Enterocolitis

Necrotizing enterocolitis (NEC) is an inflammatory necrosis of the intestine that results in significant morbidity and mortality in premature infants (see Table 14.1) [1, 2]. About 5–10% of infants born weighing less than 1500 g develop NEC resulting in over 25,000 cases annually; 10–30% of affected babies will succumb to the disease, rendering NEC the leading cause of death in these vulnerable infants [2, 3]. Despite years of research, the exact etiology of NEC remains elusive; however, it is presumed that the pathophysiology of this disease is multi-factorial. Immaturity of the mucosal host defense in a vulnerable host (the premature infant), substrate provision by early enteral feeding, administration of antibiotics altering the intestinal flora and promoting virulent bacterial colonization, hypoxia/intestinal ischemia due to perinatal stress, and an exaggerated inflammatory immune reaction are all thought to contribute to the development of epithelial cell injury and a weakened mucosal defense system that allow for the onset of NEC in preterm infants [3].

The clinical presentation of NEC is highly variable. Bilious emesis is present in 75% of cases, and guaiac positive stools or hematochezia is common. Infants may progress from periods of mild illness to periods of severe, life-threatening sepsis. Current treatment of NEC is primarily supportive; bowel rest, total parenteral nutrition, antibiotics, volume resuscitation, and ionotropic support as indicated. The optimal time for operative intervention is prior to bowel necrosis or perforation; however, there is no specific marker for these impending events. Indication

Table 14.1
Pediatric surgical disorders presenting with diarrhea

Etiology	Age	Type of diarrhea	Unique lab value	Recommended imaging
Necrotizing enterocolitis	Preterm infants	Guaiac positive stools/hematochezia		Abdominal plain film
Intussusception	3 months to 3 years	"Currant jelly stool"		Ultrasound, barium or air enema
Malrotation with midgut volvulus	Birth to 1 year	Guaiac positive stool/hematochezia		Upper GI, ultrasound
Perforated appendicitis	Child to adult	Non-bloody diarrhea		Abdominal CT with IV, oral, rectal contrast
Short bowel syndrome	Birth to adult	Non-bloody diarrhea		
Inflammatory Bowel Disease	Child to adult	Ileocolic disease: non-bloody diarrhea		Colonoscopy, barium enema
Crohn's disease		Colonic: bloody, mucoid diarrhea		
Ulcerative colitis		Diarrhea mixed with blood + stool		

Table 14.1
(continued)

Etiology	Age	Type of diarrhea	Unique lab value	Recommended imaging
Neuroblastoma/VIPoma	1–4 years	Secretory, watery diarrhea	Urine VMA, HVA, serum VIP	CT, MRI, MIBG scan
Verotoxigenic *E. coli* and hemolytic uremic syndrome	5 years	Bloody diarrhea	Stool Shiga toxin, blood culture	Abdominal plain film, colonoscopy
Post-transplant lymphoproliferative disease	Child to adult	Diarrhea (occasionally bloody)	Bone marrow biopsy	CT, PET scan
Colocutaneous fistula after PEG placement	Child to adult	Osmotic diarrhea, stool in PEG tube		Contrast study of PEG tube
Juvenile polyposis coli	Child to 20 years	Diarrhea, sometimes bloody, protein-losing enteropathy		Colonoscopy

for operation is pneumoperitoneum, while relative indications include clinical deterioration, persistent acidosis, progressive thrombocytopenia, erythema of the bowel wall, portal venous gas, and the presence of a fixed intestinal loop. The principles of operation are excision of gangrenous bowel and exteriorization of viable ends with preservation of bowel length. In the very low birth weight preemie, an alternative to laparotomy is peritoneal drain placement. Overall, whether children with NEC undergo exploratory laparotomy or placement of a peritoneal drain, survival is not affected [4]. Gastrointestinal continuity is re-established when the child attains a body mass of 2–2.5 kg. The mortality rate for infants requiring surgery ranges from 20 to 50% [5, 6]. Necrotizing enterocolitis is a major cause of short bowel syndrome (SBS) in children (discussed later in the chapter).

Intussusception

Intussusception, a condition in which a segment of intestine is drawn into the lumen of more proximal bowel, occurs in 1–3 per 1000 live births in the United States making it the most common cause of pediatric small bowel obstruction [7]. It most commonly presents in infants that are 5–9 months of age (range 3 months to 3 years) [7] and is most frequently ileocolic [8]. The etiology of intussusception is unclear. Unlike in adults where most cases of intussusception have a pathologic lead point (often a cancer), intussusception in children is thought to be idiopathic, due to hypertrophy of Peyer's patches secondary to a recent or current infection [7, 7]. However, intussusception with a pathologic lead point including a Meckel's diverticulum, intestinal polyps, enteric duplication cysts, or lymphoma has also been detected in children [9].

Clinically, children with intussusception present with crampy abdominal pain, intervening periods of lethargy, vomiting, and bloody, mucous-rich diarrhea often termed "currant jelly stool." One in 10 children will have diarrhea before the signs and symptoms of intussusception become obvious. Occasionally, clinicians are able to palpate an elongated mass in the right upper quadrant or epigastrium corresponding to the intussusceptum, associated with an empty right lower quadrant (Dance's sign). Abdominal ultrasound is highly sensitive and specific for making the diagnosis of intussusception, and it usually demonstrates the target or pseudokidney signs [10]. Hydrostatic reduction of the intussusception is preformed with barium or air. The main contraindication to hydrostatic reduction is peritonitis, including gangrenous intestine which is an indication for immediate operative management. Reduction is considered complete when there is reflux of barium or insufflation of air into the terminal ileum. Review of the literature notes that failure of hydrostatic reduction and the need for surgical intervention are higher in patients who present with greater than 24 h of symptoms [11]. Typically, exploratory laparotomy via a right lower quadrant incision is performed. The intussusception is delivered into the wound, and the intussusceptum is gently milked, reducing the intussusception. If gangrenous bowel and/or a pathologic lead point are detected, the area is resected and repaired primarily. An appendectomy is generally preformed. The recurrence rate following operative intervention is approximately 3%, which is lower than the 5–7% recurrence rate following hydrostatic reduction.

Malrotation with Midgut Volvulus

Midgut volvulus results from abnormal intestinal rotation and fixation during embryogenesis. Normal rotation and fixation anchor the small and large intestine preventing twisting on itself. The broad base of the mesentery, extending from the ileocecal junction and extending obliquely to the ligament of Treitz, stabilizes the small bowel. When rotation and fixation are complete at 12 weeks of gestation, the duodenum is fixed securely in the retroperitoneum behind the superior mesenteric vascular pedicle, and the ascending and descending colon are fixated to their respective sides of the abdomen. If fixation does not occur, the small bowel is suspended by the narrow stalk of the superior mesenteric vessels and is susceptible to volvulus. The incidence of malrotation is estimated at 1/6000 live births; acute midgut volvulus occurs in 67% of patients with malrotation and is present in 50% of patients who come to surgery for rotational abnormalities. Most patients with midgut volvulus present within the first week of life (30%), 50% present within the first month of life, and 90% within the first year [12].

Infants with malrotation and midgut volvulus typically present with bilious vomiting; however, with intestinal necrosis, the vomitus may become bloody. Guaiac positive stool, hematochezia, or bloody diarrhea may occur early .With progression to transmural necrosis, the patient may present with peritonitis, respiratory failure, hypotension, and acidosis [13]. Older children with malrotation may present with chronic midgut volvulus, a history of recurrent abdominal pain from intermittent episodes of partial midgut volvulus. The partial obstruction results in lymphatic and venous obstruction resulting in abdominal pain, bilious emesis, diarrhea, and weight loss [14].

There are no pathognomonic findings for malrotation or midgut volvulus on plain films. Abdominal films may demonstrate a paucity of intestinal gas with several air fluid levels if midgut volvulus is present due to resorption of intraluminal air and the accumulation of fluid

Chapter 14 / Surgical Conditions Presenting with Diarrhea 243

within the bowel lumen [13]. When malrotation is suspected, the definitive imaging study is an upper GI. The diagnostic findings of malrotation include absence of the normal positioning of the duodenojejunal junction at the ligament of Treitz with the duodenum and proximal jejunum descending on the right side of the abdomen. If volvulus is present, the contrast may abruptly taper into a corkscrew or bird's beak appearance at the second portion of the duodenum. Ultrasound may be utilized to assess the relative relationship of the superior mesenteric vessels, with reversal of the normal orientation being present in malrotation. Ultrasound may also show the classic "whirlpool sign" which has been shown to be highly sensitive for midgut volvulus secondary to malrotation [15].

Emergent laparotomy is required for malrotation with midgut volvulus. The presence of chylous ascites indicates lymphatic obstruction from a volvulus; bloody ascitic fluid indicates vascular compromise. The procedure includes complete evisceration of the bowel and mesentery to assess for bowel viability. If present the volvulus is reduced. Correction of the malrotation, Ladd's procedure, includes dividing Ladd's bands, the abnormal peritoneal folds that may compress the duodenum. This maneuver also broadens the mesenteric pedicle to prevent recurrent volvulus. Necrotic intestine is resected. If ischemia is present, and bowel viability is questioned, a second-look laparotomy is performed 24–48 h after the initial operation to assess for vascular recovery. Alternatively, a coil-spring transparent silo may be placed at the time of the initial operation to allow for continuous inspection of the bowel and monitoring of vascular recovery. At the conclusion of Ladd's procedure, the small bowel is positioned on the right and the colon on the left. An appendectomy is performed, as future diagnosis of appendicitis may be difficult given the new location of the cecum [13]. The mortality rate for operative correction of malrotation ranges from 3 to 9%. Recurrent volvulus is rare, occurring in less than 10% of children; however, midgut volvulus accounts for 18% of cases of short gut syndrome in the pediatric population.

Perforated Appendicitis

Appendicitis is the most common surgical emergency in children [16]. The diagnosis of appendicitis in children remains challenging because of its varied presentations, delays in seeking medical care, and the difficulties in obtaining an accurate history and physical examination. The mistakes made in the diagnosis of appendicitis are sometimes due to failure to realize the variability in the position of the appendix or failure to recognize that appendicitis can mimic many other intra-abdominal processes. The most important pathologic factor in appendicitis is obstruction of the appendiceal lumen. In children, obstruction is commonly due to extrinsic compression from lymphoid hyperplasia. Fecaliths, small elements of condensed, hardened stool, can become impacted at the appendiceal orifice resulting in luminal obstruction [16].

Appendicitis classically presents with periumbilical pain, anorexia, vomiting, and fever. The symptoms of perforated appendicitis include anorexia with vomiting, severe, generalized abdominal pain, fever (>38°C), and diarrhea. After perforation, diarrhea is a much more common presenting symptom of appendicitis, and studies have shown that 50% of missed cases of appendicitis initially presented with diarrhea [16]. Non-verbal children may present with right hip pain mimicking a septic hip. Appendicitis in children less than 3 years of age is characterized by delays in diagnosis and perforation. Diarrhea as a presenting symptom has been reported in 33–46% of children in this age group. In differentiating appendicitis from gastroenteritis, the diarrhea with appendicitis is culture-negative and limited to the release of small amounts of loose stool in contrast to the voluminous watery stool seen associated with enteritis [17]. Children less than 5 years of age, with their sparse omentum, are less capable of "walling off" the perforation and often present with generalized peritonitis. The overall goal of management is to diagnose acute appendicitis before perforation occurs. The risk of perforation is higher in children than adults. This has been shown to be related to delay in presentation to the surgeon rather than specific physiologic differences in children [18].

In an effort to avoid the consequences of missed diagnosis, when the history and physical examination are equivocal, radiologic studies are obtained to confirm the diagnosis of appendicitis. Ultrasound has a sensitivity of 75–90% and a specificity of 86–100% with an overall accuracy of 90–94%. CT scans may be useful in atypical patients with undiagnosed abdominal symptoms, patients in whom satisfactory ultrasound examinations are not possible (e.g., obese or immunologically suppressed children), or patients lacking localizing physical findings. CT scans may also be useful in patients with perforated appendicitis to distinguish phlegmon from abscess or to plan therapeutic interventions such as percutaneous, transrectal, or transvaginal abscess drainage. CT findings consistent with acute appendicitis include visualization of a distended appendix with a diameter greater than 6 mm and/or the appearance of peri-appendiceal inflammatory changes. Treatment of choice is early appendectomy performed open or laparoscopically. The standard approach to perforated appendicitis has been limited laparotomy, with drainage of an abscess if present, and appendectomy. It has

Chapter 14 / Surgical Conditions Presenting with Diarrhea

been argued that given the inflammation involving the cecum and surrounding bowel, this approach can be complicated by greater blood loss, increased risk of bowel injury, and subsequent development of postoperative abdominal and/or pelvic abscess by entering an established abscess. Alternative approaches depend upon whether the mass is a phlegmon or an abscess, as determined by ultrasound or CT. If the mass is determined to be a phlegmon, intravenous antibiotics and volume resuscitation without immediate laparotomy are a safe and effective treatment provided the patient demonstrates clinical improvement (e.g., resolution of fever, leukocytosis, and abdominal pain). Elective interval appendectomy can be planned 6 weeks later, generally with postoperative hospital stay of 1 day. Laparotomy is indicated if clinical improvement does not occur after 24 h of non-operative management. If an abscess is identified, after volume resuscitation and intravenous antibiotics, drainage by percutaneous, transvaginal, or transrectal routes may be performed. With clinical improvement, antibiotic therapy is continued until the patient is afebrile and the leukocytosis and abdominal tenderness have resolved. Elective interval appendectomy can be planned 6 weeks later, generally with a postoperative hospital stay of 1 day. The ability to safely and accurately distinguish perforated from non-perforated acute appendicitis is imperative to the institution of conservative management [19].

CHRONIC DIARRHEAL DISORDERS IN PEDIATRICS

Short Bowel Syndrome

Diarrhea is a common symptom in children with short bowel syndrome. SBS is defined as the presence of insufficient intestinal absorptive capacity to maintain normal enteral nutrition [20, 21]. The reported incidence is unknown due to the variation of definition. The mortality in children with SBS is 37.5% with the major causes of death being liver failure due to parenteral nutrition and sepsis [22]. The two most common causes of SBS are NEC and midgut volvulus.

The factors influencing intestinal function in SBS include the total length of remaining small intestine, the type of intestine remaining (jejunum vs. ileum), the presence of an ileocecal valve, and the presence of the colon. Extensive ileal resection results in deficiencies of vitamin B_{12} and the fat-soluble vitamins, and diarrhea. The diarrhea is due to the large fluid volumes being presented to the colon due to decreased transit time and loss of absorptive surface area. With loss of the terminal ileum, high concentrations of bile acids (principally absorbed in the terminal ileum) pass into the colon instead of entering the enterohepatic circulation. Colonic bacteria deconjugate bile salts, increasing the free bile salt pool stimulating colonic secretory activity resulting in diarrhea. The relative bile salt deficiency impairs fat absorption resulting in steatorrhea. Absorptive capacity is also impacted by the presence of a functional colon. The ileocecal valve functions to increase the pressure gradient between the ileum and the colon preventing reflux of colonic fluid containing high concentrations of bacteria. An intact ileocecal valve is associated with improved absorption given the delay in transit time and increased nutrient contact time [20].

The loss of significant small bowel length results in anatomic and physiologic changes referred to as intestinal adaptation. This process begins immediately after resection and can take 2 years to complete. The initial treatment of SBS involves the use of parenteral nutrition with the slow introduction of enteral feedings as tolerated. Children are typically maintained on proton pump inhibitors and H_2 blockers to reduce gastric acid secretion. Further, anti-motility agents and octreotide (to reduce the volume of GI secretions by slowing intestinal transit time and increasing water and sodium absorption) are also utilized. Antibiotics decrease the potential for bacterial overgrowth in the setting of dysmotility [20]. Cholestyramine, a bile acid sequestrant, decreases stool losses by exchanging chloride ions for bile acids creating non-absorptive complexes excreted in the feces.

Surgical options in the treatment of SBS are designed to slow transit time or increase the length and surface area of the intestine in order to increase nutrient and fluid absorption [20]. These procedures include intestinal tapering, reversed small bowel segments [23–26], colonic interposition [27, 28], construction of intestinal valves to disrupt the normal motility of the small intestine and prevent retrograde reflux of intestinal contents [29, 30], and electrical pacing of the small intestine. Two well-described and validated procedures for increasing the length of small intestine in children with SBS are the longitudinal intestinal lengthening and tailoring procedure (LILT) and the serial transverse enteroplasty procedure (STEP). Both have been shown to lengthen remaining bowel and aid in weaning children from TPN [22, 31–34]. Despite the success of lengthening procedures, small bowel transplant may be the only option in patients with small intestinal failure to adapt, patients who are unable to be maintained on enteral feeds with TPN dependence and resulting liver failure, and in patients who no longer have central venous access [20]. Two-thirds of small bowel transplants are performed in children and are often performed as a combined small intestine and liver transplant due to the high rate of SBS-associated liver failure [20]. Transplants allow 50–70% of patients to be successfully weaned from TPN with the success of weaning being higher in children than adults [20].

Chapter 14 / Surgical Conditions Presenting with Diarrhea

Inflammatory Bowel Disease: Crohn's Disease and Ulcerative Colitis

The inflammatory bowel diseases (IBD), Crohn's disease and ulcerative colitis, can be differentiated from each other based on clinical, radiologic, endoscopic, and pathologic criteria, but in 10% of cases the findings are non-specific and categorized as "indeterminate colitis." See also Chapter 3 for a more detailed discussion of IBD.

The presentation of Crohn's disease varies depending upon the age of the child, which segment of the gastrointestinal tract involved, and the chronicity of the inflammation. Crohn's disease may involve the entire gastrointestinal tract; in children, the most common location is ileocolonic (42%), diffuse small bowel (28%), isolated colonic and anorectal (31%). The presentation may be vague resulting in a delay in diagnosis. Diarrhea is frequently seen in patients with ileocolic involvement and may not always be bloody. Perianal Crohn's disease should be suspected in children with chronic diarrhea and multiple, recurrent, or atypical perianal fistulae or abscesses. Isolated colonic Crohn's disease may mimic ulcerative colitis, presenting with bloody, mucoid diarrhea.

There is no curative therapy for Crohn's disease; rather treatment is designed to palliate symptoms [35]. Medical treatment includes antibiotics (for perianal disease, enterocutaneous fistulae, and active colonic disease), aminosalicylates, corticosteroids, azathiopurine/6-mercaptopurine, methotrexate, and immunomodulators (infliximab, an anti-TNF antibody). Overall, 80% of all patients diagnosed with Crohn's disease will eventually require surgery. Indications for surgical management include failure of medical management: (1) complications of steroid/drug therapy including growth failure; (2) persistent symptoms despite maximal medical therapy and complications such as perforation, excessive or uncontrolled bleeding, fistula formation, stricture formation with obstruction, sepsis, and toxic megacolon.

Ulcerative colitis involves the rectum with frequent extension in a contiguous pattern proximally without skip areas. It may present insidiously with persistent diarrhea with blood and mucus mixed in the stool. Unlike Crohn's disease, because ulcerative colitis is limited to the colon, surgery is curative. Indications for surgical management include hemorrhage, perforation, toxic megacolon or failure of medical management, persistent symptoms, growth failure, delayed puberty, and histologic dysplasia.

Tumors

Paraneoplastic syndromes are caused by the remote humoral effects of a tumor and not by local effects or metastases. These syndromes (see also Chapter 15) may be the first clinical symptom of a tumor. Secretory diarrhea is seen in the watery diarrhea, hypokalemia, and achlorhydria syndrome (WHDA), first described by Verner and Morrison in 1958 in association with pancreatic islet cell tumors in adults [36].

Vasoactive intestinal peptide (VIP) producing tumors can be divided into two groups: pancreatic endocrine tumors and neurogenic tumors. Neuroblastomas arise from the sympathetic nervous system and predominantly composed of adrenergic neurons involved in catecholamine synthesis. A small fraction of involved neurons possess cholinergic neurotransmission capabilities including secretion of vasoactive peptide (VIP) and VIPoma formation. The development of WDHA syndrome [37] in association with neuroblastoma, ganglioneuroblastoma, and ganglioneuroma has been described in 80 cases in the literature [38, 39]. Diarrhea may precede the tumor diagnosis or occur secondarily after chemotherapy with tumor differentiation [37]. The diagnosis of neuroblastomas includes measuring urinary catecholamine metabolites, vanillylmandelic acid (VMA), homovanillic acid (HVA), and baseline serum VIP levels with the presenting symptom of diarrhea [37]. Treatment of neuroblastomas associated with VIP secretion is essentially identical to treatment for more typical neuroblastomas. Surgical resection of localized disease has demonstrated efficacy in controlling the tumor and the associated diarrhea.

Non-neurogenic tumors associated with VIP secretion and diarrhea include pancreatic non-beta cell hyperplasia and pancreatoblastoma [40].

Verotoxigenic Escherichia coli and Post-diarrheal Hemolytic Uremic Syndrome

Verotoxigenic *E. coli* infection (see also Chapter 1) occurs in six per million children less than 5 years old and 1.74 per million children greater than 5 years old [41]. Hemolytic uremic syndrome (HUS) is a microangiopathy characterized by thrombocytopenia, hemolytic anemia, and acute renal failure that occurs in 30–40% of these children, with a mortality rate of approximately 5% during the acute phase of infection [41]. The disease is acquired predominantly by ingestion of incompletely cooked hamburgers, unpasteurized milk, and water contaminated by *E. coli* [41]. Children typically present with crampy abdominal pain, vomiting, abdominal distention, and diarrhea that is initially watery but becomes bloody [42]. These symptoms usually precede the development of HUS by 5–7 days and are due to the production of the Shiga toxin by the *E. coli* [48, 49]. This

Chapter 14 / Surgical Conditions Presenting with Diarrhea 249

toxin causes a microangiopathy resulting in multisystem organ failure. Gut manifestations include ischemia, necrosis, perforation, rectal prolapse, intussusception, colonic necrosis, hemorrhagic colitis, and stricture [41, 43]. Neurologic sequelae include seizures, stroke, and cerebral edema. Diagnosis is made by stool sample for Shiga toxin and blood culture for the presence of antibody. Abdominal plain films may show dilation, thumbprinting characteristic of ischemia, or ascites. Colonoscopy typically reveals friable, ulcerated bowel covered with a gray-pseudomembrane [42].

Management of verotoxic *E. coli* infection and HUS is initially conservative. The development of renal failure may require the placement of a peritoneal dialysis catheter [43, 44]. Surgery is indicated for perforation, peritonitis, toxic megacolon, acidosis unresponsive to dialysis, or obstruction [42, 44]. Renal transplant has been necessary for irreversible renal failure [43].

Post-transplant Lymphoproliferative Disease

Post-transplant lymphoproliferative disease (PTLD) is a complication of both solid organ and bone marrow transplant that results in a heterogeneous group of tumors that include both hyperplasias and neoplasias [45]. Eighty-five percent of cases are associated with Epstein–Barr virus (EBV) reactivation or primary infection from the donor organ [46, 47]. The incidence varies depending on the type of transplant performed. After heart, lung, and small bowel transplants there is a 5–20% incidence of PTLD; after kidney transplant there is only a 1–3% incidence [45, 46]. It is presumed that this difference is due to the increased immunosuppression after heart, lung, and small bowel transplant as compared to after kidney transplant [45]. In addition, there is a direct variation in disease incidence with the type of immunosuppressant utilized and the presence of EBV infection [48]. PTLD is most commonly diagnosed in the first year after transplant [45, 48]; however, there is no difference in survival between those people who are diagnosed early after transplant (3 months) as compared to later (greater than 12 months) [45]. Given the variability of disease site, presentation and clinical course are quite variable. The most common sites of involvement are extranodal (liver, lung, kidney, bone marrow, and spleen) with the gastrointestinal tract being the most common site of clinical presentation due to an increased propensity for ulceration and perforation [48]. The majority of patients present with fever, lymphadenopathy, diarrhea or bloody stool, bowel obstruction due to mass effects, weight loss, anorexia, and lethargy. The diagnosis is typically made by CT imaging and bone marrow biopsy; however, positron emission tomography

(PET) scanning is being used more frequently to diagnose and monitor response to treatment with CT-PET scans being more accurate than either CT or PET scan alone [48].

Treatment for PTLD involves reduction or withdrawal of immunosuppression; however, this intervention must be balanced with the subsequent risk of rejection. Surgical excision of the lesion or possible bowel resection may be required for ulceration, obstruction secondary to mass effect, or hemorrhage [48]. Chemotherapy has been shown to be associated with remission rates from 30 to 80% and a long-term survival of 20–60% [46]. Alternatively, rituximab, interferon therapy, and infusion of autologous EBV-specific cytotoxic T lymphocytes have also been shown to be advantageous in treating patients with PTLD [46]. Mortality rates from PTLD are quite high with a range of 60–100% being reported in the literature. The mortality rate from PTLD varies by the type of organ transplant with a reported 40% mortality after renal transplant and 50% mortality after heart transplant [45]. Overall, mortality rates have been shown to decrease when definitive local therapy (surgery or radiation) combined with immunosuppression reduction is utilized [48].

Colocutaneous Fistula After Percutaneous Endoscopic Gastrostomy Tube Placement

Percutaneous endoscopic gastrostomy (PEG) tube placement was introduced in 1980 as a less invasive alternative to open gastrostomy tube placement. The procedure is successful in 95% of patients [49]. The most common indication for PEG insertion is dysphagia associated with neurologic impairment [49]. Overall, there is a 2–3% incidence of colocutaneous fistula after PEG insertion [50]. Gastrocolocutaneous fistula after PEG placement in a child has also been reported [51]. These patients present with severe osmotic diarrhea [50]. A contributing factor to this complication may be the abnormal body habitus of the child due to contractures or scoliosis. The mechanism of misplacement may occur during the initial PEG procedure: the needle passes through the colon that is positioned between the stomach and the abdominal wall and the gastrostomy appliance does not pass beyond the colon; or the gastrostomy tube passes into the stomach and then retracts into the colon [52]. The complication may be recognized later at the time of appliance change which may result in the migration of the tube from the stomach to the colon. The misplacement of the tube into the colon should be considered when there is recurrent severe diarrhea of undigested food or fecal contents in the gastrostomy appliance or the sudden onset of

Chapter 14 / Surgical Conditions Presenting with Diarrhea 251

transient diarrhea within minutes after tube feedings. The diagnosis is made by performing a contrast study of the PEG tube. In most cases, the fistula will close with simple removal of the PEG tube; however, if the fistula has matured, surgical repair may be necessary [53].

Juvenile Polyposis Coli

Juvenile polyposis coli, a rare condition with autosomal dominant inheritance, was first described in 1964. Affected patients typically have between 50 and 200 hamartomatous polyps distributed throughout their entire colon and they usually develop symptoms, including anemia due to gastrointestinal bleeding, diarrhea, rectal prolapse, intussusception, and less commonly, protein-losing enteropathy, prior to the age of 15 [54]. Symptoms typically present prior to the development of malignancy [54]. While the malignant potential for a solitary juvenile polyp is quite low, patients with juvenile polyposis coli have a malignant potential that ranges from 17 to 65% [54]. Management includes genetic counseling, annual colonoscopy with polypectomy, and evaluation for subtotal vs. total colectomy if high-grade dysplasia or invasive adenocarcinoma is detected on pathology or if the polyps are not able to be completely resected endoscopically [54].

SURGICAL DISORDERS PRESENTING WITH DIARRHEA IN ADULTS

Intestinal Ischemia

Several different syndromes of inadequate blood flow to the bowel result in diarrhea (see Table 14.2). Generally, the bowel is able to tolerate a wide range in perfusion and has the remarkable capacity to adapt to less than adequate blood flow. The incidence of ischemic bowel doubles with age every 5 years such that up to 217 per 100,000 people over the age of 85 have some degree of intestinal ischemia [55].

The etiology of intestinal ischemia can be divided into three general categories: presplanchnic, e.g., decreased mesenteric blood flow due to heart failure, hypovolemia, hemorrhage; splanchnic, e.g., decreased blood flow at the local level due to thrombosis, embolus, trauma, compression, and medications; and postsplanchnic, e.g., venous disease, hypercoagulable syndromes, and cirrhosis [55]. Injury to the gut occurs by both ischemia and reperfusion and results in four distinct clinical presentations: acute mesenteric ischemia, chronic mesenteric ischemia, mesenteric venous thrombosis, and ischemic colitis.

Table 14.2

Adult surgical conditions presenting with diarrhea

Etiology	Age	Type of diarrhea	Unique lab value	Recommended imaging
Intestinal ischemia	>60 years			CT/CT angiography
Acute (AMI)		Diarrhea (often bloody)		
Chronic (CMI)		Diarrhea (often bloody)		
Mesenteric venous thrombosis (MVT)		Melena + diarrhea		
Ischemic colitis		Passage of blood that may be associated with diarrhea		
C. difficile colitis	Adult	Watery diarrhea	Stool cytotoxin/ELISA	CT scan (colonoscopy in non-acute setting)
Carcinoid/carcinoid syndrome	>65 years	Explosive secretory diarrhea	24 h urine 5-HIAA, plasma chromogranin A	CT scan
Gastrinoma	50 years	Voluminous secretory diarrhea	Fasting gastrin level >1000 pg/ml, basal acid output >15 Eq/g, gastric pH < 3, secretin stimulation test >200 pg/ml over basal	CT scan, somatostatin receptor scintigraphy, MRI, EUS if pancreatic lesion
Vipoma	Adult	Secretory, watery diarrhea	Fasting serum VIP >500 pg/ml	CT scan, somatostatin receptor scintigraphy
Somatostatinoma	>50 years	Steatorrhea + diarrhea	Serum somatostatin	CT/MRI
Medullary thyroid cancer	50–60 years	Diarrhea	Serum calcitonin, serum CEA, FNA cytology, 24 h urine VMA, catecholamines, metanephrines, serum Ca	Neck ultrasound
Chronic pancreatitis	>50 years	Diarrhea, steatorrhea		CT scan, ERCP/EUS

Chapter 14 / Surgical Conditions Presenting with Diarrhea

Acute Mesenteric Ischemia (AMI)

Acute mesenteric ischemia (AMI) is a life-threatening disease with reported mortality ranging between 30 and 90% depending on etiology [55]. AMI can have four presentations: (1) embolic occlusion of the superior mesenteric or celiac arteries (50%), (2) acute thrombosis of the celiac or mesenteric arteries (25%), (3) non-occlusive mesenteric ischemia (NOMI) (20%), and (4) mesenteric venous thrombosis (5%). Acute thromboembolic occlusion of the superior mesenteric artery (SMA) is associated with a 93% mortality [55]. The classic presentation of patients with acute mesenteric ischemia is the acute onset of mid-abdominal pain that is disproportional to the physical exam and may be associated diarrhea. Patients with embolic occlusion have a history of atrial fibrillation or recent myocardial infarction [55]. Patients with AMI secondary to SMA thrombosis typically have other manifestations of diffuse atherosclerotic occlusive disease. NOMI is due to mesenteric vasospasm or vasoconstriction and is seen in patients undergoing treatment for systemic illnesses such as sepsis or cardiogenic shock. The pain is less acute and is a waxing and waning pattern in quality. Patients presenting with mesenteric venous thrombosis present with non-specific complaints of abdominal pain associated with diarrhea [55].

Contrast angiography remains the gold standard for imaging the visceral vessels. Non-invasive modalities to diagnose AMI include CT angiography and MR angiography. CT is helpful in assessing for bowel for necrosis and other etiologies of abdominal pain. Delayed views are the diagnostic test of choice for mesenteric venous thrombosis. The treatment of acute mesenteric ischemia depends upon the etiology and patient presentation. The therapeutic goals include restoring pulsatile blood flow to the abdominal viscera, resection of non-viable intestine, and when intestinal viability is questioned, a "second-look" laparotomy.

Chronic Mesenteric Ischemia (CMI)

Chronic mesenteric ischemia (CMI) results from chronic gut hypoperfusion via the main intestinal arteries that cannot be compensated by collateral splanchnic arterial inflow. Mesenteric atherosclerotic lesions located proximally and focally are generally the cause of CMI [55]. Non-atherosclerotic etiologies include arterial fibrodysplasia, connective tissue disease, and inflammatory arteritis secondary to abdominal radiation [55]. Patients with CMI characteristically describe crampy, postprandial abdominal pain (intestinal angina) and demonstrate behavioral patterns that limit oral intake (food fear), weight loss, and diarrhea. Symptoms are often more insidious than those seen with acute ischemia due to the ability of the colon to develop collateral flow in the setting of chronic ischemia.

Contrast angiography remains the gold standard in diagnosis of CMI; CT angiography and MR angiography have been shown to correlate well with angiography findings [56]. Treatment of CMI involves restoration of arterial perfusion by relieving proximal stenoses or occlusions in the mesenteric arteries using either open surgical reconstruction or catheter-directed endovascular angioplasty or stenting techniques.

Mesenteric Venous Thrombosis (MVT)

Mesenteric venous thrombosis (MVT) most commonly occurs in individuals between 50 and 60 years of age, and like mesenteric arterial ischemia may have an acute and chronic form [56]. Acute MVT involves thrombosis of the larger mesenteric veins, and patients typically present with severe abdominal pain, nausea, vomiting, melena and diarrhea. Patients with chronic MVT present with vague abdominal pain with associated symptoms that fluctuate over time. A predisposing etiology can be determined in 60–80% of patients and include factor 5 Leiden deficiency, cancer, oral contraceptive use, recent surgery (especially splenectomy), venous stasis, inflammation, abdominal trauma, peritonitis, and portal hypertension [57, 58]. Treatment of MVT is generally systemic anticoagulation [57]. The presence of peritonitis mandates an exploratory laparotomy; up to 30% of patients with MVT require exploration for resection of necrotic bowel. Patients with MVT should be assessed for an underlying hypercoagulable etiology that could necessitate lifelong anticoagulation.

Ischemic Colitis

The most common form of intestinal ischemia, ischemic colitis, represents 50–60% of all cases of gastrointestinal ischemia [55, 56]. Generally, 90% of cases occur in patients over 60 years old [59]; however, 10–20% of patients are younger than 40 years of age [60]. The etiologies of ischemic colitis are diverse and include systemic shock (hypovolemic, septic, neurogenic), cardiogenic shock (heart failure, recent coronary artery bypass grafting), major arterial occlusion (aortic dissection, embolic, thrombotic), surgical (aneurysmectomy, colectomy), small artery occlusion (diabetes, atherosclerosis), vasculitis (systemic lupus erythematosus, polyarteritis nodosa, thromboangiitis obliterans, sickle cell disease), inflammatory (pancreatitis, diverticulitis), hypercoagulable states (malignancy, factor deficiencies, e.g., protein S, protein C, antithrombin III), colonic obstruction, and medications including antibiotics, vinca alkaloids, taxanes,

Chapter 14 / Surgical Conditions Presenting with Diarrhea

vasopressors, diuretics, statins, non-steroidal anti-inflammatory agents, estrogens, and some laxatives [55, 59–62]. The clinical presentation depends upon the extent of the ischemia. Most patients with non-gangrenous colonic ischemia present with the acute onset of mild, crampy abdominal pain. During the first 24 hours, the patient commonly passes blood, either bright red or maroon, that may be associated with diarrhea. Blood loss is minimal; profuse bleeding should prompt determining another source. Severe ischemia, transmural infarction, or perforation may result in the development of a leukocytosis, metabolic acidosis, and septic shock [61].

Colonoscopy is the traditional gold standard for the diagnosis of ischemic colitis; it has greater sensitivity for detecting mucosal changes and allows for biopsy. Colonoscopy is preferable to flexible sigmoidoscopy because the area of ischemia will be proximal to the splenic flexure in 30–40% of patients [62]. Colonoscopy is contraindicated in the presence of peritonitis due to an increased risk of perforation [55]. CT scan is often the primary diagnostic imaging study in these patients, and in the setting of ischemic colitis, non-specific colonic wall thickening, pneumatosis, fat stranding, and portal venous gas may be observed. Ultrasound may detect colonic abnormalities and color Doppler can detect patency of mesenteric veins and absent or diminished bowel wall flow in 80% of cases [55]. The role of contrast angiography is limited being that most ischemic colitis is the result of non-occlusive or venous disease rather than arterial insufficiency. Those patients with known predisposing factors, e.g., hypercoagulable state, cardiac thrombus, or evidence of arterial insufficiency on CT may benefit from angiography and thrombolytic therapy [62].

Treatment of ischemic colitis depends upon the severity of presentation. In 60–80% of patients, acute colonic ischemia will resolve in 24–48 h with non-operative management. Endoscopic and radiographic findings may persist for up to 2 weeks; ischemia resulting in ulceration may take as long as 6 months to completely resolve. In 20% of patients, the colonic ischemia will progress and surgery will be indicated. The associated mortality rate of these patients is 60% [55]. Areas of transmural infarction are resected; primary anastomosis is generally contraindicated and the bowel ends are left in the abdomen if a "second-look" is planned or exteriorized as a stoma with Hartmann pouch [61]. Depending upon the etiology of colonic ischemia re-vascularization may be indicated [61]. Incomplete healing after resolution of the acute episode may result in chronic segmental colitis characterized by persistent diarrhea, protein loss, bleeding, or stricture formation with obstructive symptoms [62].

Clostridium difficile Colitis

Systemic treatment with antibiotics results in disruption of normal colonic flora such that aggressive pathologic bacteria are able to grow. The administration of clindamycin, cephalosporins, and fluoroquinolones have all been shown to foster an environment that permits *C. difficile* overgrowth [63]. *C. difficile* infection has multiple clinical presentations ranging from the asymptomatic carrier state to severe diarrhea and pseudomembranous colitis to severe life-threatening fulminant colitis with perforation [64]. *C. difficile* is the most common nosocomial infectious diarrhea in adults, with an incidence of 3 million infections in the United States yearly [63–66]. Annually, 13.1 per 1000 surgical inpatients will be infected with *C. difficile* [64]. Infected patients with simple colitis typically report abdominal pain and watery diarrhea. In the setting of fulminant colitis, in addition to diarrhea, patients will also demonstrate fever, hypotension, abdominal distention, and leukocytosis [63]. Multiple centers have reported an increased prevalence of hypervirulent strains of *C. difficile* that have led to greater disease severity, increased reliance on intensive care monitoring, and increased need for surgical intervention [64, 66]. Presumably this increase in hypervirulent strains accounts for the observation that mortality within 30 days of diagnosis of *C. difficile* infection has increased from 4.7% in 1991 to 13.8% in 2003 [63]. Factors associated with a more complicated clinical course include patient age over 65, leukocyte count greater than 20×10^9 cells/l, acquisition of the infection while hospitalized, renal failure, and immunosuppression [63].

The diagnosis of *C. difficile* infection should be considered in any patient with recent antibiotic administration and diarrhea. The gold standard for *C. difficile* diagnosis is a stool cytotoxin assay; however, this test may take up to 3 days to yield results, so most centers rely on ELISA stool tests. Typically the ELISA is repeated three times to account for the increased false-negative rate as compared to the cytotoxin assay [63]. Abdominal CT scan demonstrates colonic wall thickening and dilation; however, CT findings do not correlate well with the clinical severity of disease [63]. Colonoscopy or flexible sigmoidoscopy may demonstrate the pathognomonic pseudomembranes associated with *C. difficile* infection; generally clinical presentation and CT scan results are sufficient [64].

In the setting of simple *C. difficile* colitis medical management includes discontinuing the offending antimicrobial agent, and oral metronidazole or vancomycin should be administered. If the patient is unable to tolerate oral intake, intravenous metronidazole may be provided; vancomycin is effective only in the oral form [63]. If clinical improvement is not observed within 24–48 h of the initiation of medical

Chapter 14 / Surgical Conditions Presenting with Diarrhea   257

management, a surgical consultation in warranted. Ten percent of patients with *C. difficile* colitis will require surgery, specifically total abdominal colectomy with end ileostomy [65, 72]. The decision to perform a colectomy on a patient with fulminant *C. difficile* colitis is based on surgical judgment rather than specific criteria. The reported mortality rate for fulminant *C. difficile* colitis is between 30 and 80% [67]; however, this may be decreased by half when surgical intervention is undertaken prior to the development of septic shock [66]. Aggressive surgical management has also been shown to be advantageous by researchers who investigated whether the mortality rate of patients with fulminant *C. difficile* colitis admitted to a surgical service differed compared to those admitted to a non-surgical service. Interestingly, the authors that found that those patients admitted to a non-surgical service had a 3.4-fold higher mortality rate compared to those patients admitted to a surgical service [66].

CHRONIC DIARRHEAL DISORDERS IN ADULTS

Both children and adults share the diagnoses of Crohn's disease, ulcerative colitis, and short bowel syndrome. This section will address the chronic diarrheal disease etiologies that occur predominantly in adults. The reader is referred to the pediatric section for review of the surgical conditions that present with diarrhea that occur in both children and adults.

Tumors

Multiple tumors secrete bioactive substances that cause diarrhea, including carcinoid tumors, gastrinomas, vasoactive intestinal peptidomas, somatostatinomas, and medullary cancer of the thyroid.

Carcinoid/Carcinoid Syndrome

Carcinoid tumors are morphologically and biochemically diverse tumors capable of synthesizing various bioactive substances including serotonin, histamine, and prostaglandins. Their behavior is determined by their site of origin; 64% are localized to the midgut. Typically, carcinoids present in adults age 65 or older [68]. Symptoms of midgut carcinoids include vague abdominal pain due to intestinal obstruction, mass effect, intussusception, or hypermotility, and diarrhea. The carcinoid syndrome occurs in the presence of hepatic metastases. Carcinoid syndrome-associated diarrhea is an explosive, episodic, secretory diarrhea linked to serotonin secretion. Pellagra, characterized by dermatitis, dementia, and diarrhea, may occur with carcinoid syndrome with diversion of dietary tryptophan to tumor hormone production depleting nicotinic acid stores [68]. Plasma chromogranin A is measured as a screening test, and it is elevated in 80% of patients with carcinoid tumors [68]. The biochemical diagnosis is made with a 24-h urine collection measuring 5-hydroxyindoleactic acid (5-HIAA) which is 75% sensitive for primary tumors and 100% sensitive for metastatic disease. Diagnostic imaging includes abdominal CT scan to evaluate the extension of the primary lesion, metastasis, and vessel involvement. Radiolabeled somatostatin analogue (octreotide) scintigraphy localizes primary and metastatic tumors expressing somatostatin receptors. Surgical resection is the most effective treatment with primary tumor location, size, and presence/absence of metastatic disease determining operative management [68]. It is necessary to prevent the development of carcinoid crisis secondary to anesthesia and surgical stress with the preoperative administration of octreotide. Gross resection has been shown to result in symptom-free survival for many years, but the recurrence of liver metastasis occurs in 85% of patients, so lifelong surveillance with laboratory and radiologic follow-up is required [68].

Gastrinomas/Zollinger–Ellison Syndrome

Gastrinomas are gastrin-secreting duodenal or pancreatic neuroendocrine tumors. Zollinger–Ellison syndrome (ZES) is characterized by severe peptic ulceration in association with gastric acid hypersecretion and non-beta islet cell tumors of the pancreas [69]. ZES is rare and occurs in a sporadic form in 80% of cases and familial as part of the multiple endocrine neoplasia syndrome type 1 (MEN-1) [68, 69]. Gastrinoma is the most common functional neuroendocrine tumor in patients with MEN-1 syndrome. The most common symptoms are heartburn, dysphagia, and diarrhea. A secretory diarrhea occurs in up to 40% of patients with ZES; diarrhea is the only presenting complaint in 20% of cases. The secretory diarrhea is caused by hypersecretion of gastric acid resulting in a low intraluminal pH that damages the intestinal mucosa and inactivates various pancreatic enzymes resulting in malabsorption and steatorrhea [69].

Vasoactive Intestinal Peptide Tumor (VIPoma)

VIPomas are rare lesions with an annual incidence of 1 in 10 million patients in the United States [69]. These tumors secrete vasoactive intestinal peptide which stimulates secretion of intestinal fluid and inhibits intestinal absorption of sodium, chloride, potassium, and

Chapter 14 / Surgical Conditions Presenting with Diarrhea

water resulting in the clinical WDHA syndrome of watery diarrhea, hypokalemia, and achlorhydria (WDHA).

Somatostatinoma

Somatostatinomas, tumors that produce excessive somatostatin, create a syndrome of symptoms including diabetes, cholelithiasis, and steatorrhea [69, 70]. Diabetes results due to the inhibitory effects of somatostatin on insulin release. Cholelithiasis results due to decreased gallbladder contractility and CCK release in the presence of elevated somatostatin. Steatorrhea results secondary to somatostatin-induced inhibition of pancreatic enzyme secretion.

Medullary Thyroid Cancer

Medullary thyroid cancer, a cancer arising from calcitonin secreting, parafollicular cells of the thyroid, accounts for 5% of all thyroid malignancies. Twenty-five percent of cases occur as a component of multiple endocrine neoplasia syndrome type 2a or type 2b (MEN-2a or MEN-2b) due to a mutation in the RET proto-oncogene. Diarrhea frequently results in patients with medullary thyroid cancer due to the tumors ability to secrete calcitonin, carcinoembryonic antigen (CEA), histamidases, prostaglandins, and serotonin which work collectively to increase intestinal mobility, impair luminal water absorption, and alter intestinal electrolyte flux.

Chronic Pancreatitis

Etiologies of chronic pancreatitis include alcohol consumption, choledocolithiasis, cigarette smoking, hyperparathyroidism resulting in hypercalcemia, hyperlipidemia, and pancreas divisum [71]. Severe destruction of the pancreas may occur resulting in inadequate endocrine and exocrine function. When exocrine capacity falls below 10% of normal, diarrhea, specifically steatorrhea (bulky, loose, foul smelling, floating stool), may result due to severe enzyme deficiency [72].

REFERENCES

1. Anand RJ, et al. The role of the intestinal barrier in the pathogenesis of necrotizing enterocolitis. Shock 2007; 27(2):124–133.
2. Kliegman RM. Models of the pathogenesis of necrotizing enterocolitis. J Pediatr 1990; 117(1 Pt 2):S2–S5.
3. Jilling T, et al. The roles of bacteria and TLR4 in rat and murine models of necrotizing enterocolitis. J Immunol 2006; 177(5):3273–3282.

4. Moss RL, et al. Laparotomy versus peritoneal drainage for necrotizing enterocolitis and perforation. N Engl J Med 2006; 354(21):2225–2234.
5. Tudehope DI. The epidemiology and pathogenesis of neonatal necrotizing enterocolitis. J Paediatr Child Health 2005; 41(4):167–168.
6. Lee JS and RA Polin Treatment and prevention of necrotizing enterocolitis. Semin Neonatol 2003; 8(6):449–459.
7. Applegate KE. Intussusception in children: evidence-based diagnosis and treatment. Pediatr Radiol 2009; 39(Suppl 2):S140–S143.
8. Bergman K, Mones R, Matuozzi W. Idiopathic cecocolic intussusception in a 16-year-old boy. Pediatr Surg Int 2009; 25(9):819–821.
9. Lu SJ, Goh PS. Traumatic intussusception with intramural haematoma. Pediatr Radiol 2009; 39(4):403–405.
10. Hryhorczuk AL, Strouse PJ. Validation of US as a first-line diagnostic test for assessment of pediatric ileocolic intussusception. Pediatr Radiol 2009; 39(10):1075–1079.
11. Lehnert T, et al. Intussusception in children – clinical presentation, diagnosis and management. Int J Colorectal Dis 2009; 24(10):1187–1192.
12. Fonkalsrud E. Rotational anomalies and volvulus. In O'Neill J, Grossfeld JL, Fonkalsrud EW, Coran AG, Calmadone AA, eds. Principles of pediatric surgery. Philadelphia, PA: Mosby, 2003, pp. 477–458.
13. Millar MR, et al. Application of 16S rRNA gene PCR to study bowel flora of preterm infants with and without necrotizing enterocolitis. J Clin Microbiol 1996; 34(10):2506–2510.
14. Imamoglu M, et al. Rare clinical presentation mode of intestinal malrotation after neonatal period: malabsorption-like symptoms due to chronic midgut volvulus. Pediatr Int 2004; 46(2):167–170.
15. Patino MO, Munden MM. Utility of the sonographic whirlpool sign in diagnosing midgut volvulus in patients with atypical clinical presentations. J Ultrasound Med 2004; 23(3):397–401.
16. Reynolds SL. Missed appendicitis in a pediatric emergency department. Pediatr Emerg Care 1993; 9(1):1–3.
17. Horowitz JR, GM, Jaksic T, Lally KP. Importance of diarrhea as a presenting symptom of appendicitis in very young children. Am J Surg 1997; 173: 80–82.
18. Appendix and Meckel diverticulum. In: Oldham KT, Colombani P, Foglia RP, eds. Surgery of infants and children: scientific principles and practice. Philadelphia, PA: Lippincott-Raven, 1997, pp. 1215–1228.
19. Weiner DJ, Katz A, Hirschl RB, et al. Interval appendectomy in perforated appendicitis. Pediatr Surg Int 1995; 10:82–85.
20. Buchman AL, Scolapio J, Fryer J. AGA technical review on short bowel syndrome and intestinal transplantation. Gastroenterology 2003; 124(4):1111–1134.
21. Wales PW. Surgical therapy for short bowel syndrome. Pediatr Surg Int 2004; 20(9):647–657.
22. Modi BP, et al. First report of the international serial transverse enteroplasty data registry: indications, efficacy, and complications. J Am Coll Surg 2007; 204(3):365–371.
23. Gibson LD, Carter R, Hinshaw DB. Segmental reversal of small intestine after massive bowel resection. Successful case with follow-up examination. JAMA 1962; 182:952–954.
24. Thomas JF, Jordan GL Jr. Massive resection of small bowel and total colectomy: use of reversed segment. Arch Surg 1965; 90:781–786.

Chapter 14 / Surgical Conditions Presenting with Diarrhea 261

25. Fink WJ, Olson JD. The massive bowel resection syndrome. Treatment with reversed intestinal segments. Arch Surg 1967; 94(5):700–706.
26. Poth EJ. Use of gastrointestinal reversal in surgical procedures. Am J Surg 1969; 118(6):893–899.
27. Garcia VF, et al. Colon interposition for the short bowel syndrome. J Pediatr Surg 1981; 16(6):994–995.
28. Glick PL, et al. Colon interposition: an adjuvant operation for short-gut syndrome. J Pediatr Surg 1984; 19(6):719–7125.
29. Waddell WR, et al. A simple jejunocolic "valve". For relief of rapid transit and the short bowel syndrome. Arch Surg 1970; 100(4):438–444.
30. Ricotta J, et al. Construction of an ileocecal valve and its role in massive resection of the small intestine. Surg Gynecol Obstet 1981; 152(3):310–314.
31. Bianchi A, Intestinal loop lengthening – a technique for increasing small intestinal length. J Pediatr Surg 1980; 15(2):145–151.
32. Devine RM, Kelly KA. Surgical therapy of the short bowel syndrome. Gastroenterol Clin North Am 1989; 18(3):603–618.
33. Kim HB, et al. Serial transverse enteroplasty (STEP): a novel bowel lengthening procedure. J Pediatr Surg 2003; 38(3):425–429.
34. Javid PJ, et al. Serial transverse enteroplasty is associated with successful short-term outcomes in infants with short bowel syndrome. J Pediatr Surg 2005; 40(6):1019–1023; discussion 1023–1024.
35. Lichtenstein GR, Hanauer SB, Sandborn WJ. Management of Crohn's disease in adults. Am J Gastroenterol 2009; 104(2):465–483; quiz 464, 484.
36. Wildhaber B, NF, Bergstrasser E, Stallmach T, Sacher P. Paraneoplastic syndromes in ganglioneuroblastoma: contrasting symptoms of constipation and diarrhea. Euro J Pediatr 2003; 162:511–513.
37. Bourdeaut F, et al. VIP hypersecretion as primary or secondary syndrome in neuroblastoma: a retrospective study by the Societe Francaise des Cancers de l'Enfant (SFCE). Pediatr Blood Cancer 2009; 52(5):585–590.
38. Bourgois B, et al. Intractable diarrhoea revealing a neuroblastoma hypersecreting the vasoactive intestinal peptide. Arch Pediatr 2004; 11(4):340–343.
39. Campus R, et al. Intractable diarrhea and neuroblastoma: report of a clinical case. Pediatr Med Chir 2000; 22(1):47–48.
40. Quak SH, et al. Vasoactive intestinal peptide secreting tumours in children: a case report with literature review. Aust Paediatr J 1988; 24(1):55–58.
41. de Buys Roessingh AS, et al. Gastrointestinal complications of post-diarrheal hemolytic uremic syndrome. Eur J Pediatr Surg 2007; 17(5):328–334.
42. Siegler RL, et al. A 20-year population-based study of postdiarrheal hemolytic uremic syndrome in Utah. Pediatrics 1994; 94(1):35–40.
43. Masumoto K, et al. Colonic stricture secondary to hemolytic uremic syndrome caused by Escherichia coli O-157. Pediatr Nephrol 2005; 20(10):1496–1499.
44. Tapper D, et al. Lessons learned in the management of hemolytic uremic syndrome in children. J Pediatr Surg 1995; 30(2):158–163.
45. Nalesnik MA. The diverse pathology of post-transplant lymphoproliferative disorders: the importance of a standardized approach. Transpl Infect Dis 2001; 3(2):88–96.
46. Bakker NA, et al. Presentation and early detection of post-transplant lymphoproliferative disorder after solid organ transplantation. Transpl Int 2007; 20(3):207–218.
47. McDiarmid SV, et al. Prevention and preemptive therapy of posttransplant lymphoproliferative disease in pediatric liver recipients. Transplantation 1998; 66(12):1604–1611.

48. Chia SC, Chau YP, Tan YM. Late-onset post-transplant lymphoproliferative disease presenting as massive occult gastrointestinal haemorrhage. Singapore Med J 2008; 49(5):e117–e120.
49. Okutani D, Kotani K, Makihara S. A case of gastrocolocutaneous fistula as a complication of percutaneous endoscopic gastrostomy. Acta Med Okayama 2008; 62(2):135–138.
50. Jensen SW, Eriksen J, Kristensen K. Severe diarrhea after the original well-functioning percutaneous endoscopic gastrostomy tube was replaced by a Mic-Key button. Ugeskr Laeger 2006; 168(10):1038–1039.
51. Chen Y, Ni YH, Lai HS. Gastrocolocutaneous fistula in a child with congenital short bowel syndrome: a rare complication of percutaneous endoscopic gastrostomy. J Formos Med Assoc 2004; 103(4):306–310.
52. Friedmann R, Feldman H, Sonnenblick M. Misplacement of percutaneously inserted gastrostomy tube into the colon: report of 6 cases and review of the literature. JPEN J Parenter Enteral Nutr 2007; 31(6):469–476.
53. Yamazaki T, et al. Colocutaneous fistula after percutaneous endoscopic gastrostomy in a remnant stomach. Surg Endosc 1999; 13(3):280–282.
54. Chow E, Macrae F. A review of juvenile polyposis syndrome. J Gastroenterol Hepatol 2005; 20(11):1634–1640.
55. Paterno F, Longo WE. The etiology and pathogenesis of vascular disorders of the intestine. Radiol Clin North Am 2008; 46(5):877–885, v.
56. Rego A, et al. Attenuation of vascular relaxation and cyclic GMP responses by cyclosporin A. J Pharmacol Exp Ther 1990; 252(1):165–170.
57. Herbert GS, Steele SR. Acute and chronic mesenteric ischemia. Surg Clin North Am 2007; 87(5):1115–1134, ix.
58. Thomas DP, Roberts HR. Hypercoagulability in venous and arterial thrombosis. Ann Intern Med 1997; 126(8):638–644.
59. Theodoropoulou A, Koutroubakis, IE. Ischemic colitis: clinical practice in diagnosis and treatment. World J Gastroenterol 2008; 14(48):7302–7308.
60. Taourel P, et al. Imaging of ischemic colitis. Radiol Clin North Am 2008; 46(5):909–924, vi.
61. Steele SR. Ischemic colitis complicating major vascular surgery. Surg Clin North Am 2007; 87(5):1099–1114, ix.
62. *Clostridium difficile* colitis. In: Cameron J, ed. Current surgical therapy, 9th edn. Philadelphia, PA: Mosby, 2008, pp. 186–188.
63. Jaber MR, et al. Clinical review of the management of fulminant clostridium difficile infection. Am J Gastroenterol 2008; 103(12):3195–3203; quiz 3204.
64. Malkan AD, Pimiento JM, Maloney SP, et al. Unusual manifestations of *Clostridium difficile* infection. Surg Infect (Larchmt) 2010; 11(3):333–337.
65. Adams SD, Mercer DW. Fulminant Clostridium difficile colitis. Curr Opin Crit Care 2007; 13(4):450–455.
66. Sailhamer EA, et al. Fulminant Clostridium difficile colitis: patterns of care and predictors of mortality. Arch Surg 2009; 144(5):433–439; discussion 439–440.
67. Ali SO, Welch JP, Dring RJ. Early surgical intervention for fulminant pseudomembranous colitis. Am Surg 2008; 74(1):20–26.
68. Akerstrom G, Hellman P. Surgical aspects of neuroendocrine tumours. Eur J Cancer 2009; 45(Suppl 1):237–250.
69. Mansour JC, Chen H. Pancreatic endocrine tumors. J Surg Res 2004; 120(1):139–161.
70. Doherty GM. Rare endocrine tumours of the GI tract. Best Pract Res Clin Gastroenterol 2005; 19(5):807–817.

71. Frey CF. Role of subtotal pancreatectomy and pancreaticojejunostomy in chronic pancreatitis. J Surg Res 1981; 31(5):361–370.
72. DiMagno EP, Go VL, Summerskill WH. Relations between pancreatic enzyme outputs and malabsorption in severe pancreatic insufficiency. N Engl J Med 1973; 288(16):813–815.

15 Chronic Diarrheal Disorders due to Endocrine Neoplasms

Tanvi Dhere, MD, Julia Massaad, MD and Shanthi V. Sitaraman, MD, PhD

CONTENTS

INTRODUCTION
GASTRINOMAS
CARCINOID
VIPOMAS
SOMATOSTATINOMAS
GLUCAGONOMAS
SYSTEMIC MASTOCYTOSIS AND OTHER
    RARE CAUSES OF NEUROENDOCRINE
    TUMORS RESULTING IN DIARRHEA
REFERENCES

Summary

Endocrine neoplasms of the gut are a rare cause of chronic diarrhea and account for <1% of patients who present with chronic diarrhea. However, diarrhea associated with endocrine neoplasms can cause significant morbidity and mortality, and clinicians should recognize the diarrheal syndromes associated with endocrine neoplasms. This chapter discusses pathophysiology, diagnostic tests, and treatment options for diarrhea associated with endocrine neoplasms.

Key Words: Chronic diarrhea, Secretory diarrhea, Neuroendocrine tumors

From: *Diarrhea, Clinical Gastroenterology*
Edited by: S. Guandalini, H. Vaziri, DOI 10.1007/978-1-60761-183-7_15
© Springer Science+Business Media, LLC 2011

INTRODUCTION

Endocrine neoplasms of the gut are rare tumors that secrete excess amounts of autocoids or gastrointestinal peptides which can result in a wide range of signs and symptoms, including diarrhea. These tumors may be sporadic or associated with familial syndromes such as multiple endocrine neoplasia I (MEN I) or Wermer's syndrome. Although the reported frequency of neuroendocrine tumors (Fig. 15.1) is approximately 0.5–1.5% of autopsy specimens, less than 1 per 100,000 persons are symptomatic. Neuroendocrine tumors account for <1% of chronic diarrhea [1]. Routine testing for gastrointestinal peptides is not recommended in the workup of patients with chronic diarrhea. One study showed the positive predictive value of the test to be <2% with false positives being 45% [2]. Table 15.1 lists the endocrine tumors associated with diarrhea and related syndrome findings.

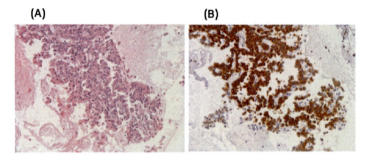

Fig. 15.1. a Well-differentiated neuroendocrine tumor. **b** Synaptophysin stained neuroendocrine tumor.

GASTRINOMAS

Gastrinomas are rare neuroendocrine tumors that involve primarily the pancreas and duodenum and can result in Zollinger–Ellison syndrome (ZES). Gastrinomas are the most common type of pancreatic neuroendocrine tumors and account for 70% of all functioning neuroendocrine tumors [3]. The mean age of onset is about 41 years old but there is a delay in diagnosis by about 5–6 years. The majority of these tumors are sporadic but 20–25% of them are familial and associated with the MEN I syndrome.

Clinical Presentation

The hallmark symptoms of these tumors include abdominal discomfort, diarrhea, and GERD. The majority of patients diagnosed with

Chapter 15 / Chronic Diarrheal Disorders due to Endocrine Neoplasms 267

Table 15.1
Neuroendocrine tumors and associated syndrome findings

Tumor	Percentage of patients with diarrhea	Syndrome findings
Gastrinoma	75	Diarrhea/steatorrhea, abdominal pain, GERD, ulcer
Carcinoid	10	Flushing, diarrhea
VIPoma	100	Secretory diarrhea, hypokalemia, achlorhydria
Somatostatinoma	10	Diabetes, hypochlorhydria, cholelithiasis, diarrhea/steatorrhea, anemia, weight loss
Glucagonoma	15 – 20	Diabetes, DVT, depression, dermatitis
Mastocytosis	43	No associated syndrome

gastrinomas present with abdominal pain or diarrhea. Heartburn and reflux are the initial symptoms in 44%. Prominent gastric folds are found in 94% of patients [4]. Gastrinomas are characterized by recurrent ulcers which typically occur in the duodenum but may occur in the jejunum. About 75% of patients present with watery diarrhea. This is thought to be due to mechanical irritation and trauma of the duodenum and jejunum due to acidified contents and volume overload on the small intestine due to increased gastric acid secretion. Steatorrhea may be present as well due to inactivation of pancreatic lipase by gastric acid secretion.

Approximately 50–60% of gastrinomas are malignant. The presence of liver metastases is the most important predictor of overall survival, resulting in a 5-year survival rate of 20–30% [5].

Diagnosis

Hyergastrinemia (greater than 150 pg/ml) serves as a hallmark for diagnosis of ZES. However, hypergastrinemia may be the result of other disorders, including chronic atrophic gastritis, *Helicobacter pylori* infection, and antral G-cell hyperplasia. Elevated gastrin levels are also seen in 25% of patients taking proton pump inhibitors (PPI). Also, false-positive secretin stimulation test for gastrinoma have been associated with the use of PPI [6]. However, it is rare to see values that approach the levels seen in ZES or chronic atrophic gastritis [7]. Despite this,

PPI therapy should be stopped for at least 2 weeks prior to checking gastrin levels and performing secretin stimulation testing. Basal acid output can also be measured with levels greater than 15 mmol/h prior to surgery being associated with the presence of gastrinomas.

Most ZES patients do not have gastrin levels that are >1000. Provocative tests with the infusion of secretin or calcium may be required. When secretin is used, gastrin levels are increased by at least 200 pg/ml after 2–10 min of infusion with gradual return to baseline values [6]. The combination of hypergastrinemia along with hyperchlorhydria suggests ZES.

If there is a high suspicion of gastrinoma based on clinical presentation and labs, imaging workup should be the next step. Obtaining an octreotide scan or somatostatin receptor scintigraphy aids in identifying a gastrinoma. If this test is negative, a CT or MRI may be obtained. However, tumors less than 1 cm are often not visualized with CT. If the previous radiologic examinations are negative, an endoscopic ultrasound may be performed to help establish the diagnosis. If all of the above are negative, an angiogram with arterial stimulation with secretin combined with venous sampling may be obtained.

Treatment

Apart from surgical resection of the incipient tumor, symptoms from gastrinomas including diarrhea are often alleviated with the use of high-dose proton pump inhibitors. Doses of omeprazole 80–100 mg or pantoprazole 40–160 mg are employed. Once control of gastric output has been established, the dose of proton pump utilized is significantly reduced. The goal of treatment is to achieve a gastric pH >4 and a basal acid output reduction of 10 mEq H^+ per hour in order to relieve symptoms as well as prevent cytotoxic effects on mucosa secondary to elevated acid levels.

In patients that present with sporadic gastrinomas without hepatic metastases and in whom the risk of surgery is negligible, an operative exploration with duodenotomy is recommended. Intraoperative ultrasound may also be used to help localize gastrinomas. Surgical exploration results in a 95% detection rate for gastrinomas [8]. The goal of surgery is not only to provide cure and symptom improvement but also to prevent malignant progression [9].

In patients with MEN I, the role of surgery is more complicated as these patients tend to have multifocal disease and approximately 50% present with metastases to the liver, lymph nodes, or elsewhere. Also, the multifocal neoplasms may be secreting nonfunctioning peptides and as such, the ability to localize functional gastrinomas becomes more

Chapter 15 / Chronic Diarrheal Disorders due to Endocrine Neoplasms   269

difficult, thereby resulting in a lower cure rate. When surgery is considered, neck exploration for resection of parathyroid hyperplasia should be performed. Hyperparathyroidism is present in more than 95% of patients with MEN I and resection of parathyroid hyperplasia has been shown to reduce the effects of hypergastrinemia [10].

Cytotoxic chemotherapy with the use of streptozotocin with or without 5-fluorouracil along with doxorubicin is used in advanced cases for patients that are not surgical candidates. The use of chemotherapy in gastrinomas has been shown to reduce tumor burden as well as decrease gastrin levels, resulting in diarrheal and other symptom improvement [10].

CARCINOID

Carcinoid tumors are the most common neuroendocrine tumors with a prevalence of 1–2/100,000. In addition, the incidence of these tumors is on the rise [11]. The majority of carcinoids originate in the gastrointestinal tract while carcinoids of the lungs and bronchi are less common. Because of the indolent nature of the majority of these tumors, the average time from onset of symptoms to obtaining a diagnosis is about 9 years [12]. Five-year survival rate is 67.2% regardless of the site of tumor.

The three main areas of gastrointestinal origin of carcinoid are the foregut (stomach, duodenum, pancreas, bronchial), midgut (jejunum–right colon), and hindgut (transverse colon–rectum). The incidence of carcinoid varies according to the site of origin. The ileum is the most common site, followed then by the rectum, colon, stomach, appendix, lungs, and bronchi.

Clinical Presentation

Symptoms of carcinoid vary depending on location as well as release of hormonally active compounds. Classically, patients present with flushing and diarrhea, which is referred to as carcinoid syndrome, which occurs most commonly with metastatic disease. Most carcinoids, however, are small indolent tumors. Those that occur in the foregut may present atypically due to secretion of other hormones aside from serotonin. Those that occur in the midgut (the small intestine) may present with carcinoid syndrome if there is concomitant metastatic and bulky retroperitoneal adenopathy. This is due to the high levels of serotonin produced by these tumors. Hindgut carcinoids rarely produce symptoms unless the disease is more advanced. Other symptoms include mild abdominal discomfort and intestinal obstruction.

Carcinoid syndrome, which occurs more often with midgut tumors associated with metastatic liver disease, is a predictor of poor survival as the presence of this syndrome indicates more advanced disease. The syndrome occurs in only about 10% of patients with carcinoid tumor [13]. It may be precipitated by exertion or by eating foods rich in tyramine, such as blue cheese and chocolate, or by drinking alcohol. Carcinoid syndrome is a result of serotonin (5-hydroxytryptamine) released by the tumors into the systemic circulation that bypass metabolism in the liver. The product leads to excitation of smooth muscle as well as vascular dilation resulting in diarrhea, flushing, hypotension, and bronchospasm. About two-thirds of these patients may also have evidence of carcinoid heart disease, which results in fibrous thickening of the endocardium of the right heart.

Carcinoid crisis refers to a life-threatening event that may be precipitated by stressful events such as anesthesia and surgery. The overwhelming release of biologically active compounds leads to flushing, diarrhea, tachycardia, arrhythmias, bronchospasm, and altered mental status.

Diagnosis

For those patients presenting with carcinoid syndrome, the urinary levels of the major serotonin metabolite 5-hydroxyindoleacetic acid (5-HIAA) levels may be measured. The test has a diagnostic sensitivity of 70% and a specificity of 88–100%. Serum chromogranin A levels, which are more sensitive than 5-HIAA, may be measured as well in those patients whom carcinoid tumor is suspected. The sensitivity approaches 80% and specificity approaches 95%. OctreoScans have a sensitivity of 80–90% and may be the initial imaging diagnostic test in localizing carcinoid lesions. However, the addition of octreotide to standard SPECT/CT imaging provides higher diagnostic value and more reader confidence through the ability to identify lesions, determine physiologic activity, and gain additional anatomic information (Fig 15.2) [14]. Endoscopic ultrasound may also be used.

Treatment

Apart from surgical resection, the mainstay of treatment of diarrhea associated with carcinoid syndrome is octreotide or lanreotide, which both avidly bind to somatostatin receptor subtype 2. They both are equally effective in the treatment of carcinoid-associated diarrhea and must be administered by multiple subcutaneous injections or by continuous intravenous infusion. The slow-release depot intramuscular

Chapter 15 / Chronic Diarrheal Disorders due to Endocrine Neoplasms   271

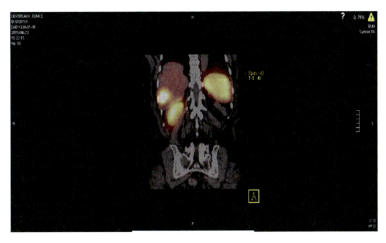

Fig. 15.2. Octreoscan with SPECT/CT in female with metastatic carcinoid. Uptake noted in gastric antrum and right hepatic lobe.

formulation of both medications, however, can be administered every 4 weeks [15]. The interval may be decreased depending on the patient's symptoms. If one somatostatin analogue fails, the other analogue should be administered for treatment of carcinoid syndrome. A new somatostatin analogue, pasireotide, which has a broader binding affinity for somatostatin receptors, is currently being studied in clinical trials [16]. Despite continuous treatment with octreotide, failure may occur. Attempts of treating carcinoid-associated diarrhea have included the use of serotonin receptor antagonists, such as cyproheptadine and methysergide [17]. Despite the reduction in diarrhea, severe central nervous side effects as well as risk of retroperitoneal fibrosis with the use of methysergide preclude the use of these treatments long term. Successful treatment with the use of ondansetron has been found to be effective for carcinoid-related diarrhea; however, no randomized trials are available [18]. Alpha 2 receptor agonists have been used as well as an adjunct treatment for carcinoid syndrome [19].

Surgical treatment for localized carcinoid tumors varies depending on the size of the lesion as well as the location. The risk for metastases is the least for appendiceal tumors and greatest for rectal primaries, which are the least associated with carcinoid syndrome.

Patients with limited metastases to the liver may be surgically managed [20]. Other options include hepatic artery embolization (HAI) or ligation with or without interferon/chemotherapy [21]. Liver transplantation continues to be a consideration in patients with liver-only metastases [22]. Long-acting somatostatin analogues lanreotide or depot octreotides may also be considered, although the biochemical response far outweighs the tumor response rates. For patients with more systemic spread, chemotherapy, interferon alpha, along with long-acting somatostatin analogues, may be used to treat diarrhea and other symptoms. Another novel approach that is currently under investigation includes the use of peptide receptor radionuclide therapy (PRRT) for treatment of metastatic unresectable neuroendocrine tumors. The results thus far have been promising for the treatment of somatostatin receptor-positive endocrine tumors [23].

Treatment response can be assessed with monitoring of biomarkers, most notably 5-HIAA. Reductions in tumor size on cross-sectional imaging may also be used to determine treatment efficacy.

VIPOMAS

Vipomas are rare islet cell tumors, the majority of which occur in the pancreas. The annual incidence of these tumors is 1 in 10,000,000 individuals [24]. The most common clinical presentation is profuse watery diarrhea associated with hypokalemia, hyperglycemia, hypercalcemia, achlorhydria, and flushing, a syndrome previously referred to as "pancreatic cholera." VIPomas have a high malignant potential and at least 60% of these tumors have metastasized by the time of diagnosis [25]. Most VIPomas are solitary tumors but can be part of the MEN 1 syndrome in 1% of the cases [26]. The overall 5-year survival rate for patients with pancreatic VIPomas is 68.5%.

Clinical Presentation

Elevated VIP levels can lead to excessive fluid and chloride secretion, thus leading to the profuse secretory diarrhea associated with VIPomas. Large amounts of potassium and bicarbonate are excreted in the stool which can lead to life-threatening cardiovascular arrhythmias, acidosis, and volume depletion. Typically, patients have more than 3 l of stool per day, so a stool volume <700 ml/day rules out a VIPoma [27]. Other manifestations of VIPomas include flushing, hypercalcemia, and hyperglycemia [28].

Diagnosis

The diagnosis of VIPoma is suggested by a fasting plasma VIP level of more than 200 pg/ml in the presence of secretory diarrhea [29]. The diarrhea persists despite fasting and has a low osmolality <50 mosm/kg and a high sodium concentration [30]. Laxative abuse and the Zollinger–Ellison syndrome can present similar to VIPomas with severe secretory diarrhea and an elevated fasting VIP level. Because most VIPomas present at a mean size >3 cm and are highly vascular, radiologic evaluation will confirm the presence of the tumor in the majority of cases, as well as document the presence or absence of metastatic disease. Other imaging modalities used to localize VIPomas include endoscopic ultrasound, somatostatin receptor scintigraphy, and MRI [31, 32].

Treatment

The mainstay of therapy of VIPoma is aggressive correction of fluid and electrolyte abnormalities. Medical therapy including octreotide ameliorates many of the clinical manifestations of the disease including diarrhea, dehydration, and hypokalemia [33]. Interferon alpha is used as an alternative therapy or add-on therapy in patients who respond poorly to octreotide despite the lack of widespread acceptance particularly due to its potential side effects which include fatigue, depression, thyroid dysfunction, and myelosuppression [34].

Medical therapy such as the use of somatostatin analogues often target the elevated VIP levels and help alleviate the diarrhea, but the only hope for cure is with surgical therapy. Surgical options include palliative or curative modalities. The literature reports a 44–50% resectability rate of VIPomas, with a 10% "resectable for cure" rate [35]. If curative resection is not feasible, then palliative resection should be considered if the patient is an acceptable surgical candidate [36].

Other treatment modalities for metastatic disease have been suggested including cytotoxic chemotherapy and organ targeted therapy [37]. Given the frequent metastatic spread of VIPomas to the liver, multiple liver targeted therapies have proven to be promising including hepatic arterial embolization and radiofrequency ablation [38]. When feasible, surgical resection of hepatic metastasis remains the treatment of choice. Orthotopic liver transplantation for hepatic metastasis is an investigational approach at this point in time [39]. The role of these treatment modalities continues to be undetermined at this point in time, with concern for a high recurrence rate in the limited published literature [40].

SOMATOSTATINOMAS

Somatostinomas are one of the rarest pancreatic endocrine tumors. These tumors possess somatostatin immunoreactivity but are not always associated with a functional syndrome. The majority of the tumors are sporadic but rarely may be associated with neurofibromatosis type 1, MEN I, and von Hippel–Lindau syndromes.

Somatostatinoma syndrome, which occurs in close to 10% of patients with somatostatinomas, is associated with markedly elevated levels of somatostatin, diabetes of recent onset, hypochlorydria, gallbladder disease, diarrhea or steatorrhea, anemia, and weight loss [41]. The most common symptoms include diabetes and gallbladder disease. Diarrhea is present in 37% of patients with the syndrome. Steatorrhea is present in 47%.

Approximately 53–84% of all tumors show evidence of metastatic spread at the time of diagnosis [42]. The mean 5-year survival rate of metastatic disease is about 60%. Patients without metastases have an excellent prognosis with close to 100% 5- year survival rates.

The pathophysiology of somatostatinoma syndrome can be largely explained by the hormone's inhibitory action. Somatostatin inhibits release of gastrointestinal hormones, stimulated acid and pancreatic secretion, and intestinal absorption of amino acids, sugars, and calcium. Diarrhea and steatorrhea are a result of the inhibition on secretion of pancreatic enzymes and bicarbonate as well as inhibition of absorption of lipids [41].

The diagnosis of somatostatinomas begins with radiologic imaging, such as MRI or octreotide scan, to localize and evaluate the extent of the tumor. EUS may be used to localize small submucosal somatostatinomas that may be located in the duodenum or pancreatic head that are not otherwise visualized using standard imaging techniques. A real-time intraoperative ultrasound should be used during exploratory surgery to help localize the primary tumor and evaluate for metastatic disease. Elevated plasma levels of somatostatin-like immunoreactivity (SLI) concentrations are associated with the clinical syndrome [43].

Medical treatment for somatostatinomas includes octreotide, which aids in diminishing symptoms of diabetes and diarrhea as well as decreasing metastatic tumor burden [44]. Patients also may be malnourished and require hyperalimentation along with correction of nutritional deficiencies. Oral hypoglycemics are used to control blood sugars in the setting of diabetes. If imaging shows resectability, patients may benefit from surgical resection of the tumor. Metastatic disease may benefit from chemotherapeutic agents including combination therapy with 5-fluorouracil and streptozotocin or doxorubicin. For patient with hepatic metastases, HAI or chemoembolization is an option for treatment. Cytoreductive surgical resection of liver metastases can be performed in patients without extensive spread. Interferon alpha is used as well to control clinical symptoms [45]. When surgery is performed, a cholecystectomy is also completed in lieu of the risk of cholelithiasis.

GLUCAGONOMAS

Glucagonomas are rare pancreatic endocrine tumors that are also associated with diarrhea. The average time from the first manifestation to diagnosis is about 2 years and the prevalence is close to 1 in 20 million people.

The syndrome associated with these tumors is often referred to as the "4-D" syndrome. Diabetes, deep venous thromboses, depression, and dermatitis represent the D's [46]. The classic rash is termed necrolytic migratory erythema, which is a pruritic red rash involving the pretibial, perioral, and intertriginous areas [47]. Diarrhea is present in 15–20% of patients. Glucagonomas are also a part of the MEN 1 syndrome in rare cases.

Diagnosis is made by elevated levels of plasma glucagons (>500 pg/ml). Decreased levels of zinc, amino acids, and essential fatty acids may also be found. SRS may be used in localization as well as long-term follow-up.

Medical therapy is similar to the other gastro-entero-pancreatic neuroendocrine tumors and includes octreotide to suppress glucagon production, which alleviates diarrhea [48]. A combination of streptozocin and doxorubicin is often used for metastatic or recurrent disease to control symptoms [49]. When surgery is performed, a distal pancreatectomy with resection of lymph nodes as well as liver metastases is completed. This is possible in only 30% of glucagonoma cases. Symptoms, including diarrhea, improve rapidly after resection; however, there is a high probability of repeat resection for recurrent metastases [50].

Other options for liver metastases include the use of chemotherapy, HAI, and percutaneous or intraoperative radio frequency ablation. Liver transplantation is also a possibility for treatment; however, this is rarely performed [37].

The prognosis for patients with glucagonomas includes a 5-year survival rate of 50% without resection. However, most patients have evidence of metastases at the time of presentation.

SYSTEMIC MASTOCYTOSIS AND OTHER RARE CAUSES OF NEUROENDOCRINE TUMORS RESULTING IN DIARRHEA

Systemic mastocytosis (SM) is a rare disease with abnormal proliferation and infiltration of mast cells in at least one extracutaneous organ. Gastrointestinal symptoms are present in 14–85% of patients due to effects of mast cell mediators as well as direct infiltration of mast cells into the GI tract. Diarrhea or steatorrhea is found in 43% of patients. It is due to direct mucosal injury and edema, gastric acid hypersection, and altered bowel motility. Protein losing enteropathy is present in some cases. Other GI symptoms include abdominal pain, nausea, vomiting, and bloating [51]. Triggers for mast cell release and induction of symptoms include exposure to NSAIDS, opiates, and penicillin.

The diagnosis of mastocytosis is made by identification of mast cells in various organs. There is no curative therapy for aggressive SM. However, cytoreductive therapy with use of combination of interferon alpha, prednisolone, cladribine, and specific KIT tyrosine kinase inhibitors are often used [52, 53]. During treatment, the risk of mast cell activation and mediator release may be life-threatening; it is imperative to utilize histamine receptor antagonists as prophylaxis.

Other rarer neuroendocrine causes of diarrhea include medullary thyroid cancer and calcitonin-secreting pancreatic endocrine tumors.

Medullary thyroid cancers (MTC) are derived from parafollicular or C cells, which are part of the APUD (amine precursor and uptake decarboxylation) system [54]. They secrete calcitonin but have the ability to also secrete other hormones such as serotonin, which may be the cause of diarrhea in patients afflicted with these cancers.

For diagnosis, fine needle aspiration of the thyroid is first performed and confirmed by high serum levels of calcitonin; a level less than 10 pg/ml virtually excludes medullary thyroid cancer. An octreotide scan, which is the most sensitive test, may be performed.

Treatment is total thyroidectomy with central neck lymph node dissection. Standard chemotherapy or radiation therapy has little effect for metastatic disease. Vandetanib, which is an oral selective inhibitor of RET, has shown reduction in calcitonin levels in metastatic hereditary MTC [55]. Diarrheal symptoms respond to octreotide as well.

Survival for MTC varies according to the extent. For localized disease, the 10-year survival rate is 95%. For patients with distant metastases, the 10-year survival rate is close to 45%.

Fewer than 20 case reports of *calcitonin secreting pancreatic endocrine tumors* have been published. About half of the cases were symptomatic, with the predominant complaints being diarrhea or flushing [56, 57]. The diagnosis rests with radiologic examinations as well as findings on exploratory laparotomy. Unfortunately, most cases are malignant. Treatment is similar to other endocrine tumors in that surgery is the backbone of treatment. Pancreatic resection may be performed for tumors that are isolated. Pancreatic resection along with resection of liver metastases may be considered for patients who present with more extensive disease [58].

REFERENCES

1. Schiller LR. Diarrhea and malabsorption in the elderly. Gastroenterol Clin N Am 2009; 38:481–502.
2. Schiller LR, Rivera LM, Santangelo WC, et al. Diagnostic value of fasting plasma peptide concentrations in patients with chronic diarrhea. Dig Dis Sci 1994; 39:2216–2122.
3. Jensen RT, Niederle B, Mitry E, et al. Gastrinoma (duodenal and pancreatic). Neuroendocrinology 2006; 84(3):173–182.
4. Roy PK, Venzon DJ, Shojamanesh H, et al. Zollinger-Ellison syndrome: clinical presentation in 261 patients. Medicine 2000; 79:379–411.
5. Imamura M, Komoto I, Ota S. Changing treatment strategy for gastrinoma in patients with Zollinger-Ellison syndrome. World J Surg 2006; 30:1–11.
6. McGulgan JE, Wofe MM. Secretin injection test in the diagnosis of gastrinoma. Gastroenterology 1980; 79:1324–1331.
7. Bonapace ES, Fisher RS, Parkman HP. Does fasting serum gastrin predict gastric acid suppression in patients on PPI? Dig Dis Sci 2000; 45:34–39.
8. Norton JA, Doppman JL, Jensen RT. Curative resection in Zollinger-Ellison syndrome: results of a 10 year prospective study. Ann Surg 1992; 215:8–18.
9. Norton JA, Fraker DL, Alexander HR. Surgery increases survival in patients with gastrinoma. Ann Surg 2006; 244:410–419.
10. Norton JA. Gastrinoma: advances in localization and treatment. Surg Oncol Clin Am 1998; 7:845–861.
11. Ghevariya V, Malieckal A, Ghevariya N, et al. Carcinoid tumors of the gastrointestinal tract. South Med J 2009; 102(10):1032–1040.
12. Modlin IM, Lye KD, Kidd M. A 5-decade analysis of 13,715 carcinoid tumors. Cancer 2003; 97:934–959.
13. Jensen R, Doherty GM. Carcinoid tumors and the carcinoid syndrome. In: DeVita VT Jr, Hellman S, Rosenberg SA, eds. Cancer: principles and practice of oncology, 7th edn. Philadelphia: Lippincott Williams and Wilkins, 2005, pp. 1559–1574.
14. Wong KK, Cahill JM, Frey KA, et al. Incremental value of 111-in pentetreotide SPECT/CT fusion imaging of neuroendocrine tumors. Acad Radiol 2010; 17(3):291–297.
15. O'Toole D, Ducreux M, Bommelaer G, et al. Treatment of carcinoid syndrome: a prospective crossover evaluation of lanreotide versus octreotide in terms of efficacy, patient acceptability, and tolerance. Cancer 2000; 88(4):770–776.
16. Modlin IM, Pavel M, Kidd M, et al. Review article: somatostatin analogs in the treatment of gastro-entero-pancreatic neuroendocrine (carcinoid) tumors. Aliment Pharmacol Ther 2010;31(2):169–188.
17. Moertel CG, Kvols LK, Rubin J. A study of cyproheptadine in the treatment of metastatic carcinoid tumor and the malignant carcinoid syndrome. Cancer 1991; 67(1):33–36.
18. Platt AJ, Heddle RM, Rake MO, et al. Ondansetron in carcinoid syndrome. Lancet 1992; 339(8806):1416.
19. Schwörer H, Münke H, Stöckmann F, et al. Treatment of diarrhea in carcinoid syndrome with ondansetron, tropisetron, and clonidine. Am J Gastroenterol 1995; 90(4):645–648.
20. Yao KA, Talamonti MS, Nemcek A, et al. Indications and results of liver resection and hepatic chemoembolization for metastatic gastrointestinal neuroendocrine tumors. Surgery 2001; 130:677–682.

21. Gupta S, Yao JC, Ahrar K, et al. Hepatic artery embolization and chemoembolization for treatment of patients with metastatic carcinoid tumors: the MD Anderson experience. Cancer J 2003; 9:261–267.
22. Bechstein WO, Neuhaus P. Liver transplantation for hepatic metastases of neuroendocrine tumors. N Y Acad Sci 1994; 733:507–514.
23. van Essen M, Krenning EP, Kam BL, et al. Peptide-receptor radionuclide therapy for endocrine tumors. Nat Rev Endocrinol 2009; 5(7):382–393.
24. Ghaferi A, Chojnacki K, Long W, et al. Pancreatic VIPomas: subject review and one institutional experience. J Gastrointest Surg 2008; 12:382–393.
25. Friesen SR. Update on the diagnosis and treatment of rare neuroendocrine tumors. Surg Clin North Am 1987; 67:379.
26. Smith S, Branton S, Avino A, et al. Vasoactive intestinal polypeptide secreting islet cell tumors: a 15-year experience and review of the literature. Surgery 1998; 124:1050–1055.
27. Krejs G. VIPoma syndrome. Am J Med 1987; 82(suppl 5B):37–48.
28. Grier J. WDHA syndrome: clinical features, diagnosis, and treatment. Southern Med J 1995; 88(1):22–25.
29. Delcore R, Friesen S. Gastrointestinal Neuroendocrine Tumors. J Am Coll Surg 1994;178:187–211.
30. Mansour J, Chen H. Pancreatic Endocrine Tumors. J Surg Research 2004; 120:139–161.
31. Legmann P, Vignaux O, Dousset B, et al. Pancreatic tumors: comparison of dual-phase helical CT and endoscopic sonography. Am J Roentgenol 1998; 170(5):1315–1322.
32. Theoni RF, Mueller-Lisse UG, Chan R, et al. Detection of small functional islet cell tumors in the pancreas: selection of MR imaging sequences for optimal sensitivity. Radiology 2000; 214(2):483–490.
33. Lamberts S, Van Der Lely A, De Herder W, et al. Octreotide. N Eng J Med 1996; 334(4):246–254.
34. Faiss S, Ulrich-Frank P, Bohmig M, et al. Prospective, randomized, multi-center trial on the antiproliferative effect of lantreotide, interferon alpha, and their combination for therapy of metastatic neuroendocrine gastropancreatic tumors: The International Lantreotide and Interferon Alpha Study Group. J Clin Oncol 2003; 21(14):2689–2696.
35. Thompson GB, Van Heerden JA, Grant CS, Carney JA, Ilstrup DM. Islet cell carcinomas of the pancreas: a twenty year experience. Surgery 1988; 104:1011–1017.
36. Thompson NW, Eckhauser FE. Malignant islet cell tumors of the pancreas. World J Surg 1984; 8:940–951.
37. Abood G, Go A, Malhotra D, et al. The surgical and systemic management of neuroendocrine tumors of the pancreas. Surg Clin North Am 2009; 89(1): 249–266.
38. Marlink RG, Lockich JJ, Robins JR, et al. Hepatic arterial embolization for metastatic hormone-secreting tumors: technique, effectiveness, and complications. Cancer 1990; 65:2227–2232.
39. Le Treut P, Delpero J, Dousset B, et al. Results of liver transplantation in the treatment of metastatic neuroendocrine tumors: a 31 case French multicentric report. Ann Surg 1997; 225(4):355–364.
40. Soga J, Yakuwa Y. Vipoma/diarrheogenic syndrome: a statistical evaluation of 241 reported cases. J Exp Clin Cancer Res 1998; 17(4):389–400.
41. Krejs GJ, Orci L, Conlon JM, et al. Somatostatinoma syndrome. Biochemical, morphologic and clinical features NEJM 1979; 301:285–292.

Chapter 15 / Chronic Diarrheal Disorders due to Endocrine Neoplasms 279

42. Vinik A. Strodel WE, Eckhauser FE, et al. Somatostatinomas, PPoma, neurotensi-nomas. Semin Oncol 1987; 14:263.
43. Farr CM, Price HM, Bezmalinovic Z. Duodenal somatostatinoma with congenital pseudoarthrosis. J Clin Gastro 1991; 13:195–197.
44. Arnold R, Trautmann ME, Creutzfeldt W, et al. Somatostatin analogue octreotide and inhibition of tumour growth in metastatic endocrine gastroenteropancreatic tumors. Gut 1996; 38:430–438.
45. Nesi G, Marcucci T, Rubio CA, et al. Somatostatinoma: clinico-pathological features of three cases and literature reviewed. Gastroenterol Hepatol 2008; 23(4):521–526.
46. Stacpoole PW. The glucagonoma syndrome: clinical features, diagnosis, and treatment. Endocrine Rev 1981; 2:347–361.
47. van Beek AP, de Haas ERM, van Vloten WA. The glucagonoma syndrome and necrolytic migratory erythema: a clinical review. Eur J Endocrinol 2004; 151(5): 531–537.
48. Bouin M, Aoust LD. Clinical response of an atypical glucagonoma treated with a long-acting somatostatin analog. Gastroenterol Clin Biol 2002; 26:926–929.
49. Carvajal C, Azabache V, Lobos P, et al. Glucagonoma: evolution and treatment. Rev Med Chil 2002; 130:671–676.
50. Hellman P, Andersson M, Rastad J, et al. Surgical strategy for large or malignant endocrine pancreatic tumors. World J Surg 2000; 24:1353–1360.
51. Jensen RT. GI abnormalities and involvement in systemic mastocytosis. Hematol Oncol Clin North Am 2000; 14:579–623.
52. Valent P, Akin C, Sperr WR, et al. Aggressive systemic mastocytosis and related mast cell disorders: current treatment options and proposed response criteria. Leuk Res 2003; 27:635–641.
53. Shah NP, Lee FY, Luo R, et al. Dasatinib inhibits KITD816V, an imatinib-resistant activating mutation that triggers neoplastic grown in most patients with systemic mastocytosis. Blood 2006; 108:286–291.
54. Kebebew E, Ituarte PH, Siperstein AE, et al. Medullary thyroid carcinoma: clinical characteristics, treatment, prognostic factors, and a comparison of staging systems. Cancer 2000; 88:1139–1148.
55. Ryan AJ, Wedge SR. ZD6474: a novel inhibitor of VEGFR and EGFR tyrosine kinase activity. Br J Cancer 2005; 92:s6–s13.
56. Fleury A, Flejou JF, Sauvanet A, et al. Calcitonin-secreting tumors of the pancreas: about six cases. Pancreas 1998; 16:545–550.
57. Mullerpatan PM, Joshi SR, Shah RC, et al. Calcitonin-secreting tumor of the pancreas. Dig Surg 2004; 21:321–324.
58. Jarufe NP, Coldham C, Orug T, et al. Neuroendocrine tumors of the pancreas: predictors of survival after surgical treatment. Dig Surg 2005; 22:157–162.

16 Diarrhea from Enterotoxins

Gianluca Terrin, MD, PhD and Roberto Berni Canani, MD, PhD

CONTENTS

INTRODUCTION
INCREASING CL⁻ SECRETION
REDUCING CL⁻ ABSORPTION
DECREASING NA⁺ ABSORPTION
IMPAIRMENT OF WATER INTESTINAL
  TRANSPORT
THERAPEUTIC STRATEGIES
REFERENCES

Summary

Diarrhea determined by enterotoxins is an important public health problem worldwide. A number of microorganisms can cause diarrhea by producing and secreting enterotoxins that affect the absorptive and/or secretory processes of the enterocyte without causing considerable acute inflammation or mucosal destruction. Our knowledge of diarrheal diseases determined by enterotoxins has expanded enormously over the past decade. The chapter reviews various aspects of diarrhea induced by enterotoxins, including its management.

Key Words: Intestinal transport, *Vibrio cholerae*, CFTR, CLCA, DRA, Congenital chloride diarrhea, NHE, SGLT1, Cholera toxin, Aquaporin, TDH, ETEC, Heat-stable enterotoxin, NSP4, Rotavirus, Tat, HIV-1, Virotoxin, EPEC, Therapy, Oral rehydration solution, Zinc

From: *Diarrhea, Clinical Gastroenterology*
Edited by: S. Guandalini, H. Vaziri, DOI 10.1007/978-1-60761-183-7_16
© Springer Science+Business Media, LLC 2011

Abbreviations

AQP	aquaporins
CFTR	cystic fibrosis transmembrane regulator
CLCA	Ca^{2+}-activated Cl^- channel
CT	cholera toxin
DRA	downregulated in adenoma (DRA)
ER	endoplasmic reticulum
EPEC	enteropathogenic *E. coli*
ETEC	enterotoxigenic *Escherichia coli*
GM1	ganglioside
LT	heat-labile enterotoxin
NHE	Na^+/H^+ exchangers
NSP4	non-structural protein 4
ORS	oral rehydration solution
PKA	protein kinase A
SGLT1	sodium/glucose cotransporter 1
ST	heat-stable enterotoxin
Tat	transactivator factor peptide
VIP	vasointestinal peptide

INTRODUCTION

A number of microorganisms cause diarrhea by producing and secreting enterotoxins that affect the absorptive and/or secretory processes of the enterocyte without causing considerable acute inflammation or mucosal destruction [1]. In addition to the typical microbial causes of enterotoxin-induced diarrhea, such as *Vibrio cholerae*, several enterotoxin-producing organisms, such as *Staphylococcus aureus*, *Clostridium perfringens*, and *Bacillus cereus*, have preformed toxins that survive cooking and cause food poisoning without intestinal colonization [1, 2]. Patients with enterotoxin-induced diarrhea generally have few systemic signs or symptoms such as abdominal cramping, nausea, or vomiting, and fever is frequently absent [3, 4]. They do typically present with high volume of watery stools. Our knowledge of infectious diarrheal diseases has expanded enormously over the past decade, particularly with regard to understanding the pathogenesis. An overview of the pathogenesis of the enterotoxin-induced diarrhea is shown in Figs. 16.1, 16.2, 16.3, and 16.4 and is discussed further below.

Enterotoxins can elicit diarrhea through the following mechanisms:

i. Increasing Cl^- secretion through cystic fibrosis transmembrane regulator (CFTR) or Ca^{2+}-activated Cl^- channel (CLCA) (Fig. 16.1).

Chapter 16 / Diarrhea from Enterotoxins

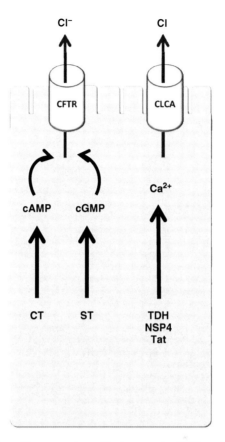

Fig. 16.1. Increasing Cl⁻ secretion. Cholera toxin (CT) or heat-labile toxin (LT) produced by enterotoxigenic *Escherichia coli* (ETEC) stimulates Cl⁻ secretion by cystic fibrosis transmembrane regulator (CFTR) via cAMP. ETEC secretes also a heat-stable (ST) enterotoxin able to trigger an increase in the intracellular levels of cGMP leading to stimulation of Cl⁻ secretion via CFTR. Thermostable direct hemolysin (TDH) produced by *Vibrio parahaemolyticus*, non-structural protein 4 (NSP4) from *Rotavirus*, and transactivator factor peptide (Tat) from *HIV-1* are able to mobilize intracellular Ca^{2+} leading to Cl⁻ secretion by Ca^{2+}-activated chloride channel (CLCA).

ii. Decreasing Cl⁻ absorption through inhibition of the Cl⁻/OH⁻ exchanger called downregulated in adenoma (DRA) (Fig. 16.2).
iii. Decreasing Na^+ uptake by inhibition of Na^+/H^+ exchangers (NHE) or by downregulation of Na^+/glucose cotransporter 1 (SGLT1) (Fig. 16.3).
iv. Inhibiting water channels or aquaporins (AQPs) (Fig. 16.4).

We will review here the basic pathophysiology of these processes and then present therapeutic strategies.

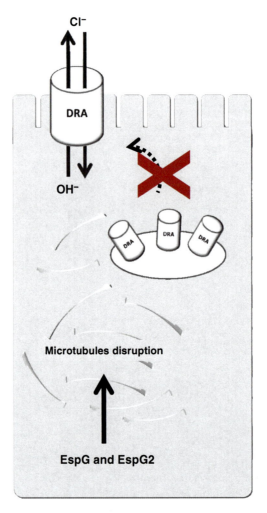

Fig. 16.2. Reducing Cl$^-$ absorption. Effector proteins EspG and EspG2 from enteropathogenic *Escherichia coli* (EPEC) disrupt microtubules, leading to misfolding of the Cl$^-$/OH$^-$ exchanger downregulated in adenoma (DRA) at the apical side of enterocyte.

INCREASING CL$^-$ SECRETION

Some enterotoxins trigger signaling molecules such as cyclic AMP (cAMP), cyclic GMP (cGMP), or intracellular Ca^{2+}, which, in turn, activate apical Cl$^-$ channels leading to an increase in secretion of Cl$^-$ and consequently of water (Fig. 16.1) [1, 3]. The typical model of this pathway is diarrhea induced by *V. cholerae*. All vibrio strains

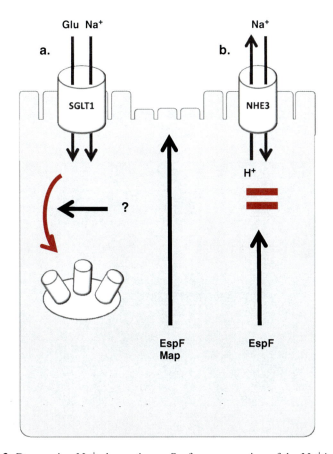

Fig. 16.3. Decreasing Na$^+$ absorption. **a** Surface expression of the Na$^+$/glucose cotransporter named SGLT1 is decreased by enteropathogenic *Escherichia coli* (EPEC) effector proteins Map and EspF, through internalization of apical SGLT1 into intracellular vesicles and flattening of microvilli. Also nonstructural protein 4 (NSP4) from *Rotavirus* and transactivator factor peptide (Tat) from *HIV-1* are able to elicit a similar effect. **b** EPEC regulates also apical NHE isoforms, decreasing NHE3 activity through EspF toxin.

produce the same enterotoxin, but different species had differences in their antibiotic susceptibility. Although cholera toxin (CT) can affect the whole intestine, cholera is largely caused by toxin activity in the proximal small intestine [5–7]. Cholera toxin consists of two subunits, a single toxic active A subunit and a B subunit pentamer, which is responsible for binding of the toxin to the intestinal epithelial cell via a ganglioside (GM1) receptor present on the brush border membrane [7]. The bound toxin is internalized into the intestinal

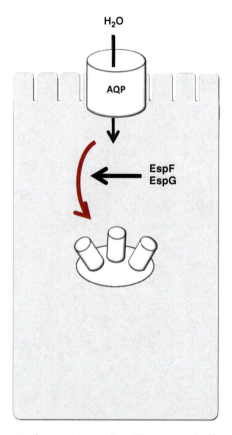

Fig. 16.4. Impairment of water absorption. The secreted effector proteins EspF and EspG by enteropathogenic *Escherichia coli* (EPEC) reduce the number of aquaporin (AQP) channels at the apical and lateral membranes, and presumably cause a decrease in water absorption.

epithelial cell, through either caveolin-coated vesicles, clathrin-coated vesicles, or the so-called Arf6 endocytic pathway [8]. The internalization and toxicity of CT is dependent on cell type, shifting from clathrin- to caveolin-mediated uptake as cells mature [9]. One explanation for the increased sensitivity of neonates to CT-induced diarrhea is the development-associated alterations in membrane phospholipids and consequent changes in endocytosis and signaling pathways [9, 10]. In intestinal epithelial cells, maturation of membrane phospholipids and association of membrane proteins with lipid rafts shift the endocytic process from a rapid clathrin-dependent mechanism to the slow and regulated caveola-mediated pathway [10]. Thus, clathrin-mediated uptake is predominant early in the life, whereas in adult uptake is mediated by caveolae and shows dependence on GM1 and

Chapter 16 / Diarrhea from Enterotoxins

lipid rafts [10]. After entering the cell, CT is routed in a retrograde manner through the Golgi apparatus into the endoplasmic reticulum (ER) [10–12]. A specific amino acid sequence, KDEL, which is located within the A2 subunit of the toxin, mirrors an epitope that is present in proteins that are typically retained in the ER and results in CT translocation from the Golgi to the ER by a shuttle protein known as ERD2 [13, 14]. Cholera toxin co-opts the ER-associated degradation (ERAD) pathway to subsequently gain entry into the host cell cytosol. The ERAD pathway ensures that proteins transiting through the ER for secretion are properly folded. Cholera toxin mimics a misfolded protein and is retrotranslocated into the cytosol, where typical ERAD targets would be degraded by the proteasome. At ER level the A subunit is then cleaved into two peptides, A1 and A2. Instead, the A1 peptide of CT goes on to ADP-ribosylate adenylate cyclase, leading to production of cAMP, which activates protein kinase A (PKA) (Fig. 16.1). Protein kinase A then phosphorylates the regulatory domain of CFTR, leading to Cl^- secretion [15]. In addition, CT stimulates enterochromaffin cells to release serotonin, which in turn stimulates the release of vasointestinal peptide (VIP) from local enteric neurons, also producing diarrhea [16].

Also heat-labile enterotoxin (LT), produced by enterotoxigenic *Escherichia coli* (ETEC) and closely biologically and antigenically related to CT, induces diarrhea activating cAMP through ADP ribosylation of Gs [17]. Similar to CT, the B subunit of LT is made up of five identical subunits. However, in addition to the high affinity of heat-labile enterotoxin for GM1, this enterotoxin also has binding affinity for various receptors in the human intestine, including polylactosaminoglycan-containing receptors or glycoproteins [18]. However, ETEC can secrete also another peptide named heat-stable (ST) enterotoxin able to bind guanylate cyclase C and to trigger an increase in the intracellular levels of cGMP [18]. There are two major STs, although only one of these, STa, is associated with human disease. ST activates enterocyte cGMP and also leads to the stimulation of Cl^- secretion via CFTR (Fig. 16.1). *Yersinia enterocolitica*, *Citrobacter freundii*, non-O1 vibrios, and other vibrio species elaborate highly homologous ST [19–22]. These enterotoxins act in a manner similar to that of *E. coli* ST. There is a direct evidence of interspecies transfer of the ST plasmid to other non-*E. coli* bacterial strains. In addition, enteroaggregative *E. coli* (EAEC) produce a low molecular weight ST named EAEC heat-stable enterotoxin 1 (EAST1) [23]. The role of EAST1 is not clear but might also stimulate secretion. These EAEC strains have been epidemiologically associated with infantile acute and persistent diarrhea in developing countries [24].

Several toxins produced by bacteria (i.e., *Vibrio parahaemolyticus* thermostable direct hemolysin, TDH) or by viruses (the virotoxins elaborated by *Rotavirus* and *HIV-1*) induce a direct secretory effect in the enterocytes modifying intracellular Ca^{2+} concentrations (Fig. 16.1) [25–27]. *V. parahaemolyticus* thermostable direct hemolysin causes an increase in intracellular Ca^{2+} through a protein kinase C (PKC)-dependent manner [26], but direct regulation of CLCA activity by PKC has not been studied. The pathogenesis of diarrhea induced by *Rotavirus*, the major cause of infantile gastroenteritis worldwide, is multifactorial. But in the first phases of intestinal infection, the virus may cause secretory diarrhea via the activity of non-structural protein 4 (NSP4) enterotoxin, which alters intracellular Ca^{2+} mobilization in epithelial cells [27, 28]. Mobilization of Ca^{2+} leads to Cl^- secretion by the CLCA [28]. Elevation of ionized Ca^{2+} leads to age-dependent halide ion movement across the plasma membrane. Altered Ca^{2+} mobilization may signal other Ca^{2+}-sensitive cellular processes such as cation channels and ion and solute transporters to increase fluid secretion while curtailing fluid absorption [29]. These primary Ca^{2+}-dependent steps appear to be cyclic nucleotide independent. A secondary component appears to involve the enteric nervous system and may be cyclic nucleotide dependent [30]. Also the transactivator factor peptide (Tat) produced by *HIV-1* is able to induce intestinal ion secretion by a similar mechanism [31].

REDUCING CL⁻ ABSORPTION

Enteropathogenic *E. coli* (EPEC) is able to decrease the levels of apical Cl^-/OH^- exchanger called DRA, inhibiting absorption of Cl^- [32]. This process depends on the injection of effector proteins into the host cytosol by a type III secretion system (T3ss) [32]. The injected effector proteins EspG and EspG2 disrupt microtubules [32], leading to misfolding of the DRA at the apical level of the enterocyte (Fig. 16.2). In EPEC-infected cells DRA is displaced from the cell surface into sub-apical membrane vesicles. This blocks one route of apical Cl^- absorption, which has been previously implicated in congenital chloride diarrhea a rare and severe form of chronic diarrhea with prenatal onset [33].

DECREASING NA⁺ ABSORPTION

All pathogens that stimulate Cl^- secretion through cAMP can modulate Na^+ absorption through an inhibition of both apical intestinal NHE isoforms (NHE2 and NHE3) [34, 35]. The effect of CT on NHE2 is post-translational, whereas the effect on NHE3 is post-transcriptional [35]. The effector protein EspF produced by EPEC is able to inhibit NHE3 activity through a mechanism that involves activation of phospholipase C and Ca^{2+} (Fig. 16.3) [35].

EPEC alters also SGLT1 function [36]. SGLT1 is active only in the presence of glucose. Oral rehydration solution (ORS) relies on the presence of glucose and SGLT1 to drive Na^+ into cells and restore fluid balance [37]. Interestingly, clinical evidences suggest that EPEC-mediated diarrhea is typically less severe than that caused by *V. cholerae*, but is refractory to oral rehydration therapy [36, 37]. EPEC alters SGLT1 activity by two distinct mechanisms [36, 37]. The first is associated with the formation of attaching and effacing lesions, by the bacteria leading to the effacement of microvilli (Fig. 16.3). The second means of altering SGLT1 is specific and occurs more rapidly. The mechanism by which this occurs is still unclear (Fig. 16.3).

Also the virotoxins produced by *Rotavirus* (NSP4) or by *HIV-1* (Tat) can inhibit Na^+ absorption. These virotoxins impair Na^+-solute symport activities by blocking SLGT1, hence contributing to diarrhea [38] (Fig. 16.3). As SGLT1 supports water absorption in the postprandial state under physiological conditions, the inhibition of this system could also be a cause of *Rotavirus*-induced malabsorptive osmotic diarrhea [39].

IMPAIRMENT OF WATER INTESTINAL TRANSPORT

Experimental evidences suggest a possible role of water channel named AQP in the pathogenesis of diarrhea [40, 41]. Correlation between the internalization of AQPs 2 and 3 with peak fluidity of stool was demonstrated [40, 41]. Probably AQP have a role in the early stages of EPEC infection. Infection of mice with *Citrobacter rodentium*, a murine pathogen closely related to EPEC and EHEC, resulted in decreased AQPs staining at the apical and lateral membranes, causing a decrease in water absorption. The secreted effector proteins EspF and EspG were implicated in this phenotype (Fig. 16.4).

THERAPEUTIC STRATEGIES

In all cases of enterotoxin-induced diarrhea, the attention to fluid and electrolyte replacement is fundamental. Oral rehydration solution is the first-line therapy for the management of all subjects with diarrhea [42]. In the last years, the World Health Organization (WHO), the

United Nations Children's Fund (UNICEF), and the European Society for Pediatric, Gastroenterology Hepatology and Nutrition (ESPGHAN) released recommendations for the use of a new lower osmolarity solution in the treatment of diarrhea [43–45]. However, ORS neither reduces the severity nor the duration of diarrhea. Over the years, several substrates and substances that affect transepithelial fluid transport have been added to ORS in the attempt to enhance efficacy, but conclusive clinical data about their effect are scanty. Studies and meta-analyses indicate that Zn^{2+}-fortified ORS reduces diarrhea duration and severity in children with acute diarrhea [45–49]. Zinc is now included in the WHO essential medicine list for diarrhea treatment, and in the 2008 Copenhagen Consensus, a group of leading global economists, ranked Zn^{2+} supplementation as the most effective intervention for advancing human development. Clinical trials, reviews, and meta-analyses have demonstrated that Zn^{2+} reduces diarrhea duration, stool output, and stool frequency. Zinc is widely used in the treatment of acute gastroenteritis in developing countries where it has been estimated that it is responsible for saving more than 400,000 lives a year. Moreover, a universal Zn^{2+}-containing super-ORS has been proposed by various authors. Finally, experimental evidences suggest that Zn^{2+} is able to limit diarrhea elicited by cAMP and Ca^{2+}, but not by a cGMP-mediated mechanism [28].

Available data in children with acute diarrhea do support the continuation of oral feeding during the illness [45]. Table 16.1 provides recommendations for the therapy in the main form of enterotoxin-induced diarrhea. Drugs to improve symptoms, particularly antimotility drugs, such as loperamide, can reduce the number of stools passed and may be useful in controlling the stool rate with watery diarrhea. They should not be used in children because of the possible risk of paralytic ileum [44].

Racecadotril, a drug active on the metabolism of particular proabsorptive neuropeptides (i.e., enkephalins), has been proposed for the treatment of childhood diarrhea particularly in *Rotavirus*-induced acute and persistent diarrhea. But definitive data on the efficacy in all forms of enterotoxin-mediated diarrhea and in adult patients are still lacking [50].

The value of antibiotic therapy in uncomplicated acute diarrhea has not been established. Therapy with an antimicrobial drugs is useful in selected cases of diarrhea caused by enterotoxins (see Table 16.1) [51]. Patient populations who should be considered for empiric antibiotic therapy include subjects with bacteremia and extraintestinal manifestations, elderly patients, patients with diabetes, patients with cirrhosis, immunocompromised patients, patients with cancer receiving

Chapter 16 / Diarrhea from Enterotoxins 291

Table 16.1
Main pathogens responsible for enterotoxin-induced diarrhea

Enteropathogen	Clinical and epidemiologic features	Diagnosis	Treatment*	
			Children	Adults
Vibrio cholerae 01	Acute dehydrating diarrhea in endemic regions	Stool culture in special salt-containing media (TCBS) with study of isolates for O1 serotype	Erythromycin (30 mg/kg/day PO q8h for 3 days); or azithromycin (10 mg/kg/day PO q24h for 3 days)	Doxycycline (300 mg/day PO q24h); or tetracycline (500 mg/day PO q6h for 3 days); or erythromycin (250 mg/day PO q8h); or azithromycin (500 mg/day PO q24h for 3 days).
Non-choleric vibrios	Watery diarrhea often with dysenteric characteristics; associated with shellfish and seafood	Stool culture in special salt-containing media (TCBS)	None or azithromycin (10 mg/kg/day PO q24h for 3 days) or ceftriaxone (50 mg/kg/day EV/IM q24h for 3 days)	None or ciprofloxacin (750 mg/day PO q24h for 3 days); or azithromycin (500 mg/day PO q24h for 3 days)

Table 16.1
(continued)

Enteropathogen	Clinical and epidemiologic features	Diagnosis	Treatment*	
			Children	Adults
Enterotoxigenic *Escherichia coli*	Acute watery diarrhea; cause of nearly half of cases of traveler's diarrhea, important cause of diarrhea in children in developing regions; growing cause of foodborne disease in the United States	Stool culture for *E. coli*, followed by assay for heat-labile cholera-like enterotoxin and heat-stable enterotoxins by ELISA, DNA hybridization, or PCR methods	Azithromycin (10 mg/kg/day PO q24h for 3 days);or ceftriaxone (50 mg/kg/day PO q24h for 3 days)	Ciprofloxacin (500–750 mg PO q12h or 400 mg IV q12h for 1–3 days); azithromycin (1000 mg/day PO in a single dose); or rifaximin (200 mg/day PO q8h for 3 days)
Enteropathogenic *E. coli*	Classic types cause hospital nursery outbreaks and pediatric diarrhea worldwide; atypical types may be more important causes of diarrhea in children and adults but remain largely unstudied in most populations	Virulence assays have largely replaced serotyping, including demonstration of focal attachment to HEp-2 cells, DNA probe for enteroadherence factor, or PCR to identify bundle-forming pili and intimin	Symptomatic treatment alone	Symptomatic treatment alone

Chapter 16 / Diarrhea from Enterotoxins 293

Organism	Clinical manifestations	Diagnosis	Treatment	
Yersinia enterocolitica	Acute watery diarrhea, may cause fever and dysentery and a pseudo-appendicitis condition; seen most commonly in northern countries (e.g., Scandinavia and Canada) but is seen worldwide as a cause of acute diarrhea, with animal reservoir including swine and cattle	Organism identified in selective gram-negative media such as MacConkey agar incubated at 25–28°C	Sulfamethoxazole and trimethoprim (<2 months: do not administer; >2 months: 150 mg TMP/m^2/day PO q12h for 3 days), or ceftriaxone (<7 days: not established, >7 days: 25–50 mg/kg/day IV/IM: not to exceed 125 mg/day; infants and children: 50–75 mg/kg/day IV/IM divided q12h; not to exceed 2 g/day; for 3 days)	Ciprofloxacin (500 mg PO q12h or 400 mg IV q12h for 3–5 days), sulfamethoxazole and trimethoprim (160 mg TMP/800 mg SMZ PO q12h for 3 days), or ceftriaxone (1 g IV qd for 3 days)
Staphylococcus aureus	Foodborne outbreak of vomiting lasting ≤12 h, with an incubation period of 2–7 h	Characteristic clinical manifestations; food may be cultured for *Staphylococcus* or enzyme immunoassay may be performed for enterotoxin in food	Symptomatic treatment alone	Symptomatic treatment alone

Table 16.1
(continued)

Enteropathogen	Clinical and epidemiologic features	Diagnosis	Treatment*	
			Children	Adults
Clostridium perfringens	Potentially very large foodborne outbreaks of watery diarrhea without fever or vomiting; incubation period of 8–14 h	Confirmed in foodborne outbreaks by detecting $\geq 10^6$ *C. perfringens* spores/g of feces in affected persons or $\geq 10^5$ organisms/g in food	Symptomatic treatment alone	Symptomatic treatment alone
Bacillus cereus	Foodborne outbreaks of gastroenteritis; two syndromes resembling *S. aureus* with vomiting after 2–7 h or *C. perfringens* disease with watery diarrhea after 8–14 h	Confirmed in foodborne outbreaks by detecting $>10^5$ organisms in food	Symptomatic treatment alone	Symptomatic treatment alone
Rotavirus	Most important cause of childhood viral gastroenteritis worldwide particularly in winter. Vomiting and high fever (>39°C) could precede diarrhea	Antigens in the stools by ELISA	Probiotics (*Lactobacillus* GG $1–2 \times 10^{10} – 1 \times 10^{11}$ CFU/day orally for 5 days), racecadotril (1.5 mg/kg/day PO q8 for 5 days), human serum immunoglobulin (300 mg/kg/day PO)	Symptomatic treatment alone

chemotherapy, and health-care workers who are at an increased risk of person-to-person spread.

Selected probiotic strains, such as *Lactobacillus GG* (LGG), are included in recent guidelines for the treatment of acute gastroenteritis in children and are particularly useful in *Rotavirus* infections [45, 52]. In severe hospitalized children with *Rotavirus* infection the oral administration of serum human immunoglobulins is effective to limit the severity and duration of diarrhea [53].

REFERENCES

1. Giannella RA. Infectious enteritis and proctocolitis and food poisoning. In: Feldman M, ed. Sleisenger and Fordtran's gastrointestinal and liver disease, 8th edn. Philadelphia: WB Saunders; 2006. pp. 2333–2391.
2. Kimura J, Abe H, Kamitani S, Toshima H, et al. Clostridium perfringens enterotoxin interacts with claudins via electrostatic attraction. J Biol Chem 2010; 285: 401–408.
3. Thielman NM Guerrant RL. Clinical practice. Acute infectious diarrhea. N Engl J Med 2004; 350:38–47.
4. Musher DM, Musher BL. Contagious acute gastrointestinal infections. N Eng J Med 2004; 351:2417–2428.
5. Dhar U, Bennish ML, Khan WA, et al. Clinical features, antimicrobial susceptibility and toxin production in Vibrio cholerae O139 infection: comparison with V. cholerae O1 infection. Trans R Soc Trop Med Hyg 1996; 90:402–405.
6. Basu A, Garg P, Datta S, et al. Vibrio cholerae 0139 in Calcutta, 1992–1998: incidence, antibiograms, and genotypes. Emerg Infect Dis 2000; 6: 139–142.
7. Shogomori H, Futerman AH. Cholera toxin is found in detergent insoluble rafts/domains at the cell surface of hippocampal neurons but is internalized via a raft-independent mechanism. J Biol Chem 2001; 276:9182–9188.
8. Massol RH Massol RH, Larsen JE, Fujinaga Y, et al. Cholera toxin toxicity does not require functional Arf6- and dynamin-dependent endocytic pathways. Mol Biol Cell 2004; 15:3631–3641.
9. Lu L, Khan S, Lencer W, Walker WA. Endocytosis of cholera toxin by human enterocytes is developmentally regulated. Am J Physiol Gastrointest Liver Physiol 2005; 289 :G332–G341.
10. Lu L, Bao Y, Khan A, et al. Hydrocortisone modulates cholera toxin endocytosis by regulating immature enterocyte plasma membrane phospholipids. Gastroenterology 2008; 135:185–193.
11. Lencer WI, de Almeida JB, Moe S, et al. Entry of cholera toxin into polarized human intestinal epithelial cells. Identification of an early brefeldin A sensitive event required for A1-peptide generation. J Clin Invest 1993; 92:2941–2951.
12. Orlandi PA, Curran PK, Fishman PH. Brefeldin A blocks the response of cultured cells to cholera toxin. Implications for intracellular trafficking in toxin action. J Biol Chem 1993; 268:12010–12016.
13. Pelham HR, Roberts LM, Lord JM. Toxin entry: how reversible is the secretory pathway? Trends Cell Biol 1992; 2:183–185.

14. Lencer WI, Constable C, Moe S, et al. Targeting of cholera toxin and Escherichia coli heat labile toxin in polarized epithelia: role of COOH-terminal KDEL. J Cell Biol 1995; 131:951–962.
15. Vanden Broeck D, Horvath C, De Wolf MJ. Vibrio cholerae: cholera toxin. Int J Biochem Cell Biol 2007; 39:1771–1775.
16. Mourad FH, O'Donnell LJ, Dias JA, et al. Role of 5-hydroxytryptamine type 3 receptors in rat intestinal fluid and electrolyte secretion induced by cholera and Escherichia coli enterotoxins. Gut 1995; 37:340–345.
17. Moss J, Richardson SH. Activation of adenylate cyclase by heat-labile E. coli enterotoxin. J Clin Invest 1978; 62:281–285.
18. Evans DG, Silver RP, Evans DJ Jr, et al. Plasmid-controlled colonization factor associated with virulence in *Escherichia coli* enterotoxigenic for humans. Infect Immun 1975; 12:656–667.
19. Saha S, Chowdhury P, Mazumdar A, et al. Role of *Yersinia enterocolitica* heat-stable enterotoxin (Y-STa) on differential regulation of nuclear and cytosolic calcium signaling in rat intestinal epithelial cells. Cell Biol Toxicol 2009; 25:297–308.
20. Guarino A, Giannella R, Thompson MR. Citrobacter freundii produces an 18-amino-acid heat-stable enterotoxin identical to the 18-amino-acid *Escherichia coli* heat-stable enterotoxin (ST Ia). Infect Immun 1989; 57:649–652.
21. Begum K, Ahsan CR, Ansaruzzaman M, Dutta DK, Ahmad QS, Talukder KA. Toxin(s), other than cholera toxin, produced by environmental non O1 non O139 *Vibrio cholerae*. Cell Mol Immunol 2006; 3:115–121.
22. Navaneethan U, Giannella RA. Mechanisms of infectious diarrhea. Nat Clin Pract Gastroenterol Hepatol 2008; 5:637–647.
23. Herold S, Karch H, Schmidt H. Shiga toxin-encoding bacteriophages-genomes in motion. Int J Med Microbiol 2004; 294:115–121.
24. Weintraub A. Enteroaggregative *E. coli*: epidemiology, virulence, and detection. J Med Microbiol 2007; 56:4–8.
25. Takahashi A, Sato Y, Shiomi Y, et al. Mechanisms of chloride secretion induced by thermostable direct haemolysin of Vibrio parahaemolyticus in human colonic tissue and a human intestinal epithelial cell line. J Med Microbiol 2000; 49: 801–810.
26. Fuller CM, Benos DJ. Electrophysiological characteristics of the Ca^{2+}-activated Cl^- channel family of anion transport proteins. Clin Exp Pharmacol Physiol 2000; 27:906–910.
27. Lundgren O, Svensson L. Pathogenesis of Rotavirus diarrhea. Microbes Infect 2001; 3:1145–1156.
28. Berni Canani R, Secondo A, Passariello A, et al. Zinc inhibits calcium-mediated and nitric oxide-mediated ion secretion in human enterocytes. Eur J Pharmacol 2010; 25:266–270.
29. Morris, AP, Estes, MK. Microbes and microbial toxins: paradigms for microbial-mucosal interactions. VIII. Pathological consequences of rotavirus infection and its enterotoxin. Am J Physiol Gastrointest Liver Physiol 2001; 281:G303.
30. Lundgren, O, Peregrin, AT, Persson, K, et al. Role of the enteric nervous system in the fluid and electrolyte secretion of rotavirus diarrhea. Science 2000; 287:491.
31. Berni Canani R, Ruotolo S, Buccigrossi V, et al. Zinc fights diarrhoea in HIV-1-infected children: in-vitro evidence to link clinical data and pathophysiological mechanism. AIDS 2007; 21:108–110.
32. Gill RK, Borthakur A, Hodges K, et al. Mechanism underlying inhibition of intestinal apical Cl^-/OH^- exchange following infection with enteropathogenic E. coli. J Clin Invest 2007; 117; 428–437.

Chapter 16 / Diarrhea from Enterotoxins

33. Berni Canani R, Terrin G, Cirillo P, et al. Butyrate as an effective treatment of congenital chloride diarrhea. Gastroenterology 2004; 127:630–634.

34. Subramanya SB, Rajendran VM, Srinivasan P, et al. Differential regulation of cholera toxin-inhibited Na-H exchange isoforms by butyrate in rat ileum. Am J Physiol Gastrointest Liver Physiol 2007; 293:G857–G863.

35. Hecht G, Hodges K, Gill RK, et al. Differential regulation of Na^+/H^+ exchange isoform activities by enteropathogenic E. coli in human intestinal epithelial cells. Am J Physiol Gastrointest Liver Physiol 2004; 287:G370–G378.

36. Dean P, Maresca M, Schuller S, et al. Potent diarrheagenic mechanism mediated by the cooperative action of three enteropathogenic Escherichia coli-injected effector proteins. Proc Natl Acad Sci 2006; 103:1876–1881.

37. Nataro JP, Kaper JB. Diarrheagenic Escherichia coli. Clin. Microbiol Rev 1998; 11:142–201.

38. Berni Canani R, De Marco G, Passariello A, et al. Inhibitory effect of HIV-1 Tat protein on the sodium-D-glucose symporter of human intestinal epithelial cells. AIDS 2006; 20:5–10.

39. Halaihel N, Liévin V, Alvarado F, et al. Rotavirus infection impairs intestinal brush-border membrane Na (+) solute cotransport activities in young rabbits. Am J Physiol Gastrointest Liver Physiol 2000; 279:G587–G596.

40. Preston GM, Agre P. Isolation of the cDNA for erythrocyte integral membrane protein of 28 kilodaltons: member of an ancient channel family. Proc Natl Acad Sci 1991; 88:1110–1114.

41. Guttman, J. A. et al. Aquaporins contribute to diarrhoea caused by attaching and effacing bacterial pathogens. Cell Microbiol 2007; 9:131–141.

42. Lee YS, Lin HJ, Chen KT. McKittrick-Wheelock syndrome: a rare cause of life-threatening electrolyte disturbances and volume depletion. J Emerg Med 2010; Epub ahead of print Jan 21.

43. Borenshtein D, Fry RC, Groff EB. Diarrhea as a cause of mortality in a mouse model of infectious colitis. Genome Biol 2008; 9:R122.

44. WHO Library Cataloging-in-Publication Data Diarrhoea: Why children are still dying and what can be done. The United Nations Children's Fund (UNICEF)/World Health Organization (WHO) 2009. http://www.unicef.org/health/files/Final_Diarrhoea_Report_October_2009_final.pdf. Accessed February 1, 2010.

45. Guarino A, Albano F, Ashkenazi S, et al, for the ESPGHAN/ESPID. Evidence-Based Guidelines for the Management of Acute Gastroenteritis in Children in Europe Expert Working Group. European Society for Paediatric Gastroenterology, Hepatology, and Nutrition/European Society for Paediatric Infectious Diseases evidence-based guidelines for the management of acute gastroenteritis in children in Europe: executive summary. J Pediatr Gastroenterol Nutr 2008; 46: 619–621.

46. Atia AN, Buchman AL. Oral rehydration solutions in non-cholera diarrhea: a review. Am J Gastroenterol 2009; 104:2596–2604.

47. Berni Canani R, Ruotolo S. The dawning of the "zinc era" in the treatment of pediatric acute gastroenteritis worldwide? J Pediatr Gastroenterol Nutr 2006; 42:253–255.

48. Hoque KM, Sarker R, Guggino SE, et al. A new insight into pathophysiological mechanisms of zinc in diarrhea. Ann N Y Acad Sci 2009; 1165: 279–284.

49. Passariello A, Terrin G, Ruotolo S, et al. New hypotonic oral rehydration solution containing zinc and prebiotics for the management of children with acute gastroenteritis. Dig Liv Dis 2008; 40:A 66.

50. Baldi F, Bianco MA, Nardone G, et al. Focus on acute diarrhoeal disease. World J Gastroenterol 2009; 15:3341–3348.
51. Pawlowski SW, Warren CA, Guerrant R. Diagnosis and treatment of acute or persistent diarrhea. Gastroenterology 2009; 136:1874–1886.
52. Guarino A, Lo Vecchio A, Berni Canani R. Probiotics as prevention and treatment for diarrhea. Curr Opin Gastroenterol 2009; 25:18–23.
53. De Marco G, Bracale I, Buccigrossi V, et al. Rotavirus induces a biphasic entero-toxic and cytotoxic response in human-derived intestinal enterocytes, which is inhibited by human immunoglobulins. J Infect Dis 2009; 200:813–819.

17 Factitious Diarrhea

Erica N. Roberson, MD and Arnold Wald, MD, MACG, AGAF

CONTENTS

INTRODUCTION
EPIDEMIOLOGY
CLINICAL PRESENTATION
DIAGNOSTIC EVALUATION
STOOL STUDIES
LAXATIVE SCREENS
COLONOSCOPY
ROOM SEARCHES
STOOL CHARACTERISTICS
  OF FACTITIOUS DIARRHEA
MANAGEMENT
CONCLUSIONS
REFERENCES

Summary

Factitious diarrhea is an intentionally self-inflicted disorder which is motivated either internally by assuming a sick role or externally by money, health benefits, etc. The keys to diagnosis are suspicion and use of readily available stool and urine tests. Since factitious diarrhea is not uncommon and many tests used to evaluate chronic diarrhea are invasive and expensive, it is reasonable to perform a series of basic studies to evaluate for factitious diarrhea early in such an evaluation. Surreptitious laxative use is the most common etiology

From: *Diarrhea, Clinical Gastroenterology*
Edited by: S. Guandalini, H. Vaziri, DOI 10.1007/978-1-60761-183-7_17
© Springer Science+Business Media, LLC 2011

of factitious diarrhea and can present with volume depletion and an altered biochemical profile. Magnesium-containing laxatives will cause osmotic diarrhea; a high stool osmolar gap and stool magnesium level of more than 90 Meq/L will be present. Stimulant laxatives may cause non-gap diarrhea and can easily be detected in the urine. Any osmolality less than normal (290 mOsmol/kg) indicates dilutional diarrhea, usually the addition of urine or water to stool. All cases of factitious diarrhea should be well documented in the medical record to avoid future unnecessary testing.

Key Words: Factitious disorder (Munchausen syndrome), Malingering, Munchausen by proxy (Polle syndrome), Factitious diarrhea, Diarrhea, Laxatives, Bisacodyl, Senna, Magnesium salt, Anthraquinones, Melanosis coli (f), Sodium picosulfate, Ipecac, Stool osmotic gap, Osmolarity stool, Thin layer chromatography, Dilutional diarrhea, Osmotic diarrhea, Stool osmolality, Non-gap diarrhea, Miralax

INTRODUCTION

A factitious disorder, previously called Munchausen syndrome, is an intentional, self-inflicted disorder in which a patient fabricates an illness [1]. Munchhausen by proxy, also known as Polle syndrome, is a variant of Munchausen syndrome in which a caregiver, often the mother, induces illness in a child. Factitious disorders are motivated by nothing other than assuming the sick role, thus differentiating it from malingering when a patient is externally motivated by money, medical benefits, etc. Patients with factitious disorders are characteristically women who are willing and interested in diagnostic evaluations of their diarrhea. Often, a stressful event may have occurred prior to the instigation of their factitious disorders. Malingerers are often men who are disinclined to undergo assessment for their diarrhea and may have an anti-social personality disorder [2].

Patients with both factitious disorders and malingering may present to a health-care provider with obscure chronic diarrhea. Children with Munchausen by proxy may present with diarrhea after receiving laxatives without their knowledge. Hereafter, these entities will be referred to as factitious diarrhea. Such diarrhea is often characterized by a variable clinical course and symptoms out of proportion to physical signs. Factitious diarrhea can be easily diagnosed with simple stool and urine tests. The key to the diagnosis lies in considering that it may be present and then testing for it.

EPIDEMIOLOGY

Often patients with factitious diarrhea work in a health-care system and are women; nevertheless, several recent series have noted that up to 40% of such patients are men [3]. Among patients with chronic obscure diarrhea, up to 17% have factitious diarrhea and as many as 4% of new patients seen on an outpatient basis by gastroenterologists have factitious diarrhea [4, 5]. The most common cause of factitious diarrhea is laxative use; dilution of stool with water or urine is found in only 15% of cases [4]. Factitious diarrhea has also been reported in patients with an established cause of diarrhea (i.e., celiac disease) and therefore should remain in the differential diagnosis of any patient with refractory diarrhea [6]. Of interest, several cases have been reported in patients with ileostomies [7].

CLINICAL PRESENTATION

Persons with factitious diarrhea present with variable clinical courses. General symptoms may include lethargy, muscle weakness, dehydration, and malnutrition. Often, diarrhea is watery and excessive. Most patients do not report bloody diarrhea, although there are case reports of patients who have added blood to their stool [8]. Nocturnal diarrhea has been reported, in contrast to its rarity in functional bowel disorders. Associated symptoms may include abdominal cramping, nausea, and urgency but fever is absent. Physical signs of chronic volume depletion such as weight loss and orthostatic hypotension may be evident in persons who surreptitiously use laxatives to excess.

DIAGNOSTIC EVALUATION

Two factors are essential to making an early diagnosis of factitious diarrhea: suspicion and easily obtainable stool and urine tests. Patients with factitious diarrhea often have had a prior extensive workup for their symptoms and may have been seen by several physicians. Although it is reasonable to rule out more common etiologies of chronic diarrhea first (see Chapter 18), early evaluation for factitious diarrhea may avoid excessive and invasive testing.

Clues to surreptitious laxative use include evidence of volume depletion and altered biochemical profiles. Biochemical findings may include hypokalemia and hypochloremic metabolic alkalosis. Chronic volume depletion results in elevated renin levels and secondary hyperaldosteronism, further exacerbating chronic potassium loss by accentuating colon and kidney potassium excretion [9]. Potassium depletion initiates hypochloremia metabolic alkalosis by (1) impairing chloride absorption and stimulating hydrogen secretion in the colon and (2) facilitating renal tubular bicarbonate reabsorption [9]. Hypocalcemia is usually seen only with chronic ingestion of phosphate-containing laxatives. Persons using magnesium-containing laxatives may have mildly elevated magnesium despite chronic diarrhea. Patients who dilute their stools with water or urine will not have evidence of volume depletion or biochemical abnormalities. Hospitalizing a suspected patient to monitor weight, input, and output may facilitate the evaluation of the clinical situation. For example, no change in body weight despite a high stool output in excess of oral intake is consistent with a diagnosis of factitious diarrhea due to dilution of stools.

STOOL STUDIES

Since factitious diarrhea is not uncommon and many tests used to evaluate chronic diarrhea are invasive and expensive, it is reasonable to perform a series of stool studies to evaluate for factitious diarrhea early in the evaluation. Such an approach is cost-effective and may avoid unnecessary harm for the patient [10]. Initial negative stool studies should be repeated as surreptitious laxative use is often intermittent. Stool studies are relatively inexpensive and noninvasive tests that enable characterization of diarrhea, an otherwise essentially subjective symptom. A stool collection should be obtained for at least 24 h on an outpatient or inpatient basis; normal stool characteristics are shown in Table 17.1. Stool volume in factitious diarrhea can exceed 1 L/day, distinguishing it from functional disorders which have normal or minimally increased stool volume [9]. Fecal fat is usually normal (<6 g/24 h) although fecal fat outputs of up to 9 g/24 h have been reported in factitious diarrhea [9]. The pH level of stool has minimal utility except in malabsorptive syndromes where a low pH (<5.5) is found. However, pH can be acidic due to bacterial breakdown of carbohydrates during prolonged storage of stools and therefore should be performed only on fresh or refrigerated stools.

The stool osmolar gap is calculated by subtracting two times the sum of stool sodium and potassium from 290 mOsm/kg. Using 290 mOsm/kg, which is equivalent to plasma osmolality, avoids calculating an artificially high osmolar gap as stool osmolality increases with prolonged storage due to the breakdown of carbohydrates. An osmolar gap of less than 50 mOsm/kg indicates a non-gap

Table 17.1
Representative stool studies in chronic diarrhea

Diagnosis	Stool weight/24 h	Stool electrolytes (mmol/L)		Creatinine or urea	Stool osmolality (mOsmol/kg)	Stool osmolar gap (mOsmol/kg)
		Na^+	K^+			
Normal	100–200 g	30–40	70–90	—	290	50
Osmotic	>500 g	30	30	—	290	>80
Secretory	>1000 g	100	40–60	—	290	<50
Dilution with water	>500 g	Low	Low	—	150	<50
Dilution with urine	>500 g	High	Low	Present	Variable	Variable

diarrhea. Alternatively, an unmeasured osmotically active substance may cause an osmotic diarrhea, indicated by an osmolar gap larger than 80 mOsm/kg.

Measuring stool osmolality is useful to establish a diagnosis of dilutional diarrhea (Table 17.1). As mentioned earlier, stool osmolality approximates plasma osmolality as the small and large intestines can neither concentrate nor dilute intraluminal contents. Therefore, any osmolality less than normal osmolality (290 mOsmol/kg) indicates the addition of a hypotonic substance, frequently urine or water. The presence of creatinine or urea in stool is diagnostic of dilution with urine. Although bacterial fermentation can raise stool osmolality in stored specimens to some extent, a stool osmolality greater than 600 mOsmol/kg suggests the addition of a hypertonic liquid.

LAXATIVE SCREENS

Negative laxative screens should be repeated as surreptitious laxative use may be intermittent and unpredictable. Simple stool tests can easily detect some laxatives. For example, the addition of sodium hydroxide will turn the stool red in the presence of phenolphthalein and blue-purple with bisacodyl [5]. These tests have a low sensitivity and a negative result should not be viewed as conclusive.

Although testing of blood can be used to identify laxatives and their metabolites, urine testing is a better strategy because concentrations are far greater. Mass spectrometry, gas chromatography, and thin layer chromatography (TLC) have been used to screen both urine and stool for laxatives. Frequently, a "laxative panel" can be ordered, but the laxatives that are included in such panels should be specified. For example, the laxative panel by NMS Labs (Willow Grove, Pennsylvania) tests for anthraquinones, magnesium, bisacodyl, oils, oxyphenisatin, phenolphthalein, and phosphorus. However, newer laxatives, such as polyethylene glycol 3350, are not included because polyethylene glycol is not absorbed from the intestines. Magnesium is frequently not a part of such laxative screens and may need to be ordered separately. Magnesium-containing laxatives will result in levels greater than 100 mmol/L if used alone. As these agents are sometimes used in combination with other laxatives, a lower threshold value of 50 mmol/L should be considered positive.

The repeated use of ipecac, associated with the development of intestinal pseudo-obstruction, has been reported in a patient with Munchausen-by-proxy who presented with diarrhea, nausea, and vomiting. Ipecac administration can be diagnosed by detecting emetine in urine or stool using high-pressure chromatography with fluorescence

(National Medical Services, Willow Grove, PA) [11]. As emetine is slowly removed from the body (35% remains after 30 days), it can easily be detected long after the last administration.

COLONOSCOPY

Prolonged use of anthraquinone-containing laxatives may result in melanosis coli, a brown-black discoloration of the colon mucosa which develops within 4 months of use [9]. The rectum and sigmoid colon are affected, but discoloration is more intense in the proximal colon (Fig. 17.1) [9]. Biopsies will show pigmented macrophages in the lamina propria; such pigmentation is caused by incorporation of damaged organelles in lysosomes, forming lipofuscin [9].

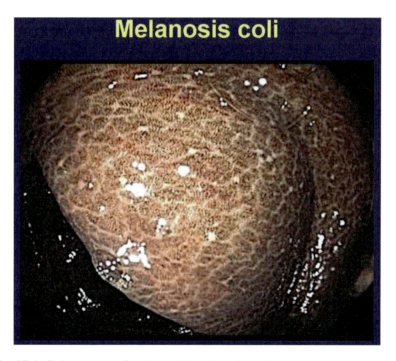

Fig. 17.1. Colonoscopy of patient with melanosis coli

ROOM SEARCHES

Searching the hospital rooms and/or belongings has been proposed as a reasonable action in the case of suspected factitious diarrhea [9]. Patients may go to extreme measures to hide their laxatives as exemplified by a case report of laxatives which were hidden in a cutout bible

[2]. However, due to significant legal concerns, this procedure should only be undertaken with written consent by the patient.

STOOL CHARACTERISTICS OF FACTITIOUS DIARRHEA

Osmotic Diarrhea

Osmotic diarrhea is characterized by the presence of an osmotic gap (Table 17.2). Magnesium compounds, found in several over-the-counter agents, including certain antacids, magnesium hydroxide, and magnesium citrate, are a common cause of factitious diarrhea reported in the literature [3, 5]. Oral magnesium results in osmotic diarrhea, often with stool magnesium levels of greater than 100 mmol/L. Clinically, a cutoff value of 50 mmol/L has been suggested as magnesium-containing laxatives are often used with other agents to produce lower levels of stool magnesium [4]. However, only magnesium levels of up to 26 mmol/L

Table 17.2
Causes of factitious diarrhea

Osmotic diarrhea
    Magnesium (hydroxide, citrate, sulfate)
    Sodium phosphate (PhosphoSoda)
    Sodium sulfate (Glauber's salt)
    Polyethylene glycol 3350 (Miralax®)
Non-gap diarrhea
    Phenolphthalein (banned 1997)
    Castor oil (ricinoleic acid)
    Anthraquinones
        Senna
        Cascara
        Rhubarb
        Frangula
        Aloe
        Danthron (banned 1987)
    Oxyphenisatin (banned 1973)
    Bisacodyl
    Sodium picosulfate (not yet available in the United States)
Dilutional diarrhea
    Added ingredients include
        Water
        Urine
        Blood

have been reported in stool without ingestion of magnesium-containing laxatives [5]. Of note, magnesium is more soluble at an acidic pH; therefore, magnesium concentrations will be artificially high in stool samples which have not been stored properly or analyzed in a timely fashion [5]. A single dose (125 mmol magnesium sulfate) can result in a stool concentration of 68 mmol/L (range 38–110) [4]. Magnesium cannot be detected using thin layer chromatography and often needs to be ordered separately from the laxative screen.

Polyethylene glycol 3350 (Miralax$^®$) can theoretically result in an osmotic diarrhea. This agent was only recently (2006) made available over the counter and no case reports have yet described factitious diarrhea from polyethylene glycol (PEG). PEG is poorly absorbed and greater than 99% of oral doses are found in stool effluents [12]. PEG can be detected in stool using liquid–liquid extraction and turbidimetric analysis; small doses (<1% ingested) can be detected in urine using high-performance liquid chromatography [12, 13]. Although PEG has been used historically for decades in intestinal perfusion studies, no commercially available test for PEG is available at this time.

Theoretically, phosphorus and sulfate could cause factitious osmotic diarrhea. In a study of healthy volunteers, a single dose of 105 mmol/L sodium phosphate resulted in a mean stool phosphorus concentration of 182 mg/dL (range 31–417). Abuse of over-the-counter sodium sulfate (Glauber's salt) is minimal and factitious diarrhea from such agents has been rarely reported [5]. Phosphorus, but not sulfate, is frequently included in laxative screens.

Non-gap Diarrhea

Stool osmolality will be normal in diarrhea due to stimulant laxatives with a low osmolar gap and high sodium (Table 17.1). Anthraquinones and bisacodyl are commonly used laxatives that cause non-gap diarrhea. Anthraquinone laxatives include senna, cascara, rhubarb, frangula, and aloe (Table 17.2) and are used by about 50% of patients with factitious diarrhea [14]. All over-the-counter anthraquinone preparations currently contain senna; however, cascara and other anthraquinones are contained in many products which are available in health food stores. Danthron is another anthraquinone that was removed from the US market in 1987 after hepatic and intestinal tumors were noted in laboratory animals. Metabolites of anthraquinones consist primarily of rhein, which can be detected in urine up to approximately 32 h after ingestion, although some reports have found rhein 72 h after senna ingestion [15]. Most labs use thin layer chromatography to detect rhein. When negative, repeat tests may be necessary as a recent report described a high false-negative rate for the current thin layer chromatography procedure [14]. Ingestion of rhubarb of up to 85 g did not give positive thin layer chromatography results [5].

Other stimulant laxatives primarily consist of bisacodyl and sodium picosulfate. Bisacodyl, the common metabolite for both forms, can also be found in both urine and stool and has been found in urine up to 52 h after ingestion [15]. Although some studies have proposed that urine is superior to other bodily fluids in detecting bisacodyl, a recent study found higher sensitivity for stool than urine after one dose of the laxative (91% versus 73%) [14]. Of particular concern in the evaluation of factitious diarrhea are reports of high false-positive rates with the current thin layer chromatography test for bisacodyl [14]. Such a test must therefore be interpreted with caution before confronting a patient with surreptitious laxative abuse.

Castor oil, an extract of the seed from *Ricinus communis*, is an over-the-counter laxative that will cause a non-gap diarrhea. Although abuse is not frequently reported in the literature, most laxative screens do test for castor oil. Other stimulant laxatives removed from the US market include oxyphenisatin and phenolphthalein. Oxyphenisatin was removed in 1973 after reports of liver failure and phenolphthalein was banned in 1997 after reports of cancer in rodent models [16]. Many laxative panels still screen for both of these agents.

Dilutional Diarrhea

As stool osmolality can never be less than that of plasma, a low osmolality can only result by adding a hypotonic solution to the stool specimen. In this situation, it should be confirmed that the testing laboratory did not add water to a formed stool in order to obtain an osmolality (personal observation). Agents most frequently used by patients include urine and water; differentiation is made by the presence of creatinine and urea in the former. A very high stool osmolality (greater than 600 mmol/kg) may be a clue to stool diluted with hypertonic solutions, such as tomato juice and blood [17]. An osmolality of less than 600 mmol/kg often indicates prolonged storage and therefore carbohydrate breakdown.

MANAGEMENT

Confrontation is often unfruitful as frequently, patients adamantly deny the use of such agents. Such denial may not be deliberate because patients may internally "block" such information [9]. As confrontation will result in shame and "shattered self-image," health-care providers must be understanding and supportive in their approach [2]. While no studies have shown that psychological evaluation and treatment are beneficial, it is often recommended to patients, although frequently declined. In such cases, the health-care provider should document such findings in the medical record.

CONCLUSIONS

Factitious diarrhea is not an uncommon disorder seen in clinical practice. Easy, inexpensive, and noninvasive stool studies and laxative screens should be performed early when evaluating chronic diarrhea to prevent unnecessary and invasive diagnostic tests.

REFERENCES

1. American Psychiatric Association. American Psychiatric Association. Task Force on DSM-IV. Diagnostic and statistical manual of mental disorders: DSM-IV, 4th edn. Washington DC: American Psychiatric Association, 1994.
2. Savino AC, Fordtran JS. Factitious disease: clinical lessons from case studies at Baylor University Medical Center. Proc Bayl Univ Med Cent 2006; 19(3): 195–208.
3. Phillips SF. Surreptitious laxative abuse: keep it in mind. Semin Gastrointest Dis 1999; 10(4):132–137.
4. Phillips S, Donaldson L, Geisler K, Pera A, Kochar R. Stool composition in factitial diarrhea: a 6-year experience with stool analysis. Ann Intern Med 1995; 123(2):97–100.
5. Duncan A, Cameron A, Stewart MJ, Russell RI. Diagnosis of the abuse of magnesium and stimulant laxatives. Ann Clin Biochem 1991; 28(Pt 6):568–573.
6. Keswani RN, Sauk J, Kane SV. Factitious diarrhea masquerading as refractory celiac disease. South Med J 2006; 99(3):293–295.
7. Pollok RC, Banks MR, Fairclough PD, Farthing MJ. Dilutional diarrhoea: under-diagnosed and over-investigated. Eur J Gastroenterol Hepatol 2000; 12(6): 609–611.
8. Duncan A, Forrest JA. Surreptitious abuse of magnesium laxatives as a cause of chronic diarrhoea. Eur J Gastroenterol Hepatol 2001; 13(5):599–601.
9. Ewe K, Karbach U. Factitious diarrhoea. Clin Gastroenterol 1986; 15(3):723–740.
10. Bytzer P, Stokholm M, Andersen I, Klitgaard NA, Schaffalitzky de Muckadell OB. Prevalence of surreptitious laxative abuse in patients with diarrhoea of uncertain origin: a cost benefit analysis of a screening procedure. Gut 1989; 30(10): 1379–1384.
11. Santangelo WC, Richey JE, Rivera L, Fordtran JS. Surreptitious ipecac administration simulating intestinal pseudo-obstruction. Ann Intern Med 1989; 110(12): 1031–1032.
12. Schiller LR, Santa Ana CA, Porter J, Fordtran JS. Validation of polyethylene glycol 3350 as a poorly absorbable marker for intestinal perfusion studies. Dig Dis Sci 1997; 42(1):1–5.
13. Ryan CM, Yarmush ML, Tompkins RG. Separation and quantitation of polyethylene glycols 400 and 3350 from human urine by high-performance liquid chromatography. J Pharm Sci 1992; 81(4):350–352.

14. Shelton JH, Santa Ana CA, Thompson DR, Emmett M, Fordtran JS. Factitious diarrhea induced by stimulant laxatives: accuracy of diagnosis by a clinical reference laboratory using thin layer chromatography. Clin Chem 2007; 53(1):85–90.
15. Beyer J, Peters FT, Maurer HH. Screening procedure for detection of stimulant laxatives and/or their metabolites in human urine using gas chromatography-mass spectrometry after enzymatic cleavage of conjugates and extractive methylation. Ther Drug Monit 2005; 27(2):151–157.
16. Kotha P, Rake MO, Willatt D. Liver damage induced by oxyphenisatin. Br Med J 1980; 281(6254):1530.
17. Zimmer KP, Marquardt T, Schmitt GM. More on factitious diarrhea. J Pediatr Gastroenterol Nutr 2002; 35(4):584–585.

18 Chronic Idiopathic Diarrhea

Lawrence R. Schiller, MD

CONTENTS

INTRODUCTION
WHAT IS THE DEFINITION OF DIARRHEA?
WHAT CONSTITUTES CHRONIC DIARRHEA?
DIFFERENTIAL DIAGNOSIS
AVAILABLE TESTS
WHAT CONDITIONS SHOULD BE
  CONSIDERED IN THE DIFFERENTIAL
  DIAGNOSIS OF DIARRHEA OF OBSCURE
  ETIOLOGY?
WHAT IS THE CHARACTERISTIC HISTORY
  AND COURSE OF SPORADIC CHRONIC
  IDIOPATHIC SECRETORY DIARRHEA?
BRAINERD DIARRHEA
POTENTIAL ETIOLOGIES
MANAGEMENT OF CHRONIC IDIOPATHIC
  SECRETORY DIARRHEA
REFERENCES

Summary

Chronic diarrhea is defined as passage of loose stools for more than 4 weeks. In most instances the cause of chronic diarrhea can be discovered and treated effectively. A few less common causes also play a role: laxative abuse, small bowel bacterial overgrowth, and even bile acid malabsorption. Rarer syndromes account for a much smaller percentage of chronic diarrheas but may be more difficult to identify

From: *Diarrhea, Clinical Gastroenterology*
Edited by: S. Guandalini, H. Vaziri, DOI 10.1007/978-1-60761-183-7_18
© Springer Science+Business Media, LLC 2011

and treat. In a small number of patients, a cause for chronic diarrhea cannot be found and they are said to have chronic idiopathic secretory diarrhea, a fairly homogeneous disorder that can be sporadic or epidemic. This disorder can be diagnosed after excluding other causes of chronic diarrhea; it is associated with moderate weight loss and gradually subsides after 1.5–3 years. A sensible approach to the patient with chronic diarrhea of unexplained cause is based on a comprehensive history, focusing on the stool characteristics (watery, bloody, fatty), the occurrence of weight loss, aggravating and mitigating factors (with special emphasis on the diet); on a thorough physical examination and on the careful use of selected laboratory investigations such as complete blood count, comprehensive metabolic panel, thyroid tests, and of course stool tests such as bacterial cultures and extensive search for parasites; electrolytes, pH, occult blood test, leukocytes (or lactoferrin/calprotectin) and fat assessment. Subsequent analysis will depend on the findings from history, physical exam, and stool analysis and may or may not include more aggressive investigations such as CT enterography, small bowel followthrough radiograms, and videocapsule enteroscopy. Additional tests may have to be occasionally utilized, including plasma peptides (chromogranin, gastrin, calcitonin, VIP, somatostatin) and urine chemistry tests (5-HIAA, metanephrines, histamine).

Key Words: Chronic diarrhea, Osmotic diarrhea, Secretory diarrhea, Brainerd diarrhea, Idiopathic diarrhea, Stool tests

INTRODUCTION

Chronic diarrhea is a common complaint. In the United States it has been estimated that 3–5% of the population has loose stools for more than 4 weeks per year [1] and an even higher proportion (28%) has been reported to have frequent, loose, or urgent bowel movements at least 25% of the time [2]. For many of these individuals the cause of chronic diarrhea is apparent or readily diagnosed. Common causes include drugs, previous surgery on the gastrointestinal tract (e.g., gastric surgery, cholecystectomy, intestinal resection), inflammatory bowel disease, carbohydrate malabsorption, and celiac disease. Irritable bowel syndrome with diarrhea affects about 5% of the population, and while abdominal pain is the predominant symptom, diarrhea is an important component [3]. Other conditions, such as laxative abuse, bile acid malabsorption, and small bowel bacterial overgrowth, may be more difficult to detect, but need to be considered.

When a careful and complete evaluation of the patient fails to determine a cause for diarrhea, the diarrhea can be said to be *idiopathic*.

Chapter 18 / Chronic Idiopathic Diarrhea

While it might seem that this category would include many different disorders – some of which might be "new" or previously unrecognized conditions, most patients with chronic idiopathic diarrhea have remarkably similar histories and courses, suggesting that they may share a common condition [4].

WHAT IS THE DEFINITION OF DIARRHEA?

Diarrhea has both common and scientific definitions (Table 18.1, see also Chapter 1). Most patients seem to identify loose stool consistency as the key feature of diarrhea [5]. Stool consistency varies widely between individuals and sometimes in individuals from day-to-day. The descriptions used by patients to identify stools as being diarrhea may range from soft or unformed stools to pourable watery stools. Other patients identify unusually frequent stools as diarrhea, even if the stools are formed. For most diarrheal diseases, both diminished stool consistency and excessive frequency occur concurrently. Some patients confuse fecal incontinence with diarrhea and will report incontinence as severe diarrhea.

Physicians tend to emphasize increased stool frequency as the key definition for diarrhea, rarely mentioning consistency at all. Because of these potential discrepancies, it is important for the treating physician to understand exactly what the patient means by the complaint of "diarrhea" and not assume that it matches his/her definition.

Scientists tend to define diarrhea as excessive stool weight (or volume). Normal stool weight varies with the amount and type of fiber consumed [6]. In the United States the cutoff used to distinguish

Table 18.1
Definitions of diarrhea

Patient-based
  Loose stool consistency
  Frequent bowel movements
  (Fecal incontinence)

Physician-based
  Frequent bowel movements
  Loose stool consistency
  Increased stool weight

Scientist-based
  Stool weight (>200 g/24 h or >10 ml/kg/day in infants and young children)
  Stool frequency (>2 bowel movements/day)
  Decreased stool viscosity

---

diarrhea from normal often is set at 200 g/24 h (roughly the mean + 2 standard deviations). This does not take into consideration the facts that women produce somewhat less stool each day than men and that diets vary widely in fiber content from person to person. Moreover, no patient has any concept of his/her stool weight before seeing the physician and few clinicians measure stool weight as part of a routine evaluation of diarrhea. Other measurable definitions used by scientists include stool frequency (normally 3 per week to 2 per day) and (less commonly) stool viscosity. These varying definitions may lead to misunderstandings when patients, physicians, and scientists use the same term ("diarrhea") to describe symptoms.

WHAT CONSTITUTES *CHRONIC* DIARRHEA?

The duration of diarrhea may be an important clue to etiology. Most viral and bacterial diarrheas run their courses over 2 weeks, even without treatment [7]. Protozoal diarrheas may last longer, typically up to 4 weeks in patients with intact immune systems. Diarrhea lasting more than 4 weeks is less likely to be infectious in etiology. Thus a practical distinction among acute (up to 2 weeks), persistent (2—4 weeks), and chronic (>4 weeks) diarrhea can be used to predict the likelihood of an infectious etiology and the probable type of infection. This distinction is arbitrary. Some authors consider diarrhea to be chronic after 2 weeks and others after 2 months.

In addition to duration, the consistency of loose stools is a key characteristic of chronic diarrhea. Patients with variable stool consistency (i.e., sometimes fluid, sometimes formed) are more likely to have irritable bowel syndrome (IBS-M, irritable bowel syndrome with mixed stool form) or diet-induced diarrhea (e.g., lactose intolerance) than any of the other potential causes of chronic diarrhea.

DIFFERENTIAL DIAGNOSIS

Diarrhea that lasts more than 4 weeks can have a number of potential etiologies (Table 18.2) [1]. Although infection is less likely than in acute diarrhea or persistent diarrhea, a recognizable pathogen still may be present and should be sought with appropriate bacterial cultures, determination of *Clostridium difficile* toxin, protozoal stool antigen tests, and microscopic examination of stools for ova and parasites.

When there is no likely diagnosis for the cause of chronic diarrhea after obtaining a history, it is worthwhile attempting to categorize the type of diarrhea as watery (with secretory and osmotic subtypes),

Table 18.2
Differential diagnosis of chronic diarrhea by diarrhea category

Watery diarrhea
  Osmotic diarrhea
    Carbohydrate malabsorption
    Osmotic laxatives (e.g., Mg^{2+}, PO_4^{3-}, SO_4^{2-})
  Secretory diarrhea
    Bacterial toxins
    Congenital syndromes (e.g., congenital chloridorrhea)
    Ileal bile acid malabsorption
    Inflammatory bowel disease
      Crohn's disease
      Microscopic colitis
        Collagenous colitis
        Lymphocytic colitis
      Ulcerative colitis
    Diverticulitis
    Medications and poisons
    Disordered motility/regulation
      Diabetic autonomic neuropathy
      Amyloidosis
      Irritable bowel syndrome
      Postsympathectomy diarrhea
      Postvagotomy diarrhea
    Endocrinopathies
      Addison's disease
      Carcinoid syndrome
      Gastrinoma
      Hyperthyroidism
      Mastocytosis
      Medullary carcinoma of the thyroid
      Pheochromocytoma
      Somatostatinoma
      VIPoma
    Idiopathic secretory diarrhea
      Epidemic chronic idiopathic secretory diarrhea (Brainerd diarrhea)
      Sporadic chronic idiopathic secretory diarrhea
    Laxative abuse (stimulant laxatives)
    Neoplasia
      Colon carcinoma
      Lymphoma
      Villous adenoma
    Vasculitis

Table 18.2
(continued)

Inflammatory diarrhea
  Diverticulitis
  Infectious diseases
    Invasive bacterial infections (e.g., tuberculosis, yersinosis)
    Invasive parasitic infections (e.g., amebiasis, strongyloides)
    Pseudomembranous colitis
    Ulcerating viral infections (e.g., cytomegalovirus, herpes simplex virus)
  Inflammatory bowel disease
    Crohn's disease
    Ulcerative colitis
    Ulcerative jejunoileitis
  Ischemic colitis
  Neoplasia
    Colon cancer
    Lymphoma
  Radiation colitis

Fatty diarrhea
  Malabsorption syndromes
    Mesenteric ischemia
    Mucosal diseases (e.g., celiac disease, Whipple's disease)
    Short bowel syndrome
    Small intestinal bacterial overgrowth
  Maldigestion
    Inadequate luminal bile acid concentration
    Pancreatic exocrine insufficiency

inflammatory, or fatty in order to simplify the differential diagnosis and extent of testing (Table 18.2) [1]. This can be done by visual inspection of an aliquot of stool, measurements of stool sodium and potassium concentrations (to determine fecal osmotic gap), assessment of stool pH, and testing for fecal occult blood, fecal leukocytes (either by microscopy or a surrogate test such as fecal lactoferrin or calprotectin), and stool fat (either by microscopy with Sudan stain or direct measurement).

Watery diarrhea typically is pourable and contains no blood, pus, or fat. It can be further categorized as secretory or osmotic by calculation of the fecal osmotic gap (FOG) [8]. This can be estimated by the following formula:

$$FOG = 290 - 2 \times \left([Na^+] + [K^+]\right),$$

Chapter 18 / Chronic Idiopathic Diarrhea 317

where 290 represents the osmolality of luminal contents within the intestine and [Na$^+$] and [K$^+$] are the sodium and potassium concentrations in stool water, respectively. The measured cation concentration is doubled to account for unmeasured anions. (Measured stool osmolality should *not* be used because it largely reflects bacterial metabolism in vitro, not intraluminal osmolality.) As calculated, the FOG represents unmeasured osmoles and is high (>100 mosm/kg) when a poorly absorbed substance is present (i.e., osmotic diarrhea) and is low (<50 mosm/kg) when electrolytes account for most of stool osmolality (i.e., secretory diarrhea). Osmotic diarrheas are due to ingestion of poorly absorbed substances, such as lactose in a lactase-deficient individual, mannitol, magnesium, phosphate, or sulfate. Secretory diarrheas caused by incomplete electrolyte absorption or excess electrolyte secretion have a broad differential diagnosis (Table 18.2) [1].

Inflammatory diarrhea is characterized by blood and pus in the stool. It is caused by inflammatory processes, such as colitis or Crohn's disease, and by some neoplasms. Fecal leukocytes are the hallmark of inflammatory diarrhea, mostly colonic in location, and can be assessed by stool microscopy or by measurement of leukocyte enzymes in stool, such as lactoferrin or calprotectin.

Fatty diarrhea has excess fat in the stool due to maldigestion or malabsorption problems, such as pancreatic exocrine insufficiency or celiac disease. Steatorrhea can be assessed by quantitative stool collection or more simply by fecal microscopy with the use of Sudan stain [9].

Once the type of diarrhea is categorized and the differential diagnosis is pared down, directed testing can usually lead to a diagnosis. For example, in a patient with blood and pus in the stool, colonoscopy with mucosal biopsies may find evidence of inflammatory bowel disease. Categorizing the type of diarrhea also can limit the type of tests done. For example, a patient without steatorrhea does not need tests for pancreatic exocrine insufficiency or other causes of fat malabsorption or maldigestion.

AVAILABLE TESTS

Table 18.3 shows minimal evaluation sets for patients with various types of chronic diarrhea [1]. Not all the suggested tests should be conducted once a diagnosis is reached, but the patient should not be labeled as having idiopathic diarrhea until they are all completed and fail to give an answer.

Table 18.3
Evaluation of chronic diarrhea

In all patients
- Comprehensive history
  - Onset
  - Pattern
  - Epidemiology
  - Stool characteristics (watery, bloody, fatty)
  - Fecal incontinence
  - Abdominal pain
  - Weight loss
  - Aggravating factors (including diet)
  - Mitigating factors (including previous treatments)
  - Previous evaluation
  - General medical history (possible systemic diseases, drugs)
  - Psychiatric assessment (for factitious diarrhea)
- Physical examination
  - General condition (nutritional status, evidence for dehydration)
  - Skin, thyroid, cardiovascular system
  - Anorectal exam
- Routine laboratory tests
  - Complete blood count
  - Comprehensive metabolic (chemistry) panel
  - Thyroid tests
- Stool analysis (either quantitative collection or spot collection)
  - Stool electrolytes, pH
  - Fecal occult blood test, stool leukocytes (or lactoferrin/calprotectin)
  - Fat assessment (quantitative or estimate from Sudan stain)

Secretory diarrhea
- Exclude infection
  - Bacterial culture
  - Protozoal examinations (microscopy, stool antigen tests)
  - Unusual pathogens (herpes virus, cytomegalovirus, cyclospora, cryptosporidia, microsporidia, tuberculosis)
- Exclude structural disease
  - CT enterography, small bowel follow-through radiograms
  - Capsule enteroscopy
  - Endoscopy with small bowel biopsy, aspirate for quantitative culture
  - Colonoscopy with biopsies
- Additional tests
  - Plasma peptides (chromogranin, gastrin, calcitonin, VIP, somatostatin)
  - Urine chemistry tests (5-HIAA, metanephrines, histamine)
  - Cosyntropin stimulation test (for adrenal insufficiency)
  - Serum protein electrophoresis, immunoglobulins
  - Empiric trial of bile acid binder

Chapter 18 / Chronic Idiopathic Diarrhea

Table 18.3
(continued)

Osmotic diarrhea
  If low pH (suggesting carbohydrate malabsorption)
    Dietary review
    Breath hydrogen test (lactose) or lactose tolerance test
  Fecal magnesium output

Inflammatory diarrhea
  Exclude structural disease
    CT enterography, small bowel follow-through radiograms
    Capsule enteroscopy
    Endoscopy with small bowel biopsy, aspirate for quantitative culture
    Colonoscopy with biopsies
  Exclude infection
    Bacterial culture
    Protozoal examinations (microscopy, stool antigen tests)
    Unusual pathogens (herpes virus, cytomegalovirus, cyclospora,
      cryptosporidia, microsporidia, tuberculosis)

Fatty diarrhea
  Exclude structural disease
    CT enterography, small bowel follow-through radiograms
    Capsule enteroscopy
    Endoscopy with small bowel biopsy, aspirate for quantitative culture,
      endoscopic ultrasound examination of pancreas
    Serological tests for celiac disease (anti-tissue transglutaminase or
      anti-endomysial antibodies)
  Tests for pancreatic exocrine insufficiency
    Secretin test
    Stool chymotrypsin or elastase activity
    Empiric trial of pancreatic enzyme treatment

WHAT CONDITIONS SHOULD BE CONSIDERED IN THE DIFFERENTIAL DIAGNOSIS OF DIARRHEA OF OBSCURE ETIOLOGY?

Our experience in evaluating 193 patients referred to Baylor University Medical Center, Dallas, with chronic diarrhea that had evaded diagnosis or failed management was summarized in a paper published in 1994 [10]. To be included in this group of patients with difficult-to-diagnose diarrhea, patients had to have had continuous diarrhea lasting more than 1 month, with negative microbiological studies, no evidence of structural gastrointestinal disease or endocrine disease, and no history of gastrointestinal surgery or radiation therapy. Eleven diagnoses were commonly found in this group (Table 18.4). In most instances the diagnosis could have been made with a more careful evaluation [1].

Table 18.4
**Common diagnoses in patients with diarrhea
of obscure origin**

Bile acid-induced diarrhea
Carbohydrate malabsorption
Chronic idiopathic secretory diarrhea
Fecal incontinence
Functional diarrhea, irritable bowel syndrome
Iatrogenic diarrhea (drugs, surgery, radiation)
Microscopic colitis
Pancreatic exocrine insufficiency
Peptide-secreting tumors
Small intestinal bacterial overgrowth
Surreptitious laxative ingestion

A more recent survey of 62 patients with chronic watery diarrhea in Spain identified a specific cause for chronic diarrhea in 50 patients with additional testing [11]. Diagnoses included bile acid malabsorption in 28, sugar malabsorption in 10, gluten-sensitive enteropathy in 10, and combined bile acid and sugar malabsorption in 2. All patients with an identified diagnosis responded to specific therapy. Twelve patients had no further diagnosis made.

During the course of earlier investigations, a group of patients with chronic idiopathic secretory diarrhea was identified [4]. These patients had chronic secretory diarrhea and no diagnosis had been reached after an intensive evaluation. While it might be assumed that these patients had a variety of conditions, they had a characteristic history and course that leads to the conclusion that they all have the same disorder, chronic idiopathic secretory diarrhea.

WHAT IS THE CHARACTERISTIC HISTORY AND COURSE OF SPORADIC CHRONIC IDIOPATHIC SECRETORY DIARRHEA?

All of these patients had been in good health and suddenly developed profound watery diarrhea that often was severe enough to produce dehydration and weight loss in the first weeks of illness [4]. They had no blood in the stools and had little if any abdominal pain, cramping, nausea, or vomiting. In many cases, the diarrhea began after travel to a local lake or recreational area, raising the question of an infectious etiology. However, fellow travelers rarely became ill and household contacts never became ill with chronic diarrhea. There were no common epidemiological exposures that could be traced.

Each patient had an extensive evaluation, including blood tests, stool cultures, stool examination for ova and parasites, colonoscopy and endoscopy with mucosal biopsies, quantitative stool collection, laxative screening, quantitative culture of jejunal aspirate, small bowel radiography and computerized tomography, and serum levels of peptides known to be secreted by tumors that cause diarrheal syndromes. All had therapeutic trials of bile acid binders and antibiotics. The evaluations were negative and therapeutic trials were not helpful. Diarrhea usually could be mitigated by the use of opiate antidiarrheals.

All patients had a complete and lasting remission that occurred from 7 to 31 months after onset. The offset was gradual, usually taking each patient several months to return to normal. When contacted months to years later neither recurrent diarrhea nor irritable bowel syndrome had developed.

BRAINERD DIARRHEA

Another diarrheal condition with a similar time course and evolution – but a different epidemiological background – is Brainerd diarrhea. This epidemic form of chronic secretory diarrhea was first reported as an outbreak associated with milk ingestion in Brainerd, Minnesota, in 1984 [12, 13]. Since that time, several outbreaks have been reported, often in confined settings, such as aboard cruise ships, or associated with a point source, such as a restaurant, associated with potentially contaminated food and drink [14–18].

The clinical course is identical to the pattern described above for sporadic idiopathic secretory diarrhea, with watery diarrhea lasting for months to years followed by complete clinical remission. Reports of these outbreaks describe relatively normal evaluations, including detailed microbiological testing in some cases, and poor response to empiric antibiotic therapy. One review of mucosal biopsy specimens from patients involved in an outbreak on a cruise ship in the Galapagos Islands showed evidence of colonic epithelial lymphocytosis similar – but not identical – to that seen with microscopic colitis in 20 of 22 patients. These specimens differed from microscopic colitis in that there were no surface degenerative changes as in lymphocytic colitis and there was no thickened collagen layer as in collagenous colitis.

Three had focal active colitis as seen frequently in patients with acute infectious colitis.

POTENTIAL ETIOLOGIES

The occurrence of outbreaks of chronic idiopathic secretory diarrhea strongly suggests an infectious cause for this condition and perhaps for sporadic chronic idiopathic secretory diarrhea as well. Despite detailed investigation of several of these outbreaks by the Centers for Disease Control (CDC) even while they were ongoing, no pathogen has been identified [17].

This has several implications. First, if chronic idiopathic secretory diarrhea is due to a microbe, the pathogen is unlikely to be a currently recognized cause of diarrhea, since these organisms were sought as part of the investigation of the outbreaks. The pathogen may be a new type of organism or may be a known organism that utilizes a new mechanism to cause diarrhea. Second, the pathogen is unusual in that it causes diarrhea that lasts more than a month. As mentioned earlier, most microbial diarrheas last less than 4 weeks in immunocompetent individuals. Third, the pathogen is resistant to antibiotics frequently used to treat infectious diarrhea, such as fluoroquinolones and metronidazole.

Alternate etiologies for a point source outbreak of diarrhea could be ingestion of some sort of toxin or poison, but this seems unlikely. Toxigenic diarrheas like cholera have a limited duration because irreversibly intoxicated enterocytes are shed after a few days by normal processes of apoptosis at the villous tips. One would need to postulate ongoing exposure to the toxin or poison, which seems unlikely.

Thus the etiology of both sporadic chronic idiopathic secretory diarrhea and epidemic chronic idiopathic secretory diarrhea (Brainerd diarrhea) remains unknown and perplexing.

MANAGEMENT OF CHRONIC IDIOPATHIC SECRETORY DIARRHEA

When patients first develop chronic idiopathic secretory diarrhea, they may develop dehydration and electrolyte depletion that may need to be addressed with intravenous fluids or oral rehydration solution.

Evaluation should proceed as outlined in Table 18.3 with the precise order of tests determined by the presentation, results of previous tests, and the effectiveness of therapeutic trials with drugs such as bile acid binders. Only after a complete evaluation can the diarrhea truly be said to be idiopathic.

Chapter 18 / Chronic Idiopathic Diarrhea

Therapy is non-specific. Stool output can be reduced with opiate antidiarrheal drugs. If standard agents such as loperamide or diphenoxylate do not produce adequate results, more potent opiates such as codeine, morphine, or opium may need to be utilized. These more potent drugs should be started at low doses and titrated up to an effective level [19].

Patients with chronic idiopathic secretory diarrhea may be comforted by the knowledge that their problem eventually will clear on its own. Unlike the onset of the condition, the offset of the disorder is gradual, often taking several months [4].

REFERENCES

1. Fine KD, Schiller LR. AGA technical review on the evaluation and management of chronic diarrhea. Gastroenterology 1999; 116:1464–1486.
2. Chang JY, Locke GR 3rd, Schleck CO, Zinsmeister AR, Talley NJ. Risk factors for chronic diarrhea in the community in the absence of irritable bowel syndrome. Neurogastroenterol Motil 2009; 21:1060–1087. Epub 2009 May 21.
3. Hungin APS, Chang L, Locke GR, Dennis EH, Barghout V. Irritable bowel syndrome in the United States: prevalence, symptom patterns and impact. Aliment Pharmacol Ther 2005; 21:1365–1375.
4. Afzalpurkar RG, Schiller LR, Little KH, Santangelo WC, Fordtran JS. The self-limited nature of chronic idiopathic diarrhea. N Engl J Med 1992; 327: 1849–1852.
5. Wenzl HH, Fine KD, Schiller LR, Fordtran JS. Determinants of decreased fecal consistency in patients with diarrhea. Gastroenterology 1995; 108:1729–1738.
6. Tucker DM, Sandstead HH, Logan GM jr, Klevay LM, Mahalko J, Johnson LK, Inman L, Inglett GE. Dietary fiber and personality factors as determinants of stool output. Gastroenterology 1981; 81:879–883.
7. Pawlowski SW, Warren CA, Guerrant R. Diagnosis and treatment of acute or persistent diarrhea. Gastroenterology 2009; 136:1874–1886.
8. Eherer AJ, Fordtran JS. Fecal osmotic gap and pH in experimental diarrhea of various causes. Gastroenterology 1992; 103:545–51.
9. Fine KD, Ogunji F. A new method of quantitative fecal fat microscopy and its correlation with chemically measured fecal fat output. Am J Clin Path 2000; 113:528–534.
10. Schiller LR, Rivera LM, Santangelo WC, Little KH, Fordtran JS. Diagnostic value of fasting plasma peptide concentrations in patients with chronic diarrhea. Dig Dis Sci 1994; 39:2216–2222.
11. Fernandez-Banares F, Esteve M, Salas A, et al. Systematic evaluation of the causes of chronic watery diarrhea with functional characteristics. Am J Gastroenterol 2007; 102:2520–2528.
12. Centers for Disease Control. Chronic diarrhea associated with raw milk consumption—Minnesota. MMWR Morb Mortal Wkly Rep 1984; 33:521–522, 527–528.
13. Osterholm MT, MacDonald KL, White KE, et al. An outbreak of a newly recognized chronic diarrhea syndrome associated with raw milk consumption. JAMA 1986; 256:484–490.

14. Martin DL, Hoberman LJ. A point source outbreak of chronic diarrhea in Texas: no known exposure to raw milk. JAMA 1986; 256:469.
15. Parsonnet J, Trock SC, Bopp CA, et al. Chronic diarrhea associated with drinking untreated water. Ann Intern Med 1989; 110:985–991.
16. Mintz ED, Weber JT, Guris D, et al. An outbreak of Brainerd diarrhea among travelers to the Galapagos Islands. J Infect Dis 1998; 177:1041–1045.
17. Kimura AC, Mead P, Walsh B, et al. A large outbreak of Brainerd diarrhea associated with a restaurant in the Red River Valley, Texas. Clin Infect Dis 2006; 43:55–61.
18. Vugia DJ, Abbott S, Mintz ED, et al. A restaurant-associated outbreak of Brainerd diarrhea in California. Clin Infect Dis 2006; 43:62–64.
19. Schiller LR. Review article: anti-diarrhoeal pharmacology and therapeutics. Aliment Pharmacol Ther 1995; 9:87–106.

19 Irritable Bowel Syndrome

Arnold Wald, MD, MACG, AGAF

CONTENTS

INTRODUCTION
CLINICAL MANIFESTATIONS
DIAGNOSTIC CRITERIA
DIAGNOSTIC APPROACH
TREATMENT
MEDICATIONS
SUMMARY AND RECOMMENDATIONS
REFERENCES

Summary

Irritable bowel syndrome (IBS) is a gastrointestinal syndrome characterized by chronic abdominal pain and altered bowel habits in the absence of an organic cause. One of the four subtypes is IBS with diarrhea, defined as loose or watery stools ≥25% of bowel movements and hard or lumpy stools ≤25% of bowel movements. The diagnostic approach to patients with IBS symptoms and no "alarm" signs includes a complete history and physical examination and a limited number of diagnostic studies to rule out organic illness.

The focus of treatment should be on symptom relief and addressing the patient's concerns. The most important component is the establishment of a strong, therapeutic physician–patient relationship. Other elements include pateient education, dietary modifications, pharmacologic agents and, in selected patients, behavioral treatments such as cognitive behavioral therapy, hypnotherapy, and dynamic psychotherapy.

From: *Diarrhea, Clinical Gastroenterology*
Edited by: S. Guandalini, H. Vaziri, DOI 10.1007/978-1-60761-183-7_19
© Springer Science+Business Media, LLC 2011

Key Words: Irritable bowel syndrome (IBS), Diarrhea, Manning criteria, Rome criteria for IBS, Celiac disease, Placebo response, Physician–patient relationship, Antispasmodic agents, Tricyclic agents, Antidepressants, Loperamide, Serotonin 3 receptor antagonists, Cognitive behavioral therapy, Hypnosis

INTRODUCTION

Irritable bowel syndrome (IBS) is a gastrointestinal syndrome characterized by chronic abdominal pain and altered bowel habits in the absence of any organic cause. It is the most commonly diagnosed gastrointestinal condition with prevalence in North America estimated from population-based studies to be approximately 10–15% [1, 2].

IBS affects men and women of all ages. However, younger patients and women are more likely to be diagnosed with IBS. A systematic review estimated that there is an overall 2:1 female predominance in North America [2].

Although only about 15% of those affected actually seek medical attention [2, 3], the number of patients is still so large that IBS in its various forms comprises 25–50% of all referrals to gastroenterologists. IBS also accounts for a significant number of visits to primary care physicians and is the second highest cause of work absenteeism after the common cold. IBS has been associated with increased health-care costs, with some studies suggesting annual direct and indirect costs of up to $30 billion [4].

CLINICAL MANIFESTATIONS

Patients with IBS present with a wide array of symptoms which include both gastrointestinal and extraintestinal complaints. However, the symptom complex of chronic abdominal pain and altered bowel habits remains the main characteristic of IBS [5].

Chronic Abdominal Pain

Abdominal pain in IBS is usually described as a crampy sensation with variable intensity and periodic exacerbations. The pain is generally located in the lower abdomen, often on the left side; however, the location and character of the pain can vary widely [5]. The severity of the pain may range from mildly annoying to debilitating.

Some clinical features associated with pain are not compatible with the syndrome and should prompt an investigation for organic diseases. These include the following: (1) pain associated with anorexia, malnutrition, or weight loss is rare in IBS unless there is a concurrent major

Chapter 19 / Irritable Bowel Syndrome 327

psychologic illness; (2) pain that is progressive, awakens the patient from sleep, or prevents sleep is not characteristic of IBS.

Altered Bowel Habits

By definition, patients with IBS complain of altered bowel habits and it is important to elicit a careful history of the volume, frequency, and consistency of the patient's stools. Patients with IBS complain of diarrhea, constipation, alternating diarrhea and constipation, or normal bowel habits alternating with either diarrhea and/or constipation.

Diarrhea

Diarrhea is usually characterized as frequent loose stools of small to moderate volume. Stools generally occur during waking hours, most often in the morning or after meals. Most bowel movements are preceded by lower abdominal cramps and urgency even to the point of fecal incontinence and may be followed by a feeling of incomplete evacuation. Approximately one-half of all patients with IBS complain of mucus discharge with stools.

Large volume diarrhea, bloody stools, nocturnal diarrhea, and greasy stools are not associated with IBS and suggest an organic disease. A subgroup of patients describe an acute viral or bacterial gastroenteritis which then leads to a subsequent disorder characteristic of diarrhea-predominant IBS, called post-infectious IBS [6].

Constipation

Constipation may last from days to months, with interludes of diarrhea or normal bowel function. Patients may also experience a sense of incomplete evacuation even when the rectum is empty.

Other Gastrointestinal Symptoms

Upper gastrointestinal symptoms, including gastroesophageal reflux, intermittent dyspepsia, nausea, and non-cardiac chest pain, are common in patients with IBS [5]. Patients with IBS also frequently complain of abdominal bloating and increased gas production in the form of flatulence or belching.

DIAGNOSTIC CRITERIA

In the absence of a biologic disease marker, efforts have been made to standardize the diagnosis of IBS using symptom-based criteria. This concept originated in 1978 when Manning et al. formulated a symptom

Table 19.1
Symptom complex suggestive of irritable bowel syndrome

Rome III criteria for IBS	Manning criteria for IBS
Recurrent abdominal pain or discomfort[a] at least 3 days per month in the last 3 months associated with two or more of the following: 1. Improvement with defecation 2. Onset associated with a change in frequency of stool 3. Onset associated with a change in form (appearance) of stool	1. Pain relieved by defecation 2. More frequent stools at the onset to pain 3. Looser stools at the onset of pain 4. Visible abdominal distension 5. Passage of mucus 6. Sensation of incomplete evacuation

[a]Discomfort means an uncomfortable sensation not described as pain.

complex suggestive of IBS (Table 19.1) [7]. These symptoms included relief of pain with bowel movements, looser and more frequent stools with onset of pain, passage of mucus, and a sense of incomplete emptying. A later report substantiated the usefulness of these symptoms in 361 outpatients: 81 had IBS, 101 had organic gastrointestinal disease, and 145 were controls [8]. The following results were noted: (1) the likelihood of IBS was proportional to the number of Manning's criteria; (2) the sensitivity and specificity to discriminate IBS from organic gastrointestinal disease were 58 and 74%, respectively; (3) the sensitivity and specificity to discriminate IBS from all patients without IBS were 42 and 85%, respectively.

In an effort to standardize clinical research protocols, an international working team published a consensus definition in 1992 called the Rome criteria, which was revised in 1999 and again in 2005 [5]. IBS was defined as a functional group of bowel disorders in which abdominal pain is associated with defecation or a change in bowel habit and with features of disordered defecation. Four subtypes of IBS were recognized by the most recent iteration called the Rome III criteria: (1) *IBS with constipation* (hard or lumpy stools $\geq 25\%$ and loose (mushy) or watery stools $< 25\%$ of bowel movements); (2) *IBS with diarrhea* (loose (mushy) or watery stools $\geq 25\%$ and hard or lumpy stools $< 25\%$ of bowel movements); (3) *Mixed IBS* (hard or lumpy stools $\geq 25\%$ and loose (mushy) or watery stools $\geq 25\%$ of bowel movements); and (4) *Unsubtyped IBS* (insufficient abnormality of stool consistency to meet the above subtypes).

The Rome criteria for IBS have been criticized for their overemphasis on abdominal pain and failure to emphasize postprandial urgency, abdominal pain, and/or diarrhea. As a result, some investigators continue to use the Manning criteria or a combination of both.

A number of studies have assessed the accuracy of the Rome and Manning criteria in a variety of practice settings. Although the overall sensitivity and specificity are high, results in individual studies have been variable, providing a rationale for ongoing studies to further refine these criteria [9]. Furthermore, the predictive values of the criteria depend upon the prevalence of IBS and organic disease in the individual practice setting.

Considering the available data and the above limitations, a consensus statement issued by the American Gastroenterological Association recommends that the diagnosis of IBS should be based upon the identification of positive symptoms consistent with the condition (as summarized by the Rome criteria) and excluding, in a cost-effective manner, other conditions with similar clinical presentations [10].

DIAGNOSTIC APPROACH

Many physicians place great importance on the exclusion of organic causes of symptoms compatible with IBS. However, to avoid unnecessary and costly testing, the diagnosis of IBS can be made on the basis of classic symptoms in most patients (see Table 19.2). Emphasis should be placed upon identifying a symptom complex compatible with IBS and then using prudent, but not exhaustive, diagnostic testing except in those patients with atypical symptoms or laboratory abnormalities such as anemia or electrolyte disturbances. The Rome and Manning criteria provide guidelines to identify patients with suspected IBS. A 2009 position statement issued by the American College of Gastroenterology (ACG) suggests that specific testing be guided by the clinical setting [1].

Table 19.2

**Diagnostic approach to patients with symptoms
of irritable bowel syndrome (no "alarm" signs)**

Complete history and physical examination
Complete blood count
Stool hemoccult
Routine colon cancer screening at ages ≥ 50 years

ACG Functional GI Disorders Task Force (2002).

The first step in diagnosis is a careful assessment of the patient's symptoms. A non-judgmental series of open-ended questions helps to establish a caring physician–patient relationship. A careful history may identify dietary factors and medications that mimic or exacerbate symptoms of IBS. Examples include lactose [11], sorbitol [12], and magnesium containing antacids that may cause diarrhea.

Initial Diagnostic Studies

There is limited evidence to support the routine performance of specific diagnostic testing in patients without alarm features and in those without diarrhea. Nevertheless, some amount of testing is usually performed. In patients who have symptoms suggestive of IBS based upon the Rome III criteria and no alarm symptoms or signs on the history and physical examination, a limited number of diagnostic studies can be used to rule out organic illness in the majority of patients with IBS and diarrhea:

- Routine laboratory studies such as a complete blood count are normal in IBS. A normal C-reactive protein is useful to exclude an underlying inflammatory conditions causing diarrhea.
- In patients who have risk factors for a parasitic infection (such as recent foreign travel to a developing country), three separate and fresh stools to be examined for ova and parasites are suggested.
- A 24-h stool collection may sometimes be useful if an osmotic or secretory diarrhea or malabsorption is suspected; stool weight in excess of 300 g/day or increased fecal fat is unlikely in IBS (see Chapter 9).
- Serum testing for celiac disease using IgA antibody to tissue transglutaminase (tTG) is recommended in patients in whom celiac disease is a consideration. In a meta-analysis of 14 studies focusing on unselected adults who met diagnostic criteria for IBS, celiac disease was four times as likely to be present as controls without IBS; the absolute proportion of patients who fulfilled criteria for IBS and had celiac disease was approximately 4% [13] (see Chapter 12).
- Routine flexible sigmoidoscopy and biopsy have a low diagnostic yield and are not cost-effective in IBS, although they may help to reassure an anxious patient. We occasionally perform this procedure in younger patients with persistent diarrhea to exclude inflammatory bowel disease [14]. The ACG position statement emphasizes that routine use of colon cancer screening tools is recommended for all patients $\geq$50 years old, including IBS patients [1]. Mucosal biopsies should be performed in those with persistent and continuous diarrhea to exclude microscopic colitis (see Chapter 5).

This limited diagnostic approach rules out organic disease in over 95% of patients with IBS and diarrhea. Stated differently, less than 5%

of patients with organic disease will be incorrectly diagnosed with IBS using this diagnostic strategy.

Thus, normal diagnostic studies at this point in the evaluation suggest that it is reasonable to begin a trial of symptomatic therapy. Patients should be re-evaluated in 3–6 weeks to assess the response to treatment. Persistent symptoms do not mean that the diagnosis was incorrect. However, a more extensive evaluation should be considered in patients who have had no change or progression of symptoms.

Other Diagnostic Studies

It may be reasonable to consider additional diagnostic studies in patients who do not respond to general treatment measures. The diagnostic evaluation depends upon the predominant symptoms: patients with predominant diarrhea should have a workup similar to other patients with chronic diarrhea (see Chapter 27).

TREATMENT

General Principles

Because IBS is a chronic and incurable condition, the focus of treatment should be on relief of symptoms and addressing the patient's concerns. An important question to ask is why the patient is seeking help at this time. Recent exacerbating factors (medications, dietary changes), concerns about serious illness, stressors, hidden agenda (disability claims, requests for opiates), or psychiatric comorbidity are critical to establish when developing an optimum therapeutic strategy.

Therapeutic Relationship

The most important component of treatment lies in the establishment of a therapeutic physician–patient relationship. The doctor should be non-judgmental, establish realistic expectations with consistent limits, and involve the patient in treatment decisions. Patients with established, positive physician interactions have fewer IBS-related follow-up visits [15].

The importance of therapeutic relationship in IBS was emphasized in a study that investigated the components of placebo effect and patient–provider interaction in 262 patients with IBS [16]. Group 1 was assigned to a wait list only, whereas group 2 received sham acupuncture with little interaction with a health-care provider. Group 3 received sham acupuncture but had much more interaction with their health-care provider. At both 3 and 6 weeks, the level of improvement in group 3 was significantly higher than group 2, which in turn was significantly higher than group 1. The conclusion was that the benefits of placebo are significant in IBS and the patient–health-care provider interaction is a key part of that effect.

Patient Education

Education about the proposed mechanisms of IBS helps to validate the patient's illness experience and sets the basis for therapeutic interventions. Patients should be informed of the chronic and benign nature of IBS that the diagnosis (if well established) is not likely to be changed and that he/she should have a normal life span.

Dietary Modification

A careful dietary history may reveal patterns of symptoms related to dairy and gas-producing foods. Given the similarity that may occur in symptoms of IBS and lactose intolerance, an empiric trial of a lactose-free diet should be considered in patients suspected of having irritable bowel syndrome [17]. Similar symptoms may arise from excessive consumption of fructose-containing beverages in patients predisposed to fructose intolerance [18].

Exclusion of foods that increase flatulence such as beans, onions, celery, carrots, raisins, bananas, apricots, prunes, brussel sprouts, wheat germ, pretzels, and bagels should be considered in patients who complain of gas. Underlying visceral hyperalgesia in IBS may explain the exaggerated discomfort experienced with consumption of gas-producing foods.

Whether elimination of other specific foods is beneficial is unclear. While it is possible that food allergy or intolerance may have a role in the development of symptoms, there are no reliable means to identify such individuals. Testing for serum immunoglobulins directed at specific dietary antigens (and eliminating responsible foods) has been proposed but the relationship between the results of such testing and improvement of symptoms require additional study before such an approach can be recommended.

An increase in the intake of fiber is often recommended, either through diet or the use of commercial supplements. However, not all authorities agree; for example, a decrease in fiber intake to 12 g/day (particularly insoluble fiber such as bran) was suggested in a British guideline, because of the potential of fiber to exacerbate symptoms [19]. A recent placebo-controlled study found that soluble fiber (psyllium) but not insoluble fiber (bran) was beneficial in IBS in primary care practices [20].

The proposed beneficial effect of fiber's mechanisms of action include the following: enhancement of water-holding properties of the stool, formation of gels to provide lubrication, bulking of the stool, and binding of agents such as bile. Despite their widespread use, a systematic review that included 13 randomized controlled trials found no convincing evidence that the commonly used bulking agents were more effective than placebo at relieving global IBS symptoms [21]. Indeed, some patients may experience increased bloating and gaseousness due to colonic metabolism of non-digestible fiber.

MEDICATIONS

Pharmacologic agents are only an adjunct to treatment in IBS. Furthermore, the drugs chosen vary depending on the patient's major symptoms. Thus, diarrhea-predominant IBS is treated differently from constipation-predominant disease.

Antispasmodic Agents

Antispasmodic agents are the most frequently used pharmacologic agents in the treatment of IBS. Certain antispasmodics (hyoscine, cimetropium, pinaverium, and peppermint oil) provide short-term relief but long-term efficacy has not been demonstrated [20, 21].

The antispasmodic agents include those that directly affect intestinal smooth muscle relaxation (e.g., mebeverine and pinaverine) and those that act via their anticholinergic or antimuscarinic properties (e.g., dicyclomine and hyoscyamine) [1]. Their selective inhibition of gastrointestinal smooth muscle reduces stimulated colonic motor activity and may be beneficial in patients with postprandial abdominal pain, gas, bloating, and fecal urgency.

A meta-analysis of 23 controlled trials of smooth muscle relaxants found that they were more effective than placebo (risk difference for global improvement of 22% and overall pain improvement of 53 versus 41%) [22]. In contrast, weak evidence for a benefit on abdominal pain and global assessment of symptoms was suggested in a second meta-analysis [23]. A systematic review confirmed the support for short-term use for some antispasmodics [1].

Administration of these medications in the treatment of IBS should be on an as-needed basis and/or in anticipation of stressors with known exacerbating effects. Typical doses include dicyclomine (20 mg orally four times daily as needed) and hyoscyamine (0.125–0.25 mg orally or sublingual three to four times daily as needed) or sustained release hyoscyamine (0.375–0.75 mg orally every 12 h).

Antidepressants

Some antidepressants are thought to have analgesic properties which are believed to be independent of their mood improving effects and may therefore be beneficial in patients with neuropathic pain. The postulated mechanisms of pain modulation with tricyclic antidepressants (TCAs) and serotonin reuptake inhibitors (SSRIs) in IBS are facilitation of endogenous endorphin release, blockade of norepinephrine reuptake leading to enhancement of descending inhibitory pain pathways, and blockade of the pain neuromodulator, serotonin. Tricyclic agents, via their anticholinergic properties, also slow intestinal transit time and may be especially beneficial in diarrhea-predominant IBS [24].

Several meta-analyses have evaluated the role of various antidepressants in patients with functional gastrointestinal disorders and IBS. One meta-analysis that included 12 placebo-controlled trials of antidepressants in functional gastrointestinal disorders concluded that tricyclic agents were associated with improvement in symptoms [25]. A systematic review confirmed that TCAs and SSRIs were more effective than placebo at relieving global IBS symptoms and appeared to reduce abdominal pain [1]. Finally, a later meta-analysis that included 12 placebo-controlled trials of antidepressants in patients with IBS concluded that they were significantly more effective than placebo (RR of symptoms persisting 0.66, 95% CI 0.57–0.78) [26]. Treatment effects were similar for SSRIs and tricyclic antidepressants.

Improvement in pain with TCAs occurs at lower doses than required for treatment of depression. As a result, if an antidepressant is chosen for the treatment of IBS, low doses should be administered initially and titrated to pain control or tolerance. Because of their delayed onset of action, 3–4 weeks of therapy should be attempted before considering treatment insufficient and increasing the dose. Examples of medications used for this purpose include amitriptyline, imipramine, nortriptyline, and desipramine (10–50 mg at bedtime). The initial dose should be adjusted based upon tolerance and response. Paroxetine and fluoxetine (20 mg orally daily), sertraline (100 mg orally daily), or other antidepressant medications can be considered if depression is a cofactor [25].

There are less published experience with other antidepressants such as SSRIs or serotonin norepinephrine reuptake inhibitors (SNRIs), although they are used clinically. Results of the few published trials (mainly with SSRIs) have been inconsistent [26–28], although as noted above, a meta-analysis concluded that overall treatment effects were similar to tricyclic antidepressants.

Antidiarrheal Agents

In diarrhea-prone patients with IBS, the stools characteristically are loose and frequent but of normal total daily volume. A systematic review identified three controlled trials evaluating loperamide in the treatment of IBS [29]. All were of short duration, enrolled a small number of patients, and did not use standardized criteria to identify patients. Overall, the trials suggested that loperamide was more effective than placebo for treatment of diarrhea, but not for treatment of global IBS symptoms or abdominal pain. Patients who consistently develop diarrhea after meals may benefit from taking a dose about 45 min before meals. Patients who are fearful of leaving the house because of possible urgent diarrhea should take 2 mg loperamide approximately 1 h before doing so. Loperamide should be used cautiously in those with symptoms alternating between diarrhea and constipation.

Benzodiazepines

Anxiolytic agents are of limited usefulness in IBS because of the risk of drug interactions, habituation, and rebound withdrawal. Furthermore, benzodiazepines may lower pain thresholds by stimulating gamma aminobutyric acid (GABA), thereby decreasing brain serotonin. They may, however, be useful for short-term (less than 2 weeks) reduction of acute situational anxiety that may be contributing to symptoms.

5-Hydroxytryptamine (Serotonin) 3 Receptor Antagonists

5-Hydroxytryptamine-3 receptor antagonists (such as alosetron, cilansetron, ondansetron, and granisetron) modulate visceral afferent activity from the gastrointestinal tract and may improve abdominal pain. A meta-analysis that included 14 randomized controlled trials in IBS (involving alosetron or cilansetron) found a benefit in global improvement in IBS and relief of abdominal pain and discomfort [30].

Alosetron was developed for use in IBS with diarrhea based upon its favorable effects on colonic motility and secretion and afferent neural systems. In clinical trials, the drug was most effective in female patients in whom diarrhea was predominant. However, the drug was subsequently found to be associated with ischemic colitis and serious complications related to severe constipation, prompting the Food and Drug Administration (FDA) to remove it from the market in the United States. Evaluation of post-marketing data and demand from a subset of patients who had responded to treatment has prompted the FDA to make the drug available under tight control.

Antibiotics

Scattered reports have suggested that some patients with IBS improve with antibiotic treatment [31, 32]. Most of the improvement has been with bloating but not for abdominal pain or altered bowel habits. The mechanisms leading to benefit are unclear but may be due to suppression of gas-producing bacteria in the colon. Such studies do not prove the hypothesis that bacterial overgrowth in the small intestine underlies the symptoms of most patients with IBS.

Furthermore, in one report, lactulose breath testing (the method used for suggesting bacterial overgrowth in some of these studies) did not discriminate patients with IBS from healthy controls. Thus, the relationships between bacterial overgrowth, benefits of antibiotics in patients with IBS, and methods to test for bacterial overgrowth in IBS require further study before this approach can be recommended.

Psychosocial Therapies

Behavioral treatments may be considered for motivated patients who associate symptoms with stressors, although their benefits remain controversial [33, 34]. Hypnosis, biofeedback, and psychotherapy help to reduce anxiety levels, encourage health promoting behavior, increase patient responsibility and involvement in the treatment, and improve pain tolerance.

A systematic review of 25 controlled studies concluded that psychological interventions are of marginal clinical significance and with unclear durability of benefit [35]. However, another review concluded that cognitive behavioral therapy, dynamic psychotherapy, and hypnotherapy are each more effective than usual care in relieving global symptoms of IBS [1].

Alternative Therapies

Multiple alternative forms of therapy for IBS have been suggested, such as herbs, probiotics, acupuncture, and enzyme supplementation [36]. Their role remains uncertain.

SUMMARY AND RECOMMENDATIONS

Treatment of IBS varies with the severity and type (diarrhea versus constipation predominant) of symptoms that are present.

Mild Symptoms

Patients with mild or infrequent symptoms usually have little or no functional impairment or psychologic disturbance. Thus, treatment should focus upon the general measures described above (such as establishment of the physician–patient relationship, patient education, reassurance, dietary modification, and, if bloating is not a major factor, fiber supplementation) rather than specific pharmacologic therapy.

Moderate Symptoms

Patients with moderate symptoms of IBS experience disruptions of normal daily activities due to exacerbations of symptoms; these patients may also demonstrate psychologic impairment.

This author often monitors patients' symptoms for several weeks to help identify precipitating factors, such as lactose intolerance, excess caffeine, or specific stressors. Modifications in diet, behavioral changes, and psychotherapy may improve the clinical outcome.

Randomized controlled trials evaluating specific pharmacologic agents have demonstrated their superiority compared with placebo. However, there have been few controlled trials evaluating specific strategies such as the duration for which these drugs should be used in conjunction with other types of treatment (such as fiber therapy), how long they should be used alone, or whether they should be given continuously or episodically. This author often not only uses pharmacologic intervention to control symptom flares but also uses continuous pharmacologic therapy (such as tricyclic antidepressant drugs) for periods of months or years. The choice of specific therapies is based mainly upon symptoms and response to empiric trials.

Intractable Symptoms

A small subset of patients with IBS present to tertiary care centers with severe, unrelenting symptoms that are often associated with underlying psychiatric impairment and frequent health-care utilization. I often suggest behavioral modification and the use of psychoactive drugs in such patients [37].

REFERENCES

1. American College of Gastroenterology IBS Task Force. An evidence-based position statement on the management of irritable bowel syndrome. Am J Gastroenterol 2009; 104:S1–S35.
2. Thompson WG, Irvine EJ, Pare P, et al. Functional gastrointestinal disorders in Canada: first population based survey using Rome II criteria with suggestions for improving the questionnaire. Dig Dis Sci 2002; 47:225–235.
3. Ford AC, Forman D, Bailey AG, et al. Irritable bowel syndrome: a 10 year natural history of symptoms and factors that influence consultation behavior. Am J Gastroenterol 2008; 103:1229–1239.

4. Sandler RS, Everhart JE, Donowitz M, et al. The burden of selected digestive diseases in the United States. Gastroenterology 2002; 122:1500–1511.
5. Longstreth GF, Thompson WG, Chey WD, et al. Functional bowel disorders. Gastroenterology 2006; 130:1480–1491.
6. Spiller R, Garsed K. Postinfectious irritable bowel syndrome. Gastroenterology 2009; 136:1979–1988.
7. Manning AP, Thompson WG, Heaton KW, Morris AF. Towards a positive diagnosis of the irritable bowel. Br Med J 1978; 2:653–654.
8. Talley NJ, Phillips SF, Melton LJ, et al. Diagnostic value of the Manning criteria in irritable bowel syndrome. Gut 1990; 31:77–81.
9. Vanner SJ, Depew WT, Paterson WG, et al. Predictive value of the Rome criteria for diagnosing the irritable bowel syndrome. Am J Gastroenterol 1999; 94:2912–2917.
10. American Gastroenterological Association medical position statement: irritable bowel syndrome. Gastroenterology 2002; 123:2108–2131.
11. Suarez FL, Savaiano DA, Levitt MD. A comparison of symptoms after the consumption of milk or lactose-hydrolyzed milk by people with self reported severe lactose intolerance. N Engl J Med 1995; 333:1–4.
12. Hyams JS. Sorbitol intolerance: an unappreciated cause of functional gastrointestinal complaints. Gastroenterology 1983; 84:30–33.
13. Ford AC, Chey WD, Talley NJ, et al. Yield of diagnostic tests for celiac disease in individuals with symptoms suggestive of irritable bowel syndrome: systematic review and meta analysis. Arch Intern Med 2009; 169:651.
14. Cash BD, Schoenfeld P, Chey WD. The utility of diagnostic tests in irritable bowel syndrome patients: a systematic review. Am J Gastroenterol 2002; 97:2812–2819.
15. Owens DM, Nelson DK, Talley NJ. The irritable bowel syndrome: Long term prognosis and the physician-patient relationship. Ann Intern Med 1995; 122:107–112.
16. Kaptchuk TJ, Kelley JM, Conboy LA, et al. Components of placebo effect: randomized control trial in patients with irritable bowel syndrome. Br Med J 2008; 336:999–1103.
17. Bohmer DJ, Tuynman HA. The effect of a lactose restricted diet in patients with a positive lactose tolerance test, earlier diagnosed as irritable bowel syndrome: A 5 year follow up study. Eur J Gastroenterol Hepatol 2001; 13:941–944.
18. Choi YK, Johlin FC Jr., Summers RW, et al. Fructose intolerance: an under recognized problem. Am J Gastroenterol 2003; 98:1348–1353.
19. Dalrymple J, Bullock I. Diagnosis and management of irritable bowel syndrome in adults in primary care: summary of NICE guidance. Br Med J 2008; 336:556.
20. Ford AC, Talley NJ, Spiegel BMR, et al. Effect of fibre, antispasmodics and peppermint oil in the treatment of irritable bowel syndrome: systematic review and meta-analysis. Br Med J 2008; 337:a2313
21. Bijkerk CJ, Muris JW, Whorwell PJ, Knottnerus JA, Hoes AW. Soluble or insoluble fibre in irritable bowel syndrome in primary care? Randomised placebo controlled trial. Br Med J 2009; 339:b3154
22. Poynard T, Regimbeau C, Beenhamou Y. Meta analysis of smooth muscle relaxants in the treatment of irritable bowel syndrome. Aliment Pharmacol Ther 2001; 15:355–361.
23. Quartero A, Meineche-Schmidt V, Muris J, et al. Bulking agents, antispasmodic and antidepressant medication for the treatment of irritable bowel syndrome. Cochrane Database Syst Rev 2005; 18(2):CD003460.

Chapter 19 / Irritable Bowel Syndrome

24. Clouse RE, Lustman PJ, Geisman RA, Alpers DH. Antidepressant therapy in 138 patients with irritable bowel syndrome: a five year clinical experience. Aliment Pharmacol Ther 1994; 8:409–416.
25. Jackson JL, O'Malley PG, Tomkins G, et al. Treatment of functional gastrointestinal disorders with antidepressant medications: a meta analysis. Am J Med 2000; 108:65–72.
26. Ford AC, Talley NJ, Schoenfeld PS, et al. Efficacy of antidepressants and psychological therapies in irritable bowel syndrome: systematic review and meta analysis. Gut 2009; 58:367–378.
27. Tack J, Broekaert D, Fischler B, et al. A controlled crossover study of the selective serotonin reuptake inhibitor citalopram in irritable bowel syndrome. Gut 2006; 55:1095–1103.
28. Vahedi H, Merat S, Rashidioon A, et al. The effect of fluoxetine in patients with pain and constipation predominant irritable bowel syndrome: a double blind randomized controlled study. Aliment Pharmacol Ther 2005; 22:381–385.
29. Efskind PS, Bernklev T, Vatn MH. A double blind placebo controlled trial with loperamide in irritable bowel syndrome. Scand J Gastroenterol 1996; 31:463–468.
30. Andresen V, Montori VM, Keller J et al. Effects of 5-hydroxytryptamine (Serotonin) type 3 antagonists on symptom relief and constipation in non-constipation irritable bowel syndrome: a systematic review and meta-analysis of randomized controlled trials. Clin Gastroenterol Hepatol 2008; 6:545–555.
31. Sharara AI, Aoun E, Abdul-Baki H, et al. A randomized double blind placebo controlled trial of rifaximin in patients with abdominal bloating and flatulence. Am J Gastroenterol 2006; 101:326–333.
32. Pimentel M, Park S, Mirocha J, et al. The effect of a nonabsorbed oral antibiotic (rifaximin) on the symptoms of the irritable bowel syndrome: a randomized trial. Ann Intern Med 2006; 145:557–563.
33. Lackner JM, Jaccard J, Krasner SS, et al. Self administered cognitive behavior therapy for moderate to severe irritable bowel syndrome: clinical efficacy, tolerability, feasibility. Clin Gastroenterol Hepatol 2008; 6:899–906.
34. Lackner JM, Jaccard J, Krasner SS, et al. How does cognitive behavior therapy for irritable bowel syndrome work? A mediational analysis of a randomized clinical trial. Gastroenterology 2007: 133:433–444.
35. Zijdenbos IL, de Wit NJ, van der Heijden GJ, et al. Psychological treatments for the management of irritable bowel syndrome. Cochrane Database Syst Rev 2009;CD006442.
36. Spanier JA, Howden CW, Jones MP. A systematic review of alternative therapies in the irritable bowel syndrome. Arch Intern Med 2003; 163:265–274.
37. Tabas G, Beaves M, Wang J, et al. Paroxetine to treat irritable bowel syndrome not responding to high fiber diet: a double blind, placebo controlled trial. Am J Gastroenterol 2004; 99:914–920.

20 Functional Diarrhea (Non-specific Chronic Diarrhea, Toddler Diarrhea)

Roberto Gomez, MD
and Marc A. Benninga, MD, PhD

CONTENTS

INTRODUCTION
TERMINOLOGY
DEFINITION ACCORDING TO THE "ROME
 III CRITERIA"
EPIDEMIOLOGY
CLINICAL EVALUATION
DIFFERENTIAL DIAGNOSIS
PATHOPHYSIOLOGY
MOTILITY
INFECTION
BACTERIAL OVERGROWTH
PROSTAGLANDINS
BILE ACID MALABSORPTION
FECAL MICROBIOTA
THERAPY
PHARMACOLOGICAL TREATMENT
CONCLUSION
REFERENCES

From: *Diarrhea, Clinical Gastroenterology*
Edited by: S. Guandalini, H. Vaziri, DOI 10.1007/978-1-60761-183-7_20
© Springer Science+Business Media, LLC 2011

Summary

Functional diarrhea (FD) or non-specific chronic diarrhea (NSCD) is considered as the most frequent cause of chronic diarrhea without failure to thrive in toddlers. According to the Rome III classification, this clinical entity is defined as a daily painless, recurrent passage of three or more, large, unformed stools during a period of at least 4 weeks, with an absence of alarm signs such as failure to thrive if caloric intake is adequate, abdominal pain, or blood in the stool and emesis. The clinical history is the key point to identify patients with FD. Minimal blood and stool tests may help to differentiate between the causes of diarrhea such as infection, celiac disease, and inflammatory conditions. The pathophysiology of FD is not well understood. Starch, fructose, and sorbitol malabsorption have been implicated as important nutritional substances in the development of FD. In the same hand, parental factors are important in the perpetuation of functional diarrhea and induction of complications such as malnutrition. Functional diarrhea in childhood is a self-limiting disease and therefore no treatment is necessary. The recognition that dietary factors play a key role in the majority of these children has focused awareness upon the dietary intervention of this FGID.

Key Words: Functional diarrhea, Toddler's diarrhea, Unspecific diarrhea, Chronic diarrhea

INTRODUCTION

Functional diarrhea (FD) or non-specific chronic diarrhea (NSCD) is considered as the most frequent cause of chronic diarrhea without failure to thrive in toddlers. This functional disorder not only occurs in toddlers or children but is also frequently present in the adult population. Generally the syndrome is associated with normal growth and intestinal absorption. The etiology and pathophysiology is poorly understood, but it is believed to be secondary to abnormalities in the gastric and intestinal motility after ingestion of beverages containing fructose as a predominant carbohydrate. The differential diagnosis is wide, but this entity can be easily recognized clinically. The diagnostic workup typically is unremarkable. Usually the patient recovers without squeals or complications.

TERMINOLOGY

Several denominations have been used in reference of functional diarrhea. The term "non-specific diarrhea" is often used due to the non-specific etiology that causes this disease [1, 2]. "Irritable bowel syndrome of infancy" due to similar characteristics of this syndrome with diarrhea-predominant irritable bowel syndrome D-(IBS) with the main difference that there is no pain involved in functional diarrhea [3]. The other term used "toddlers diarrhea" is of course due to the age of presentation which frequently ranges between 6 months and 3 years [1]. As stated in the introduction, functional diarrhea is also a very frequent cause of persistent diarrhea in adults [4] (see also Chapters 18 and 19).

DEFINITION ACCORDING TO THE "ROME III CRITERIA"

Functional diarrhea (FD) in toddlers according to the Rome III classification is defined as a daily painless, recurrent passage of three or more, large, unformed stools during a period of at least 4 weeks, in children between the ages of 6 and 36 months. Passage of these unformed stools occurs during waking hours. Furthermore, there is an absence of alarm signs such as failure to thrive if caloric intake is adequate, abdominal pain, or blood in the stool and emesis [5].

EPIDEMIOLOGY

Functional diarrhea is a common condition and has been estimated as the most frequent cause of diarrhea in toddlers without the presence of failure to thrive. Recently an Italian prospective cohort study was performed to determine the prevalence of different functional gastrointestinal disorders. A total of 9660 patients aged from birth to 12 years were enrolled by 13 primary care pediatricians from the Campania region of the Italian National Health Service [6]. A total of 2% met the strict criteria for at least one functional gastrointestinal disorder (FGID). Of these 194 children, 3.6% fulfilled the criteria for functional diarrhea resulting in a total prevalence of 0.07%. The prevalence of FD in children has not been established among different races and regions in the world. A recent study among Afro-American children living in the United States revealed a prevalence of FGID of 19%; however, data concerning FD were lacking in this study [7].

CLINICAL EVALUATION

The clinical history is the key point to identify patients with FD; generally, the toddler is unperturbed by the bowel movements that usually occur during waking hours and playtime. In these children both the defecation frequency and stool consistency markedly differ from healthy children. FD children have four to more than ten times daily runny or watery stools, whereas the defecation pattern of healthy toddlers is between two and four times per day [8]. The stools of FD children are light colored and foul smelling. Typically, the first stool of the day is of normal amount and has a formed or semi-formed consistency. During the day, stools become less solid with each defecation. Undigested remnants almost always are present. Importantly, defecation does not occur at night. Mother usually denies symptoms such as pain, abdominal distension, emesis, presence of bloody stools, whereas the patient does not exhibit signs of dehydration and usually drinks plenty of fluids.

Apart from these characteristics, medical history taking should aim at the assessment of the age diarrhea started and events accompanying it. Special attention should be paid to detailed dietary history and focus on the "four F's": fiber, fluid, fat, and fruit juices. Indeed, often times it is found in these children that the diet may be poor in fiber or fat, while excessive in fluid and sugary beverages intake. Furthermore, a complete history about family diseases such as inflammatory bowel disease, cystic fibrosis, celiac disease, pancreatic insufficiency, food allergies should be obtained to direct better the interrogatory. It is also important to address any history of allergic reactions during the addition of complementary food, milk intolerance, or specific intolerance to juices, sorbitol, and fructose-enriched beverages. A history of recent enteric infections, laxative, or antibiotic use is also an important point to consider.

By definition, these children present with normal heights and weights. They appear healthy and happy; they eat well and are normally active. Studies about the incidence or prevalence of hyperactivity in children with FD have not been published. Thus, the growth usually is not affected in a child with FD, unless the calorie amount in the diet is restricted, crucial point during the clinical history as explained above. Failure to thrive may also significantly deviate the diagnosis, due to the broad differential diagnosis of intestinal malabsorption and failure to thrive and may lead to perform an extended workup that usually turns unremarkable.

DIFFERENTIAL DIAGNOSIS

Protracted enteritis, generally secondary to an acute viral or bacterial gastroenteritis, causes with secondary disaccharidase deficiency and bacterial overgrowth that usually runs together with this syndrome and is absent in FD. Ova and parasites should be excluded. Presence of

Giardia can mimic FD, with the difference that *Giardia* can induce mucosal injury, malabsorption, and abdominal pain, not present in FD. Celiac disease has an increased prevalence in patients from a European background and is becoming more frequent in the United States, should be ruled out as well, due to the wide spectrum of symptoms than can mimic FD. Pancreatic insufficiency is another key point in the differential diagnosis; the prevalence of diarrhea in cystic fibrosis raises and is almost invariably associated with severe failure to thrive [9]. Congenital sucrose isomaltase deficiency, a rare autosomal recessive disease, mimics FD by presenting with chronic intermittent diarrhea with normal growth in children generally with ethnic background from Canada, Greenland, or Eskimo's origin [10, 11]. Other rare diseases presented with diarrhea such as immunodeficiency, protein-losing enteropathy, autoimmune enteropathy, Inflammatory bowel disease should also be taken into consideration.

Basic laboratories may help to differentiate between the causes of diarrhea: blood test included white/red cell count to rule out neutropenia, lymphopenia, and anemia; sedimentation rate and CRP to exclude inflammation. Serum electrolytes are important to analyze potential impact of the disease on the acid–base and electrolyte balance; serum albumin will help to exclude protein-losing enteropathy or malnutrition. Stool test for guaiac or occult blood, pH and reducing substances, and the presence of ova and parasite and *Giardia* antigen.

Other specialized tests like anti-endomysial antibodies with Ig-A determination, stool fat quantification and fecal elastase determination, sweat test may have a possible diagnostic role specially if there is an associated failure to thrive. If protein-losing enteropathy is suspected, a fecal alpha-1 antitrypsin determination may be of benefit.

Special studies such as breath test, upper endoscopy with disaccharidase determination, colonoscopy with biopsy, and pancreatic stimulation test are normally not indicated unless there is a strong suspicion of presence of congenital disaccharidase deficiency, celiac disease, or an inflammatory condition.

Antro-duodenal or colonic manometric studies are not indicated in FD. These procedures have been used in research, but they seem to be of little or no clinical benefit. Furthermore, both motility studies are not easy to perform, are invasive, and generally do not alter the management, given the benign nature of the disease.

PATHOPHYSIOLOGY

The pathophysiology of FD is not well understood. Many factors to explain this syndrome have been proposed: abnormalities in gastric and duodenal motility after fructose ingestion, different stool composition in terms of microbiota, fluid content and bile acids, bacterial overgrowth, fructose and carbohydrate malabsorption. Parental factors may play an important role in the perpetuation of this syndrome as well.

MOTILITY

Several gastrointestinal motility abnormalities have been described in patients with FD.

Gastric Motility

The gastric emptying rate for carbohydrate beverages is primarily determined by the volume, the caloric content, and the osmolality of the fluid ingested [12]. For instance, gastric emptying is faster for a fructose solution than for an isocaloric glucose or galactose solution [8]. This is possibly due to the greater inhibitory feedback associated with the introduction of glucose in the duodenum. The smooth muscle cells of the distal two-thirds of the stomach exhibit a cyclic recurrent electric activity that is characterized by regular depolarization of the cellular membranes. Electrogastrography (EEG) is a non-invasive technique which allows study of the pattern of the electric activity and frequency of the gastric contraction and effect of meal and different conditions on this pattern. Using EGG, Moukarzel and Sabri showed that gastric myoelectric activity in FD patients differs from healthy subjects in whom the EGG's pattern and breath hydrogen production significantly change after ingestion of pear (fructose and sorbitol) or grape (glucose) juices [13]. Postprandial period dominant power (PDP) and running spectrum total power (RSTP) were higher ($p < 0.02$) in the pear juice group than in the grape juice group, suggesting higher antral myoelectric activity after ingestion of the pear juice. In volunteers, ingestion of pear juice induced elevation of the breath hydrogen in 57% of them, while grape juice only resulted in an increase of breath hydrogen in 4% of them. These results suggested the presence of an increased myoelectric activity induced by fructose and sorbitol; and possibly faster gastric emptying and malabsorption of the juices containing these carbohydrates compared to a predominant glucose juice [13]. Another study performed in toddlers with FD showed a non-significant decrease in the gastric emptying rate, performed with $^{13}CO_2$ glycine after ingestion of apple juice with and without pulp. However, there was a significant elevation of the breath hydrogen in the ones who ingested juice without pulp suggesting that a different amount of soluble fibers contained in the juice may also have an effect by modulating gastric emptying and absorption of fructose [14].

Small Bowel Motility

The migrating motor complex (MMC) characterizing the small bowel fasting motility pattern is interrupted by a meal and replaced by postprandial activity in healthy children and adults. During the postprandial state the effect of meals especially of fat and some hormones such as insulin, CCK induce a disturbance of phase III of the MMC with a consequent decrease on intestinal transit [15, 16]. By using antro-duodenal manometry it has been shown that, unlike healthy controls, intraduodenally instilled dextrose failed to interrupt the phase III of MMC in children with functional diarrhea [8]. Failure to interrupt MMC results in diminished small bowel transit time and increased colonic delivery of bile salts, fluids, and possibly incompletely absorbed nutrients, such as fatty acids. In the early 1980s Jonas et al. already showed that sodium and bile acid concentrations were elevated in the extractable water phase of stools from toddlers with FD [17]. As an interesting analogy a parallel phenomenon occurs in patients with diarrhea-predominant IBS in which abnormalities in the amplitude, velocity, and propagation of MMC have been described suggesting the presence of these abnormalities as a possible mechanism for the development of diarrhea [18–20]. This abnormality in the small bowel motility in IBS-D is not well understood and is presumed to be associated with the presence of small bowel overgrowth, frequently associated with this syndrome [21–23].

INFECTION

Parasitic and bacterial infections have been suggested as possible precipitating factors for the development of functional diarrhea [2]. There is a well-known association between several gastrointestinal infectious processes and FGID in children. In a series of children with a known history of bacterial gastroenteritis, defined as a presence of bacterial pathogens in stool cultures, the relative risk of having an FGID was 3.2 (95% CI: 1.2–7.9). The main symptom was abdominal pain; also loose stools were reported in 8 out of 44 patients with a history of positive cultures. Furthermore, post-infectious irritable bowel syndrome (PI-IBS) has been widely described in adults and presents as frequent episodes of abdominal pain and diarrhea up to 6 months after an acute episode of gastroenteritis in a previously healthy individual [24]. In PI-IBS there is an activation of the immune system leading to mucosal inflammation, explained by the persistence of colonic mucosal abnormalities such as increased number of intraepithelial lymphocytes, lamina propia T lymphocytes, and calprotectin positive macrophages and increased number of mast cells in the terminal ileum [25, 26]. Studies done specifically in functional diarrhea in adults showed a significant association between a history of bacterial gastroenteritis and the development of PI-IBS. Out of 108 patients with a positive history of bacterial gastroenteritis, 9 developed FD while just 2 of 201 controls developed FD, OR 9.05 (95% CI 1.9–42.6). The most frequent pathogens associated with PI-IBS were *Campylobacter, Salmonella, Shigella, E. coli*, and *Aeromonas sobria* [27]. In another study 47% of the patients developed irritable bowel syndrome-associated diarrhea following a previous history of *Giardia lamblia* infection.

BACTERIAL OVERGROWTH

The presence of small bowel bacterial overgrowth (SBBO) has also been associated with the development of diarrhea in irritable bowel syndrome (D-IBS). This condition mimics the symptoms of functional diarrhea. An abnormal elevation of hydrogen during a glucose breath test was demonstrated in a substantial number of patients with this condition. The reversal of symptoms after treatment of SBBO strongly suggests an association of SBBO and D-IBS [28, 29]. To date, no studies have been performed in children with functional diarrhea to evaluate the presence of SBBO.

PROSTAGLANDINS

Diarrhea is a frequent symptom in patients exhibiting elevation of prostaglandins. A significant elevation of the prostaglandin $PGF\alpha$ was demonstrated in children with FD compared with controls [30]. As a possible effect an indirect evidence of increased intestinal secretion has been reported in FD due to an increased activity of the Na^+–K^+-ATPase and adenylate cyclase [31]. In a proportion of patients, there was a good clinical response to aspirin (a prostaglandin synthetase inhibitor or loperamide (an opiate analogue)) [28]. Aspirin therapy decreased plasma prostaglandin levels but loperamide had only little effect. These results are interesting in view of the normal jejunal secretion in children with FD, and because of the action of prostaglandins on adenylate cyclase activation and intestinal secretion.

BILE ACID MALABSORPTION

Bile acid malabsorption has been proposed as a cause of functional diarrhea in adults. Using the method of the 75-seleno-homocholic acid-taurine test (SehCAT) several authors demonstrated that 40–60 % of

Chapter 20 / Functional Diarrhea

patients with chronic functional diarrhea have evidence of bile acid malabsorption, responding favorably to the use of cholestyramine [32, 33]. In toddlers with FD, daily stool determination of fat and bile acids was not different when compared with controls; however, an abnormal elevated concentration of bile salts in the watery phase of the stool was obtained in the group of patients with functional diarrhea. These findings suggest that a secretory component may be present in patients with functional diarrhea [17]. The diagnosis of bile acid malabsorption is difficult without the SehCAT. We were unable to find studies in toddlers using this latter method, leading us to presume that the association between bile acid malabsorption and functional diarrhea in toddlers or children remains to be a question. New lights in the diagnosis of bile acid malabsorption are offered by Walters et al. who measured the levels of fibroblast growth factor 19 (FGF19), which is produced in the ileum in response to bile acid absorption and regulates hepatic bile acid synthesis. They showed that patients with bile acid malabsorption have reduced serum FGF19. The authors suggested a mechanism whereby impaired FGF19 feedback inhibition causes excessive bile acid synthesis that exceeds the normal capacity for ileal absorption, producing bile acid diarrhea [34].

FECAL MICROBIOTA

It is well known that the frequency, form, consistency, and composition of feces are changed in a variety of gastrointestinal diseases. Bacteria comprise more than 90% of the fecal mass and are always involved in these alterations. Swidsinski et al. quantitatively assessed the biostructure of fecal microbiota in healthy subjects and patients with chronic idiopathic diarrhea by using in situ hybridization [35]. Compared to healthy adults, they demonstrated that the assembly of fecal microbiota in idiopathic diarrhea was markedly different, characterized by mucus depositions within feces; mucus septa and striae; marked reduction in concentrations of habitual *Eubacterium rectale*, *Bacteroides*, and *Faecalibacterium prausnitzii* groups; and increased concentrations of occasional bacteria. Furthermore, they showed an improvement in all parameters for diarrhea after treatment with the probiotic yeast *Saccharomyces boulardii*. Most of these changes persisted after cessation of therapy. The structural organization of fecal microbiota in healthy subjects was stable and unaffected by *S. boulardii*. To date there is evidence that *S. boulardii* is beneficial for the treatment of acute gastroenteritis and the prevention of antibiotic-associated diarrhea in children [36] (see also Chapter 27). However, no data are available with respect to the effect of *S. boulardii* in children with functional diarrhea.

Role of Nutrition: Carbohydrate Consumption and Malabsorption

Starch, fructose, and sorbitol malabsorption have been implicated as important nutritional substances in the development of FD. Modified starch (MS) chemically treated to introduce ester groups or to cross-link starch chains of amylopectin is present in a great variety of foods especially in baby food and is used to increase stability and texture and to prevent gel formation during the storage of food. MS can produce elevation of breath hydrogen and induce the presence of loose stools; this phenomena is aggravated by adding sorbitol and/or fructose [37]. Fructose is a six-carbon sugar that is present naturally in table sugar, apples, pear, peaches, prunes honey, and many food sweeteners. Fructose absorption is carrier mediated and consequently has a limited absorption depending on GLUT-5 transporter and is absorbed mainly in the small intestine [38]. Also fructose is absorbed by passive diffusion by solvent drag promoted by glucose [39]. Carbohydrate content varies in different juices; apple and pear juices contain high fructose–glucose ratio and sorbitol while grape and orange contain equivalent quantities of both sugars and no addition of sorbitol [40, 41]. The absorption of fructose and sorbitol from apple and pear juice is very limited inducing diarrhea and abdominal pain, while the absorption of fructose/glucose from grape and orange juice is better tolerated [42–45]. After consuming a large dose of fructose, several gastrointestinal symptoms have been reported in adult volunteers. An elevation of hydrogen and methane was reported after a dose of 25 g fructose and presence of symptoms included diarrhea after a dose of 50 g [46]. Both irritable bowel syndrome and FD in children have been associated with pear and apple juice carbohydrate malabsorption, with a complete resolution of the symptoms after refrain from these particular juices [47].

Psychosocial and Parental Factors

Childhood stressors such as family problems, physical or sexual abuse, changing school or homes, or loss of family or friends are able to induce disordered gastrointestinal motility. Parental factors in the perpetuation of functional diarrhea and induction of complications such as malnutrition are invariable secondary to the level of anxiety, generated by the symptoms and the lack of abnormal workup. Environmental studies have shown that families of patients with FD exhibited increased levels of stress compared to matched controls and suggested that decreasing anxiety levels will positively contribute to the management [48, 49]. Parental adherence to the management is frequently a problem: in fact, due to some cultural backgrounds, parents may fail to appreciate that the administration of sugar-loaded beverages in response to diarrhea can actually worsen the disease [50]. Furthermore, it has been often believed by anxious mothers that diarrhea is induced by certain type of food intolerance and consequently a diverse variety of exclusion and restrictive diets are given to the child, sometimes to the deleterious point of impairing his/her growth gain and inducing malnutrition [2].

THERAPY

Functional diarrhea in childhood is a self-limiting disease and therefore no treatment is necessary. Intensive support, education, and reassurance of parents by the physician are crucial at the beginning of nutritional or medical interventions. Reassurance of the parents regarding the benign nature and good outcome of the disease helps decreasing the level of anxiety and increases adherence to therapy. Furthermore, it helps to avoid unnecessary interventions such as ominous malnutrition trying to control diarrhea [51].

Dietary Intervention

The recognition that dietary factors play a key role in the majority of these children has focused awareness upon the dietary intervention of this FGID. Increase of the fiber intake should be encouraged by the (re)introduction of whole meal bread and fruits. Fluid intake must be within normal limits. Furthermore, a high fat content diet is recommended, to slow gastric emptying. The effect of fat may be mediated by its action on receptors at different sites in the stomach and small bowel. Infusion of a fatty solution or hyperosmotic glucose into the duodenum relaxes the fundus, facilitating redistribution of food from the distal to the proximal stomach, whereas the tone of the pylorus and phasic pyloric contractions increase, interrupting the flow from the stomach to the duodenum [52]. Fat should be increased to at least 35–40% of total energy intake [2]. Finally, carbonated, sugar-loaded beverages, fruit juices, punches, sodas should be avoided. Avoidance of fruit juices can induce remission in some of the patients. In those cases, cloudy apple juice may be a safe alternative [14]. The role of beverages enriched with complex carbohydrates such as maltodextrines and glucose polymers is unclear and has not been studied.

PHARMACOLOGICAL TREATMENT

Enzymes

It is hypothesized that a subgroup of patients with functional diarrhea is symptomatic because of a high sucrose intake in their diets or due to unrecognized partial or complete deficiency of intestinal sucrase–isomaltase (SIMD). The use of enzymes which promote the absorption of monosaccharides has been proposed in a small subgroup of patients with FD. A trial of sacrosidase (β, D-fructofuranoside fructohydrolase) derived from the yeast *Saccharomyces cerevisiae* has been used in eight patients with FD improving the frequency and characteristics of stools in 50 % of them. The authors concluded that the improvement was due to the high sucrose intake rather than having a possible primary SIMD, with consequent malabsorption of sucrose [53].

Probiotics

The use of probiotics has been extensively studied in the treatment of acute diarrhea in children [54–56] (see also Chapter 27). In these studies, probiotics appeared to be safe in healthy children. Even in immune compromised or seriously ill children, significant complications were rare. Different probiotic strains showed to be effective in reducing the risk of antibiotic-acquired diarrhea and in reducing the duration of acute infectious diarrhea. Until now no studies have been performed using any probiotic strain in the treatment of functional diarrhea in young children. However, a study in adults with chronic non-specific diarrhea showed reestablishment of the fecal microbiota with the use of *S. boulardii*. The frequency of stools improved in 70% of the patients and in 45% of them a complete resolution of the diarrhea was accomplished [35].

Anticholinergic Agents

Loperamide, an opioid receptor agonist that inhibits peristaltic movement by reducing the release of acetylcholine and prostaglandin during distension in vitro is a well-known therapy to decrease the number of days of diarrhea in conditions like infectious gastroenteritis, functional diarrhea, traveler's diarrhea, and FGIDs such as diarrhea-predominant IBS in adults [30, 57, 58]. Although there have been no randomized controlled trials evaluating the use of loperamide in functional diarrhea in children, many pediatric gastroenterologists have found that loperamide produces symptomatic relief in this specific patient group. This anticholinergic medication has been approved by the FDA for children over 2 years; however, side effects are more frequent in patients less than 3 years.

Binding Resins

The use of cholestyramine has been proved to help patients with bile acid malabsorption and functional diarrhea [32]. Cholestyramine is a quaternary ammonium anion exchange resin, with a strong affinity for bile salts. The polymer binds the negative carboxyl groups on the bile salts and prevents them to flow into the colon [59].

CONCLUSION

Although functional diarrhea is the most common cause of diarrhea in toddlers, this well-recognized disorder remains poorly understood. However, these children recover spontaneously, and usually no treatment other than effective reassurance for the parents is necessary.

REFERENCES

1. Walker-Smith JA. Toddler's diarrhoea. Arch Dis Child 1980; 55:329–330.
2. Cohen SA, Hendricks KM, Mathis RK, et al. Chronic nonspecific diarrhea: dietary relationships. Pediatrics 1979; 64:402–407.
3. Davidson M, Waserman R. The irritable colon of childhood (chronic nonspecific diarrhea syndrome). J Pediatr 1966; 69:1027–1038.
4. Drossman DA, Li Z, Andruzzi E, et al. U.S. householder survey of functional gastrointestinal disorders. Prevalence, sociodemography, and health impact. Dig Dis Sci 1993; 38:1569–1580.
5. Hyman PE, Milla PJ, Benninga MA, et al. Childhood functional gastrointestinal disorders: neonate/toddler. Gastroenterology 2006; 130:1519–1526.
6. Miele E, Simeone D, Marino A, et al. Functional gastrointestinal disorders in children: an Italian prospective survey. Pediatrics 2004; 114:73–78.
7. Uc A, Hyman PE, Walker LS. Functional gastrointestinal disorders in African American children in primary care. J Pediatr Gastroenterol Nutr 2006; 42: 270–274.
8. Kneepkens CM, Hoekstra JH. Chronic nonspecific diarrhea of childhood: pathophysiology and management. Pediatr Clin North Am 1996; 43:375–390.
9. Vanderhoof JA. Chronic diarrhea. Pediatr Rev 1998; 19:418–422.
10. Treem WR. Congenital sucrase-isomaltase deficiency. J Pediatr Gastroenterol Nutr 1995; 21:1–14.
11. Baudon JJ, Veinberg F, Thioulouse E, et al. Sucrase-isomaltase deficiency: changing pattern over two decades. J Pediatr Gastroenterol Nutr 1996; 22:284–288.
12. Moore JG, Christian PE, Brown JA, et al. Influence of meal weight and caloric content on gastric emptying of meals in man. Dig Dis Sci 1984; 29:513–519.
13. Moukarzel AA, Sabri MT. Effect of gastric myoelectric activity on carbohydrate absorption of fruit juice in children. J Clin Gastroenterol 2000; 30:162–169.

14. Hoekstra JH, van den Aker JH, Ghoos YF, et al. Fluid intake and industrial processing in apple juice induced chronic non-specific diarrhoea. Arch Dis Child 1995; 73:126–130.
15. Schang JC, Dauchel J, Sava P, et al. Specific effects of different food components on intestinal motility. Electromyographic study in dogs. Eur Surg Res 1978; 10:425–432.
16. De Wever I, Eeckhout C, Vantrappen G, Hellemans J. Disruptive effect of test meals on interdigestive motor complex in dogs. Am J Physiol 1978; 235: E661–E665.
17. Jonas A, Diver-Haber A. Stool output and composition in the chronic non-specific diarrhoea syndrome. Arch Dis Child 1982; 57:35–39.
18. Wang SH, Dong L, Luo JY, et al. A research of migrating motor complex in patients with irritable bowel syndrome. Zhonghua Nei Ke Za Zhi 2009; 48:106–110.
19. Schmidt T, Hackelsberger N, Widmer R, et al. Ambulatory 24-hour jejunal motility in diarrhea-predominant irritable bowel syndrome. Scand J Gastroenterol 1996; 31:581–589.
20. Small PK, Loudon MA, Hau CM, et al. Large-scale ambulatory study of postprandial jejunal motility in irritable bowel syndrome. Scand J Gastroenterol 1997; 32:39–47.
21. Posserud I, Stotzer PO, Bjornsson ES, et al. Small intestinal bacterial overgrowth in patients with irritable bowel syndrome. Gut 2007; 56:802–808.
22. Barbara G, Stanghellini V, Brandi G, et al. Interactions between commensal bacteria and gut sensorimotor function in health and disease. Am J Gastroenterol 2005; 100:2560–2568.
23. Pimentel M, Soffer EE, Chow EJ, et al. Lower frequency of MMC is found in IBS subjects with abnormal lactulose breath test, suggesting bacterial overgrowth. Dig Dis Sci 2002; 47:2639–2643.
24. Saps M, Pensabene L, Di Martino L, et al. Post-infectious functional gastrointestinal disorders in children. J Pediatr 2008; 152:812–816.
25. Spiller RC. Postinfectious irritable bowel syndrome. Gastroenterology 2003; 124:1662–1671.
26. Barbara G, De Giorgio R, Stanghellini V, et al. New pathophysiological mechanisms in irritable bowel syndrome. Aliment Pharmacol Ther 2004; 20 Suppl 2:1–9.
27. Parry SD, Stansfield R, Jelley D, et al. Does bacterial gastroenteritis predispose people to functional gastrointestinal disorders? A prospective, community-based, case-control study. Am J Gastroenterol 2003; 98:1970–1975.
28. Pimentel M, Chow EJ, Lin HC. Eradication of small intestinal bacterial overgrowth reduces symptoms of irritable bowel syndrome. Am J Gastroenterol 2000; 95:3503–3506.
29. Parodi A, Dulbecco P, Savarino E, et al. Positive glucose breath testing is more prevalent in patients with IBS-like symptoms compared with controls of similar age and gender distribution. J Clin Gastroenterol 2009; 43:962–966.
30. Dodge JA, Hamdi IA, Burns GM, Yamashiro Y. Toddler diarrhoea and prostaglandins. Arch Dis Child 1981; 56:705–707.
31. Tripp JH, Muller DP, Harries JT. Mucosal (Na^+-K^+)-ATPase and adenylate cyclase activities in children with toddler diarrhea and the postenteritis syndrome. Pediatr Res 1980; 14:1382–1386.
32. Eusufzai S. Bile acid malabsorption in patients with chronic diarrhoea. Scand J Gastroenterol 1993; 28:865–868.

33. D'Arienzo A, Maurelli L, Di Siervi P, et al. The 75-seleno-homocholic acid-taurine test (SeHCAT). A useful method for detecting the idiopathic malabsorption of bile salts in chronic functional diarrhea. Clin Ter 1989; 130:11–16.

34. Walters JR, Tasleem AM, Omer OS, et al. A new mechanism for bile acid diarrhea: defective feedback inhibition of bile acid biosynthesis. Clin Gastroenterol Hepatol 2009; 7:1189–1194.

35. Swidsinski A, Loening-Baucke V, Verstraelen H, Osowska S, Doerffel Y. Biostructure of fecal microbiota in healthy subjects and patients with chronic idiopathic diarrhea. Gastroenterology 2008; 135:568–579.

36. Vandenplas Y, Brunser O, Szajewska H. Saccharomyces boulardii in childhood. Eur J Pediatr 2009; 168:253–265.

37. Lebenthal-Bendor Y, Theuer RC, Lebenthal A, et al. Malabsorption of modified food starch (acetylated distarch phosphate) in normal infants and in 8-24-month-old toddlers with non-specific diarrhea, as influenced by sorbitol and fructose. Acta Paediatr 2001; 90:1368–1372.

38. Riby JE, Fujisawa T, Kretchmer N. Fructose absorption. Am J Clinical Nutr 1993;58: 748S-753S.

39. Skoog SM, Bharucha AE. Dietary fructose and gastrointestinal symptoms: a review. Am J Gastroenterol 2004; 99:2046–2050.

40. Hyams JS, Etienne NL, Leichtner AM, Theuer RC. Carbohydrate malabsorption following fruit juice ingestion in young children. Pediatrics 1988; 82: 64–68.

41. Hardinge MG, Swarner JB, Crooks H. Carbohydrates in foods. J Am Diet Assoc 1965; 46:197–204.

42. Kneepkens CM, Vonk RJ, Fernandes J. Incomplete intestinal absorption of fructose. Arch Dis Child 1984; 59:735–738.

43. Perman JA, Barr RG, Watkins JB. Sucrose malabsorption in children: noninvasive diagnosis by interval breath hydrogen determination. J Pediatr 1978; 93:17–22.

44. Hyams JS. Chronic abdominal pain caused by sorbitol malabsorption. J Pediatr 1982; 100:772–773.

45. Hyams JS, Leichtner AM. Apple juice. An unappreciated cause of chronic diarrhea. Am J Dis Child 1985; 139:503–505.

46. Rao SS, Attaluri A, Anderson L, Stumbo P. Ability of the normal human small intestine to absorb fructose: evaluation by breath testing. Clin Gastroenterol Hepatol 2007; 5:959–963.

47. Moukarzel AA, Lesicka H, Ament ME. Irritable bowel syndrome and nonspecific diarrhea in infancy and childhood--relationship with juice carbohydrate malabsorption. Clin Pediatr 2002; 41:145–150.

48. Dutton PV, Furnell JR. Toddler's diarrhoea: individual variation with environmental change. Child Care Health Dev 1987; 13:297–301.

49. Dutton PV, Furnell JR, Speirs AL. Environmental stress factors associated with toddler's diarrhoea. J Psychosom Res 1985; 29:85–88.

50. Li ST, Klein EJ, Tarr PI, Denno DM. Parental management of childhood diarrhea. Clin Pediatr 2009; 48:295–303.

51. Lloyd-Still JD. Chronic diarrhea of childhood and the misuse of elimination diets. J Pediatr 1979; 95:10–13.

52. Rao SSC, Schulze-Delrieu K. The stomach, pylorus and duodenum In: Ed Kumar D, Wingate D, eds. An illustrated guide to gastrointestinal motility. London: Churchill Livingstone, 1993, pp. 373–393.

53. Rahhal RM B, WP. Sucrosidase Trial in Chronic nonspecific Diarrhea in Children. Open Pediatr Med J 2008; 2:35–38.

54. Guandalini S. Probiotics for children: use in diarrhea. J Clin Gastroenterol 2006; 40:244–248.
55. Sarker SA, Sultana S, Fuchs GJ, et al. Lactobacillus paracasei strain ST11 has no effect on rotavirus but ameliorates the outcome of nonrotavirus diarrhea in children from Bangladesh. Pediatrics 2005; 116:e221–e228.
56. Billoo AG, Memon MA, Khaskheli SA, et al. Role of a probiotic (Saccharomyces boulardii) in management and prevention of diarrhoea. World J Gastroenterol 2006; 12:4557–4560.
57. di Bosco AM, Grieco P, Diurno MV, et al. Binding site of loperamide: automated docking of loperamide in human mu- and delta-opioid receptors. Chem Biol Drug Des 2008; 71:328–335.
58. Baker DE. Loperamide: a pharmacological review. Rev Gastroenterol Disord. 2007; 7 Suppl 3:S11–S18.
59. Thompson WG. Cholestyramine. Can Med Assoc J 1971; 104:305–309.

21 Diarrhea Related to Non-neoplastic Endocrine Diseases

Ashwani K. Singal, MD,
Nischita K. Reddy, MD,
and Don W. Powell, MD

CONTENTS

INTRODUCTION
DIABETIC DIARRHEA
DIARRHEA RELATED TO HYPER-
   AND HYPO-FUNCTION OF THE
   THYROID GLAND
DIARRHEA RELATED TO ADRENAL GLAND
DIARRHEA RELATED TO IMMUNE
   DYSFUNCTION, POLYENDOCRINOPATHY,
   ENTEROPATHY, X-LINKED SYNDROME
   (IPEX)
REFERENCES

Summary

Diarrhea may result from either neoplastic (e.g., gastrinoma, VIPoma, medullary carcinoma of the thyroid) or non-neoplastic dysfunction of the endocrine glands. This chapter deals with diarrhea due to hyper- or hypofunction of the endocrine pancreas, thyroid, adrenal gland, or congenital immune-related disease affecting several endocrine glands. The epidemiology, clinical features, diagnosis, and treatment of the diarrhea of these non-neoplastic endocrine diseases

From: *Diarrhea, Clinical Gastroenterology*
Edited by: S. Guandalini, H. Vaziri, DOI 10.1007/978-1-60761-183-7_21
© Springer Science+Business Media, LLC 2011

are covered here. Although some of these diarrheal syndromes are rare, some (e.g., diabetic diarrhea and the diarrhea of hyperthyroidism) are common because of the prevalence of the underlying disease.

Key Words: Non-neoplastic endocrinal diarrhea, Diabetic diarrhea, Celiac disease, Diabetes mellitus, Sorbitol, Bile acid malabsorption, Lymphocytic colitis, Pancreatic insufficiency, Diabetic microangiopathy, Autonomic neuropathy, Intestinal fluid and electrolyte transport, Intestinal motility, Bacterial overgrowth, Anorectal dysfunction, Fecal incontinence, Loperamide, Clonidine, Somatostatin, Thyrotoxicosis, Steatorrhea, Coefficient of fat absorption, Ulcerative colitis, Propylthiouracil, Beta blockers, Addison's disease, Autoimmune polyglandular syndrome, APS type I, APS type II, John F Kennedy, IPEX, Polyendocrinopathy, FOXP3, Cyclosporine, Tacrolimus, Bone marrow transplantation

INTRODUCTION

Endocrine or hormonal diarrhea is an important cause of chronic diarrhea comprising neoplastic and non-neoplastic causes (Table 21.1). This chapter will focus on diarrhea related to non-neoplastic endocrine

causes. Although some diarrheas related to endocrine disorders are rare, some are more common because of the prevalence of the respective endocrine disorder.

DIABETIC DIARRHEA

Diabetics experience GI symptoms more frequently compared to non-diabetics in the general population [1–4]. In one survey, up to 76% of diabetic outpatients reported at least one GI symptom with constipation being the commonest and reported in 60% cases [2]. Diarrhea has been reported among 8–22% of diabetics [2–4]. The prevalence may be underestimated given the lack of prospective epidemiologic studies. Cross-sectional studies have reported a higher prevalence in type I diabetes mellitus (T_1DM) compared to type 2 diabetes mellitus (T_2DM) (5.2% vs. 0.4%; $p < 0.01$) [5]. Whether the prevalence of diarrhea in diabetics is increased with poorly controlled diabetes is not entirely clear. In one population-based study, there was a direct correlation between the number of GI symptoms and the self-reported glycemic control [3]. However, in another community-based study, upper GI symptoms but not the diarrhea was related to glycemic control [4]. The reason for an increase in prevalence of GI symptoms with poor glycemic control is

Chapter 21 / Diarrhea Related to Non-neoplastic Endocrine Diseases

not entirely clear. However, this has been shown to be likely related to effect of blood sugar levels on the motility of the GI tract including the small bowel [6]. There are no data on the osmotic process contributing to diarrhea by diffusion of glucose into the GI lumen or by the metabolism of glucose to short chain fatty acids with resultant osmotic diarrhea.

Definition of Diabetic Diarrhea

The term "diabetic diarrhea" was introduced by Bragen et al. in 1936 to describe unexplained diarrhea in diabetics. This was more clearly defined by Whalen et al. and Malins and Mayne in the 1960s [7–9]. It includes all three components of the definition of diarrhea, i.e., increased frequency, watery consistency, and increased weight >200 g/day.

Causes of Diarrhea in Diabetes Mellitus

RELATED OR ASSOCIATED WITH DIABETES MELLITUS

Drug/diet induced: Metformin administration is the most common cause of diarrhea in diabetics [1]. Dietary food containing sorbitol,

Table 21.1
Causes of endocrinal diarrhea

Neoplastic causes
Carcinoid syndrome
Gastrinoma
Somatostatinoma
VIPoma
Medullary carcinoma of thyroid
Mastocytosis[a]
Non-neoplastic causes
Diabetes mellitus
Thyroid disorders
– Thyrotoxicosis
– Hypothyroidism
Adrenal gland disorders
– Addison's disease
– Autoimmune polyglandular syndromes type I and II
X-linked immune deficiency with polyendocrinopathy and diarrhea (IPEX)

[a]Although mastocytosis is not due to neoplasia of an endocrine organ, the role of systemic mediators in the cause of diarrhea is similar to the other neoplastic endocrine diseases.

medication elixirs, and laxative use should be explored as other potential causes. The diagnosis is made by response to withdrawal of the offending agent.

Celiac disease (CD): The prevalence of concomitant CD is reported to be 1–7.8% among T_1DM [10–28] (Table 21.1). Wide variation in the reported prevalence may be attributed to the study population (children vs. adults); type of screening test used; sample size; and percentage of cases with biopsy confirmation. Prevalence is higher among adults with a longer duration of diabetes [10, 29]. The prevalence of CD among diabetics is similar in the USA and Europe and may even be higher in the USA (Table 21.2). Sharing a common histocompatibility gene HLA-DQB1 between the two diseases as well as several shared non-HLA gene loci may explain this association [30].

The diagnosis of associated CD in diabetics is important for adequate management of the diabetics. The clinical distinction is difficult as symptoms in CD may be similar to the GI symptoms in diabetics. Diagnosis requires serology and small bowel biopsy. The index of suspicion is heightened by (a) gastrointestinal symptoms preceding onset of diabetes; (b) frequent episodes of hypoglycemia; (c) associated malabsorption with anemia, hypocalcaemia, or low serum folate levels; (d) absence of neuropathy in patients with diabetic diarrhea; and (e) presence of constitutional symptoms.

All patients with T_1DM should be screened for CD [31]. Although the awareness is increasing over the last decade, the screening frequency in 2006 was reported at only around 70% [29]. It has been shown that annual screening for CD in T_1DM increases the cumulative frequency of the diagnosis of CD from 3.7% at the time of diagnosis of T_1DM to 10% at 5 years of follow-up [28]. This is corroborated by the increased prevalence of CD in T_1DM in adults as compared to children (Table 21.2).

Bile acid malabsorption: Though not well studied, there appears to be increased excretion of bile acids in the stool in 15% of diabetics with diarrhea as demonstrated by a bile acid breath test [32]. Unfortunately, there is inconsistent efficacy of cholestyramine in treating patients with diabetic diarrhea [33].

Lymphocytic colitis: In a retrospective study on 199 Swedish patients with lymphocytic colitis, 40% had some sort of autoimmune disease including diabetes mellitus, thyroid disease, or CD [34].

Pancreatic insufficiency: The prevalence of chronic pancreatitis is increased in diabetics. Mild exocrine pancreatic insufficiency has been reported among 20–70% of diabetics [35]. This is postulated to be due to inhibition of pancreatic enzymes by high levels of glucagon. Structural and inflammatory damage to the pancreas may be suspected

Table 21.2
Celiac disease in type 1 diabetes mellitus[a]

Adults

Author	Sample size	Screening test used	Biopsy (%)	Frequency of CD (%)
Sjoberg et al. [10]	848	AGA, EMA	50	2.6
Cronin et al. [11]	101	EMA	100	4.9
Talal et al. [12]	185	EMA	55	6.4
Sategna-Guidetti et al. [14]	383	EMA	83	2.6
Collin et al. [15]	195	ARA	100	4.1
Page et al. [17]	767	AGA	67	2
Rensch et al. [25]	47	EMA	100	6.4
De Vitis et al. [27]	639	AGA, EMA	NA	7.8
Pooled prevalence[b] (95% CI)				4.1 (2.6–6.4)

Children and adolescents

Author	Sample size	Screening test used	Biopsy (%)	Frequency of CD (%)
Maki et al. [13]	215	ARA	100	2.3
Koletzko et al. [16]	1032	AGA	53	1.1–1.3
Savilahti et al. [18]	201	ARA, AGA, biopsy	100	3.5
Sigurs et al. [19]	436	AGA, ARA	95	4.6
Cacciari et al. [20]	146	AGA	100	3.4
Barera et al. [21]	498	AGA	73	3.2
Gadd et al. [22]	180	AGA	100	2.2
Rossi et al. [23]	211	EMA	30	1.4
Verge et al. [24]	273	AGA, EMA	100	1.8
Saukkonen et al. [26]	776	ARA, AGA	100	2.4
Larsson et al. [28]	300	EMA	100	3.3
Pooled prevalence[b] (95% CI)				2.6 (2.0–3.4)

[a]Diagnosis of type 1 diabetes mellitus required anti-islet antibodies or low serum C-peptide or multiple autoimmunity diseases. Clinical diagnosis was made if two or more of the following present: age of onset <35 years, requirement of insulin within 3 years, and BMI <25 in women or <27 in men.

[b]Calculated using random effects meta-analysis model.

AGA – antigliadin antibodies, ARA – antireticulin antibodies, EMA – endomysial antibodies; CI – confidence interval.

with (a) pain as a dominant symptom, (b) history of alcohol abuse, (c) presence of pancreatic calcification, and (d) increasing insulin sensitivity and occurrence of frequent hypoglycemic episodes. Diagnosis is made by secretin–cholecystokinin stimulation test and measuring the pancreatic exocrine secretion or response to therapeutic trial of oral pancreatic enzymes.

Diabetic microangiopathy: The presence of hyalinized periodic acid Schiff (PAS) positive, thick vessel walls of the small bowel was reported on duodenal biopsy in a patient with T_1DM and chronic diarrhea using monoclonal antibodies against type IV collagen [36]. However, these changes are not always seen in patients with diabetic diarrhea and are also unable to explain the intermittent nature of symptoms [9, 37, 38]. Moreover, thickening of vessel walls and microangiopathy is a nonspecific finding and is commonly seen in patients with long-standing diabetes mellitus. Therefore, the clinical significance of this finding is not clear and intestinal biopsy is not recommended for making the diagnosis of diabetic diarrhea.

ASSOCIATED WITH AUTONOMIC NEUROPATHY

Autonomic neuropathy is thought to be a major pathologic factor contributing to diarrhea in diabetics. This idea is supported by the presence of other manifestations of autonomic neuropathy in diabetic patients with diarrhea [39], the occurrence of diarrhea after use of ganglion blocking agents or with infiltrative diseases of the ganglia [40], and the demonstration of degenerative nerve changes in patients with diabetic diarrhea [41]. Neuropathy may cause diarrhea by altering fluid and electrolyte transport or by altering motility.

Intestinal fluid and electrolyte transport abnormalities: Alpha adrenergic receptors mediate fluid and electrolyte absorption in the small bowel [42]. Loss of this adrenergic tone in diabetics may result in increased net fluid and electrolyte secretion. This is corroborated by the observation of impaired net fluid absorption in non-diabetic rats with chemical sympathectomy and in rats made diabetic with streptozotocin [42]. This pathophysiologic syndrome has been labeled as idiopathic or true diabetic diarrhea. Its diagnosis is made by (a) its characteristic clinical features (Table 21.3), (b) exclusion of other causes (Fig. 21.1), and (c) response to either octreotide and/or clonidine [43, 44]. Measurement of intestinal secretions is a research procedure available only in a few centers. Among all patients with diabetic diarrhea, impaired autonomic function was the cause in 62% of T_1DM and 16% of T_2DM [5].

Table 21.3
Clinical characteristics of true diabetic diarrhea

- Occurrence in a patient with type 1 diabetes of long-standing duration
- Features of chronic secretory diarrhea, i.e., diarrhea persisting on 24–48 h of fasting with no osmotic gap in stool
- Intermittent episodes of diarrhea
- Brown voluminous watery stools
- Nocturnal severity of symptoms
- Associated peripheral neuropathy with autonomic component such as orthostasis, anhidrosis, retrograde ejaculation, urinary symptoms, and abnormal papillary responses
- Frequent response to agents such as clonidine or somatostatin

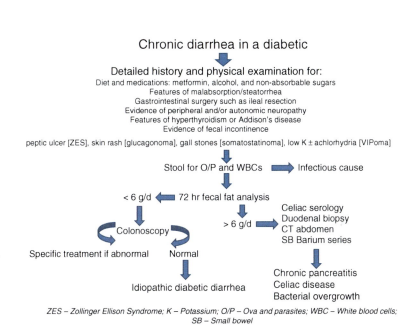

Fig. 21.1. Diagnostic approach to chronic diarrhea in a patient with diabetes mellitus.

Intestinal motility abnormalities: Increased GI motility with fast transit and abnormal migratory motor complexes is described in diabetics [45–50]. All these patients had associated peripheral and autonomic neuropathy. Whether this abnormal motility pattern exists in patients without neuropathy is not entirely clear. Moreover, the abnormal motility does not correlate with the presence of symptoms

[46]. Conflicting data also exist with demonstration of increased [47] as well as slow motility [48] in patients with diabetes mellitus and diarrhea. Further, inability to link the abnormal motility to the gastrointestinal symptoms and diarrhea limits the acceptance of the abnormal GI motility as the primary mechanism of diarrhea in this disease.

Abnormalities of intestinal motility may be demonstrated by manometry, orocecal transit time, or radioisotopic methods. Orocecal transit time measurement by the demonstration of excretion of hydrogen in breath after ingestion of 14C xylose is the most available technique. Measurement of GI motility may be helpful to guide the use of prokinetic or antimotility agents for the treatment of diarrhea.

Bacterial overgrowth: Diabetics with slow intestinal motility may develop bacterial overgrowth. The diagnosis is supported by jejunal aspirates demonstrating $>10^5$ aerobic or anaerobic organisms/ml, 14C xylose breath test, or response to a therapeutic trial of broad-spectrum antibiotics.

Anorectal dysfunction and incontinence: Anal sphincter dysfunction has been described in diabetics with chronic diarrhea especially among patients with peripheral neuropathy [2]. These patients have fecal incontinence as a major symptom, although this is not true diarrhea. Anorectal manometry shows the sphincter dysfunction to be limited to internal anal sphincter with preserved function of the external anal sphincter [51].

Approach to the Diabetic Patient with Chronic Diarrhea

Detailed history and physical examination is the first step in approaching all patients with diarrhea (Fig. 21.1). Focus should be on (a) duration of diarrhea; (b) features of malabsorption such as greasy foul smelling stools, weight loss, anemia, and peripheral edema; (c) evidence of fecal incontinence; (d) use of sorbitol containing compounds, laxatives, and drugs such as metformin especially eliciting the temporal relationship between the onset of diarrhea and introduction of either of these agents; (e) abdominal pain; (f) history of alcoholism; (g) presence of other autoimmune diseases; (h) symptoms of peripheral and autonomic neuropathy; and (i) type and duration of diabetes. Diarrhea in diabetics may or may not respond to fasting. It must be remembered that hormonal diarrhea due to certain neoplastic causes may have associated diabetes, e.g., glucagonoma, somatostatinoma, and VIPoma. However, the duration of diabetes in these conditions usually will be short. In contrast, diabetic diarrhea usually develops in patients with long-standing diabetes mellitus (mean 17 years; 2–45 years of age) [52].

Chapter 21 / Diarrhea Related to Non-neoplastic Endocrine Diseases   365

Complete blood count and comprehensive biochemical examination are performed as screening tests for malabsorption (anemia, hypocalcaemia, and hypoproteinemia), infection leukocytosis, and electrolyte/fluid deficits. Stool samples are sent for ova/parasites and WBC's for an infectious etiology. Celiac serology should be obtained for T_1DM patients. Colonoscopy is then indicated if the initial workup is non-contributory and there are features suggestive of a colonic origin of diarrhea. Although sigmoidoscopy can pick up a large percentage of colonic causes of diarrhea, colonoscopy is preferred for taking random mucosal biopsies from left and right sides of the colon to exclude microscopic or collagenous colitis and for ileal intubation with biopsies to exclude Crohn's disease [53]. If the qualitative stool fat test is positive, next step should be to check for quantitative stool fat excretion (Fig. 21.1). Normal fat excretion is <6 g/day on a diet with 100 g fat per day. Because up to 14 g/day of fat excretion can occur just because of motility or secretory dysfunction of the small bowel, which frequently happens in diabetics [54], a true diagnosis of steatorrhea among diabetics is most reliable if the fat excretion is >14 g/day. Specific tests are then performed for small bowel, pancreatic, or celiac disease. Patients with symptoms suggestive of fecal incontinence can be diagnosed more firmly with anorectal manometry. If the etiology of diarrhea is still unexplained, the patient is diagnosed to have diabetic diarrhea (Table 21.3).

Treatment of Diabetic Diarrhea

Effective management is crucial as there is a significant impact of GI symptoms in diabetics on the quality of life (QOL) [55]. It has been shown that the QOL scores in these patients get worse with increasing number of symptoms. Moreover, the condition can be fatal among infants with type 1 diabetes and secretory diabetic diarrhea [56].

Initial attempts should be to restore fluid and electrolyte status. Adequate control of blood sugar levels should be assured, although there are no clear data whether this is really helpful. Symptomatic control of diarrhea can be achieved using opiates such as codeine or better still, loperamide. It is unclear whether opiates are efficacious by their clear action on the muscle or by their reported action of reducing intestinal secretions [57, 58]. Loperamide is given orally in a dose of 2–4 mg after each bowel movement to a maximum of 12–24 mg/day. It should be assured that the patient does not have an infectious etiology or severe colitis as use of these agents in these situations has a potential for prolonging bacterial clearance or precipitating toxic megacolon. Specific treatment is attempted based on the pathogenetic mechanism identified (Table 21.4).

Table 21.4

Mechanisms, criteria for diagnosis, and treatment of diarrhea in diabetics

Mechanism	Diagnosis	Treatment
Iatrogenic (metformin, sorbitol)	History	Removal of the offending agent
Bile acid malabsorption	SECHAT breath test[a]	Cholestyramine
Celiac disease	Anti-endomysial antibody or anti-TTG screening and small bowel biopsy	Gluten-free diet
Lymphocytic colitis	Colonoscopy with random biopsy	5-ASA and/or budesonide
Increased intestinal secretions	Stool electrolytes	Clonidine
		Somatostatin or octreotide
Fast intestinal transit	OCTT by D-xylose breath test	Loperamide
Bacterial overgrowth	Jejunal aspirate for bacterial culture	Broad-spectrum antibiotics[b]
Anorectal dysfunction with incontinence	Anorectal manometry	Biofeedback training exercises
		Loperamide

[a]If unavailable, trial of cholestyramine may be the only option.
[b]Ideally given on a rotating basis for 10–14 days every month to avoid bacterial resistance; OCTT – orocecal transit time.

True or idiopathic diabetic diarrhea can be treated with clonidine, which decreases intestinal secretions and thus has therapeutic role in control of diarrhea [59]. The drug is given orally in a dose of 0.1–0.6 twice a day. As an adrenergic agonist, it acts on the α-2 adrenergic receptors of the enterocytes (Fig. 21.2) which are hypersensitive as a result of loss of adrenergic tone in diabetics with autonomic neuropathy (denervation hypersensitivity) [43]. Restoring adrenergic tone results in net fluid and electrolyte absorption and improvement in diarrhea. The drug is occasionally limited by orthostasis and hypotension and should be used with caution in elderly and those susceptible to falls [59]. In this respect, topical subcutaneous application of clonidine (clonidine patch)

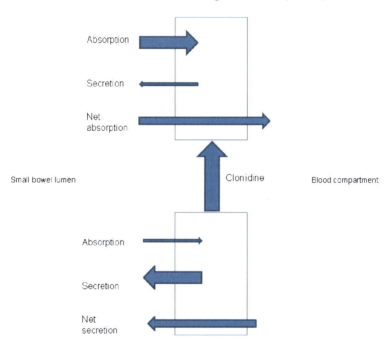

Fig. 21.2. Water and electrolyte transport in the small bowel. **a** In the normal state with intact adrenergic innervations, alpha adrenergic tone mediates net absorption. **b** In the presence of diabetic autonomic neuropathy and loss of adrenergic innervation, there is net secretion of water and electrolytes due to loss of adrenergic tone. Clonidine, an alpha-2 agonist, restores this adrenergic tone (denervation hypersensitivity) resulting in net absorption of water and electrolytes.

is useful with control of diarrhea and is less likely to cause orthostatic symptoms [60].

Somatostatin is an endogenous gastrointestinal hormone secreted from the D cells of the gastric antrum. Its synthetic octapeptide analog, octreotide, is given as subcutaneous injection to treat diarrhea due to VIPomas, carcinoid syndrome, and AIDS [61]. Given as 50 μg subcutaneous injection twice a day, it has been successful for symptomatic control in patients with diabetic diarrhea [39, 62]. The exact mechanism of action is unclear. However, slowing of the intestinal motility, improved net absorption of fluids and electrolytes, and suppression of diarrheogenic hormones have been postulated [63].

DIARRHEA RELATED TO HYPER- AND HYPO-FUNCTION OF THE THYROID GLAND

Diarrhea in Thyrotoxicosis

Symptoms of thyrotoxicosis are known to occur not only with hyperthyroidism (Grave's disease and toxic goiter) but also with inappropriate exogenous administration of thyroid hormones. GI symptoms in thyrotoxicosis are often subtle and often ignored by the patients [64]. Hyperphagia is the most common symptom, but diarrhea has been reported in about 20% of cases [65, 66]. Absence of pain, weight loss out of proportion to diarrhea, hyperphagia with increased appetite, and presence of other typical features of thyrotoxicosis (tachycardia, proptosis, moist palms, hypertonic reflexes, and fine tremors) raise the suspicion for thyrotoxicosis as the underlying etiology.

MECHANISMS OF DIARRHEA

Although the exact mechanism of diarrhea in thyrotoxicosis is unknown, there are many proposals (Table 21.5). The most commonly accepted mechanism is altered motility with a rapid intestinal transit. Barium studies have shown small bowel intestinal transit of 1–3 h in patients with thyrotoxicosis compared to 8–10 h in the normal population [67]. Although barium examination is simple and readily available, assessing the orocecal transit time by measuring pulmonary hydrogen excretion after administration of non-absorbable and bacterially metabolized carbohydrate such as lactulose is more reliable [68].

Even using the breath test, abnormal motility has not been consistently linked to the symptoms of diarrhea. Abnormal GI motility is noted in 90% of patients with thyrotoxicosis, but only 20% of these patients have symptomatic diarrhea [69]. However, in symptomatic patients, this may play an important role. With achievement

Chapter 21 / Diarrhea Related to Non-neoplastic Endocrine Diseases 369

Table 21.5
Mechanisms of diarrhea in thyroid disorders

A. Thyrotoxicosis

Steatorrhea associated
Hyperphagia and fast intestinal transit
Bile acid and lactose malabsorption
Associated celiac disease

Non-steatorrhea associated
Secretory diarrhea
Associated lymphocytic colitis
Associated inflammatory bowel disease

B. Hypothyroidism
Slow intestinal transit and bacterial overgrowth

of euthyroid status, motility is restored to normal with disappearance of diarrhea [70].

Steatorrhea has been described in 46–60% of patients with thyrotoxicosis [71, 72]. This has been shown to be related to thyrotoxicosis as it normalizes with achievement of euthyroid status. However, steatorrhea is unrelated to the thyroid disease severity, body mass index, and daily fat intake [71]. Pancreatic and small bowel functions have been consistently shown to be normal in these patients and do not explain the steatorrhea [71, 72]. The proposed mechanism of steatorrhea is linked to hyperphagia resulting in increased fat ingestion causing increased fat excretion. The coefficient of fat absorption (g fat intake – g fecal loss/g fat intake × 100) or COFA does not rise in parallel to the increased intake leading to steatorrhea [72]. However, the validity of this concept was not reproduced in another study [71]. Additional mechanisms postulated are bile acid malabsorption [73] and lactose malabsorption [74].

Diarrhea due to increased intestinal secretion is described in T3 hyperthyroidism [75]. This responds well to treatment of thyrotoxicosis and is thought to be mediated through increased intestinal cAMP signaling. Thyroid disease may be associated with ulcerative colitis (UC) or celiac disease (CD) [76]. Common haplotypes and autoimmunity may explain this association. Iodine deficiency and consequent goiter have been described in patients with UC [77]. Prevalence of hyperthyroidism in UC is reported at 3.8% compared to 0.8% in the general population [77]. Presence of thyrotoxicosis makes the management of UC difficult due to malabsorption of therapeutic anti-inflammatory drugs as a result of fast intestinal transit [78]. Based on prospective follow-up, the prevalence of thyroid abnormalities has been described in 14% of patients with CD [79]. Patients with both diseases usually present at a later age, with thyroid dysfunction presenting first in 70% of cases [79]. Lack of response of CD to gluten-free diet and an associated high MCV raise suspicion of concomitant thyroid disease.

Diarrhea in Hypothyroidism

Constipation is a more frequent symptom in hypothyroidism. However, diarrhea is rarely reported. The mechanism of diarrhea has been postulated to be secondary to bacterial overgrowth as a result of reduced gastrointestinal motility with consequent stasis [80].

Treatment of Thyroid Gland-Related Diarrhea

As for diabetic diarrhea, the maintenance of fluid/electrolyte and nutritional status takes the priority in management. Adequate control of thyroid status should be assured. Specific treatment for diarrhea can be accomplished by two means. Propylthiouracil and carbimazole have been shown to improve orocecal transit and improvement in diarrhea with attainment of euthyroid status [70, 81]. However, antithyroid drugs take a few weeks for their efficacy. In this respect, beta blockers are useful especially for severe diarrhea requiring faster relief. Beta blockers act by blocking the beta adrenergic receptors and in turn decreasing the intestinal secretions secondary to inhibition of enterocyte cAMP levels [82]. This is a class effect with all beta blockers having equal efficacy. Specific treatment must also take into consideration other rare mechanisms such as bile acid malabsorption, celiac disease, and lymphocytic colitis. Broad-spectrum antibiotics are useful for patients with hypothyroidism provided bacterial overgrowth is demonstrated.

DIARRHEA RELATED TO ADRENAL GLAND

Addison's Disease

This disease with its clinical syndrome was described by Thomas Addison in 1855 [83]. Deficiency of cortisol and aldosterone, the hormones secreted from the adrenal gland, could be due to the diseases of the adrenal gland itself (primary adrenal insufficiency or Addison's disease) or secondary to pituitary disease (secondary adrenal insufficiency). The most common cause of the primary disease is autoimmune destruction of the gland. Clinical features are non-specific with tiredness, weakness, and dizziness occurring in almost all the cases

Chapter 21 / Diarrhea Related to Non-neoplastic Endocrine Diseases   371

[84]. Pigmentation of the knuckles and skin is a classic sign but is seen in less than 10% of cases [85, 86]. GI symptoms occur frequently and are reported in 56% cases of Addison's disease. Rarely, they may be the presenting manifestations [84]. Although gastrointestinal symptoms usually consist of nausea, vomiting, and anorexia, diarrhea has been reported to occur in about 20% of cases [87, 88].

The mechanism of diarrhea with Addison's disease (AD) is not clearly known. Most patients have chronic secretory diarrhea. Steatorrhea with fat malabsorption is described and responds to corticosteroid replacement [89]. Associated CD is described in 8–12% of patients with AD [90–92]. Although presence of common HLA-DR3 and HLA-DQ2 with the two diseases explains this association, other environmental and genetic factors also play a role [93]. CD can antedate the diagnosis of AD in 50% of cases [91–93]. AD occurs as a component of autoimmune polyglandular syndrome (APS) in about 50% of cases (see below) [91].

It is recommended that all patients with AD be screened for associated CD [94]. Symptoms of CD are usually non-specific or very subtle [91]. The suspicion is increased in the presence of chronic diarrhea, inability to adequately control AD with corticosteroid replacement due to poor absorption of steroids, and presence of other endocrine problems [91]. Treatment of Addison's disease is with replacement of the deficient hormones. Definite treatment depends on characterization of the cause, i.e., whether this is primary or secondary to pituitary disease. It must be remembered that occurrence of significant abdominal pain and/or intractable vomiting during the clinical course of these patients usually signifies the onset of acute Addison's crisis and should be recognized and treated appropriately to avoid a bad outcome.

Diarrhea Related to Autoimmune Polyglandular Syndromes

About half of patients with AD have other concomitant diseases such as diseases of thyroid gland, diabetes mellitus, or pernicious anemia [84]. The term polyendocrine syndrome is a misnomer as many of these patients have non-endocrine disorders (Table 21.6).

AUTOIMMUNE POLYENDOCRINE SYNDROME (APS) TYPE I

It is clinically recognized by a triad of muco-cutaneous candidiasis, autoimmune hypoparathyroidism, and AD (Table 21.6). This syndrome is due to mutation of autoimmune regulator (AIRE) gene located on short arm of chromosome 21. The disease manifests during infancy and the prevalence increases with age. Diarrhea in these patients is related to fat malabsorption; mechanism(s) of which are not clearly known.

Table 21.6
Autoimmune polyendocrine syndromes

Feature	Autoimmune polyendocrine syndrome type 1	Autoimmune polyendocrine syndrome type 2
Inheritance	Monogenic (AIRE gene on chromosome 21)	Polygenic (HLA-DR3 and HLA-DR-4 associations)
Prevalence	Rare	Common
Age	Infancy	20–60 years
Gender predominance	Either	Females
Immune deficiency	Susceptibility to candidiasis due to absence of spleen	No immune deficiency
Endocrine diseases	Addison's disease	Addison's disease
	Hypoparathyroidism	Autoimmune thyroid disease
	Type 1 diabetes mellitus	Type 1 diabetes mellitus
Other diseases	Muco-cutaneous candidiasis	Celiac disease
	Pernicious anemia	Vitiligo
	Myopathy	Primary hypogonadism
		Myasthenia gravis

Modified with permission from Eisenbarth and Gottlieb. N Engl J Med 2004; 352: 2069.

Postulated mechanisms are severe superimposed Giardia infection, pancreatic insufficiency, and lymphangiectasia [95]. Malabsorption secondary to cholecystokinin deficiency due to absence of cholecystokinin producing cells in the small intestine has been documented [96]. Diagnosis is clinical and confirmation is with demonstration of anti-interferon antibodies. Treatment of diarrhea is symptomatic and specific treatment depends upon identification of a defined mechanism. Low fat diet and medium chain triglyceride supplementation in the diet are useful for patients deficient in cholecystokinin [96].

AUTOIMMUNE POLYGLANDULAR SYNDROME TYPE II

The more common of the two polyglandular syndromes, APS type II, occurs during adulthood with a female preponderance. The syndrome is clinically characterized by the presence of two or more diseases: AD, autoimmune thyroid disease, T_1DM, CD, primary hypogonadism, or myasthenia gravis. Diarrhea may be secondary to associated Addison's

Chapter 21 / Diarrhea Related to Non-neoplastic Endocrine Diseases 373

or celiac disease, but no specific cause has been identified in some patients with diarrhea in this disease [95]. Diagnosis is clinical and treatment is symptomatic and specifically tailored to the clinical components of the syndrome. Family members of patients with both types of polyendocrine disorders should be screened for the common diseases associated with these disorders. It has been proposed that the late President John F. Kennedy suffered from APS type II perhaps with concomitant celiac disease [97].

DIARRHEA RELATED TO IMMUNE DYSFUNCTION, POLYENDOCRINOPATHY, ENTEROPATHY, X-LINKED SYNDROME (IPEX)

This disease was first reported in 1982 with description of severe secretory diarrhea and immune deficiency in 19 male children. Most of these patients developed severe diarrhea in infancy with fatal outcome in most by school age [98]. Diarrhea is usually secondary to severe enteropathy resulting from enteral infections due to underlying immune deficiency. In addition, patients have multiple other disorders such as hypothyroidism, thrombocytopenia, hemolytic anemia, eczema or atopy, and lymphadenopathy [98]. The disorder is rare and is due to X-linked inheritance of mutated FOXP3 gene which encodes a protein named "scurfin." The scurfin protein is a transcription factor and is needed for the development of regulatory CD4+CD25+ T cells (regulatory T cells) which are necessary for maintenance of tolerance to self-tissue [99]. Recognition is important as untreated disease is fatal. Bone marrow transplantation may potentially reverse the disorder and should be considered [100]. Immune suppression is another option. Calcineurin inhibitors (cyclosporine or tacrolimus) have strong immune-suppressive action, but are limited by their potential for nephrotoxicity, especially in small children. Sirolimus, another immune suppressant, overcomes this limitation. Its successful use is reported in three children with IPEX. Sirolimus was used for 5 years in combination with methotrexate in one child and for over 15 months in combination with azathioprine in the other two children. The disease was well controlled with maintenance of remission in all these three children with IPEX [101].

ACKNOWLEDGMENTS

No financial or assistance in any other form was received.

REFERENCES

1. Powell DW. Approach to the patient with diarrhea. In: Yamada T, Alpers DH, Kalloo AN, Kaplowitz N, Owyang C, Powell DW, eds. Principles of clinical gastroenterology, 5th edn. Oxford: Wiley-Blackwell, 2008, pp. 304–360.
2. Feldman M, Schiller LR. Disorders of gastrointestinal motility associated with diabetes mellitus. Ann Intern Med 1983; 98:378–384.
3. Bytzer P, Talley NJ, Leemon M, Young LJ, Jones MP, Horowitz M. Prevalence of gastrointestinal symptoms associated with diabetes mellitus: a population-based survey of 15,000 adults. Arch Intern Med 2001; 161:1989–1996.
4. Bytzer P, Talley NJ, Hammer J, Young LJ, Jones MP, Horowitz M. GI symptoms in diabetes mellitus are associated with both poor glycemic control and diabetic complications. Am J Gastroenterol 2002; 97:604–611.
5. Lysy J, Israeli E, Goldin E. The prevalence of chronic diarrhea among diabetic patients. Am J Gastroenterol 1999; 94:2165–2170.
6. de Boer SY MA, lam WF, Schipper J, Jansen JB, Lamers CB. Hyperglycemia modulates gallbladder motility and small intestinal transit time in man. Dig Dis Sci 1997; 38:2228–2235.
7. Bragen JA, Bollman JL, Kepler EJ. The 'diarrhea of diabetes' and steatorrhea of pancreatic insufficiency. Mayo Clin Proc 1936; 11:737–742.
8. Whalen GE, Soergel KH, Geenen JE. Diabetic diarrhea. A clinical and pathophysiological study. Gastroenterology 1969; 56:1021–1032.
9. Malins JM, Mayne N. Diabetic diarrhea. A study of thirteen patients with jejunal biopsy. Diabetes 1969; 18:858–866.
10. Sjoberg K, Eriksson KF, Bredberg A, Wassmuth R, Eriksson S. Screening for coeliac disease in adult insulin-dependent diabetes mellitus. J Intern Med 1998; 243:133–140.
11. Cronin CC, Feighery A, Ferriss JB, Liddy C, Shanahan F, Feighery C. High prevalence of celiac disease among patients with insulin-dependent (type I) diabetes mellitus. Am J Gastroenterol 1997; 92:2210–2212.
12. Talal AH, Murray JA, Goeken JA, Sivitz WI. Celiac disease in an adult population with insulin-dependent diabetes mellitus: use of endomysial antibody testing. Am J Gastroenterol 1997; 92:1280–1284.
13. Maki M, Hallstrom O, Huupponen T, Vesikari T, Visakorpi JK. Increased prevalence of coeliac disease in diabetes. Arch Dis Child 1984; 59: 739–742.
14. Sategna-Guidetti C, Grosso S, Pulitano R, Benaduce E, Dani F, Carta Q. Celiac disease and insulin-dependent diabetes mellitus. Screening in an adult population. Dig Dis Sci 1994; 39:1633–1637.
15. Collin P, Salmi J, Hallstrom O, et al. High frequency of coeliac disease in adult patients with type-I diabetes. Scand J Gastroenterol. 1989; 24:81–84.
16. Koletzko S, Burgin-Wolff A, Koletzko B, et al. Prevalence of coeliac disease in diabetic children and adolescents. A multicentre study. Eur J Pediatr 1988; 148:113–117.
17. Page SR, Lloyd CA, Hill PG, Peacock I, Holmes GK. The prevalence of coeliac disease in adult diabetes mellitus. Q J Med 1994; 87:631–637.
18. Savilahti E, Simell O, Koskimies S, Rilva A, Akerblom HK. Celiac disease in insulin-dependent diabetes mellitus. J Pediatr 1986; 108:690–693.
19. Sigurs N, Johansson C, Elfstrand PO, Viander M, Lanner A. Prevalence of coeliac disease in diabetic children and adolescents in Sweden. Acta Paediatr 1993; 82:748–751.

Chapter 21 / Diarrhea Related to Non-neoplastic Endocrine Diseases   375

20. Cacciari E, Salardi S, Volta U, et al. Prevalence and characteristics of coeliac disease in type 1 diabetes mellitus. Acta Paediatr Scand 1987; 76:671–672.
21. Barera G, Bianchi C, Calisti L, et al. Screening of diabetic children for coeliac disease with antigliadin antibodies and HLA typing. Arch Dis Child 1991; 66:491–494.
22. Gadd S, Kamath KR, Silink M, Skerritt JH. Co-existence of coeliac disease and insulin-dependent diabetes mellitus in children: screening sera using an ELISA test for gliadin antibody. Aust N Z J Med 1992; 22:256–260.
23. Rossi TM, Albini CH, Kumar V. Incidence of celiac disease identified by the presence of serum endomysial antibodies in children with chronic diarrhea, short stature, or insulin-dependent diabetes mellitus. J Pediatr 1993; 123: 262–264.
24. Verge CF, Howard NJ, Rowley MJ, et al. Anti-glutamate decarboxylase and other antibodies at the onset of childhood IDDM: a population-based study. Diabetologia 1994; 37:1113–1120.
25. Rensch MJ, Merenich JA, Lieberman M, Long BD, Davis DR, McNally PR. Gluten-sensitive enteropathy in patients with insulin-dependent diabetes mellitus. Ann Intern Med 1996; 124:564–567.
26. Saukkonen T, Savilahti E, Reijonen H, Ilonen J, Tuomilehto-Wolf E, Akerblom HK. Coeliac disease: frequent occurrence after clinical onset of insulin-dependent diabetes mellitus. Childhood Diabetes in Finland Study Group. Diabet Med 1996; 13:464–470.
27. De Vitis I, Ghirlanda G, Gasbarrini G. Prevalence of coeliac disease in type I diabetes: a multicentre study. Acta Paediatr Suppl 1996; 412:56–57.
28. Larsson K, Carlsson A, Cederwall E, et al. Annual screening detects celiac disease in children with type 1 diabetes. Pediatr Diabetes 2008; 9:354–359.
29. Frohlich-Reiterer EE, Hofer S, Kaspers S, et al. Screening frequency for celiac disease and autoimmune thyroiditis in children and adolescents with type 1 diabetes mellitus – data from a German/Austrian multicentre survey. Pediatr Diabetes 2008; 9:546–553.
30. Smyth DJ, Plagnol V, Walker NM, et al. Shared and distinct genetic variants in type 1 diabetes and celiac disease. N Engl J Med 2008; 359:2767–2777.
31. Holmes GK. Screening for coeliac disease in type 1 diabetes. Arch Dis Child 2002; 87:495–498.
32. Scarpello JH, Hague RV, Cullen DR, Sladen GE. The 14C-glycocholate test in diabetic diarrhoea. Br Med J 1976; 2:673–675.
33. Merrick MV. Bile acid malabsorption. Clinical presentations and diagnosis. Dig Dis 1988; 6:159–169.
34. Olesen M, Eriksson S, Bohr J, Jarnerot G, Tysk C. Lymphocytic colitis: a retrospective clinical study of 199 Swedish patients. Gut 2004; 53: 536–541.
35. Blumenthal HT, Probstein JG, Berns AW. Interrelationship of Diabetes Mellitus and Pancreatitis. Arch Surg. 1963; 87:844–850.
36. De Las Casas LE, Finley JL. Diabetic microangiopathy in the small bowel. Histopathology 1999; 35:267–270.
37. Bennett WA, Berge KG, Sprague RG. The intestinal tract in diabetic diarrhea; a pathologic study. Diabetes 1956; 5:289–294.
38. Green PA, Berge KG, Sprague RG. Control of diabetic diarrhea with antibiotic therapy. Diabetes 1968; 17:385–387.
39. Dudl RJ, Anderson DS, Forsythe AB, Ziegler MG, O'Dorisio TM. Treatment of diabetic diarrhea and orthostatic hypotension with somatostatin analogue SMS 201-995. Am J Med 1987; 83:584–588.

40. French JM, Hall G, Parish DJ, Smith WT. Peripheral and autonomic nerve involvement in primary amyloidosis associated with uncontrollable diarrhoea and steatorrhoea. Am J Med 1965; 39:277–284.
41. Hensley GT, Soergel KH. Neuropathologic findings in diabetic diarrhea. Arch Pathol 1968; 85:587–597.
42. Chang EB, Bergenstal RM, Field M. Diarrhea in streptozocin-treated rats. Loss of adrenergic regulation of intestinal fluid and electrolyte transport. J Clin Invest 1985; 75:1666–1670.
43. Chang EB, Fedorak RN, Field M. Experimental diabetic diarrhea in rats. Intestinal mucosal denervation hypersensitivity and treatment with clonidine. Gastroenterology 1986; 91:564–569.
44. Michaels PE, Cameron RB. Octreotide is cost-effective therapy in diabetic diarrhea. Arch Intern Med. 1991; 151:2469–2473.
45. Camilleri M, Malagelada JR. Abnormal intestinal motility in diabetics with the gastroparesis syndrome. Eur J Clin Invest 1984; 14:420–427.
46. Dooley CP, el Newihi HM, Zeidler A, Valenzuela JE. Abnormalities of the migrating motor complex in diabetics with autonomic neuropathy and diarrhea. Scand J Gastroenterol. 1988; 23:217–223.
47. Keshavarzian A, Iber FL. Intestinal transit in insulin-requiring diabetics. Am J Gastroenterol 1986; 81:257–260.
48. Spengler U, Stellaard F, Ruckdeschel G, Scheurlen C, Kruis W. Small intestinal transit, bacterial growth, and bowel habits in diabetes mellitus. Pancreas 1989; 4:65–70.
49. Wegener M, Borsch G, Schaffstein J, Luerweg C, Leverkus F. Gastrointestinal transit disorders in patients with insulin-treated diabetes mellitus. Dig Dis 1990; 8:23–36.
50. Vantrappen G, Janssens J, Hellemans J, Ghoos Y. The interdigestive motor complex of normal subjects and patients with bacterial overgrowth of the small intestine. J Clin Invest. 1977; 59:1158–1166.
51. Schiller LR, Santa Ana CA, Schmulen AC, Hendler RS, Harford WV, Fordtran JS. Pathogenesis of fecal incontinence in diabetes mellitus: evidence for internal-anal-sphincter dysfunction. N Engl J Med 1982; 307:1666–1671.
52. Valdovinos MA, Camilleri M, Zimmerman BR. Chronic diarrhea in diabetes mellitus: mechanisms and an approach to diagnosis and treatment. Mayo Clin Proc 1993; 68:691–702.
53. Schiller LR, Sellin J. Diarrhea. In: Feldman M, Friedman LS, Brandt LJ, eds. Textbook of gastroenterology, 8th edn. Philadelphia, PA: Saunders, 2008, pp. 159–186.
54. Fine KD, Fordtran JS. The effect of diarrhea on fecal fat excretion. Gastroenterology 1992; 102:1936–1939.
55. Talley NJ, Young L, Bytzer P, et al. Impact of chronic gastrointestinal symptoms in diabetes mellitus on health-related quality of life. Am J Gastroenterol 2001; 96:71–76.
56. Jonas MM, Bell MD, Eidson MS, Koutouby R, Hensley GT. Congenital diabetes mellitus and fatal secretory diarrhea in two infants. J Pediatr Gastroenterol Nutr 1991; 13:415–425.
57. Powell DW. Muscle or mucosa: the site of action of antidiarrheal opiates. Gastroenterology 1981; 80:406–408.
58. Powell DW, Field M. Pharmacological approaches to treatment of secretory diarrhea. In: Field M, Fordtran JS, Schultz S, eds. Secretory diarrhea. Bethesda, MD: American Physiology Society, 1980, p. 187.

Chapter 21 / Diarrhea Related to Non-neoplastic Endocrine Diseases   377

59. Fedorak RN, Field M, Chang EB. Treatment of diabetic diarrhea with clonidine. Ann Intern Med 1985; 102:197–199.
60. Sacerdote A. Topical clonidine for diabetic diarrhea. Ann Intern Med 1986; 105(1):139.
61. Gaginella TS, O'Dorisio TM, Fassler JE, Mekhjian HS. Treatment of endocrine and nonendocrine secretory diarrheal states with Sandostatin. Metabolism 1990; 39:172–175.
62. Walker JJ, Kaplan DS. Efficacy of the somatostatin analog octreotide in the treatment of two patients with refractory diabetic diarrhea. Am J Gastroenterol 1993; 88:765–767.
63. Meyer C, O'Neal DN, Connell W, Alford F, Ward G, Jenkins AJ. Octreotide treatment of severe diabetic diarrhoea. Intern Med J 2003; 33: 617–618.
64. Middleton WR. Thyroid hormones and the gut. Gut 1971; 12:172–177.
65. Scarf M. Gastrointestinal manifestations of hyperthyroidism. J Lab Clin Med 1936; 21:1253–1258.
66. Chapman EM, Maloof F. Bizarre clinical manifestations of hyperthyroidism. N Engl J Med. 1956; 254:1–5.
67. Kim SK. Small intestine transit time in the normal small bowel study. Am J Roentgenol Radium Ther Nucl Med 1968; 104:522–524.
68. Bond JH Jr, Levitt MD, Prentiss R. Investigation of small bowel transit time in man utilizing pulmonary hydrogen (H2) measurements. J Lab Clin Med 1975; 85:546–555.
69. Shirer JW. Hypermotility of the gastrointestinal tract in hyperthyroidism. Am J Med Sci 1933; 186:73–78.
70. Tobin MV, Fisken RA, Diggory RT, Morris AI, Gilmore IT. Orocaecal transit time in health and in thyroid disease. Gut 1989; 30:26–29.
71. Goswami R, Tandon RK, Dudha A, Kochupillai N. Prevalence and significance of steatorrhea in patients with active Graves' disease. Am J Gastroenterol 1998; 93:1122–1125.
72. Thomas FB, Caldwell JH, Greenberger NJ. Steatorrhea in thyrotoxicosis. Relation to hypermotility and excessive dietary fat. Ann Intern Med 1973; 78:669–675.
73. Raju GS, Dawson B, Bardhan KD. Bile acid malabsorption associated with Graves' disease. J Clin Gastroenterol 1994; 19:54–56.
74. Szilagyi A, Lerman S, Barr RG, Stern J, Colacone A, McMullan S. Reversible lactose malabsorption and intolerance in Graves' disease. Clin Invest Med 1991; 14:188–197.
75. Culp KS, Piziak VK. Thyrotoxicosis presenting with secretory diarrhea. Ann Intern Med 1986; 105:216–217.
76. Snook JA, de Silva HJ, Jewell DP. The association of autoimmune disorders with inflammatory bowel disease. Q J Med 1989; 72:835–840.
77. Jarnerot G. The thyroid in ulcerative colitis and Crohn's disease. I. Thyroid radioiodide uptake and urinary iodine excretion. Acta Med Scand 1975; 197: 77–81.
78. Powell JR, Shapiro HA, Carbone JV. Therapeutic problems of ulcerative colitis with hyperthyroidism. Am J Gastroenterol 1968; 50:116–124.
79. Counsell CE, Taha A, Ruddell WS. Coeliac disease and autoimmune thyroid disease. Gut. 1994; 35:844–846.
80. Goldin E WD. Diarrhea in hypothyroidism: bacterial overgrowth as a possible etiology. J Clin Gastroenterol 1990; 12:98–99.

81. Papa A, Cammarota G, Tursi A, et al. Effects of propylthiouracil on intestinal transit time and symptoms in hyperthyroid patients. Hepatogastroenterology 1997; 44:426–429.
82. Bricker LA, Such F, Loehrke ME, Kavanaugh K. Intractable diarrhea in hyperthyroidism: management with beta-adrenergic blockade. Endocr Pract 2001; 7:28–31.
83. Addison T. On the constitutional and local effects of diseases of Supra-renal capsules. London Med Gaz 1855; 43:517 (abstract).
84. Nerup J. Addison's disease – clinical studies. A report for 108 cases. Acta Endocrinol (Copenh). 1974; 76:127–141.
85. Tobin MV, Aldridge SA, Morris AI, Belchetz PE, Gilmore IT. Gastrointestinal manifestations of Addison's disease. Am J Gastroenterol 1989; 84:1302–1305.
86. Dunlop D. Eighty-six cases of Addison's disease. Br Med J 1963; 2:887–891.
87. Ross EJ. Symptomatology in adrenal disease. In: Milo KW, Fowler PBS, eds. Clinical endocrinology. London: William Heinman Medical Books, 1984, pp. 425–433.
88. Oelkers W. Adrenal insufficiency. N Engl J Med 1996; 335:1206–1212.
89. Guarini G, Macaluso M. Steatorrhoea in Addison's disease. Lancet 1963; 1: 955–956.
90. A case of adult coeliac disease with Addison's disease. Presented at the Royal Postgraduate Medical School. Br Med J 1970; 2:711–716.
91. Myhre AG, Aarsetoy H, Undlien DE, Hovdenak N, Aksnes L, Husebye ES. High frequency of coeliac disease among patients with autoimmune adrenocortical failure. Scand J Gastroenterol 2003; 38:511–515.
92. O'Mahony D, O'Leary P, Quigley EM. Aging and intestinal motility: a review of factors that affect intestinal motility in the aged. Drugs Aging 2002; 19:515–527.
93. Biagi F, Campanella J, Soriani A, Vailati A, Corazza GR. Prevalence of coeliac disease in Italian patients affected by Addison's disease. Scand J Gastroenterol 2006; 41:302–305.
94. Collin P, Kaukinen K, Valimaki M, Salmi J. Endocrinological disorders and celiac disease. Endocr Rev 2002; 23:464–483.
95. Barker JM, Gottelib PA, Eisenbarth GS. The immunoendocrinopathy syndromes. In: Kronenberg HM, Melmed S, Polonsky KS, Larsen PR, eds. Williams textbook of endocrinology, 11th edn. Philadelphia, PA: Saunders Elsevier, 2008, pp. 1748–1758.
96. Hogenauer C, Meyer RL, Netto GJ, et al. Malabsorption due to cholecystokinin deficiency in a patient with autoimmune polyglandular syndrome type I. N Engl J Med 2001; 344:270–274.
97. Mandel LR. Endocrine and autoimmune aspects of the health history of John F. Kennedy. Ann Intern Med 2009; 151:350–354.
98. Powell BR, Buist NR, Stenzel P. An X-linked syndrome of diarrhea, polyendocrinopathy, and fatal infection in infancy. J Pediatr 1982; 100:731–737.
99. Hori S, Nomura T, Sakaguchi S. Control of regulatory T cell development by the transcription factor Foxp3. Science 2003; 299:1057–1061.
100. Baud O, Goulet O, Canioni D, et al. Treatment of immune dysregulation, polyendocrinopathy, enteropathy, X-linked syndrome (IPEX) by allogenic bone marrow transplantation. N Eng J Med 2001; 344:1758–1762.
101. Bindl L, Togerson T, Perroni L, et al. Successful use of the new immunesuppressor sirolimus in IPEX (immune dysregulation, polyendocrinopathy, enteropathy, X-linked syndrome). J Pediatr 2005; 147:256–259.

22 Alcohol-Related Diarrhea

Nischita K. Reddy, MD, MPH,
Ashwani Singal, MD,
and Don W. Powell, MD

CONTENTS

INTRODUCTION
CLASSIFICATION
ABSORPTION AND METABOLISM
OF ALCOHOL IN THE GUT
ETIOPATHOGENESIS OF DIARRHEA
CLINICAL PRESENTATION
TREATMENT
REFERENCES

Summary

Diarrhea related to alcohol abuse may be either acute or chronic. Acute diarrheas are the result of dietary indiscretion, transient anatomic or motility changes of the stomach or small intestine, impaired nutrient absorption, mucosal barrier function or pancreatic secretion as well as hormonal/cytokine abnormalities related to alcohol hangover. Chronic diarrheas may result from alcohol withdrawal, pancreatic or hepatobiliary dysfunction, morphologic or motility changes of the gastrointestinal tract, or macro- or micronutrient malabsorption with resulting deficiencies. Treatment of acute alcohol-related diarrhea includes ceasing alcohol ingestion, avoiding milk products, rehydration, and replacement of micronutrients, and use of antidiarrheals and NSAIDS. In addition to the above, treatment

From: *Diarrhea, Clinical Gastroenterology*
Edited by: S. Guandalini, H. Vaziri, DOI 10.1007/978-1-60761-183-7_22
© Springer Science+Business Media, LLC 2011

of chronic alcohol-related diarrheas includes assessing and treating for alcohol withdrawal, nutritional deficiencies, pancreatic or hepatobiliary dysfunction, as well as diagnosing and treating small bowel bacterial overgrowth.

Key Words: Alcohol, Ethanol, Diarrhea, Intestinal permeability, Endotoxin, Pancreatic insufficiency, Bile salt, Malabsorption, Bacterial overgrowth, Steatorrhea

INTRODUCTION

Alcohol intake leads to both transient and enduring effects on the human body. As the portal of entry into the body, the gastrointestinal system is particularly susceptible to the direct, hypertonic effects of alcohol [1]. The effects of alcohol ingestion vary depending on the nutritional status, gender, race, as well as the type and strength of alcoholic beverage.

CLASSIFICATION

Both acute and chronic ingestion of alcohol can lead to diarrhea. Acute alcohol-related diarrhea can be due to concurrent dietary indiscretion,

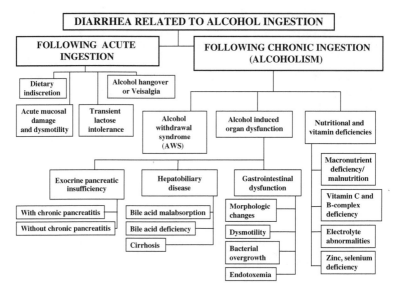

Fig. 22.1. Classification of alcohol-related diarrhea.

the noxious effect of alcohol on the gastrointestinal tract, or alcohol hangover (*veisalgia*). Alcohol hangover may occur after a single bout of drinking; alcohol withdrawal occurs usually after multiple, repeated bouts. Both can be associated with diarrhea [2]. The diarrhea of chronic alcoholism may be from alcohol withdrawal, alcohol-related organ dysfunction, nutrient deficiencies, endotoxemia, or a combination of the above (Fig. 22.1). In this chapter, we discuss the effects of alcohol on the gut, the clinical features, and treatment of alcoholic diarrhea.

ABSORPTION AND METABOLISM OF ALCOHOL IN THE GUT

Due to its inherent nature, alcohol can freely diffuse across intact membranes in the gastrointestinal tract and is distributed throughout various organs in proportion to their water content [3, 4]. Ethanol absorption is incumbent on the concentration gradient between the intestinal lumen and the mucosal capillaries, the local blood flow, and the mucosal permeability. Ethanol undergoes first-pass metabolism in the stomach and the upper small intestine [4]. In the colon, alcohol is transported from the mucosal capillaries back into the lumen where bacterial alcohol dehydrogenase converts ethanol into acetaldehyde. The concentration of acetaldehyde increases intraluminally, leading to mucosal damage, increased permeability to bacterial endotoxin with possible hepatic, pancreatic, and gastrointestinal neuromuscular injury after absorption by the portal venous system [5]. This is termed the "bacteriocolonic" pathway of ethanol oxidation [5–8]. Non-oxidative metabolism of alcohol with accumulation of toxic fatty acid ethyl esters in the pancreas, liver, heart, and adipose tissue has also been described [9].

ETIOPATHOGENESIS OF DIARRHEA

Acute and chronic alcohol intake affects the motility, morphology, barrier function, and gut microflora and interferes with the digestion, transport, and absorption of macro- and micronutrients in addition to decreasing the availability of bile acids and pancreatic enzymes [10–14] (Tables 22.1 and 22.2).

CLINICAL PRESENTATION

The most common intestinal disorders observed among alcoholics are diarrhea and malabsorption, which reverse with the cessation of alcohol and return to a normal diet within days to weeks (Table 22.1). *Binge*

Table 22.1
Pathophysiology of acute alcohol-induced diarrhea

- *Dietary indiscretion*: From concomitant use of fructose/sorbitol-containing foods, milk/dairy products or gluten intake in susceptible populations
- *Transient morphologic changes*
  Stomach: Erosions, petechiae, easy friability [18] which usually reverse with 72-h abstinence [12]
  Small intestine: Erosions due to epithelial denudation on the tips of villi, acute inflammation, and hemorrhage into the lamina propria [17–50] with increased risk of upper gastrointestinal bleeding [51]
- *Gut motility*
  Gastric emptying: Depends on the dose, concentration, and type of alcoholic beverage ingested [52]
    Lower concentrations (6% [53] or 10% [54]): No effect [55] or acceleration of emptying [54], likely due to tonic contraction of circular smooth muscle in gastric body and fundus [10]
    Red wine, irrespective of concentration, does not affect emptying [56]
    Beer (7% v/v) and white wine (7.5% v/v) accelerate gastric emptying in comparison to ethanol (7.5% v/v) [52]
    Higher concentrations (50–100%): Delayed emptying [57, 58] from increased tonic contraction of antral smooth muscle [59]
  Small intestinal motility: Intensifies duodenal [54, 60] and phase III ileal motor activity, decreases phase I jejunal activity [60], and delays the onset but prolongs the duration of interdigestive cycle [61]; shortens orocecal transit time (OCT) as measured by hydrogen-breath testing with beer (7.0% v/v) and white wine (7.5% v/v) but not ethanol (7.5% v/v) [52]
  Effects more pronounced with intraluminal compared to intravenous administration [61]
- *Nutrient absorption*
  - Impairs activity of the membrane Na^+–K^+-ATPase (sodium pump) in intestinal epithelial cells
  - Increases cAMP and decreases cGMP levels, collectively leading to active secretion of water and sodium intraluminally [62], especially with higher concentrations [63, 64]
  - Impairment of active intestinal transport of monosaccharides, fatty acids, monoglycerides [65], and L-amino acid residues [18, 62]
  - Lactose intolerance from decrease in intestinal mucosal glycolytic enzyme activity [46] and brush border lactase [66], which reverses with less than 10 days of abstinence. Effect is more pronounced in African Americans probably due to lower baseline enzyme levels [36]
  - Impairment of thiamine absorption by a third [67]
  - Folate deficiency [30]
  - Unchanged absorption of most other vitamins and minerals due to intact jejunal absorptive capacity [52]

Table 22.1
(continued)

- *Increased mucosal permeability* to macro- and micromolecules [8, 68] from destabilization of intracellular tight junctions [69]; transient endotoxemia leading to hepatic damage [7, 68]
- *Pancreatic secretion*
  - Stimulation of exocrine pancreatic secretion with simultaneous spasm of sphincter of Oddi and retention of pancreatic juices [70–72]
  - Increase in pancreatic protein concentration and decrease in bicarbonate secretion [73]
- *Alcohol hangover/veisalgia*
  - Hormonal alterations and dysregulated cytokine synthesis (excess prostaglandin E_2 and thromboxane) [19]
  - Increased antidiuretic hormone, aldosterone, cortisol levels (autonomic hyperactivity) [20]

Table 22.2
Pathophysiology of chronic alcohol-induced diarrhea

Alcohol withdrawal: Central nervous system hyperexcitability due to interaction between inhibitory GABA and excitatory NMDA receptor activity [74]

Associated with alcohol-related organ dysfunction
- *Exocrine pancreatic insufficiency* with or without chronic pancreatitis [75] (seen in 3–15% of heavy drinkers) [73, 76]
  - Exocrine secretion of lipase falls earlier compared to protease and amylase [77]
- *Bile salt malabsorption and deficiency*
  - *Bile acid malabsorption* from interrupted enterohepatic circulation [15] with *bile acid diarrhea* and eventual depletion of the bile acid pool [29]; bacterial overgrowth compounds bile acid diarrhea by disproportionately increasing toxic unconjugated bile acids [78]
  - *Deficient synthesis of bile salts*, especially in cirrhotics [40, 79]
- *Gastrointestinal tract*
  - Morphologic changes:
    Small intestine: Less evident macroscopic changes. Microscopic changes include shortening of villous height with decrease in absorptive mucosal surface area, monocytic infiltration, and goblet cell hyperplasia [11, 80]
    Eventual decrease in turnover of intestinal epithelium and crypt cells, with eventual villous atrophy [81]

Table 22.2
(continued)

Rectum: Dense mononuclear infiltration, decrease in goblet cell density, distortion of mitochondria and endoplasmic reticulum (on electron microscopy), usually reversible on abstinence [49]
- Gut motility: Altered due to change in the composition of smooth muscle contractile proteins through free radical formation, a direct toxic effect, or from the action of its metabolite, acetaldehyde [13, 14]
  Gastric emptying: Delayed compared to controls [26, 82]
  Small intestine transit: Shortening of orocecal transit (OCT) stronger phasic, propulsive contractions in individuals with diarrhea [26, 83]; prolonged OCT in those without diarrhea compared to healthy controls [26, 84, 85] due to dysfunctional activity of gut contractile proteins and vagus [84]; disruption in neuroendocrine homeostasis [84]
  Colonic transit: Dose-dependent [86] decrease in rectosigmoid transit which reverses with 10 days of abstinence [22]
- *Small bowel bacterial overgrowth* in the upper small intestine
  - Interference in nutrient absorption [6, 87]
  - Bile acid deconjugation [11, 88]
  - Increased acetaldehyde production and gram-negative endotoxemia with hepatic injury [11, 65]
  - *Increased mucosal permeability and endotoxemia* [7, 68]

Macro- and micronutrient deficiencies
- Impairment of absorption of water, electrolytes and nutrients depending on jejunoileal absorptive capacity [89]
- Decrease in D-xylose absorption depending on nutritional status and mean daily alcohol intake [62]
- No alteration in glucose and amino acid absorption [18, 62]
- Decrease in mucosal peptide hydrolysis and increase in fecal nitrogen [62] in a reversible, dose-dependent manner [90]
- Steatorrhea in individuals with and without overt exocrine pancreatic insufficiency or liver disease [62, 91]
- Pyridoxine [92], folate [30], niacin [93], and ascorbic acid [94, 95] deficiencies
- Decrease in ileal absorption of vitamin B_{12}; uncommon clinical deficiency [30, 96]
- Thiamine [67] and fat-soluble vitamin deficiencies depending on nutritional status, liver, and pancreatic disease [65]
- Hypomagnesemia, hypokalemia, and hypophosphatemia in heavy drinkers from excess urinary losses, vomiting, diarrhea, and endocrine imbalance [47, 62]
- Zinc [97, 98] and selenium [36] deficiency
- Iron overload [54]

Chapter 22 / Alcohol-Related Diarrhea 385

drinking often leads to short-lasting diarrhea with electrolyte abnormalities and hypovolemia. Hyperosmolarity of fluids or the nature of food co-ingested with alcohol [15], the inhibition of mucosal Na^+–K^+-ATPase activity, and structural damage to intestinal epithelium and microvasculature from release of inflammatory mediators [16–18] play a role in its etiopathogenesis. Patients with alcohol hangover or *veisalgia* (from the Norwegian *kveis* or "uneasiness following debauchery" and the Greek *algia* or "pain") suffer from fatigue, insomnia, diarrhea, headaches, dry mouth, malaise, and nausea in addition to autonomic hyperactivity (tremor, sweating, tachycardia, and hypertension) [2, 19]. Diarrhea is seen in 36% of patients with alcohol hangover and is the third most common presenting symptom after headache and malaise [19]. The symptoms of hangover seem to be caused by dehydration leading to elevated levels of antidiuretic hormone, dysregulated cytokine pathways, as well as the toxic effects of alcohol. Increased cardiac work and generalized slowing of cerebral activity on electroencephalography are often seen [20].

Toxic alcohol-induced diarrhea due to acute ingestions of isopropanol and diethylene glycol, either accidental or suicidal in nature, commonly present with abdominal pain, diarrhea, nausea, vomiting, and a change in mentation [21]. Although not the topic of this chapter, clinicians should suspect toxic alcohol ingestion in extremely ill alcoholics.

In contrast, *chronic alcoholics* may have diarrhea that continues for days to weeks after abstinence from alcohol withdrawal, organ dysfunction, and nutritional deficiencies. *Alcohol withdrawal syndrome* (AWS), unlike hangover, has a longer period of overall impairment (days vs. hours) [2]. AWS manifests in patients with a recent reduction or cessation in alcohol use in the setting of chronic or heavy intake with anxiety, palpitations, nausea or vomiting, diaphoresis, tremor, delirium, seizures, and rapid colonic transit manifesting as diarrhea [22]. Dehydration is often seen in this setting consequent to vomiting, diarrhea, fever, or sweating [23, 24]. In addition, alcohol-induced organ dysfunction with long-standing changes in intestinal histology and increased mucosal permeability [8,10], bacterial overgrowth [25], rapid intestinal transit from heightened propulsive contractions [26], impaired mucosal surface enzyme activity such as disaccharidase [27], as well as impaired bile and pancreatic enzyme secretion can contribute to diarrhea in chronic alcoholics [28, 29]. Chronic alcoholics often are deficient in thiamine, B_{12}, and folate [30, 31], especially when accompanied by liver disease and malnutrition. In developed countries, chronic alcoholism is one of the most common causes of pellagra (dermatitis, diarrhea, dementia, and death) from niacin deficiency [32] and scurvy from vitamin C deficiency [33, 34] among adults. Scurvy may present with diarrhea in addition to the classic features of purpuric lesions, joint pains, and bleeding gums [35].

TREATMENT

Acute Alcohol-Related Diarrhea

The most important therapy for alcohol-induced diarrhea is avoidance of alcohol (Fig. 22.2). All patients should be rehydrated and antidiarrheals such as loperamide may be used for symptom relief once active infection has been ruled out. In African Americans with suspected acute alcohol-induced diarrhea, empiric avoidance of milk and milk products may alleviate diarrhea [36]. For symptoms associated with alcohol hangover, tolfenamic acid, a prostaglandin inhibitor; Liv.52, an Indian herbal medicine; and chlormethiazole, a sedative, have shown promise in improving the overall symptomatology [20].

Chronic Alcohol-Related Diarrhea

Diarrhea and malabsorption from chronic alcohol intake usually resolve with abstinence. In patients with AWS, intravenous fluids are indicated. If dextrose-containing fluids are used, thiamine must be administered

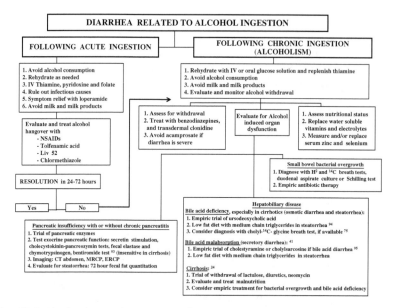

Fig. 22.2. Evaluation and treatment of patients with diarrhea in the setting of alcohol abuse.

to avoid acute Wernicke's encephalopathy. Benzodiazepines are the mainstay of treatment of AWS due to cross-tolerance with alcohol by virtue of their GABA stimulant activity [37]. In recent years, transdermal clonidine has been shown to decrease the severity of diarrhea to a greater degree in comparison to benzodiazepines [38]. However, acamprosate or calcium bisacetylhomotaurinate used in the management of alcohol withdrawal or abstinence can induce or worsen diarrhea [39].

Workup for steatorrhea and supplementation with pancreatic enzymes even without overt pancreatic or liver disease may be warranted [28, 40]. Alcoholics, especially cirrhotics, tend to have *deficient synthesis of bile acids* with decreased total bile acid pool and may present with mild steatorrhea. This is ideally treated with supplementation with ursodeoxycholic acid [41]. On the other hand, intestinal mucosal damage and bacterial overgrowth collectively lead to decreased absorption of bile salts from the ileum (*bile salt malabsorption*) and can cause watery diarrhea from the secretory effects of bile salts on the colon (bile acid diarrhea) and if severe, steatorrhea [42]. Such watery diarrhea generally responds well to bile acid binders such as cholestyramine [43]. If steatorrhea is prominent in either of these conditions, the use of medium chain triglycerides is uniformly beneficial in improving nutrition; this does not alter the course of the disease [40]. Administration of antibiotics such as ciprofloxacin [44] and polymyxin B/neomycin [45] can reduce gut aerobic flora, intracolonic acetaldehyde formation, and endotoxemia. Intestinal permeability maybe preserved by administration of L-glutamine, oats, or zinc which decrease the transfer of endotoxin to the circulation [5].

Folate deficiency is the most common hypovitaminosis in both acute and chronic alcoholics [30]. Replenishment of folate may reverse ethanol-induced inhibition of mucosal brush border enzymes and increased intestinal permeability [46], sometimes despite continued alcohol intake [47]. Replenishment of large doses of niacin (50–150 mg daily) and modest doses of oral vitamin C (66.5 mg) often can lead to dramatic improvement in the symptoms of pellagra [32] and scurvy, respectively [48]. With continued abstinence, nutritional support, and vitamin replenishment, most cases of diarrhea resolve [49].

REFERENCES

1. Cyr MG, Moulton AW. The gastrointestinal tract and pancreas. In: Barnes HN, Aronson MD, Delbanco TL, eds. Alcoholism: a guide for the primary care physician. New York, NY: Springer, 1987, pp. 127–133.
2. Swift R, Davidson D. Alcohol hangover: mechanisms and mediators. Alcohol Health Res World 1998; 22:54–60.

3. Chari ST, Teyssen S, Singer MV. What controls should be used in studies of acute effects of alcohol and alcoholic beverages on the stomach and the pancreas? Scand J Gastroenterol 1993; 28:289–295.
4. Parlesak A, Billinger MH, Schafer C, Wehner HD, Bode C, Bode JC. First-pass metabolism of ethanol in human beings: effect of intravenous infusion of fructose. Alcohol 2004; 34:121–125.
5. Purohit V, Bode JC, Bode C, et al. Alcohol, intestinal bacterial growth, intestinal permeability to endotoxin, and medical consequences: summary of a symposium. Alcohol 2008;42:349–361.
6. Hayashi M, Nishiya H, Chiba T, Endoh D, Kon Y, Okui T. Trientine, a copper-chelating agent, induced apoptosis in murine fibrosarcoma cells in vivo and in vitro. J Vet Med Sci 2007; 69:137–142.
7. Bode C, Kugler V, Bode JC. Endotoxemia in patients with alcoholic and non-alcoholic cirrhosis and in subjects with no evidence of chronic liver disease following acute alcohol excess. J Hepatol 1987; 4:8–14.
8. Bjarnason I, Peters TJ, Wise RJ. The leaky gut of alcoholism: possible route of entry for toxic compounds. Lancet 1984; 1:179–182.
9. Laposata EA, Lange LG. Presence of nonoxidative ethanol metabolism in human organs commonly damaged by ethanol abuse. Science 1986; 231: 497–499.
10. Chiba T, Phillips SF. Alcohol-related diarrhea. Addict Biol 2006; 5:117–125.
11. Persson J. Alcohol and the small intestine. Scand J Gastroenterol. 1991; 26:3–15.
12. Gottfried EB, Korsten MA, Lieber CS. Alcohol-induced gastric and duodenal lesions in man. Am J Gastroenterol 1978; 70:587–592.
13. Preedy VR. Alcohol and the gastrointestinal tract. Alcohol Clin Exp Res 1996; 20:48A–50A.
14. Preedy VR, Ohlendieck K, Adachi J, et al. The importance of alcohol-induced muscle disease. J Muscle Res Cell Motil. 2003;24:55–63.
15. Chiba T, Phillips SF. Alcohol-related diarrhea. Addict Biol 2006; 5:117–125.
16. Krasner N, Cochran KM, Russell RI, Carmichael HA, Thompson GG. Alcohol and absorption from the small intestine. 1. Impairment of absorption from the small intestine in alcoholics. Gut 1976; 17:245–248.
17. Dinda PK, Holitzner CA, Morris GP, Beck IT. Ethanol-induced jejunal microvascular and morphological injury in relation to histamine release in rabbits. Gastroenterology 1993; 104:361–368.
18. Beck IT, Dinda PK. Acute exposure of small intestine to ethanol: effects on morphology and function. Dig Dis Sci 1981; 26:817–838.
19. Harburg E, Davis D, Cummings KM, Gunn R. Negative affect, alcohol consumption and hangover symptoms among normal drinkers in a small community. J Stud Alcohol 1981; 42:998–1012.
20. Wiese JG, Shlipak MG, Browner WS. The alcohol hangover. Ann Intern Med 2000; 132:897–902.
21. Kraut JA, Kurtz I. Toxic alcohol ingestions: clinical features, diagnosis, and management. Clin J Am Soc Nephrol 2008; 3:208–225.
22. Bouchoucha M, Nalpas B, Berger M, Cugnenc PH, Barbier JP. Recovery from disturbed colonic transit time after alcohol withdrawal. Dis Colon Rectum 1991; 34:111–114.
23. Chang PH, Steinberg MB. Alcohol withdrawal. Med Clin North Am 2001; 85:1191–1212.
24. Bayard M, McIntyre J, Hill KR, Woodside J Jr. Alcohol withdrawal syndrome. Am Fam Physician 2004; 69:1443–1450.

Chapter 22 / Alcohol-Related Diarrhea

25. Bode JC, Bode C, Heidelbach R, Durr HK, Martini GA. Jejunal microflora in patients with chronic alcohol abuse. Hepatogastroenterology 1984; 31:30–34.
26. Wegener M, Schaffstein J, Dilger U, Coenen C, Wedmann B, Schmidt G. Gastrointestinal transit of solid-liquid meal in chronic alcoholics. Dig Dis Sci 1991; 36:917–923.
27. Perlow W, Baraona E, Lieber CS. Symptomatic intestinal disaccharidase deficiency in alcoholics. Gastroenterology 1977; 72:680–684.
28. Singer MV. The pancreas and alcohol. Schweiz Med Wochenschr 1985; 115: 973–987.
29. Linscheer WG. Malabsorption in cirrhosis. Am J Clin Nutr 1970; 23:488–492.
30. Lindenbaum J. Folate and vitamin B12 deficiencies in alcoholism. Semin Hematol 1980; 17:119–129.
31. Leevy CM, Moroianu SA. Nutritional aspects of alcoholic liver disease. Clin Liver Dis 2005; 9:67–81.
32. Delgado-Sanchez L, Godkar D, Niranjan S. Pellagra: rekindling of an old flame. Am J Ther 2008; 15:173–175.
33. Hirschmann JV, Raugi GJ. Adult scurvy. J Am Acad Dermatol 1999; 41:895–906.
34. Leung FW, Guze PA. Adult scurvy. Ann Emerg Med 1981;10:652–655.
35. Pimentel L. Scurvy: historical review and current diagnostic approach. Am J Emerg Med 2003;21:328–332.
36. Keshavarzian A, Iber FL, Dangleis MD, Cornish R. Intestinal-transit and lactose intolerance in chronic alcoholics. Am J Clin Nutr 1986; 44:70–76.
37. Peppers MP. Benzodiazepines for alcohol withdrawal in the elderly and in patients with liver disease. Pharmacotherapy 1996; 16:49–57.
38. Baumgartner GR, Rowen RC. Transdermal clonidine versus chlordiazepoxide in alcohol withdrawal: a randomized, controlled clinical trial. South Med J 1991; 84:312–321.
39. Sass H, Soyka M, Mann K, Zieglgansberger W. Relapse prevention by acamprosate. Results from a placebo-controlled study on alcohol dependence. Arch Gen Psychiatr 1996; 53:673–680.
40. Ros E, Garcia-Puges A, Reixach M, Cuso E, Rodes J. Fat digestion and exocrine pancreatic function in primary biliary cirrhosis. Gastroenterology 1984; 87: 180–187.
41. Salvioli G, Carati L, Lugli R. Steatorrhoea in cirrhosis: effect of ursodeoxycholic acid administration. J Int Med Res 1990; 18:289–297.
42. Powell D. Approach to the patient with diarrhea. In: Yamada T, Kalloo AN, Kaplowitz N, eds. Principles of Clinical Gastroenterology, 1st edn. New York: Wiley-Blackwell, 2008, pp. 304–359.
43. Westergaard H. Bile Acid malabsorption. Curr Treat Options Gastroenterol. 2007;10:28–33.
44. Visapaa JP, Jokelainen K, Nosova T, Salaspuro M. Inhibition of intracolonic acetaldehyde production and alcoholic fermentation in rats by ciprofloxacin. Alcohol Clin Exp Res 1998; 22:1161–1164.
45. Adachi Y, Moore LE, Bradford BU, Gao W, Thurman RG. Antibiotics prevent liver injury in rats following long-term exposure to ethanol. Gastroenterology 1995; 108:218–224.
46. Greene HL, Stifel FB, Herman RH, Herman YF, Rosenweig NS. Ethanol-induced inhibition of human intestinal enzyme activities: reversal by folic acid. Gastroenterology 1974; 67:434–440.
47. Bujanda L. The effects of alcohol consumption upon the gastrointestinal tract. Am J Gastroenterol 2000; 95:3374–3382.

48. Hodges RE, Hood J, Canham JE, Sauberlich HE, Baker EM. Clinical manifestations of ascorbic acid deficiency in man. Am J Clin Nutr 1971; 24:432–443.
49. Brozinsky S, Fani K, Grosberg SJ, Wapnick S. Alcohol ingestion-induced changes in the human rectal mucosa: light and electron microscopic studies. Dis Colon Rectum 1978; 21:329–335.
50. Dinda PK, Buell MG, Morris O, Beck IT. Studies on ethanol-induced subepithelial fluid accumulation and jejunal villus bleb formation. An in vitro video microscopic approach. Can J Physiol Pharmacol 1994; 72:1186–1192.
51. Kelly JP, Kaufman DW, Koff RS, Laszlo A, Wiholm BE, Shapiro S. Alcohol consumption and the risk of major upper gastrointestinal bleeding. Am J Gastroenterol 1995; 90:1058–1064.
52. Pfeiffer A, Hogl B, Kaess H. Effect of ethanol and commonly ingested alcoholic beverages on gastric emptying and gastrointestinal transit. Clin Investig 1992; 70:487–491.
53. Cooke AR, Birchall A. Ethanol absorption and emptying from the stomach. Gut 1969; 10:953.
54. Kaufman SE, Kaye MD. Effect of ethanol upon gastric emptying. Gut 1979; 20:688–692.
55. Cooke AR. The simultaneous emptying and absorption of ethanol from the human stomach. Am J Dig Dis 1970; 15:449–454.
56. Moore JG, Christian PE, Datz FL, Coleman RE. Effect of wine on gastric emptying in humans. Gastroenterology 1981; 81:1072–1075.
57. Barboriak JJ, Meade RC. Effect of alcohol on gastric emptying in man. Am J Clin Nutr 1970; 23:1151–1153.
58. Jian R, Cortot A, Ducrot F, Jobin G, Chayvialle JA, Modigliani R. Effect of ethanol ingestion on postprandial gastric emptying and secretion, biliopancreatic secretions, and duodenal absorption in man. Dig Dis Sci 1986; 31:604–614.
59. Sanders KM, Bauer AJ. Ethyl alcohol interferes with excitation-contraction mechanisms of canine antral muscle. Am J Physiol 1982; 242:G222–G230.
60. Robles EA, Mezey E, Halsted CH, Schuster MM. Effect of ethanol on motility of the small intestine. Johns Hopkins Med J 1974; 135:17–24.
61. Charles F, Phillips SF. Effects of ethanol, xylose, and glucose on canine jejunal motility. Am J Physiol 1995; 269:G363–G369.
62. Bode JC. Alcohol and the gastrointestinal tract. Ergeb Inn Med Kinderheilkd 1980; 45:1–75.
63. Fox JE, Bourdages R, Beck IT. Effect of ethanol on glucose and water absorption in hamster jejunum in vivo. Methodological problems: anesthesia, nonabsorbable markers, and osmotic effect. Am J Dig Dis 1978; 23:193–200.
64. Kuo YJ, Shanbour LL. Effects of ethanol on sodium, 3-O-methyl glucose, and L-alanine transport in the jejunum. Am J Dig Dis 1978; 23:51–56.
65. Bode C, Bode JC. Effect of alcohol consumption on the gut. Best Pract Res Clin Gastroenterol 2003; 17:575–592.
66. Baraona E, Pirola RC, Lieber CS. Small intestinal damage and changes in cell population produced by ethanol ingestion in the rat. Gastroenterology 1974; 66:226–234.
67. Hoyumpa AM, Jr. Alcohol and thiamine metabolism. Alcohol Clin Exp Res 1983; 7:11–14.
68. Parlesak A, Schafer C, Schutz T, Bode JC, Bode C. Increased intestinal permeability to macromolecules and endotoxemia in patients with chronic alcohol abuse in different stages of alcohol-induced liver disease. J Hepatol 2000; 32: 742–747.

Chapter 22 / Alcohol-Related Diarrhea 391

69. Draper LR, Gyure LA, Hall JG, Robertson D. Effect of alcohol on the integrity of the intestinal epithelium. Gut 1983; 24:399–404.
70. Tierney S, Qian Z, Lipsett PA, Pitt HA, Lillemoe KD. Ethanol inhibits sphincter of Oddi motility. J Gastrointest Surg 1998; 2:356–362.
71. Tiscornia OM, Gullo L, Sarles H, et al. Effects of intragastric and intraduodenal ethanol on canine exocrine pancreatic secretion. Digestion 1974; 10:52–60.
72. Tiscornia OM, Levesque D, Sarles H, et al. Canine exocrine pancreatic secretory changes induced by an intragastric ethanol test meal. Am J Gastroenterol 1977; 67:121–130.
73. Siegmund SV, Singer MV. Effects of alcohol on the upper gastrointestinal tract and the pancreas–an up-to-date overview. Z Gastroenterol 2005; 43: 723–736.
74. Littleton J. Neurochemical mechanisms underlying alcohol withdrawal. Alcohol Health Res World 1998; 22:13–24.
75. Niebergall-Roth E, Harder H, Singer MV. A review: acute and chronic effects of ethanol and alcoholic beverages on the pancreatic exocrine secretion in vivo and in vitro. Alcohol Clin Exp Res 1998; 22:1570–1583.
76. Levy P, Mathurin P, Roqueplo A, Rueff B, Bernades P. A multidimensional case-control study of dietary, alcohol, and tobacco habits in alcoholic men with chronic pancreatitis. Pancreas 1995; 10:231–238.
77. Keller J, Aghdassi AA, Lerch MM, Mayerle JV, Layer P. Tests of pancreatic exocrine function – clinical significance in pancreatic and non-pancreatic disorders. Best Pract Res Clin Gastroenterol 2009; 23:425–439.
78. Einarsson K, Bergstrom M, Eklof R, Nord CE, Bjorkhem I. Comparison of the proportion of unconjugated to total serum cholic acid and the [14C]-xylose breath test in patients with suspected small intestinal bacterial overgrowth. Scand J Clin Lab Invest 1992; 52:425–430.
79. Romiti A, Merli M, Martorano M, et al. Malabsorption and nutritional abnormalities in patients with liver cirrhosis. Ital J Gastroenterol 1990; 22:118–123.
80. Persson J, Berg NO, Sjolund K, Stenling R, Magnusson PH. Morphologic changes in the small intestine after chronic alcohol consumption. Scand J Gastroenterol 1990; 25:173–184.
81. Sjolund K, Persson J, Bergman L. Can villous atrophy be induced by chronic alcohol consumption? J Intern Med 1989; 226:133–135.
82. Willson CA, Bushnell D, Keshavarzian A. The effect of acute and chronic ethanol administration on gastric emptying in cats. Dig Dis Sci 1990; 35:444–448.
83. Keshavarzian A, Iber FL, Greer P, Wobbleton J. Gastric emptying of solid meal in male chronic alcoholics. Alcohol Clin Exp Res 1986; 10:432–435.
84. Addolorato G, Montalto M, Capristo E, et al. Influence of alcohol on gastrointestinal motility: lactulose breath hydrogen testing in orocecal transit time in chronic alcoholics, social drinkers and teetotaler subjects. Hepatogastroenterology 1997; 44:1076–1081.
85. Papa A, Tursi A, Cammarota G, et al. Effect of moderate and heavy alcohol consumption on intestinal transit time. Panminerva Med 1998; 40:183–185.
86. Berenson MM, Avner DL. Alcohol inhibition of rectosigmoid motility in humans. Digestion 1981; 22:210–215.
87. Hauge T, Persson J, Danielsson D. Mucosal bacterial growth in the upper gastrointestinal tract in alcoholics (heavy drinkers). Digestion 1997; 58: 591–595.
88. Hoyumpa AM. Mechanisms of vitamin deficiencies in alcoholism. Alcohol Clin Exp Res 1986; 10:573–581.

89. Pfeiffer A, Schmidt T, Vidon N, Pehl C, Kaess H. Absorption of a nutrient solution in chronic alcoholics without nutrient deficiencies and liver cirrhosis. Scand J Gastroenterol 1992; 27:1023–1030.
90. Dinda PK, Beck IT. Ethanol-induced inhibition of glucose transport across the isolated brush-border membrane of hamster jejunum. Dig Dis Sci 1981; 26:23–32.
91. Roggin GM, Iber FL, Kater RM, Tabon F. Malabsorption in the chronic alcoholic. Johns Hopkins Med J 1969; 125:321–330.
92. Halsted CH. Nutrition and alcoholic liver disease. Semin Liver Dis 2004; 24: 289–304.
93. Lorentzen HF, Fugleholm AM, Weismann K. Zinc deficiency and pellagra in alcohol abuse. Ugeskr Laeger 2000; 162:6854–6856.
94. Baines M. Vitamin C and exposure to alcohol. Int J Vitam Nutr Res Suppl 1982; 23:287–293.
95. Baines M. Detection and incidence of B and C vitamin deficiency in alcohol-related illness. Ann Clin Biochem 1978; 15:307–312.
96. Lindenbaum J, Lieber CS. Effects of chronic ethanol administration on intestinal absorption in man in the absence of nutritional deficiency. Ann N Y Acad Sci 1975; 252:228–234.
97. McClain CJ, Su LC. Zinc deficiency in the alcoholic: a review. Alcohol Clin Exp Res 1983; 7:5–10.
98. McClain CJ, Antonow DR, Cohen DA, Shedlofsky SI. Zinc metabolism in alcoholic liver disease. Alcohol Clin Exp Res 1986; 10:582–589.

23 Drug-Induced Diarrhea

Bincy P. Abraham, MD, MS
and Joseph H. Sellin, MD

CONTENTS

INTRODUCTION
MECHANISMS OF DRUG-INDUCED DIARRHEA
WATERY DIARRHEA
INFLAMMATORY DIARRHEA
FATTY DIARRHEA
COMPLEX DIARRHEAS
DIET
LAXATIVES
CHOLINERGICS, SERITONERGICS, AND
  OTHER NEUROMODULATORS
GASTROENTEROLOGY MEDICATIONS
DIABETES MEDICATIONS
ENDOCRINE MEDICINES
CHEMOTHERAPY AND IMMUNOMODULATORS
ANTIBIOTICS
NSAIDS
HIV MEDICATIONS
CARDIAC MEDICATIONS
MISCELLANEOUS DRUGS
CONCLUSION
REFERENCES

From: *Diarrhea, Clinical Gastroenterology*
Edited by: S. Guandalini, H. Vaziri, DOI 10.1007/978-1-60761-183-7_23
© Springer Science+Business Media, LLC 2011

Summary

Drug-induced diarrhea (DID) is common, but our understanding of the underlying mechanisms may vary from solid understanding to reasonable hypothesis to considerable conjecture. Drug-induced diarrhea is rarely an allergy, i.e., with an underlying immune mechanism, but may well be an inherent component of the pharmacologic effect of the drug, may be due to variable pharmacogenomics or be an appropriate physiologic response to the drug. Frequently, discussions of DID become lists. However, by classifying chronic diarrhea as watery, fatty, or inflammatory, one can create a framework to better understand the mechanisms of the diarrhea. In this chapter, we examine diet, laxatives, neuromodulators, diabetes medications, chemotherapy, antibiotics, HIV medications, non-steroidals, and GI medications with an emphasis on clinical relevance and underlying mechanisms in causing diarrhea.

Key Words: Drugs, Antibiotics, Laxatives, Osmotic diarrhea, Secretory diarrhea, Complex diarrheas, Chemotherapy, NSAIDs, Caffeine, Sorbitol, Fructose, Hormones

INTRODUCTION

More than 700 drugs have been implicated as causing diarrhea, accounting for approximately 7% of all drug adverse effects [1]. However, the mechanism of action by which certain drugs contribute to this adverse effect is not well known. Drug-induced diarrhea is frequently suspected in patients who develop it soon after starting a new medication, although there is usually only circumstantial evidence to support the link. The medication is usually stopped, and when the diarrhea resolves, the side effect will be attributed to that medication. The basic mechanisms are rarely investigated in these cases. Therefore, our understanding of specific drug-induced diarrheas may vary from solid understanding, to reasonable hypothesis, to considerable conjecture. Thus, in an era of evidence-based medicine, high-quality information on drug-induced diarrhea is often lacking.

For older drugs that have not undergone rigorous, randomized trials, there rarely are well-designed studies that quantify and characterize the association between a specific agent and diarrhea. The information for these drugs is derived, at best, from cohort or case–control studies. For newer drugs that have undergone clinical trials, the assessment of adverse events permits a reasonable opportunity to characterize the frequency of drug-associated diarrhea. However, even with clinical trials, there may be a considerable variability in the incidence of an adverse event such as diarrhea. This variability may depend on the different underlying disease studied, the definition of the adverse event, and the type of clinical trial. For example, most randomized clinical trials (RCTs) are short in duration, thus potentially altering an adverse effect in reference to the time a patient is exposed to the drug, compared to long-term follow-up observational studies. Also, diarrhea as an adverse event is rarely defined clearly. Thus, a minimal change in consistency and a significant increase in stool volume would both be labeled "diarrhea."

We will first consider the pathophysiology of drug-induced diarrhea in general and then review specific drugs by overall class of medication.

MECHANISMS OF DRUG-INDUCED DIARRHEA

Why some individuals develop drug-induced diarrhea and others do not is far from clear. Although an adverse event like diarrhea is frequently termed a "drug allergy," in fact, an underlying immune mechanism is rarely the case. In instances when diarrhea is an extremely frequent outcome, it may well be that the intestinal response is an inherent part of the pharmacologic effect of the drug. Diarrhea as an uncommon side effect may be due to variable pharmacogenomics. In other cases, diarrhea may be an appropriate physiologic response to the drug. On occasion, the drug may cause direct tissue injury. Finally, the probability of an individual's complaint of diarrhea may depend, in part, on baseline bowel habits.

Evidence of the mechanisms underlying the diarrhea elicited by a specific drug may be elusive and serendipitous. For example, theophylline has been a standard for eliciting intestinal secretion in basic physiology. Thus the effects of xanthine oxidase inhibitors are well understood. Similarly, as molecularly designed agents move from the bench to the bedside, there may be considerable understanding of the underlying mechanism. However, for many drugs, the purported mechanisms are based on small fragmentary studies or simple speculation. Table 23.1 lists drugs that cause diarrhea according to the frequency with which they produce this adverse effect.

In evaluating a case of suspected drug-induced diarrhea, the stool characteristics can provide some clues as to possible underlying mechanisms and potential diagnostic evaluations and therapeutic maneuvers. Diarrhea can be broadly categorized based on the following stool characteristics: (1) watery, a category that includes changes in ion transport, shortened transit time, or increased motility; (2) inflammatory; and (3) fatty. This review will examine the mechanism of drug-induced diarrhea within these broad classifications.

Table 23.1
Drugs known to cause diarrhea

Drugs that cause diarrhea in ≥20% of patients
Alpha-glucosidase inhibitors
Biguanides
Auronafin (gold salt)
Colchicine
Diacerein
Highly active antiretroviral therapy
Prostaglandins
Tyrosine kinase inhibitors

Drugs that cause diarrhea in ≥10% of patients
Antibiotics
Chemotherapeutic agents
Cholinergic drugs
Cisapride (off the market)
Digoxin
Immunosuppressive agents
Metoclopramide
Orlistat (lipase inhibitor)
Osmotic laxatives
Poorly or non-absorbable carbohydrates
Selective serotonin reuptake inhibitors
Ticlopidine

Drugs that occasionally cause diarrhea
5-Aminosalicylates (especially olsalazine)
Acetylcholinesterase inhibitors
Anticholinergics
Caffeine
Calcitonin
Carbamazepine
Chenodeoxycholic acid
Cholestyramine
Cholinesterase inhibitors
Cimetidine
Ferrous sulfate preparations (rare)
Flavanoid-related veinotonic agents
HMG-CoA reductase inhibitors
Irinotecan
Isotretinoin

Chapter 23 / Drug-Induced Diarrhea

Table 23.1
(continued)

L-Dopa-benserazide
Magnesium antacids
Methyldopa
Motilin agonists
Non-steroidal anti-inflammatory drugs
Octreotide
Penicillamine
Prebiotics
Proton pump inhibitors
Tacrine
Tegaserod (off the market)
Theophylline
Thyroid hormones

WATERY DIARRHEA

Watery diarrheas have been classified as either secretory or osmotic to explain underlying pathophysiology. However, the clinical utility of this classification has not been rigorously tested.

Osmotic diarrhea

Osmotic diarrheas can occur from intentional use of a drug as part of its inherent mechanism of action, or unintentionally. Poorly absorbed solute traps fluid in the lumen, and these unabsorbable solutes account for osmotic activity of stool water [2]. Once recognized, the treatment of osmotic diarrhea is simple. Removal of the osmotic agent usually resolves this adverse effect. Loperamide or tincture of opium can be added, especially in the case of enteral nutrition. Dose reduction or dose splitting can also help.

Secretory Diarrhea

Secretory diarrhea, on the other hand, produces voluminous stools that persist despite fasting. Drug-induced secretory diarrhea results from a medication either increasing the active secretion of ions into the intestinal lumen or from decreasing the absorption of electrolytes and nutrients from the gut lumen. The net result of either of these effects is an increase in luminal volume. In secretory diarrhea, a minimal osmotic gap is found. Specifically, drugs induce a secretory diarrhea by two main mechanisms: the inhibition of Na^+ absorption and the stimulation of Cl^-/HCO_3^- secretion. These changes may occur through either a direct effect on the transporter or changes in intracellular second messengers that alter the function of the transporter.

The treatment of watery diarrhea includes discontinuation of the offending medication. Maintaining hydration is important to prevent dehydration from the amount of fluid loss. Loperamide, lomotil, and bismuth subsalicylate can help relieve the diarrhea.

INFLAMMATORY DIARRHEA

Drug-induced inflammatory diarrheas fall into several broad categories. Perhaps the most important is the disruption of colonic flora from antibiotics and precipitation of *Clostridium difficile* colitis. Other mechanisms include the direct damage to the integrity of the mucosa that occurs with NSAIDs and polyene antibiotics, stimulation of low-grade inflammation causing microscopic colitis, disruption of the balance between proliferation and apoptosis with a resulting compromise of epithelial integrity seen with immunosuppressives and chemotherapeutic agents, and vascular compromise as occurs with ergotamine and cocaine.

Management of inflammatory diarrhea includes treatment of intercurrent infections such as CMV, antibiotic-associated colitis, dose reduction of the etiologic agent, or cautious use of empiric therapy. Loperamide, diphenoxylate, deodorized tincture of opium, and octreotide are effective for diarrhea from fluoropyridimoles [3]. Acetorphan, an enkephalinase inhibitor that blocks epithelial cyclic AMP-mediated secretion, has shown moderate activity in clinical trials in patients with irinotecan-induced diarrhea [4]. Budesonide and octreotide have been used to slow intestinal motility and decrease water and electrolyte movement through the bowel [5, 6].

FATTY DIARRHEA

Fatty diarrhea occurs in the clinical setting of weight loss and steatorrhea. This is caused by either maldigestion or malabsorption. This is probably the least common type of drug-induced diarrhea and the one least well understood. Table 23.2 lists medications that can cause this adverse effect. Highly active antiretroviral therapy has been known to cause steatorrhea, although the mechanisms have not been elucidated [7]. Treatment of drug-induced steatorrhea may require dose reduction or withdrawal of the drug. In some cases such as diarrhea due

Chapter 23 / Drug-Induced Diarrhea 399

Table 23.2
Drugs inducing steatorrhea

Aminoglycosides
Auranofin
Biguanides[a]
Cholestyramine
Colchicine
Highly active antiretroviral therapy[a]
Laxatives
Methyldopa
Octreotide
Orlistat (lipase inhibitor)[b]
Polymyxin, bacitracin
Tetracyclines

[a] $\geq$20% incidence of diarrhea.
[b] >10% incidence of diarrhea.

to metformin, continued symptoms may resolve with time even if the drug is continued, as the gastrointestinal system adjusts to the drug. Antidiarrheals such as loperamide and probiotics may help. In the case of antiretroviral drugs, soluble fiber and L-glutamine have been found to be helpful [8]. If prolonged, replacement of fat-soluble vitamins maybe needed.

COMPLEX DIARRHEAS

As it is the case with other diarrheas, the pathophysiology underlying drug-induced diarrheas is frequently multifactorial. The gastrointestinal tract is regulated through the integration of *p*aracrine, *i*mmune, *n*eural, and *e*ndocrine systems that coordinate changes in mucosal and muscular function and adapt to changing conditions [2] (see Fig. 23.1). These systems involve mechanisms that regulate mucosal permeability, intestinal transport, and the motility and metabolism of the gut [2]. Medications may influence this regulatory system through these different pathways and contribute to diarrhea.

Clinically, if drug-induced diarrhea is suspected, the simplest approach is to stop the suspected offending agent, switch to an alternative medication, and, if diarrhea persists, consider treating with an antidiarrheal agent. Novel approaches for certain drug-associated diarrheas have been shown to be effective. In some cases, diarrhea may resolve with continued use and for this reason for most examples of drug-induced diarrhea, therapeutic trials are not relevant. Only where there are no satisfactory alternatives, as is the case for some anticancer

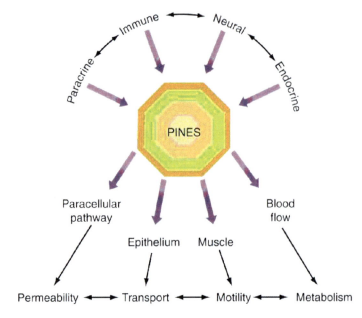

Fig. 23.1. "PINES" regulatory system in the intestine. The regulatory system of the intestine integrates *p*aracrine, *i*mmune, *n*eural, and *e*ndocrine systems and produces coordinated changes in mucosal and muscular function that permit adaptive responses to changing conditions. The regulatory system can widen or narrow the paracellular pathway that governs passive transmucosal permeation of electrolytes, accelerate or retard the transepithelial movement of nutrients and electrolytes by affecting membrane channels and pumps, relax or contract the various muscle layers in the intestine, and increase or decrease mucosal blood flow. Acting simultaneously, these mechanisms regulate mucosal permeability, intestinal transport, and the motility and metabolism of the gut (from Sellin JH (1997) Small Intestine: Functional anatomy, fluid and electrolyte absorption. In Feldman M, Schiller LR (eds) *Gastroenterology and Hepatology. The Comprehensive Visual Reference*, Vol. 7. Current Medicine, Philadelphia, p. 1.11).

therapies, is there sufficient impetus to understand the mechanisms of drug-induced diarrhea. Therefore, it is understandable why in the field of oncology there has been more significant and novel evidence in drug-induced diarrhea.

DIET

Diet in general and specific foods are not generally thought of as drugs; however, it is clear that they can have a profound effect on intestinal function and therefore should be considered in the evaluation of any diarrhea. In this age of orthorexia, in which individuals may adopt peculiar diets of all sorts, it is important to review this as a possible factor in the etiology of diarrhea.

Although lactose has been historically considered the most common culprit in diet-induced diarrhea, it has been supplanted by other dietary constituents. The most frequent offender is probably caffeine. In our hypercaffeinated society, coffee is used as a "drug" by many, causing "Starbucks® diarrhea" through increased cyclic AMP production thereby opening chloride channels and increasing fluid secretion. Caffeine administration in amounts ordinarily contained in many beverages and medications (75–300 mg) resulted in striking net secretion in the jejunum and in the ileum [9]. It is important to remember that younger individuals who may eschew coffee can consume considerable amounts of caffeine in "energy" drinks such as Red Bull™.

A healthy diet with significant amounts of fruits, vegetables, and fiber may cause a modest amount of diarrhea. As the Western diet has evolved into more and more processed foods, there have been significant changes in our nutrient intake. It is estimated that the United States consumes more high fructose corn syrup per capita than any other country. Poorly absorbed fructose, found in fruit juices and carbonated beverages, and non-absorbable sorbitol and mannitol, found in sugar-free candies and gums, may not cause diarrhea until 24–48 h after ingestion [10].

The prebiotics fructo-oligosaccharides and inulins, available in nutritional supplements and in functional foods, have been used for the treatment of antibiotic-induced diarrhea at dose ranges of 4–10 g/day [11]. When given to healthy volunteers, doses higher than 30 g daily of these prebiotics caused significant gastrointestinal discomfort (flatulence, cramping, diarrhea) through fermentation in the colon and production of an osmotic effect in the intestinal lumen [11, 12]. Splitting the dosage usually alleviates the symptoms.

Diagnosis of carbohydrate-induced diarrhea can usually be made by checking fecal pH; a pH less than 6 is highly suggestive of carbohydrate malabsorption.

Some formulas for enteral nutrition are hypertonic and may induce osmotic diarrhea by a mechanism similar to dumping syndrome. Changing to an isotonic formula or slowing the infusion rate usually resolves the diarrhea [13].

Olestra is a lipid that possesses properties of conventional fats and oils, but is neither digested nor absorbed. Olestra was approved by the FDA in January 1996 for use in snacks such as potato chips and crackers [14]. Although consumers complained of "diarrhea," a randomized control trial using higher than consumption doses showed no effect on stool frequency, but a modest stool softening effect measured by stool viscosity in subjects consuming olestra compared to controls [14].

Orlistat, used as a prescription gastrointestinal lipase inhibitor for weight loss, is now available over the counter as "alli" (2007, GlaxoSmithKline, Pennsylvania) which contains half the prescription dose. Those using this drug can have malabsorptive diarrhea if fat intake is high. Of those taking orlistat, 60–80% experience steatorrhea in a dose-related mechanism [15]. This resolves when fat intake is reduced to 45 g/day [15].

LAXATIVES

It should go without saying that a common side effect of laxatives may be diarrhea. However, with many patients consuming a polypharmacia, laxatives may often be overlooked when a patient presents with diarrhea.

The most common medications associated with osmotic diarrhea are magnesium-containing salts and laxatives such as sodium phosphates and long-chain polyethylene glycols (e.g., Miralax; Schering-Plough, Kenilworth, NJ) used for treatment of constipation and for pre-colonoscopy colon purging [3, 13]. Their cathartic action results from poor absorption in the gastrointestinal tract, leading to osmotically mediated water retention, stimulating peristalsis [13]. The usual dose of magnesium salts produces 300–600 ml of stool within 6 h [13]. Inadvertent ingestion of magnesium, with its consequent diarrhea, may occur with antacids such as Mylanta and Maalox. Switching to aluminum-containing antacids and/or antisecretory medications usually results in rapid resolution of the diarrhea.

Sodium phosphate-containing medications cause osmotic diarrhea due to the poorly absorbed phosphate. However, in contrast to magnesium-containing compounds, analysis of stool electrolytes reveals no osmotic gap because the bivalent anion binds two sodium cations [16].

Used for constipation and for the treatment of hepatic encephalopathy, lactulose is a synthetic non-absorbable disaccharide that causes an osmotic diarrhea. Because disaccharides are unabsorbable and the intestinal brush border does not possess "lactulase," lactulose reliably results in a dose-dependent diarrhea.

Lubiprostone was developed as a treatment for constipation, specifically because of its properties as a ClC2 channel opener; however, it is still unclear what specific role the ClC2 channel has in intestinal secretion.

Used as an old home remedy, castor oil is hydrolyzed in the small bowel by the action of lipases into glycerol and the active agent, ricinoleic acid, which acts primarily in the colon to stimulate secretion of fluid and electrolytes by increasing cyclic AMP and speeding intestinal transit [17, 18].

Stimulant laxatives such as diphenylmethane derivatives and anthraquinones induce a limited low-grade inflammation in the small and large bowel to promote accumulation of water and electrolytes and stimulate intestinal motility. This occurs through activation of prostaglandin-cyclic AMP and NO-cyclic GMP pathways, platelet-activating factor production, and, perhaps, inhibition of Na^+, K^+-ATPase [13]. Anthraquinone laxatives are poorly absorbed in the small bowel, are activated in the colon, produce giant migrating colonic contractions, and promote water and electrolyte secretion. Other laxatives or stool softeners such as docusate (dioctyl sodium sulfosuccinate), can cause diarrhea when taken in large quantities, by stimulating fluid secretion by the small and large intestine [19]. Clinicians should thus be aware that surreptitious use of laxative may be the cause of diarrhea in patients who present with this complaint. Table 23.3 lists a number of commonly used laxatives.

Table 23.3
Stimulant laxatives

Anthraquinones
Diphenylmethane derivatives (bisacodyl)
Oxyphenisatin – withdrawn for hepatotoxicity
Phenolphthalein – withdrawn for carcinogenicity
Ricinoleic acid (castor oil)
Sodium picosulfate – available outside the USA
Sodium dioctyl sulfosuccinate (docusate)

CHOLINERGICS, SERITONERGICS, AND OTHER NEUROMODULATORS

Drugs that modulate neurotransmission can have a profound effect on smooth muscle function and motility. Cholinergic drugs such as bethanecol, used for urinary retention and neurogenic bladder, have broad muscarinic effects via cholinergic receptors in the smooth muscle of the urinary bladder and the gastrointestinal tract [13, 20]. The effect of acetylcholine on smooth muscle the gastrointestinal tract is mediated by two types of G protein-coupled muscarinic receptors,

M_2 and M_3 in [4]. The activation of the M_3 receptor increases intracellular Ca^{2+} mediated by the G_q–PLC–IP_3 pathway [13, 21]. This results in increased gastrointestinal and pancreatic secretions, as well as increased peristalsis.

Acetylcholinesterase inhibitors, such as those used for Alzheimer's disease, allow acetylcholine to accumulate in the synaptic and neuromuscular junctions. These drugs enhance contractile effects producing diarrhea in up to 14% of patients [1, 3]. RCTs comparing donepezil to placebo for the treatment of Alzheimer's disease revealed diarrhea incidence of 15% with donepezil compared to 10% in placebo [22]. The Cochrane review on the use of donepezil over 1000 patients revealed that diarrhea occurred more frequently in donepezil-treated patients (OR 2.78, 95% CI [2.10–3.69]) [23]. In another Cochrane review of the three anticholinesterases used for Alzheimer's dementia (donepezil, galantamine, and rivastigmine), the odds ratio for diarrhea with the use of anticholinesterases in comparison to placebo was 1.91 (95% CI [1.59–2.30]) [24].

Although there is limited literature on nicotine and niacin on causing diarrhea, there is ample anecdotal evidence of smoking-induced laxation and smoking cessation is frequently associated with new-onset constipation [25].

Neostigmine, used off-label for acute colonic pseudo-obstruction (Ogilvie's syndrome) and paralytic ileus, can also cause diarrhea [13]. Irinotecan, a chemotherapeutic agent, can cause severe diarrhea from cholinergic-like syndrome through the inhibition of acetylcholinesterase [3].

Tumor-driven excesses in serotonin are a recognized cause of diarrhea, e.g., carcinoid syndrome (see Chapter 15). Therefore, it is not entirely surprising that selective serotonin reuptake inhibitors may be associated with diarrhea. In a meta-analysis of 84 randomized controlled trials of SSRIs, there was a 16% incidence of diarrhea [26]. SSRIs, especially paroxetine and sertraline, as well as carbamazepine, have also been implicated in microscopic colitis [1, 27]. Not surprisingly, anticholinergics were much more frequently associated with constipation.

Prostaglandin analogues have several therapeutic uses, including (1) ulcer prophylaxis, (2) pregnancy termination, and (3) control of pulmonary arterial hypertension [28]. Prostaglandins have potent effects on intestinal smooth muscle and fluid and electrolyte secretion; therefore, it is not surprising that diarrhea and abdominal discomfort are common side effects. More comprehensive evidence is available for misoprostol than other analogues, but diarrhea would not be an unexpected outcome for any prostaglandin. In clinical trials, an average

Chapter 23 / Drug-Induced Diarrhea

of 13% of patients (range of 14–40%) receiving conventional doses of misoprostol (400–800 µg daily) experienced diarrhea. This generally developed after 2 weeks and was often self-limited. About 2% of patients stopped the medication because of persistent diarrhea [29].

GASTROENTEROLOGY MEDICATIONS

There are a number of medications used in GI diseases that are commonly associated with diarrhea. Mesalamine compounds used in the treatment of ulcerative colitis may be associated with diarrhea, a particularly confounding side effect in patients with IBD. The most frequent offender, olsalazine, causes diarrhea in 12–25% of patients through the stimulation of bicarbonate and sodium chloride secretion in the ileum [1, 30]. Similar azo compounds sulfasalazine and mesalazine may also cause diarrhea, but less frequently. The mechanism is unclear, but may involve a direct effect on anion transporters, rather than an anti-inflammatory action [31].

Some drugs cause a secretory diarrhea by altering intracellular signaling cascades, increasing cyclic AMP, cyclic GMP, or calcium. Prostaglandin analogues can cause diarrhea through many pathways, including altered permeability, motility, electrolyte transport, and by affecting peptides that stimulate secretion [32]. Misoprostol specifically stimulates epithelial Cl^- secretion through cyclic AMP, resulting in intraluminal fluid accumulation and diarrhea, which usually occurs within the first 2 weeks of treatment [3].

A secretory type of diarrhea limited the clinical use of chenodeoxycholic acid, a bile acid initially used to dissolve cholesterol gallstones. Early studies showed that the mechanism of secretory diarrhea in chenodeoxycholic acid therapy was due to a rise in intracellular cyclic AMP levels. However, recent in vitro studies using much lower doses of bile acids suggest a mechanism involving activation of luminal K^+ channels and Cl^- secretion mediated through increased intracellular Ca^{2+} levels [33, 34]. Another dihydroxy bile acid, ursodiol causes diarrhea much less frequently. Presumably this difference is due to the alternative configuration of the hydroxyl groups compared to chenodeoxycholic acid. However, there are some reports of ursodiol causing diarrhea. A meta-analysis of ursodiol and its adverse effects revealed that diarrhea was the single most frequent adverse drug event in patients treated for gallstone disease, with an incidence of 2–9% [35]. If and when ursodiol is associated with diarrhea, there are two possible mechanisms: an increase in the secretion of all bile salts including chenodeoxycholic acid and/or luminal conversion of ursodiol to chenodeoxycholic acid by intestinal bacteria (Alan Hoffman, personal communication).

In primary biliary cirrhosis patients, on the other hand, diarrhea was rarely reported, in five large-scale RCTs. No report of ursodiol-induced diarrhea was found in the largest placebo-controlled randomized study of its use in primary sclerosing cholangitis [35]. These conflicting data highlight some of the challenges of evaluating adverse events of RCTs.

Is there a real difference in the incidence of diarrhea in gallstone disease compared to PBC/PSC? Perhaps, bile salt metabolism is different in gallstone disease, where there is an increased conversion of ursodiol to chenodeoxycholic acid which is a potent secretagogue. The gallbladder in patients with gallstones is likely to be hypo-functional and may be altered in its contractility in response to a meal or in its concentrating capacity, thus allowing more bile acid to enter the duodenum per ursodiol dose. In addition, ursodiol may be stimulatory to the inflamed bowel, while neutral or inhibitory to the bowel of patients with gallstones (Roger Soloway, personal communication). Alternatively, the design of RCTs may account for the difference: the definition of diarrhea as an adverse event, the focus on a more serious disease, or an already increased baseline bowel movement frequency in patients with PSC are possible examples of this factor.

Some have speculated that anticholinergic drugs, which most often cause constipation by reducing intestinal motility, as well as the proton pump inhibitor omeprazole, can cause a paradoxical diarrhea. Although the proposed mechanism for diarrhea is thought to be bacterial overgrowth leading to bacterial deconjugation of primary bile salts to dihydroxy bile acids causing net fluid and electrolyte secretion in the colon, there is no substantial evidence to confirm this explanation [3]. In fact, a Cochrane systemic review showed no statistically significant difference in diarrhea occurrence in patients treated with PPI for reflux disease either at maintenance dose (PPI 1.1% vs. placebo 3.3%, RR 0.34, 95% CI 0.04–3.18) or at healing dose for esophagitis (PPI 5.2% vs. placebo 2%, $p = 0.11$) [36]. A recent article suggesting a link between PPI use and small bowel bacterial overgrowth contributing to diarrhea-predominant IBS shows that there is a common assumption among gastroenterologists that PPI can cause diarrhea, that is not necessarily supported by evidence [37].

Although not as elegantly delineated as epithelial transport changes, disordered or deregulated motility can also cause diarrhea. Prokinetic agents reduce intestinal contact time between luminal fluid and the epithelium. The decreased amount of time chyme exposed to intestinal epithelium can limit absorption and ultimately lead to diarrhea [2]. Cisapride and tegaserod are 5-HT$_4$-receptor agonists that stimulate motility and accelerate gastrointestinal transit. However, both of these drugs have been removed from the market due to potential cardiotoxicity.

Cholestyramine usually causes constipation, but in doses of 24–30 g/day may cause steatorrhea [1]. Animal studies show that increasing the dietary amount of cholestyramine markedly increased the excretion of both free and esterified fat in the stool [38].

Octreotide, used as an antidiarrheal, has a paradoxical effect at higher doses, causing steatorrhea in 5–13% of patients by a possible synergistic inhibition of biliary and pancreatic function through decreased bicarbonate and lipase secretion [1, 39].

DIABETES MEDICATIONS

Diarrhea is a common occurrence in diabetes and may have many etiologies. However, one of the most frequent causes of diabetic diarrhea is medication. The biguanide metformin, used in the treatment of type II diabetes, has an effect on the brush border, reducing disaccharidase activity and leading to malabsorptive diarrhea in 10–53% of patients [21, 40].

Animal studies have found that metformin or the older biguanide phenformin inhibits intestinal glucose absorption in a dose-dependent manner through effects on mucosal and serosal glucose transfer mechanisms [41–44]. Based on a systematic review evaluating common adverse events of metformin monotherapy in type 2 diabetes mellitus, patients receiving metformin are 3.4 times more likely to develop diarrhea compared to those taking placebo ($p = 0.002$) [45]. Most cases are transient and mild, but even in severe cases, lowering the dose usually resolves the diarrhea [46]. In clinical trials, only 5% of study participants discontinued metformin because of gastrointestinal side effects [45]. There have also been cases of metformin causing late-onset chronic diarrhea in whom discontinuation of the drug resolved diarrhea [47]. Larger studies of 405 type 2 diabetics show that metformin was independently associated with chronic diarrhea with an odds ratio of 3.08 (CI 1.29–7.36, $p<0.02$) [48]. In a diabetic clinic, metformin was found to be the most common cause of diarrhea based on a questionnaire-based survey of 285 randomly selected diabetic patients [49]. Diarrhea in a diabetic patient may be related to the disease process itself; however, diabetic diarrhea usually occurs in type 1 diabetes for which metformin is not a treatment.

Acarbose and miglitol, used for the treatment of diabetes, prevent the breakdown of carbohydrates to monosaccharides by inhibition of intestinal alpha-glucosidase, causing diarrhea. In a multicenter RCT of 286 in type 2 diabetic patients comparing acarbose, tolbutamide, and tolbutamide-plus-acarbose to placebo 27% of patients taking acarbose and 35% taking acarbose + tolbutamide c/o diarrhea in comparison to 6% of patients taking placebo or tolbutamide ($p < 0.05$) [50].

Diarrhea can be minimized by starting acarbose therapy at low doses (50 mg three times daily) and, in general, tends to decrease with time [51]. In the large-scale, multinational study nvestigating different doses of acarbose (from 25 mg t.i.d. to 200 mg t.i.d), good patient tolerability and compliance were observed, even at the highest dose [52]. The study also confirmed the marked tendency for adverse effects to decline after 4–6 weeks.

Interestingly, in a postmarket surveillance study of almost 20,000 patients, which included both type 1 and 2 diabetes, only 3.2% of those taking acarbose complained of diarrhea [53]. The difference in findings between the surveillance study and the RCT may be explained by several processes: During an RCT, there may be more attention directed toward minimal changes in signs and symptoms. Acarbose-associated diarrhea is most common in the early phase of treatment. In some cases of acarbose-induced diarrhea, the symptoms may resolve over time with continued use. Finally, surveillance generally separates out those subjects who had already discontinued acarbose because of diarrhea.

The newer class of diabetes medications, GLP 1 inhibitors such as exenatide, slow gastric emptying. Diarrhea is not an infrequent side effect.

ENDOCRINE MEDICINES

Diarrhea associated with medullary carcinoma of the thyroid suggested that calcitonin may cause a secretory type of diarrhea. Calcitonin in high doses can induce a secretory diarrhea in 1–3% of patients. Studies involving intravenous infusions showed prompt and marked increase in jejunal secretion of water, sodium, chloride, and potassium, and reduced absorption of bicarbonate, which was reversed immediately with discontinuation of the infusion [54, 55]. However, in clinical practice, the use of salmon calcitonin for treatment of osteoporosis rarely causes diarrhea (Vassilopoulou-Sellin R., personal communication) [56]. This paradox highlights the variable and sometimes unpredictable pattern of drug-induced diarrhea.

Just as in thyrotoxicosis, excess levothyroxine therapy can accelerate small and large intestinal transit, causing diarrhea [57–59]. In addition to its effects on intestinal transit, levothyroxine has been implicated in bile acid malabsorption because of abnormal selenohomocholyltaurine

(SeHCAT) testing. This test can be used to diagnose bile acid malabsorption as a cause of chronic diarrhea, but it best predicts the benefit of cholestyramine in these patients [60]. However, this adverse effect of levothyroxine may be a secondary effect of increased motility.

CHEMOTHERAPY AND IMMUNOMODULATORS

Diarrhea is a common adverse effect with a wide variety of drugs used in oncology and transplant. The diarrhea is predictable and is often a rate-limiting step in treatment.

Inflammatory diarrhea can be caused by immunosuppressive and chemotherapeutic agents. The balance between absorption and secretion may be disrupted by a change in the balance between mature villus and immature crypt cells (see Fig. 23.2). This loss of intestinal epithelial homeostasis with some superficial necrosis causes an imbalance between absorptive, secretory, and motility functions of the gut contributing to diarrhea [19, 32, 61]. Epithelial apoptosis of more

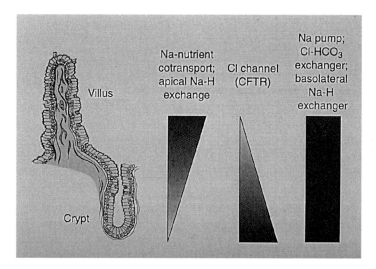

Fig. 23.2. Gradients from crypt to villus. There is a significant spatial geometry of transport proteins along the crypt–villus (crypt–surface) axis. Some transport molecules are found at relatively constant concentrations along the axis, some exhibit a greater density in the base of the crypt, and others exhibit a greater density toward the villus or surface (adapted from Sellin JH. Chapter 87: Intestinal Electrolyte Absorption and Secretion. In: Slezinger & Fordtran (eds) *Gastrointestinal and Liver Disease: Pathophysiology/ Diagnosis/Management*. 7th edn. Saunders, Philadelphia, PA. Figure 87.3, p. 1695).

than five apoptotic bodies (per 100 crypts) is considered an increase above normal. Chemotherapeutic agents, especially fluorouracil, can cause greater than 100 apoptotic bodies [27]. These agents usually cause diarrhea in a dose-related fashion. It is most commonly seen with fluoropyrimidines (fluorouracil, irinotecan, methotrexate, and cisplatin), the fluorouracil pro-drug capecitabine, and the combination treatment uracil–tegafur [1]. The patient's symptoms can range in severity from mild diarrhea to severe necrotizing enterocolitis [19].

Transplant immunosuppressives frequently cause diarrhea. This may be due to a similar apoptotic enteropathy. Mycophenolic acid may shift the balance between the pro- and antiapoptotic factors Bcl-2 and Bax, leading to changes in mucosal homeostasis, and may also alter chloride secretion (Sellin J., unpublished observations).

Irinotecan can cause acute or delayed diarrhea in 50–88% of patients. Immediate-onset diarrhea is caused by acute cholinergic effects and usually responds rapidly to atropine. The delayed-onset diarrhea usually occurs 24 h to several days after administration, can be unpredictable, occurs at all dose levels, and is worse with combination regimens with intravenous fluorouracil and leucovorin [62]. Several hypotheses have been proposed to explain the underlying mechanism. Evidence of a direct toxic effect on intestinal epithelium was provided by animal studies: Mice treated with irinotecan had intestinal wall thinning with epithelial vacuolation, vascular dilatation, an inflammatory cell infiltrate, and evidence of apoptosis in the ileum [63, 64]. These studies led to the discovery of bacterial β-glucoronidase which deconjugates the irinotecan metabolite SN38 glucuronide causing its direct effect on the intestinal epithelium [19, 65].

Multiple agents have been studied in an attempt to reverse irinotecan-induced diarrhea. In humans, the use of oral antibiotic, neomycin, which decreases β-glucuronidase activity in the intestinal lumen, resulted in good control of irinotecan-induced diarrhea in seven colorectal cancer patients [66]. The Chinese herb Hange-Shashito (TJ-14), a natural inhibitor of the β-glucuronidase activity of bacterial microflora, has also been shown to prevent the delayed diarrhea from irinotecan [67]. Probenecid, a biliary inhibitor of irinotecan and SN-38 secretion, has been shown to reduce irinotecan intestinal toxicity in mice, but no evidence has confirmed this observation in humans [68]. Oral cyclosporin (to reduce SN38 and SN38G clearance into the small bowel lumen) used with irinotecan in a phase I clinical trial prevented severe diarrhea. Only 1 patient out of 37 experienced grade 3 diarrhea, and grade 4 diarrhea did not occur [69]. At increased pH, equilibrium favors the less toxic carboxylate form of the irinotecan metabolite

SN-38. Reduced cellular damage and diarrhea was noted with bicarbonate administration in hamsters given irinotecan [70]. Phase II clinical trials also suggested benefit from sodium bicarbonate supplementation for irinotecan-induced severe delayed diarrhea [71].

Oxaliplatin combined with fluorouracil and irinotecan makes the incidence of diarrhea even more common than observed with either agent alone [62]. Diarrhea can also result from an increase in opportunistic infections: invasive bacterial infections such as tuberculosis and yersiniosis; ulcerating viral infections such as cytomegalovirus and Herpes simplex; and invasive parasitic infections such as amebiasis and strongyloides. Neutropenic enterocolitis may also complicate chemotherapy in neutropenic patients with leukemia. This is especially associated with cytosine arabinoside, cisplatin, vincristine, adriamycin, fluorouracil, and mercaptopurine [27].

Chemotherapeutic agents, besides causing inflammatory diarrhea, can damage immature epithelial cells in the crypts causing functionally compromised mature enterocytes. This effect leads to decreased nutrient absorptive capacity and potentially a malabsorptive diarrhea [3]. Rapamycin administration in rabbits showed significantly decreased jejunal and ileal villous surface areas and decreased fat and cholesterol uptake, possibly contributing to malabsorption [72].

A new class of chemotherapeutic drugs, molecularly targeted agents, have been proven to cause frequent diarrhea as frequently as their predecessors. Epidermal growth factor receptor tyrosine kinase inhibitor, erlotinib, and other tyrosine kinase inhibitors such as sorafenib, imatinib, and bortezomib cause diarrhea in up to 60% of patients [62]. Erbitux® (cetuximab), used for the treatment of EGFR-expressing, metastatic colorectal carcinoma and squamous cell carcinoma of the head and neck, and Iressa® (geftinib), used for non-small cell lung cancer, can cause diarrhea in 48–67% of patients depending on dose [73, 74]. EGF can activate PI 3-kinase and the lipid products of this enzyme inhibit calcium-dependent Cl transport in T84 human colonic epithelial cells [75, 76]. EGF-receptor inhibitors may cause diarrhea by blocking this inhibitory loop and causing secretion.

Diarrhea can be managed by loperamide, dose reduction, or treatment interruptions [62].

Sorafenib-induced diarrhea, expected in 30–43% of patients, is thought to be related to ischemic changes causing direct damage to mucosal cells. In a case report of a patient with diarrhea on sorafenib, multiple ulcers were found on colonoscopy throughout his colon [77].

Flavopiridol, a cyclin-dependent kinase inhibitor, has undergone several clinical trials as an antitumor agent, with secretory diarrhea as a dose-limiting factor. Adding cholestyramine and loperamide as a prophylactic antidiarrheal treatment allowed for use of higher doses [78]. Diarrhea may be related to flavopiridol binding to the gut mucosa acting as a modest secretagogoue. Cholestyramine, by binding flavopiridol, eases the adverse effect [79]. Pharmacogenomics may play a role in drug-induced diarrhea. For example, those with extensive hepatic glucorinidation metabolism experienced less diarrhea than others [80]. The hepatic metabolism of the drug decreases the toxic metabolites that cause intestinal secretion. In this clinical study, mild cases of diarrhea were controlled by loperamide, whereas more severe diarrhea was controlled by octreotide infusion and reduction of flavopiridol dosages in subsequent cycles [80].

ANTIBIOTICS

Antibiotics account for 25% of drug-induced diarrhea [1]. The most well-known complication is pseudomembranous colitis due to *C. difficile* (see Chapter 2), especially seen with the antibiotics clindamycin, amoxicillin, ampicillin, and cephalosporins [3]. *C. difficile* causes diarrhea by secreting enterotoxin A, which adheres to the brush border membrane of enterocytes inducing an inflammatory response, and cytotoxin B that induces direct mucosal damage [2, 61]. Diarrhea may occur a few days after antibiotic therapy is initiated and up to 8 weeks after discontinuation. In the appropriate clinical setting, diagnosis is based on detection of toxin in the stool. Endoscopy reveals raised white to yellow plaques covering a normal or moderately erythematous colonic mucosa [61]. Recently, non-antibiotic-associated community-acquired *C. difficile* infection has become more frequent with the use of acid reducing agents and immunosuppressives. Lansoprazole and, in the elderly, histamine antagonist use are reported to be significant risk factors for carriage of *C. difficile*, increasing the risk of developing pseudomembranous colitis [3, 27]. In fact, a meta-analysis to assess risk factors for recurrent *C. difficile* infection revealed that use of concomitant antacid medications increased the risk by two-fold (OR: 2.15; 95% CI: 1.13–4.08; $p = 0.019$) [81].

There has been a rise in the incidence of *C. difficile* colitis in hospitalized patients with inflammatory bowel disease [82]. This may be attributable to the use of immunosuppressives and biologic agents [83].

However, not all antibiotic-associated diarrhea is due to *C. difficile*. Antibiotic-induced shifts in the bacterial flora may result in diarrhea, presumably because of either an imbalance between different strains of bacteria, a decrease in colonic production of short chain fatty acids from fiber, or an alteration in mucosal function. Given the complexities of intestinal bacterial ecology, there is little definitive data to support these attractive hypotheses.

There are, however, some better documented mechanisms of non-*C. difficile* antibiotic-associated diarrhea. Motilin, a peptide hormone found in the gastrointestinal M cells, and in some enterochromaffin cells of the upper small bowel, is a potent contractile agent of the upper GI tract. The effects of motilin can be mimicked by macrolide antibiotics, especially erythromycin, and can cause diarrhea. In addition to its motilin agonistic effect, erythromycin at lower doses (40–80 mg) may also entail cholinergic involvement, although the mechanisms are not well understood [13].

Long-term use of oral antibacterials such as neomycin, polymyxin, and bacitracin can also cause malabsorptive diarrhea. These antibiotics damage the small intestinal mucosa, leading to a reduction of the enzyme activity of enterocytes [3, 20, 84]. They may also bind bile acids in the intestinal lumen and reduce the absorption of fat [1]. In in vitro transport studies, both neomycin and amphotericin act as membrane detergents, functionally "dissolving" the apical membrane of enterocytes or colonocytes. Administering 1 g of neomycin with a test meal to five healthy subjects caused a marked increase in fatty acid and bile acid in their aspirated intestinal contents [85]. However, a subsequent study of 2 g/day dose of neomycin given to four patients revealed no evidence of steatorrhea, although daily stool weight increased in three or four patients [86].

NSAIDS

Although physicians are attuned to the risks of NSAID-induced gastric and duodenal ulcerations, it is becoming increasingly apparent that NSAIDs may have a significant effect on the small bowel. NSAID enteropathy may present with diarrhea, GI blood loss or perforation. Through multifactorial mechanisms, diarrhea occurs in 3–9% of patients treated with the non-steroidal anti-inflammatory drugs (NSAIDs), especially the older drugs mefenamic acid and flufenamic acid [1, 87–89]. Thirty-nine percent (34 of 87) of patients in a 6-week study given meclofenamate at doses of 200–400 mg/day experienced diarrhea, including steatorrhea [21, 90].

Since NSAIDs stimulate in vitro absorption (increased Na^+ absorption and decreased Cl^- secretion), other mechanisms must be involved in diarrhea [91]. NSAIDS most likely cause diarrhea through luminal contact with the small bowel epithelium [92]. Enterocyte injury involves topical damage from ion trapping and uncoupling of oxidative phosphorylation leading to increased intestinal permeability and inflammation. This exposes the enterocytes to luminal agents (microbes, bile acids, enzymes) that cause injury and inflammation progressing to erosions and ulcers [93]. Histologic findings include prominent apoptosis and increased intraepithelial lymphocyte counts [84]. NSAIDS may double the number of apoptotic bodies normally found in the small intestine [29]. NSAIDs have been associated with both microscopic and pseudomembranous colitis. NSAIDs have also been implicated in causing collagenous colitis. Based on a case–control study of 31 patients with collagenous colitis and 31 controls, the use of NSAIDs was significantly more common in the study group (19/31) vs. (4/31) in the control group ($p < 0.02$) [94]. Ileal disease mimicking Crohn's disease has also been described.

NSAID damage to the small bowel has been assessed by both endoscopic and non-invasive techniques. Both capsule endoscopy and double balloon enteroscopy have visually documented an increased number of mucosal erosions and ulcers in the jejunum and ileum. Non-invasive methods have included indium-labeled leukocyte scans, lactulose mannitol permeability testing, and fecal calprotectin. Maiden and others have quantitatively analyzed by capsule endoscopy NSAID-induced pathology in 40 subjects taking diclofenac. Images revealed new pathology in 27 subjects (68%), with common lesions of mucosal breaks, bleeding, erythema, and denuded mucosa, with the majority having concurrent lesions [95]. These patients also had elevated fecal calprotectin (a marker for inflammation) levels from baseline. This study provides both biochemical and direct evidence of macroscopic injury to the small intestine from NSAID use [95]. In a case–control study of 105 cases of newly diagnosed colitis based on endoscopic and histologic findings, 78 patients (74%) were taking NSAIDs or salicylates prior to or during the development of their disease [96]. These studies support NSAIDs as an important class of drugs in causing enteritis and/or colitis.

Acute proctocolitis has been documented in four separate cases of NSAID etiology, with the use of flufenamic acid, mefenamic acid, naproxen, and ibuprofen. Symptoms and signs resolved in all cases with removal of the drug, but a rapid relapse occurred in three of the four patients who were subsequently rechallenged with the NSAID [97].

HIV MEDICATIONS

Virtually all protease inhibitors cause diarrhea. Ritonavir causes diarrhea in up to 52% of patients [98, 99]. Adverse effects appear to be more common in patients with more advanced HIV/AIDS and

Chapter 23 / Drug-Induced Diarrhea

in patients with higher plasma drug levels. Effects are greatest at the beginning of therapy, before ritonavir induces an increase in its own metabolism [100]. Combination therapy, especially lopinavir with ritonavir, increases the risk of diarrhea [100]. Antidiarrheal medications such as loperamide have been shown to control diarrhea. However, in vitro studies showed that several protease inhibitors inhibited lipase significantly at or below physiological concentrations [101]. Thus, the use of pancrealipase with protease inhibitors may in theory reduce or eliminate steatorrhea in these patients [100, 101].

Interestingly, in a study of 33 HIV patients who underwent evaluation for diarrhea, over 90% had steatorrhea, irrespective of HAART therapy (20/21 patients not on HAART vs. 10/12 patients on HAART) [7]. Thus, the specificity of steatorrhea secondary to HAART may be called into question.

Of the nucleoside analogue reverse transcriptase inhibitors, didanosine causes diarrhea in 17–28% of patients, especially in the buffered formulations [61]. Enteric-coated tablets decrease this incidence. Abacavir can produce diarrhea, especially in association with a hypersensitivity reaction that occurs in 3–5% of treated individuals [100, 102]. Diarrhea, among other symptoms, appears 1–4 weeks after initiation of therapy, and usually resolves within 1–2 days after discontinuation. Rechallenge with the drug, even at a decreased dose, may cause the return of symptoms within hours with increased severity [100].

CARDIAC MEDICATIONS

The Na^+ pump (Na^+, K^+-ATPase) is the final common pathway for Na^+ absorption; inhibition of the Na^+ pump blocks Na^+ (and fluid) absorption and this may cause diarrhea. Digoxin's therapeutic target is the cardiac Na^+, K^+-ATPase. However, inhibition of intestinal or colonic Na^+ pumps may cause diarrhea, most frequently at supertherapeutic drug levels, especially in elderly patients [3]. In fact, digoxin was the second commonest cause of diarrhea in a study of 100 elderly patients [103].

By reducing K^+ conductance and inhibiting calcium channels, the class I antiarrhythmic drugs quinidine and propafenone impede transepithelial Na^+ and water absorption causing diarrhea in 8–30% of patients [104].

Ticlopidine, an inhibitor of platelet aggregation, can cause diarrhea through many processes, including reported cases of lymphocytic colitis. However, increased motility is thought to be the principal mechanism based on manometric readings of jejunal motility revealing abnormal motility patterns [105].

HMG-CoA reductase inhibitors such as simvastatin, lovastatin, and pravastatin cause an inflammatory diarrhea in less than 5% of patients [1].

MISCELLANEOUS DRUGS

The phosphodiesterase inhibitor, theophylline, causes diarrhea by increasing cyclic AMP, opening chloride channels, and increasing secretion [32].

Auranofin, used previously for rheumatoid arthritis, caused secretory diarrhea in up to 74% of patients requiring discontinuation in 14% of them [3]. Severe enterocolitis has also been reported of gold therapy in over 30 cases. This adverse effect was unrelated to dosage, occurred within 3 months of beginning treatment and persisted despite withdrawal of the drug [3, 106].

Colchicine, besides causing secretory diarrhea through the inhibition of Na^+, K^+-ATPase activity, is a microtubule inhibitor and may induce diarrhea by interfering with the migration of epithelial cells from the crypt to the villus causing villous atrophy [3] and/or interfere with intracellular trafficking of specific transport proteins [32], leading to malabsorption. Three out of 12 patients evaluated for gastrointestinal effects of the long-term use of colchicine prophylaxis for recurrent polyserositis developed mild steatorrhea [107].

L-Dopa, allopurinol, and tetracycline can cause steatorrhea through changes in jejunal mucosa [21, 91]. Flutamide, the antiandrogen drug used primarily to treat prostate cancer, has been linked to microscopic colitis [1, 27]. Penicillamine has been shown in a few cases to cause acute proctosigmoiditis [87].

Isotretinoin used for acne has been associated with inflammatory diarrheas [1]. Histology from these patients often shows acute focal superficial inflammatory infiltrate of the mucosa. Multiple cases including the largest case series revealed 85 patients diagnosed with inflammatory bowel disease with prior or recent use of the drug suggesting a possible link [108]. Accutane (Roche) was recently pulled from the market; however, other brands are still available.

CONCLUSION

Ideally, decisions about diagnosis or therapy should be evidence based; however, as emphasized above, there is frequently a dearth of high-quality evidence to guide the clinician in the area of drug-induced

Chapter 23 / Drug-Induced Diarrhea 417

diarrhea. Determining the etiology of drug-induced diarrhea depends on a careful history to identify the offending agent. Any history of drug allergies or intolerances and any new prescription medications taken within the 6–8 weeks prior to symptom onset may reveal the etiology. One should always consider prescription as well as non-prescription drugs, nutritional supplements, excessive caffeine consumption, and artificial sweeteners found in diet foods as potential causes. Most cases of drug-induced diarrhea resolve spontaneously within a few days after withdrawal of the drug or with dose reduction. If diarrhea is severe or persistent, patient management should include replenishment of any fluid and electrolyte deficits with oral hydration or if warranted, with intravenous fluids. Non-specific antidiarrheal agents can reduce stool frequency and stool weight as well as decrease abdominal cramps. Opiates (loperamide, diphenoxylate with atropine), intraluminal agents (bismuth subsalicylate), and adsorbents (kaolin) also can help reduce the fluidity of bowel movements [2, 27]. A low residue diet, specific treatment as described in above sections such as antibiotics for *C. difficile* colitis, and reduction of fat intake for patients taking orlistat can also help. Probiotics as possible treatment or prevention (see Chapter 27) have not been well studied in these settings, but future studies may prove them to be useful.

REFERENCES

1. Chassany O, Michaux A, Bergmann JF. Drug-induced diarrhoea. Drug Saf 2000; 22:53–72.
2. Schiller LR, Sellin JH. Diarrhea. In: Feldman M, Friedman LS, Brandt LJ, et al., eds. Gastrointestinal and liver disease. Philadelphia, PA: Saunders, 2006, pp. 159–181.
3. Ratnaike RN, Jones TE. Mechanisms of drug-induced diarrhoea in the elderly. Drugs Aging 1998; 13:245–253.
4. Saliba F, Hagipantelli R, Misset JL, et al. Pathophysiology and therapy of irinotecan-induced delayed-onset diarrhea in patients with advanced colorectal cancer: a prospective assessment. J Clin Oncol 1998; 16:2745.
5. Lenfers BH, Loeffler TM, Droege CM, et al. Substantial activity of budesonide in patients with irinotecan (CPT-11) and 5-fluorouracil induced diarrhoea and failure of loperamide treatment. Ann Oncol 1999; 10:1251–1253.
6. Barbounis V, Koumakis G, Vassilomanolakis M, et al. Control of irinotecan-induced diarrhoea by octreotide after loperamide failure. Support Care Cancer 2001; 9:258–260.
7. Poles M, Fuerst M, McGowan I, et al. HIV-related diarrhea is multifactorial and fat malabsorption is commonly present, independent of HAART. Am J Gastroenterol 2001; 96:1831–1837.
8. Heiser CR, Ernst JA, Barrett JT, et al. Probiotics, soluble fiber and L-Glutamine (GLN) reduce nelfinavir (NFV)- or lopinavir/ritonavir (LPV/r)-related diarrhea. J Int Assoc Physicians AIDS Care (Chic Ill) 2004; 3:121–130.

9. Wald A, Back C, Bayless TM. Effect of caffeine on the human small intestine. Gastroenterology 1976; 71:738–742.
10. Fernandez-Benares F, Esteve M, Viver JM. Fructose sorbitol malabsorption. Curr Gastroenterol Rep 2009; 11(5):368–374.
11. Marteau P, Seksik P. Tolerance of probiotics and prebiotics. J Clin Gastroenterol 2004; 38:S67–S69.
12. Briet F, Achour L, Flourié B, et al. Symptomatic response to varying levels of fructo-oligosaccharides consumed occasionally or regularly. Eur J Clin Nutr 1995; 49(7):501–507.
13. Pasricha PJ. Treatment of disorders of bowel motility and water flux; antiemetics: agents used in biliary and pancreatic disease. In: Brunton LL, ed. Goodman & Gilman's the pharmacological basis of therapeutics. New York, NY: McGraw Hill; 2006, pp. 983–1008.
14. McRorie J, Zorich N, Riccardi K, et al. Effects of olestra and sorbitol consumption on objective measures of diarrhea: impact of stool viscosity on common gastrointestinal symptoms. Regul Toxicol Pharmacol 2000; 31:59–67.
15. Sjostrom L, Rissanen A, Andersen T, et al. Randomised placebo-controlled trial of orlistat for weight loss and prevention of weight regain in obese patients. Lancet 1998; 352:167–173.
16. Binder HJ. The gastroenterologist's osmotic gap: fact or fiction? Gastroenterology 1992; 103:702–704.
17. Racusen LC, Binder HJ. Ricinoleic acid stimulation of active anion secretion in colonic mucosa of the rat. J Clin Invest. 1979; 63:743–749.
18. Ramakrishna BS, Mathan M, Mathan VI. Alteration of colonic absorption by long-chain unsaturated fatty acids. Influence of hydroxylation and degree of unsaturation. Scand J Gastroenterol 1994; 29:54–58.
19. Solomon R, Cherny NI. Constipation and diarrhea in patients with cancer. Cancer J. 2006; 12:355–364.
20. Andersson KE. Current concepts in the treatment of disorders of micturition. Drugs 1988; 35:477.
21. Bateman DN. Gastrointestinal disorders. In: Davies DM, ed. Textbook of adverse drug reactions. New York, NY: Oxford University Press, 1991, pp. 230–244.
22. Pierre N, Tariot PN, Cummings JL, et al. A randomized, double-blind, placebo-controlled study of the efficacy and safety of donepezil in patients with Alzheimer's disease in the nursing home setting. J Am Geriatr Soc 2005; 49:1590–1599.
23. Birks J, Harvey RJ. Donepezil for dementia due to Alzheimer's disease. Cochrane Database Syst Rev 2006; Issue 1. Art. No.: CD001190. DOI: 10.1002/14651858.CD001190.pub2.
24. Birks J. Cholinesterase inhibitors for Alzheimer's disease. Cochrane Database Syst Rev. 2006; Issue 1. Art. No.: CD005593. DOI: 10.1002/14651858.CD005593.
25. Hajek P, Gillison F, McRobbie H. Stopping smoking can cause constipation. Addition 2003; 98(11):1563–1567.
26. Trindade E, Menon D, Topfer LA, Coloma C. Adverse effects associated with selective serotonin reuptake inhibitors and tricyclic antidepressants: a meta-analysis. CMAJ 1998; 17:159(10):1245–52.
27. Parfitt JR, Driman DK. Pathological effects of drugs on the gastrointestinal tract: a review. Human Pathol 2007; 38:527–536.
28. Mubarak KK. A review of prostaglandin analogs in the management of patients with pulmonary arterial hypertension. Respir Med 2010 Jan; 104(1):9–21. Epub 2009 Aug 15. PMID: 19683911 [PubMed – in process].

Chapter 23 / Drug-Induced Diarrhea   419

29. Pfizer. Cytotec US Prescribing Information (PDF), September 2006. http://www.pfizer.com/pfizer/download/uspi_cytotec.pdf. Retrieved 2007-03-15.
30. Kles KA, Vavricka SR, Turner JR, et al. Comparative analysis of the in vitro prosecretory effects of balsalazide, sulfasalazine, olsalazine, and mesalamine in rabbit distal ileum. Inflammatory Bowel Dis 2005; 11:253–257.
31. Pamukcu R, Hanauer SB, Change EB. Effect of disodium azodisalicylate on electrolyte transport in rabbit ileum and colon in vitro. Comparison with sulfasalazine and 5-aminosalicylic acid. Gastroenterology 1988; 95:975–981.
32. Sellin JH. The pathophysiology of diarrhea. Clin Transplant 2001; 15:2–10.
33. Mauricio AC, Slawik M, Heitzmann D, et al. Deoxycholic acid (DOC) affects the transport properties of distal colon. Pflugers Arch 2000; 439: 532–540.
34. Venkatasubramanian J, Selvaraj N, Carlos M, et al. Differences in Ca(2+) signaling underlie age-specific effects of secretagogues on colonic Cl(–) transport. Am J Physiol Cell Physiol 2001; 280:C646–C658.
35. Hempfling W, Dilger K, Beuers, U. Ursodeoxycholic acid — adverse effects and drug interactions. Aliment Pharmacol Ther 2003; 18:963–972.
36. Donnellan C, Sharma N, Preston C, Moayyedi P. Medical treatments for the maintenance therapy of reflux oesophagitis and endoscopic negative reflux disease. Cochrane Database Syst Rev 2004; issue 4. Art. No.: CD003245. DOI: 10.1002/14651858.CD003245.pub2.
37. Brennan M, Spiegel R, Chey WD, et al. Bacterial overgrowth and irritable bowel syndrome: unifying hypothesis or a spurious consequence of proton pump inhibitors? Am J Gastroenterol 2008; 103:2972–2976.
38. Harkins RW, Hagerman LM, Sarett HP Absorption of dietary fats by the rat in cholestyramine-induced steatorrhea. J Nutr 1965; 87:85–92.
39. Nakamura T, Kudoh K, Takebe K, et al. Octreotide decreases biliary and pancreatic exocrine function, and induces steatorrhea in healthy subjects. Int Med 1994; 33:593–596.
40. Berchtold P, Dahlqvist, A, Gustafson, A, et al. Effects of a biguanide (metformin) on vitamin B12 and folic acid absorption and intestinal enzyme activities. Scand J Gastroenterol 1971; 6:751.
41. Czyzyk A, Tawecki J, Sadowski J, et al. Effect of biguanides on intestinal absorption of glucose. Diabetes 1968; 17:492–498.
42. Kruger FA, Altschuld RA, Hollobaugh SL, et al. (1970) Studies on the site and mechanism of action of phenformin. II. Phenformin inhibition of glucose transport by rat intestine. Diabetes 1970; 19:50–52.
43. Ikeda T, Iwata K, Murakami H. Inhibitory effect of metformin on intestinal glucose absorption in the perfused rat intestine. Biochem Pharmacol. 2000; 59:887–890.
44. Wilcock C, Bailey CJ. Reconsideration of inhibitory effect of metformin on intestinal glucose absorption. J Pharm Pharmacol 1991; 43:120–121.
45. Saenz A, Fernandez-Esteban I, Mataix A, et al. Metformin monotherapy for type 2 diabetes mellitus. Cochrane Database Syst Rev 2005; 3. Art. No.: CD002966. DOI: 10.1002/14651858.CD002966.pub3.
46. DeFronzo RA, Goodman AM. Efficacy of metformin in patients with non-insulin-dependent diabetes mellitus. N Engl J Med 1995; 333:541–549.
47. Foss MT, Clement KD. Metformin as a cause of late-onset chronic diarrhea. Pharmacotherapy 2001; 21:1422–1424.
48. Bytzer P, Talley NJ, Jones MP, et al. Oral hypoglycaemic drugs and gastrointestinal symptoms in diabetes mellitus. Aliment Pharmacol Ther 2001; 15:137–142.

49. Dandona P, Fonseca V, Mier A, et al. Diarrhea and metformin in a diabetic clinic. Diabetes Care 1983; 6:472–474.
50. Coniff RF, Shapiro JA, Seaton TB, et al. Multicenter, placebo-controlled trial comparing acarbose (BAY g 5421) with placebo, tolbutamide, and tolbutamide-plus-acarbose in non-insulin-dependent diabetes mellitus. Am J Med 1995; 98:443–451.
51. Santeusanio F, Compagnucci P. A risk-benefit appraisal of acarbose in the management of non-insulin-dependent diabetes mellitus. Drug Safety 1994;11: 432–444.
52. Fischer S, Hanefeld M, Spengler M, et al. European study on dose-response relationship of acarbose as a first-line drug in non-insulin-dependent diabetes mellitus: efficacy and safety of low and high doses. Acta Diabetol 1998; 35:34–40.
53. Spengler M, Cagatay M. The use of acarbose in the primary-care setting: evaluation of efficacy and tolerability of acarbose by postmarketing surveillance study. Clin Invest Med 1995; 18:325–331.
54. Gray TK, Bieberdorf FA, Fordtran JS. Thyrocalcitonin and the jejunal absorption of calcium, water, and electrolytes in normal subjects. J Clin Invest 1973; 52:3084–3088.
55. Kisloff B, Moore EW. Effects of intravenous calcitonin on water, electrolyte, and calcium movement across in vivo rabbit jejunum and ileum. Gastroenterology 1977; 72:462–468.
56. Miacalcin® calcitonin-salmon. In: Physician desk reference. Montvale, NJ: Thomson PDR; 2007, pp. 2253–2254.
57. Nayak B, Burman K. Thyrotoxicosis and thyroid storm. Endocrinol Metab Clin N Am 2006; 35:663–686.
58. Wasan SM, Sellin JH, Vassilopoulou-Sellin R. The gastrointestinal tract and liver in thyrotoxicosis. In Braverman LE, Utiger RD, eds. Werner & Ingbar's the thyroid: a fundamental and clinical text. Philadelphia, PA: Lippincott Williams & Wilkins, 2005, pp. 589–594.
59. Wegener M, Wedmann B, Langhoff T, et al. Effect of hyperthyroidism on the transit of a caloric solid-liquid meal through the stomach, the small intestine, and the colon in man. J Clin Endocrinol Metab 1992; 75:745–749.
60. Raju GS, Dawson B, Bardhan KD. Bile acid malabsorption associated with Graves' disease. J Clin Gastroenterol 1994; 19:54–56.
61. Gervasio JM. Diarrhea and constipation. In: Tisdale JE, Miller DA, eds. Drug-induced diseases: prevention, detection, and management. Bethesda, MD: American Society of Health Systems Pharmacists, 2005, pp. 501–514.
62. Benson AB 3rd, Ajani JA, Catalano RB, et al. Recommended guidelines for the treatment of cancer treatment-induced diarrhea. J Clin Oncol 2004; 22:2918.
63. Ikuno N, Soda H, Watanabe M, et al. Irinotecan (CPT-11) and characteristic mucosal changes in the mouse ileum and cecum. J Natl Cancer Inst 1995; 87:1876–1883.
64. Guffroy M, Hodge, T. Re: irinotecan (CPT-11) and characteristic mucosal changes in the mouse ileum and cecum (letter; comment). J Natl Cancer Inst 1996; 88:1240–1241.
65. Goumas P, Naxakis S, Christopoulou A, et al. Octreotide acetate in the treatment of fluorouracil-induced diarrhea. Oncologist 1998; 8:50.
66. Kehrer DFS, Sparreboom A, Verweij J, et al. Modulation of irinotecan-induced diarrhea by cotreatment with neomycin in cancer patients. Clin Cancer Res 2001; 7:1136–1141.

Chapter 23 / Drug-Induced Diarrhea

67. Sakata Y, Suzuki H, Kamataki T. Preventive effect of TJ-14, a kampo (Chinese herb) medicine, on diarrhoea induced by irinotecan hydrochloride (CPT-11). Gan To Kagaku Ryoho 1994; 21:1241–1244.

68. Horikawa M, Kato Y, Sugiyama Y. Reduced gastrointestinal toxicity following inhibition of the biliary excretion of irinotecan and its metabolites by probenecid in rats. Pharm Res 2002; 19:1345–1353.

69. Chester JD, Joel SP, Cheeseman SL, et al. Phase I and pharmacokinetic study of intravenous irinotecan plus oral ciclosporin in patients with fluorouracil-refractory metastatic colon cancer. J Clin Oncol 2003; 21:1125–1132.

70. Ikegami T, Ha L, Arimori K. Intestinal alkalization as a possible preventive mechanism in irinotecan (CPT-11)-induced diarrhoea. Cancer Res 2002; 62:179–187.

71. Takeda Y, Kobayashi K, Akiyama Y, et al. Prevention of irinotecan (CPT-11)-induced diarrhoea by oral alkalization combined with control of defecation in cancer patients. Int J Cancer 2001; 92:269–275.

72. Dias VC, Madsen KL, Mulder KE, et al. Oral administration of rapamycin and cyclosporine differentially alter intestinal function in rabbits. Dig Dis Sci 1998; 43:2227–2236.

73. Erbitux® (Cetuximab) Package Insert. ImClone Systems Incorporated, New York, NY, and Bristol-Myers Squibb Company, Princeton, NJ, 2007.

74. Iressa® (geftinib) [package insert]. AstraZeneca, Wilmington, 2004.

75. Uribe JM, Keely SJ, Traynor-Kaplan AE, et al. Phosphatidylinositol 3-kinase mediates the inhibitory effect of epidermal growth factor on calcium-dependent chloride secretion. J Biol Chem 1996; 271:26588–26595.

76. Uribe JM, Gelbmann CM, Traynor-Kaplan AE, et al. Epidermal growth factor inhibits Ca2+-dependent Cl⁻ transport in T84 human colonic epithelial cells. Am J Physiol 1996; 271:C914–C922.

77. Frieling T, Heise J, Wassilew SW. Multiple colon ulcerations, perforation and death during treatment of malignant melanoma with sorafenib. Dtsch Med Wochenschr 2009; 134:e1–e2, 1464–1466.

78. Zhai S, Senderowicz AM, Sausville EA, et al. Flavopiridol, a novel cyclin-dependent kinase inhibitor, in clinical development. Ann Pharmacother 2002; 36:905–911.

79. Kahn ME, Senderowicz A, Sausville EA, et al. Possible mechanisms of diarrheal side effects associated with the use of a novel chemotherapeutic agent, flavopiridol. Clin Cancer Res 2001; 7:343–349.

80. Innocenti F, Stadler WM, Iyer L, et al. Flavopiridol metabolism in cancer patients is associated with the occurrence of diarrhea. Clin Cancer Res 2000; 6: 3400–3405.

81. Garey KW, Sethi S, Yadav Y, Dupont HL. Meta-analysis to assess risk factors for recurrent Clostridium difficile infection. J Hosp Infect. 2008; 70:298–304.

82. Rodemann JF, Dubberke ER, Reske KA, et al. Incidence of Clostridium difficile infection in inflammatory bowel disease. Clin Gastroenterol Hepatol 2007; 5:339–344.

83. Issa M, Vijayapal A, Graham MB, et al. Impact of Clostridium difficile on inflammatory bowel disease. Clin Gastroenterol Hepatol 2007; 5:345–351.

84. Price AB. Pathology of drug-associated gastrointestinal disease. J Clin Pharmacol 2003; 56:477–482.

85. Thompson GR, Barrowman J, Gutierrez L, et al. Action of neomycin on the intraluminal phase of lipid absorption. J Clin Invest 1971; 50: 319–323.

86. Sedaghat A, Samuel P, Crouse JR, et al. Effects of neomycin on absorption, synthesis, and/or flux of cholesterol in man. J Clin Invest 1975; 55:12–21.
87. D'Arcy PF, Griffin JP. Iatrogenic diseases. New York: Oxford University Press, 1986, p. 573.
88. Hill AG. Clinical trials of the fenamates. Review of flufenamic acid in rheumatoid arthritis. In Kendall PH, ed. Annuals of physical medicine (suppl.). London: Bailliere, Tindall and Cassell, 1966, pp. 87–92.
89. Holmes EL. Pharmacology of the fenamates. Experimental observations on flufenamic, mefenamic and meclofenamic acids. IV. Toleration by normal human subjects. In Kendall PH, ed. Annuals of physical medicine (suppl.). London: Bailliere, Tindall and Cassell, 1966, pp. 36–49.
90. Ward JR, Bolzan JA, Brame CL, et al. Sodium meclofenamate dose determining studies. Curr Ther Res 1978; 23(suppl.): S60–S65.
91. Langridge-Smith JE, Rao MC, Field M. Chloride and sodium transport across bovine tracheal epithelium: effects of secretagogues and indomethacin. Pflugers Arch 1984; 402:42–47.
92. Gullikson GW, Sender M, Bass P. Laxative-like effects of nonsteroidal anti-inflammatory drugs on intestinal fluid movement and membrane integrity. J Pharmacol Exp Ther 1982; 220:236–242.
93. Gupta M, Eisen G. NSAIDS and the gastrointestinal tract. Curr Gastroenterol Rep 2009; 11:345–353.
94. Riddell RH, Tanaka M, Mazzoleni G. Non-steroidal anti-inflammatory drugs as a possible cause of collagenous colitis: a case-control study. Gut 1992; 33: 683–686.
95. Maiden L, Thjodleifsson B, Theodors A, et al. A quantitative analysis of NSAID-induced small bowel pathology by capsule enteroscopy. Gastroenterology 2005; 128:1172–1178.
96. Gleeson MH, Davis AJM. Non-steroidal anti-inflammatory drugs, aspirin and newly diagnosed colitis: a case-control study. Aliment Pharmacol Ther 2003; 17:817–825.
97. Ravi S, Keat AC, Keat EC. Colitis caused by non-steroidal anti-inflammatory drugs. Postgrad Med J 1986; 62:773–776.
98. Danner SA, Carr A, Leonard JM, et al. A short-term study of the safety, pharmacokinetics, and efficacy of ritonavir, an inhibitor of HIV-1 protease. European-Australian Collaborative Ritonavir Study Group. N Engl J Med 1995; 333:1528–1533.
99. Cameron DW, Heath-Chiozzi M, Danner S, et al. Randomised placebo-controlled trial of ritonavir in advanced HIV-1 disease. The Advanced HIV Disease Ritonavir Study Group. Lancet 1998; 351:543–549.
100. Vella S, Floridia M. Antiviral therapy. In: Cohen J, Powderly WG, Berkley SF, et al., eds. Infectious diseases. New York, NY: Mosby; 2004, pp. 1387–1394.
101. Terese M, Wignot RP, Stewart KJ, et al. *In vitro* studies of the effects of HAART drugs and excipients on activity of digestive enzymes. Pharm Res 2004; 21: 420–427.
102. Kessler HA, Johnson J, Follansbee S, et al. Abacavir expanded access program for adult patients infected with human immunodeficiency virus type 1. Clin Infect Dis 2002; 34:535–542.
103. Pentland B, Pennington CR. Acute diarrhoea in the elderly. Age Ageing 1980; 9:90–92.
104. Plass H, Charisius M, Wyskovsky W, et al. Class I antiarrhythmics inhibit Na+ absorption and Cl– secretion in rabbit descending colon epithelium. Arch Pharmacol 2005; 371:492–499.

Chapter 23 / Drug-Induced Diarrhea   423

105. Guédon C, Bruna T, Ducrotté P, et al. Severe diarrhea caused by Ticlid associated with disorders of small intestine motility. Gastroenterol Clin Biol 1989; 13: 934–937.
106. Jackson CW, et. al. Gold-induced enterocolitis. Gut 1986; 27:452–456.
107. Ehrenfeld M, Levy M, Sharon P, et al. Gastrointestinal effects of long-term colchicine therapy in patients with recurrent polyserositis (familial Mediterranean fever). Dig Dis Sci 1982; 27:723–727.
108. Reddy D, Siegel CA, Sands BE, Kane S. Possible association between isotretinoin and inflammatory bowel disease. Am J Gastroenterol 2006; 101:1569–1573.

24 Runner's Diarrhea

Daniel Triezenberg, MD
and Stephen M. Simons, MD, FACSM

CONTENTS

INTRODUCTION
INCIDENCE
EXERCISE EFFECTS ON
    GASTROINTESTINAL PHYSIOLOGY
CLINICAL MANAGEMENT
RACE MANAGEMENT
TRAINING IMPLICATIONS
CONCLUSION
REFERENCES

Summary

Runners are commonly afflicted with diarrhea. Profound mechanical and physiologic gastrointestinal changes occur with exercise. These changes can contribute to "runner's trots". Medical practitioners should be alert to these running effects to better advise their active patients.

Although it may be initially compelling to attribute a single episode of running diarrhea to the exercise itself, one must always remain alert to the possibility of non-exercise causes of diarrhea merely presenting with the run. Runners may reduce chances of a disabling episode of diarrhea with some simple pre-run strategies.

Key Words: Runner's diarrhea, Athletes' GI symptoms, Mesenteric ischemia, Polycythemia, ORS, Loperamide

From: *Diarrhea, Clinical Gastroenterology*
Edited by: S. Guandalini, H. Vaziri, DOI 10.1007/978-1-60761-183-7_24
© Springer Science+Business Media, LLC 2011

INTRODUCTION

As anyone who has taken a dog for a walk knows, physical movement stimulates bowel function. More vigorous physical activity, including running, can stimulate bowel activity to the point of diarrhea. In this chapter, we will discuss the mechanisms behind this "runner's diarrhea" and some management options.

English terms for diarrhea suggest the association with running: "the runs" or "the trots."

INCIDENCE

The incidence of running-related diarrhea is at best roughly estimated. These estimates are based on self-reported questionnaires which are completed by participants at race events. Symptoms specific to diarrhea are not often differentiated from other lower GI tract symptoms such as bloating, cramping, urge to defecate, or defecation. Up to 62% of runners experience the urge to have a bowel movement during training [1–3]. Compared to non-runner controls, runners have more frequent and looser bowel movements [4]. The urge to defecate halts more runs than any other single reason to stop. The intensity of the run augments the problem and women seem to be somewhat more susceptible to this than men [5].

EXERCISE EFFECTS ON GASTROINTESTINAL PHYSIOLOGY

Medical practitioners are accustomed to normal and pathologic physiology in the resting state. However, profound physiologic changes affect all organs when subjected to intense or prolonged exercise. This section seeks to describe some of these changes as they affect the gastrointestinal system so as to help the practitioner appreciate potential clinical circumstances for active patients.

Gastrointestinal blood flow can be sharply reduced during exercise due to rapid fluid shifts and possibly ensuing dehydration. Splanchnic blood flow can be reduced by 60–70% at moderate exercise workloads and 80% at maximal workloads [6, 7]. Additionally, increased blood viscosity, erythrocyte deformability, and increased platelet aggregation may further reduce splanchnic blood flow [8]. Combined, and at higher workloads, these lead to mucosal ischemic injury which manifests as intestinal mucosal dysfunction.

Numerous changes taking place in the gastrointestinal tract may contribute to the development of running-related diarrhea. Intestinal motility, as measured by colonic transit time, can be accelerated, decelerated, or unchanged. Studies demonstrate conflicting results, possibly a reflection of varied study protocols [9]. A recent study using pH telemetry did not demonstrate any difference between symptomatic and asymptomatic athletes. The authors therefore suggested that the diarrhea experienced by the symptomatic athletes needs to be explained by an alternate mechanism [10].

Mechanical turbulence and emulsification of the bowel contents may occur from the vertical movement of running [11]. The deceleration forces that occur upon landing are estimated to be twice as much as the forces experienced by cyclists. Consequently, presuming these decelerative forces contribute to stool emulsification, runners experience more lower GI symptoms than do cyclists [2]. It is unclear exactly how much this phenomenon contributes to the development of the runner's diarrhea.

Neuroendocrine alterations are implicated to affect the GI tract. Plasma concentrations of hormones that are known to affect secretion, absorption, and motility at rest are altered during exercise. These hormones include vasoactive intestinal polypeptide, gastrin, secretin, pancreatic polypeptide, neurokinin A, pancreastatin, and motilin [12]. However it is unclear if these hormone alterations directly contribute to the clinical syndrome associated with runner's diarrhea [13].

Lower GI mucosal breech results in leak of endotoxin into the portal circulation at higher levels of exercise intensity. Increased permeability was demonstrated using a ^{51}Cr-labeled ethylenediaminetetraacetic acid marker [14]. This "leaky gut" allows for entry of lipopolysaccharides (LPS) into the portal circulation [15]. This powerful endotoxin further contributes to the release of cytokines such as tumor necrosis factor alpha, interleukin 6, C-reactive protein, and other acute-phase reactants [16].

Nutritional habits may contribute to runner's diarrhea. Sports drinks and gels containing carbohydrate concentrations exceeding 7–10% may create an osmotic gradient that either impairs proximal water absorption or attracts water across the colonic mucosal semi-permeable membrane [17]. High-fiber and high glycemic index foods may do the same thing. Caffeine is often used before long races for its effect on fat metabolism, but an inadvertent laxative effect may prevail.

CLINICAL MANAGEMENT

As a clinician taking care of a runner who is experiencing diarrhea, the most important initial question to address is whether this is "runner's diarrhea" or another condition that simply manifested in the runner

[18]. Various gastrointestinal conditions can present with diarrhea that is incidental to an episode of running. These include ischemic, infectious, and toxic etiologies. Ingested food, medication, or supplements may also cause diarrhea. Inflammatory bowel disease, biliary or pancreatic disorders, and irritable bowel syndrome are included in the differential diagnosis. Even systemic disease may present with altered colonic function.

In 2009, an algorithm was published to serve as a guide to the approach of athletes with lower GI symptoms [18].

Once the diagnosis of runner's diarrhea is made, the next step is addressing how to manage these athletes. Treatment with low doses of loperamide in addition to changing the training regimen is key.

Oral rehydration solutions designed for GI losses rather than the ones formulated for replacing sweat losses should be utilized. If a significant degree of dehydration exists, replacement should be based on laboratory evaluation of electrolytes. NSAIDs should be avoided, and advice can be given to moderate osmotic loads to the gut before and during running.

Physicians can model appropriate infection control measures such as hand washing and use of gloves.

RACE MANAGEMENT

Race coordinators should work toward providing appropriate hydration solutions that are not contaminated as well as adequate numbers of toileting facilities and good hand sanitizer. Coordinators routinely carry out measures to diminish heat-associated illnesses and should continue to follow ACSM guidelines [19].

TRAINING IMPLICATIONS

In general, an initial reduction of training intensity followed by gradual resumption of previous levels of exertion should be encouraged. Cross-training may allow continued development of aerobic capacity with fewer GI symptoms as the gut becomes conditioned to the exertion being trained for. Sports psychology approaches and mental imagery may allow peak performance with less anxiety and associated psychophysiologic GI distress.

Pre-race diets should be limited in calorie content and in the amount of osmotically active materials. Race fluids with large numbers of osmoles are not suitable for these situations, even though they might be easily digested during a non-race day event and are typically advertised as light weight sources of high-energy value.

Prior to beginning an event, an attempt to evacuate should be made. Starting a race with an adequate level of hydration is also important.

Finally, polycythemia, which may develop as a result of being trained at high altitude or by using erythropoietin, may aggravate mesenteric ischemia, which may compromise bowel perfusion and can manifest as hematochezia. It would seem prudent to avoid this additional risk.

CONCLUSION

Gastrointestinal disturbances adversely affect many runners. Numerous physiologic changes are proposed to explain these commonly experienced symptoms. Physicians caring for these recreational and occasionally elite athletes would be well advised to familiarize themselves with these running-related effects. Simple management strategies that can reduce the runner's debilitating symptoms can be recommended.

REFERENCES

1. Sullivan SN, Wong C. Runner's diarrhea. Different patterns and associated factors. J Clin Gastroenterol 1992;14(2):101–104.
2. Peters HP, Bos M, Seebregts L, et al. Gastrointestinal symptoms in long-distance runners, cyclists, and triathletes: prevalence, medication, and etiology. Am J Gastroenterol 1999;94:1570–1581.
3. Halvorsen FA, Lyng J, Glomsaker T, Ryland S. Gastrointestinal disturbances in marathon runners. Br J Sports Med 1990;24:266–268.
4. Sullivan SN, Wong C. Does running cause gastrointestinal symptoms? A survey of 93 randomly selected runners compared with controls. NZ Med J 1994;107: 328–330.
5. Riddoch C, Trinick T. Gastrointestinal disturbances in marathon runners. Br J Sports Med 1988;22(2):71–74.
6. Rowell LB, Blackmon JR, Bruce RA. Indocyanine green clearance and estimated hepatic blood flow during mild to maximal exercise in upright man. J Clin Invest 1964;43:1677–1690.
7. Clausen JP. Effect of physical training on cardiovascular adjustments to exercise in man. Physiol Rev 1977;57:779–815.
8. Vandewalle H, Lacombe C, Lelievre JC, et al. Blood viscosity after a 1-h submaximal exercise with and without drinking. Int J Sports Med 1988;9(2):104–107.
9. Strid H, Simren M. The effects of physical activity on the gastrointestinal tract. Int Sport Med J 2005;6(3):151–161.
10. Rao KA, Yazaki E, Evans DF, Carbon R. Objective evaluation of small bowel and colonic transit time using pH telemetry in athletes with gastrointestinal symptoms. Br J Sports Med 2004;38:482–487.
11. Rehrer NJ, Meijer GA. Biomechanical vibration of the abdominal region during running and bicycling. J Sports Med Phys Fitness 1991;31(2):231–234.
12. O'Connor AM, Johnston CF, Buchanan KD, et al. Circulating gastrointestinal hormone changes in marathon running. Int J Sports Med 1995;16:283-287.

13. Peters HPF, vanBerge-Henegouwen, Devries WR, et al. Potential benefits and hazards of physical activity and exercise on the gastrointestinal tract. Gut 2001;48:435–439.
14. Oktedalen O, Lunde OC, Opstad PK, Aabakken L, Kvernebo K. Changes in the gastrointestinal mucosa after long-distance running. Scand J Gastroenterol 1992;27:270–274.
15. Brok-Utne JG, Gaffin SL, Wells MT, et al. Endotoxaemia in exhausted runners after a long-distance race. S Afr Med J 1988;73:533–536.
16. Jeukendrup AE, Vet-Joop K, Stegen JHJC, et al. Relationship between gastro-intestinal complaints and endotoxaemia, cytokine release and the acute-phase reaction during and after a long-distance triathlon in highly trained men. Clin Sci 2000;98:47–55.
17. Rehrer NJ, Janssen GM, Brouns F, et al. Fluid intake and gastrointestinal problems in runners competing in a 25-km race and a marathon. Int J Sports Med 1989;10(Suppl 1):S22–S25.
18. Ho GWK. Lower gastrointestinal distress in endurance athletes. Curr Sports Med Rep 2009;8(2):85–91.
19. Armstrong LE, et al. Exertional heat illness during training and competition. MSSE 2007;39(3):556–572.

25 Evaluation of Patients with Diarrhea and Timing of Referral

Chami Amaratunge, MD and Joseph H. Sellin, MD

CONTENTS

INTRODUCTION
EVALUATION OF PATIENT WITH DIARRHEA
EVALUATION BY PRIMARY CARE
  PHYSICIANS
EVALUATION BY GASTROENTEROLOGISTS
ROLE OF ENDOSCOPY
EVALUATION FOR BILE ACID
  MALABSORPTION
EVALUATION FOR SMALL INTESTINAL
  BACTERIAL OVERGROWTH (SIBO)
REFERENCES

Summary

Diarrhea is a universal human experience, that is, a symptom and not a disease (Schiller LR, Sellin JH. Approach to a patient with symptoms and signs: diarrhea. In: Sleisenger and Fordtran's gastrointestinal and liver disease, 9th edn. Philadelphia, PA: Saunders, Elsevier, 2010, pp. 159–186). Most patients with diarrhea can be managed successfully as outpatients; however, more than 450,000 hospital admissions each year are for gastroenteritis (Schiller LR, Sellin JH. Approach to a patient with symptoms and signs: diarrhea. In: Sleisenger and Fordtran's gastrointestinal and liver disease, 9th

From: *Diarrhea, Clinical Gastroenterology*
Edited by: S. Guandalini, H. Vaziri, DOI 10.1007/978-1-60761-183-7_25
© Springer Science+Business Media, LLC 2011

edn. Philadelphia, PA: Saunders, Elsevier, 2010, pp. 159–186). The evaluation of patients with diarrhea is complex. A detailed and carefully taken history is essential to aid in the classification of diarrhea. Appropriately defining and classifying diarrhea is an essential first step that provides the clinician a framework for approaching diagnostic and therapeutic options. There are several methods to classify diarrhea and no single method of classification is ideal. The most frequently used methods of classification are as follows: by time course (acute or chronic), volume (large or small), pathophysiology (secretory or osmotic), stool characteristics (watery, fatty, inflammatory), and/or epidemiology (travel related, immune suppression, epidemic). Based on above classification methods, a rational approach can be used by the primary care physician to further manage patients with diarrhea, including when to consider referral to a gastroenterologist.

Key Words: Diarrhea management, Hospitalization, Diarrhea therapy, Patient referral

INTRODUCTION

Appropriately defining and classifying diarrhea is an essential first step that provides the clinician a framework for approaching diagnostic and therapeutic options [1]. Diarrhea can be classified in several ways (see also Chapter 1) and no single method of classification is ideal. Classifications are only helpful if they point to an efficient and effective diagnostic approach. The most frequently used methods of classification are as follows: by time course (acute or chronic), volume (large or small), pathophysiology (secretory or osmotic), stool characteristics (watery, fatty, inflammatory), and/or epidemiology (travel related, immune suppression, epidemic) (see Fig. 25.1 and Chapters 1, 2, and 18).

Diarrhea lasting for more than 4 weeks is chronic. While certain infectious agents can cause a prolonged diarrhea in immune competent patients, the etiology is usually not infectious. It has been estimated that 5–7% of the population has an episode of acute diarrhea each year and that 3–5% have chronic diarrhea that lasts more than 4 weeks [2]. This chapter will focus on chronic diarrhea, with a particular emphasis on adults. As for pediatric patients, in 2003 the Center for Disease Control (CDC) put forth new recommendations for the management of acute pediatric diarrhea in both the outpatient and inpatient settings including indication for referral [3]. Table 25.1 outlines the indications for medical evaluation of children with acute diarrhea. The report also includes information on assessment of dehydration and what steps should be taken to treat adequately (see Table 25.2).

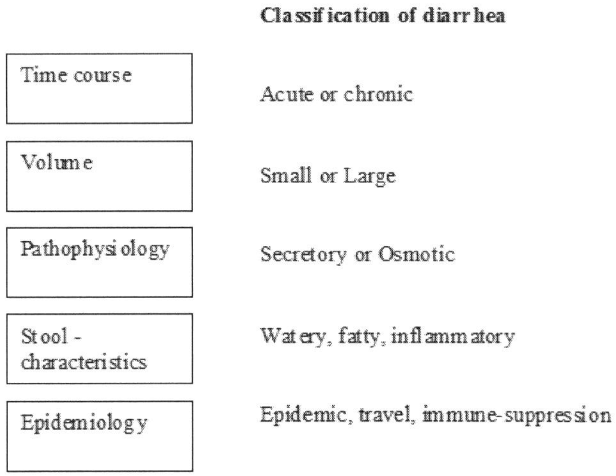

Chapter 25 / Evaluation of Patients with Diarrhea and Timing of Referral 433

Classification of diarrhea

Time course	Acute or chronic
Volume	Small or Large
Pathophysiology	Secretory or Osmotic
Stool - characteristics	Watery, fatty, inflammatory
Epidemiology	Epidemic, travel, immune-suppression

Fig. 25.1. Most frequently used method of classification of diarrhea.

Table 25.1
Indications for medical evaluation of children with acute diarrhea (adapted from [3])

Age <3 months
Weight <8 kg
History of premature birth, chronic medical conditions, or concurrent illness
Fever ≥38°C for infants <3 months or ≥39°C for children 3–36 months
Visible blood in the stool
High output diarrhea
Persistent emesis
Signs of dehydration as reported by caregiver
– sunken eyes, decreased tears, dry mucous membranes, decreased urine
    output
Mental status changes
Inadequate response to or caregiver unable to administer ORT

EVALUATION OF PATIENT WITH DIARRHEA

History

The initial approach to patient with a presenting complaint of chronic diarrhea is a carefully taken medical history. Questions should focus on discriminating among watery, inflammatory, and fatty diarrheas. Physicians should ask the relationship of diarrhea to meals, fasting,

Table 25.2
Treatment of dehydration due to diarrhea (adapted from [3])

Degree of dehydration	Rehydration therapy	Replacement of losses
Minimal or no dehydration	Not applicable	<10 kg body weight: 60–120 ml ORS for each diarrhea stool or vomiting episode >10 kg body weight: 120–140 ml ORS for each diarrheal stool or vomiting episode
Mild to moderate dehydration	ORS, 50–100 ml/kg body weight over 3–4 h	Same
Severe dehydration	Lactated Ringer's solution or normal saline in 20 ml/kg body weight intravenous amounts until perfusion and mental status improve Then administer 100 ml/kg body weight ORS over 4 h or 5% dextrose $\frac{1}{2}$ normal saline intravenously at twice maintenance fluid rates	Same, if unable to drink administer through NG tube or administer 5% dextrose $\frac{1}{4}$ normal saline with 20 mEq/l potassium chloride intravenously

urgency, and fecal incontinence. Associated symptoms of abdominal pain, fever, nausea, vomiting, and cramps should be noted. Epidemiologic clues such as travel history, sources of patient's drinking water, antibiotic use, hospitalizations, and identifiable foodborne illnesses should be elicited. Other key historical information includes patient demographics, medication history (with particular attention to over-the-counter medications), prior abdominal surgeries, prior radiation therapy, and diet. Age may shape a differential diagnosis; younger patients may raise the possibility of inflammatory bowel disease (IBD), while microscopic colitis is more likely to present in the middle-aged or elderly. Alternative and complementary medications may be important factors. Given a particular American proclivity to orthorexia, dietary history should be defined, including milk and lactose-containing products, high fructose corn syrup as found in sodas, and caffeine. Although coffee is the obvious caffeine-containing product to identify, it is important to recognize the emerging popularity of energy drinks such as Red Bull that may also be a factor in diarrhea.

The clinician should also inquire about the association of diarrhea with systemic and metabolic diseases. Both diabetes and hyperthyroidism may commonly contribute to diarrhea. However, relative zebras such as amyloidosis, IgA deficiency, or common variable immunodeficiency need to be considered. If clinical suspicion is high, the potential of secondary gain must be explored. For instance, clues such as fixation with body image should raise the possibility of laxative abuse.

A careful history can assist in distinguishing irritable bowel syndrome (IBS) from other functional and organic disorders. Classically, the major discriminants between functional and organic disease are weight loss and nocturnal diarrhea. Interestingly, the frequency of bowel movements or the presence of tenesmus is not a reliable indicator of organic disease.

Physical Examination

In patients presenting with chronic diarrhea, the physical exam does not usually help in determining a cause of diarrhea, but is beneficial in determining the severity of the illness, particularly in the pediatric age group. The presence of fever, low blood pressure, or orthostasis suggests significant volume depletion. Findings of dehydration such as dry mucus membranes and decreased skin turgor should be noted. Abdominal examination should determine the presence or absence of bowel sounds, abdominal distention, localized or generalized tenderness, masses, and enlarged liver. A detailed rectal examination can provide information regarding rectal incontinence or perhaps perianal lesions associated with Crohn's disease.

Occasionally, physical exam findings can provide clues to etiology of diarrhea. Dermatologic changes may point to an underlying etiology. Dermatitis herpetiformis indicates underlying celiac disease (see Chapter 12), whereas erythema nodosum, pyoderma gangrenosum, and psoriasis may raise the possibility of IBD (Chapter 3). Physical exam findings of hyperthyroidism such as tremor, goiter, and exopthalmosis should be documented. Lymphadenopathy might suggest acquired immune deficiency syndrome or lymphoma.

EVALUATION BY PRIMARY CARE PHYSICIANS

Diagnostic algorithms for diarrhea are based on expert opinion rather than evidence-based medicine. Recently, a largely evidence-based guideline for the treatment of children with acute diarrhea has been published [4], and the reader is referred to this publication. Most of the tests needed for a first approach to adult patients with chronic diarrhea are easily obtained by primary care physicians, while a few are best performed by gastroenterologists. Routine laboratory tests such as complete blood count and chemistries should be obtained initially. If concerned about metabolic disease, such as diabetes or hyperthyroidism, TSH and hemoglobin A1C should also be ordered. The recognition of the expanding clinical spectrum of celiac disease makes it reasonable to aggressively test for this possibility with appropriate serological testing (see Chapter 6). The etiology of anemia should be clearly defined. Vitamin B_{12} deficiency may point to ileal disease. Although a Schilling's test is the classic method to elucidate the specific mechanism of B_{12} deficiency, it is not readily available in many areas. Folate deficiency may suggest mucosal disease or small bowel bacterial overgrowth. Iron deficiency in the absence of evidence of intestinal blood loss may indicate celiac disease. The routine testing for the possibility of a neuroendocrine tumor as an etiology for chronic diarrhea is not recommended. Likewise, the value of testing for IBD serologies has not been established in the routine workup of chronic diarrhea (see Table 25.3) [5].

A hallmark of evaluation of diarrhea includes stool analysis, either with a random sample (see Fig. 25.2) or a timed collection. A timed stool collection for 48–72 h may be a logistic challenge for the patient, laboratory, and physician, but this can provide invaluable information that can guide further diagnostic studies. Patients should continue their regular activities and should consume a regular diet. Only essential medications should be taken and anti-diarrheals should be held. Stool

Table 25.3
Laboratory evaluation of chronic diarrhea: stool analysis

Test	Etiology
Stool weight >500 g	Hormone/metabolic-driven diarrhea
Fecal occult blood	Inflammation, malignancy
Fecal leukocytes	Inflammation in colon
Fecal calprotectin/lactoferrin	Inflammation in colon and/or small bowel
Stool electrolytes: Na, K,	Osmotic versus secretory diarrhea
Stool pH	Carbohydrate malabsorption
Laxative screen	Factitious diarrhea
Fecal fat/Sudan stain	Steatorrhea

Chapter 25 / Evaluation of Patients with Diarrhea and Timing of Referral 437

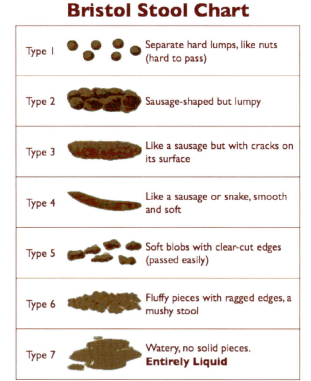

Fig. 25.2. Representative aide to classify different forms of stool.

can be collected in commercially available collection units that allow the separation of stool and urine and fits onto a commode. The stool can be analyzed for weight, sodium, potassium, magnesium, pH, fat content, and laxatives.

Stool weight may be the most useful parameter obtained from a timed stool collection. Significant increases (>1000 g) may dictate workup for a hormonally driven diarrhea. Interestingly, about 20% of timed stool collections reveal a normal weight and therefore necessarily refine the workup of diarrhea [6].

By measuring stool electrolytes and osmolarity, one can calculate an osmotic gap, osmolality that is not accounted for by the measured electrolytes. Stool osmotic gap is calculated by subtracting twice the sum of sodium and potassium concentration from 290 mOsm/kg. A significant gap (>50 mOsm) implies an osmotic diarrhea, whereas a minimal gap is consistent with a secretory diarrhea (see Table 25.4 and Fig. 25.3). Stool pH can provide information about the possibility of carbohydrate

Table 25.4
Stool osmotic gap

Stool Osmotic gap = stool osmolality $-[2 \times ([Na^+] + [K^+])]$
Stool osmolality = colonic fluid osmolality which is in equilibrium with body fluids, approximately 290 mOsm/kg

Stool osmotic gap <50 mOsm/kg → suggests secretory diarrhea
Stool osmotic gap >100 mOsm/kg → suggests osmotic diarrhea

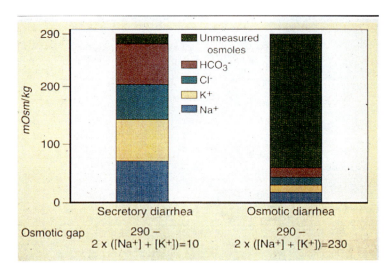

Fig. 25.3. In secretory diarrhea, almost all of the osmotic activity is accounted for by electrolytes. In osmotic diarrhea, electrolytes account for only small part of osmotic activity; unmeasured osmoles account for most of osmotic activity.

malabsorption. Carbohydrates that reach the colon are fermented by bacteria, resulting in a stool pH that is acidic, usually below 6.

Fecal fat output can be measured quantitatively by timed collection or qualitatively by Sudan stain of a random sample. Although historically, patients were put on a 100 g fat diet during this type of collection, this is rarely done these days. Steatorrhea is defined by excess fat loss in stool, greater than 7 g, which can be due to maldigestion (e.g., pancreatic insufficiency) or malabsorption, which usually point to a mucosal or luminal abnormality, most commonly celiac disease. The degree of steatorrhea and fat concentration tends to higher for maldigestion than malabsorption of fat.

The presence of fecal leukocytes signifies inflammation in the colon leading to diarrhea caused by colitis, malignancy, or infection. Accurate evaluation for fecal leukocytes requires an adept, prompt examination of the stool sample; in an outpatient setting that may not be possible. In contrast, fecal calprotectin and lactoferrin are stable non-invasive markers of inflammation in the small intestine and/or colon. Calprotectin is an abundant neutrophil protein found in both plasma and stool that is markedly elevated in infectious and inflammatory conditions, including IBD. Studies have shown that fecal calprotectin correlates well with histological inflammation as detected by colonoscopy with biopsies. Fecal calprotectin has been shown to consistently differentiate IBD from irritable bowel syndrome because it has excellent negative predictive value in ruling out IBD in undiagnosed, symptomatic patients [7, 8].

EVALUATION BY GASTROENTEROLOGISTS

Although a significant part of the workup for chronic diarrhea can be completed by a primary care physician, some diagnostic testing may be more effectively accomplished by a gastroenterologist. Endoscopy may establish a diagnosis of microscopic colitis (see Chapter 5) or inflammatory bowel disease (see Chapter 3). There has been an increasing interest in the possibility that bile acid malabsorption or small intestinal bacterial overgrowth may be important etiologic factors in chronic diarrhea. Evaluation for these abnormalities is complex, complicated, and controversial and probably should be pursued by a gastroenterologist (see Chapter 11).

ROLE OF ENDOSCOPY

Direct visualization of colonic mucosa and biopsy are helpful in ruling out inflammatory bowel disease, ischemic colitis, collagenous and microscopic colitis, and malignancy. In studies from tertiary referral centers, colonoscopy yields a diagnosis in approximately 15% of cases [9, 10]. The most common diagnoses found in large series are either inflammatory bowel disease (3–10%) or microscopic colitis (8–15%). A consensus is lacking on whether colonoscopy or flexible sigmoidoscopy should be the initial endoscopic test in patients with chronic diarrhea. The advantage of the latter is that there is no need for sedation, preparation is simpler, and it has less risk and costs. In patients with suspected inflammatory bowel disease, malignancy, and/or gross/occult bleeding, colonoscopy may be preferable. In patients over 50 years of age, the need for colon cancer screening may influence the choice of procedures. Pathologic processes such as ulcerative colitis tend to be diffuse and can be diagnosed on flexible sigmoidoscopy alone.

However, if a flexible sigmoidoscopy is non-diagnostic and symptoms persist, colonoscopy should be performed. There has yet to be a prospective randomized study of the utility of colonoscopy versus flexible sigmoidoscopy for chronic diarrhea evaluation. Clinical decision making should be individualized [11].

The role of upper gastrointestinal endoscopy (or EGD, for esophago-gastro-duodenoscopy) in the evaluation of chronic diarrhea has not been thoroughly evaluated. The most common diagnostic yield from EGD is celiac disease, but other less common enteropathies, such as food allergic or eosinophilic gastroenteropathy, amyloidosis, or Whipple's disease, may only be confirmed by small bowel biopsy. In general, a positive celiac serology should be followed with a small bowel biopsy to confirm the diagnosis before embarking on the rigors of a gluten-free diet (see Chapter 6).

EVALUATION FOR BILE ACID MALABSORPTION

The role of bile acid malabsorption in chronic diarrhea has become a matter of significant basic and clinical interest. In the setting of either ileal resection or disease, it is well established that the enterohepatic circulation is disrupted; bile acids enter the colon in increasing concentration and stimulate a secretory diarrhea [12]. However, it has been suggested that significant bile acid malabsorption may occur in the absence of obvious ileal abnormalities, i.e., idiopathic bile acid malabsorption (IBAM). This diagnosis has been based on two related observations: (i) an abnormal selenium-75-homocholic acid taurine (SeHCAT) test [13] and (ii) a favorable response to a therapeutic trial of a bile acid-binding resin.

SeHCAT is an orally administered radio-labeled synthetic bile acid. Because its ileal and hepatic transport is similar to that of cholic acid, SeHCAT has been used as an indicator of bile acid absorption and malabsorption. Bile acid malabsorption was initially reported as a rare cause of chronic diarrhea; however, after the introduction of SeHCAT as a diagnostic tool, bile acid malabsorption was reported more frequently. Because the test is not available in the United States, there has been something of a transatlantic divide in the workup for bile acid malabsorption. It has been suggested that SeHCAT test has limited value in the routine evaluation of chronic diarrhea given that some studies showing high false-positive and false-negative values. In the absence of SeHCAT testing, the diagnosis of IBAM is often made after a therapeutic trial of cholestyramine or other resins. However, the anti-diarrheal effects of cholestyramine may not be very specific [14].

One troubling aspect of the diagnosis of IBAM is the lack of credible evidence for a pathophysiologic abnormality. Although there are rare genetic abnormalities of the ileal bile acid transporter (see Chapter 9), no such defect has consistently been found in adults with a diagnosis of IBAM. The natural history of IBAM is variable and there may be frequent spontaneous resolution of the malabsorption, raising the possibility that the bile acid malabsorption may be an epiphenomenon. However, recent studies have suggested that it may be more a case of excessive bile acid synthesis rather than a defective ileal transport mechanism. The alteration in bile acid metabolism may be related to defective release of intestinal fibroblast growth factor 19 [15]. If further studies confirm this finding, it would open up an array of other tests to establish a more reliable diagnosis of IBAM and rationalize our approach to this abnormality.

EVALUATION FOR SMALL INTESTINAL BACTERIAL OVERGROWTH (SIBO)

Similar to the wave of enthusiasm for the diagnosis of IBAM in chronic diarrhea, small intestinal bacterial overgrowth has been implicated in the etiology of chronic diarrhea with increasing frequency. Because there is no widely available gold standard for the diagnosis of SIBO (see Chapter 11), tests with limited sensitivity and/or specificity have been used to establish a diagnosis of SIBO [14]. Hydrogen breath tests are particularly attractive because they are simple and non-invasive. A hydrogen signal in expired breath results from bacterial metabolism of carbohydrate. This occurs in one of two conditions: (i) malabsorption of a sugar in the small intestine with subsequent metabolism by colonic bacteria or (ii) accumulation of a significant bacterial population in the small intestine, with bacterial metabolism of a test sugar occurring before it can be fully absorbed.

Unfortunately, hydrogen breath tests may lead to both under diagnosis and, more frequently, over diagnosis of SIBO. Two test sugars are generally used: glucose and lactulose. Lactulose is particularly unreliable; because it is a non-absorbable disaccharide, it predictably reaches the colon and produces an H_2 signal. Because small bowel transit time is variable and in patients with diarrhea be as rapid as 15 min, it is not feasible to use the timing of H_2 peak to diagnose SIBO [16]. The accuracy of the breath test can be improved considerably by combining it with a nuclear medicine intestinal transit scan, which establishes a reliable, independent indicator of the position of the test sugar along the GI tract in relation to the timing of the H_2 signal [17].

REFERENCES

1. Schiller LR, Sellin JH. Approach to a patient with symptoms and signs: diarrhea. In: Sleisenger and Fordtran's gastrointestinal and liver disease. Saunders Elsevier. Philadelphia, PA. 9th edn. 2010, pp. 159–186.
2. Schiller LR, et al. Diarrhea and malabsorption in the elderly. Gastroenterol Clin N Am 2009; 38:481–502.
3. King CK, et al. Managing acute gastroenteritis among children: oral rehydration, maintenance, and nutritional therapy. MMWR Recomm Rep 2003; 52(RR-16): 1–16.
4. Guarino A, Albano F, Ashkenazi S, Gendrel D, Hoekstra JH, Shamir R, Szajewska H. ESPGHAN/ESPID evidence-based guidelines for the management of acute gastroenteritis in children in Europe. Expert Working Group. J Pediatr Gastroenterol Nutr 2008; 46(5):619–621.
5. Gupta A, Derbes C, Sellin JH. Clinical indications of the use of antineutrophil cytoplasmic antibodies and anti-Saccharomyces cerevisiae antibodies in the evaluation of inflammatory bowel disease at an Academic Medical Center. IBD J 2005; 10:898–902.
6. Sellin J, Unpublished Observations.
7. Konikoff MR, et al. Role of fecal calprotectin as a biomarker of intestinal inflammation in inflammatory bowel disease. Inflamm Bowel Dis 2006; 12(6):524–534.
8. Abraham BP, Thirumurthi S. Clinical significance of inflammatory markers. Curr Gastroenterol Rep 2009; 11(5):360–367.
9. Fine KD, et al. The prevalence, anatomic distribution, and diagnosis of colonic causes of chronic diarrhea. Gastrointest Endosc 2000; 51(3):318–326.
10. Shah RJ, et al. Usefulness of colonoscopy with biopsy in the evaluation of patients with chronic diarrhea. Am J Gastroenterol 2001; 96:1091–1095.
11. ASGE Practice Guideline. Use of Endoscopy in diarrheal illness. Gastrointest Endosc 2006; 54(6):821–822.
12. Hoffman AF, Mangelsdorf DJ, Kliewer SA. Chronic diarrhea due to excessive bile acid synthesis and not defective ileal transport. Clin Gastroenterol Hepatol 2009; 7:1151–1154.
13. Antal B, et al. The bile acid turnover rate assessed with the 75SeHCAT test is stable in chronic diarrhea but slightly decreased in healthy subjects after a long period of time. Dig Dis Sci 2008; 53:2935–2940.
14. Fan X, Sellin JH, et al. Review article: small intestinal bacterial overgrowth, bile acid malabsorption and gluten intolerance as possible causes of chronic watery diarrhea. Aliment Pharmacol Ther 2009; 29(10):1069–1077.
15. Walters JR, Tasleem AM, Omer OS, et. al. A new mechanism for bile acid diarrhea: defective feedback inhibition of bile acid biosynthesis. Clin Gastroenterol Hepatol 2009;1189–1194.
16. Bratten JR, Spanier J, Jones MP. Lactulose breath testing does not discriminate patients with irritable bowel syndrome from healthy controls. Am J Gastroenterol 2008; 103:958–963.
17. Sellin JH, Hart R. Glucose malabsorption associated with rapid intestinal transit. Am J Gastroenterol. 1992;87:584–589.

26 Empiric Treatment of Chronic Diarrhea

*Maria Soriano, MD
and Haleh Vaziri, MD*

CONTENTS

INTRODUCTION
ORAL REHYDRATION SOLUTIONS
DIETARY MODIFICATIONS
TREATMENTS BASED ON A CLINICAL
SETTING OR AFTER A SPECIFIC
DIAGNOSIS IS OBTAINED
REFERENCES

Summary

Diarrhea occurring for 4 or more weeks is deemed chronic. In an ideal world, it would be easy to identify and direct therapy to the underlying pathophysiology that is leading to chronic diarrhea, however, this is not always possible. Oral rehydration solutions play an important role in treating dehydration, which is one of the first aspects of chronic diarrhea that must be dealt with. Various medications can be used to help ameliorate the symptoms of chronic diarrhea or to treat the underlying mechanism involved. Some of these agents include silicates, bulk-forming agents, opiates, enkephalinase inhibitors, anticholinergics, somatostatin analogues, calcium channel blockers, and alpha 2- adrenergic agonists. Lastly, probiotics can be used in treating antibiotic-associated diarrhea, travelers' diarrhea, diarrhea-predominant IBS, ulcerative colitis, and in the prevention

From: *Diarrhea, Clinical Gastroenterology*
Edited by: S. Guandalini, H. Vaziri, DOI 10.1007/978-1-60761-183-7_26
© Springer Science+Business Media, LLC 2011

of pouchitis. For a more detailed discussion of the various treatment options available please refer to the corresponding chapters.

Key Words: Chronic diarrhea, Oral Redydration Solutions (ORS), Silicates, Bulk-forming agents, Opiates, Enkephalinase inhibitors, Anticholinergics, Somatostatin analogues, Calcium channel blockers, Alpha 2 adrenergic agonists, Probiotics

INTRODUCTION

The management of patients with chronic diarrhea, defined as diarrhea lasting 4 or more weeks, can be challenging. Ideally the treatment plan for chronic diarrhea should target the underlying pathophysiology. There are, however, certain circumstances in which empiric therapy can be considered including (1) prior to the completion of the diagnostic evaluation; (2) instances in which a clear diagnosis is not obtained; (3) if there is no specific treatment for the underlying condition or the specific treatment has failed [1]; (4) when a diagnosis is strongly suspected and/or the patient's comorbidities limit the diagnostic evaluation (for example, a patient who develops diarrhea after ileal resection). This chapter will review the treatment options available for patients presenting with chronic diarrhea starting with basic supportive measures, such as hydration and proceeding to specific drug therapies.

ORAL REHYDRATION SOLUTIONS

Maintaining adequate hydration or restoring hydration is the first step in the treatment of diarrheal diseases, and particularly of acute-onset diarrheas. Oral rehydration solutions (ORSs) play an important role in this regard. During the cholera pandemic it was observed that the co-administration of glucose could improve sodium absorption by the intestinal mucosa. This in turn led to the introduction of an ORS by the WHO (World Health Organization) containing sodium 90 mmol/l, potassium 20 mmol/l, and chloride 80 mmol/l. This solution has proved of paramount importance in saving thousands of lives, especially in developing countries and in cases of cholera infection, to the point that it was heralded by *The Lancet* as "potentially the most important medical advance of this century." However, subsequent research showed that a reduced osmolarity solution could be more advantageous in promoting fluid absorption, and thus in 2003, the recommended ORS was reformulated to one of reduced osmolarity, from 311 to 245 mmol/l. This was achieved by decreasing the glucose and sodium chloride concentrations (see Table 26.1). With the use of the reduced osmolarity

Table 26.1
Ingredient concentrations in the reduced osmolarity ORS

Ingredient	g/l	Molecule	mmol/l
(NaCl) Sodium chloride	2.6 (instead of 3.5)	Sodium	75
$C_6H_{12}O_6$ Glucose, anhydrous	13.5 (instead of 20)	Glucose	75
KCL Potassium chloride	1.5	Potassium Chloride	20 65
$Na_3C_6H_5O_7 \cdot 2H_2O$ Trisodium citrate, Dehydrate	2.9	Citrate	10

formula, a reduction of stool output is expected; there may, however, be the potential risk of hyponatremia, which should be monitored for in adult patients with cholera [2]. Outside of cholera, however, such solutions appear to be safe and effective [3]. Cereal-based solutions are newer preparations that may have superior efficacy [4]. Furthermore, in recent years an ORS based on amylase-resistant high amylose maize starch 50 g/l (substituted for glucose) has been tried and found very effective and superior to the low-osmolarity ORS both in children [5] and in adults [6]. It is therefore to be expected that these ORSs will receive more attention in the near future for expanded use.

In most instances of common acute-onset diarrhea in otherwise healthy adults, however, saltine crackers taken with flavored mineral water will meet the patient's hydration requirement. It is important to note that caution should be advised when treating dehydration with sports drinks as they are only effective in replacing mild electrolyte losses that typically occur during exercise and do not have an adequate amount of sodium or nutrients needed to hydrate a patient with diarrhea.

Certain fluids should be avoided when diarrhea is moderate to severe. These include coffee, secondary to its diuretic effect and most soft drinks and sweetened tea or fruit drinks, which can cause an osmotic diarrhea. Appropriate home-prepared drinks include salted rice water, vegetable or chicken soup with salt and salted yogurt-based drinks.

To prepare a homemade cereal-based ORS: $\frac{1}{2}$ cup of dry, precooked baby rice cereal can be mixed with $\frac{1}{4}$ teaspoon of salt in two cups of water.

DIETARY MODIFICATIONS

Dietary modifications can significantly alter the course of certain gastrointestinal conditions. For instance, it is evident that avoidance of lactose or gluten-containing foods can greatly benefit patients with lactose intolerance or celiac disease, respectively. Avoidance of lactose is also advised in cases of extensive small bowel damage, in which case decreasing the delivery of large amounts of lactose to the colon will reduce the subsequent colonic water retention that would normally take place.

In general, however, no dietetic restrictions are needed for most instances of *acute* diarrheas. Lactose intolerance was once thought to be a major problem in infants and children with diarrhea and a reason to delay refeeding milk-based formulas. In reality, and in spite of the common occurrence of reducing substances in the stools of infants with diarrhea, it is believed that lactose intolerance should not be a clinical concern for the vast majority of patients in developed countries, as research has demonstrated that unrestricted diets do not worsen the course or symptoms of mild diarrhea compared with ORSs or intravenous therapy alone (reviewed in [7]). The occurrence of clinically significant lactose intolerance, however, must not be completely disregarded: rarely, and more so in malnourished children, diarrhea may worsen with reintroduction of milk or "normal" formulas. If fecal pH decreases and 1% or more reducing substances are found in the stools, lactose intolerance should at that point be diagnosed and a lactose-free formula employed at least temporarily to prevent persistent diarrhea.

The remainder of this chapter focuses on the empiric treatment approach to the adult patient with *chronic* diarrhea.

TREATMENTS BASED ON A CLINICAL SETTING OR AFTER A SPECIFIC DIAGNOSIS IS OBTAINED

As illustrated in Chapter 25, certain treatments can be implemented in the appropriate clinical setting prior to subjecting the patient to an extensive workup (for example, pancreatic enzyme supplementation in a patient with chronic pancreatitis or the use of bile acid-binding resins after ileal surgery). In other instances, therapy should be initiated only after a specific diagnosis is made (for example, instituting a gluten-free diet after the diagnosis of celiac disease; prescribing clonidine in a patient having "diabetic diarrhea"; starting octreotide for a neuroendocrine tumor-associated diarrhea; administering antibiotics in small

Chapter 26 / Empiric Treatment of Chronic Diarrhea

bowel bacterial overgrowth; or initiating budesonide in a patient with collagenous colitis).

Empiric treatment can be considered if no specific cause is identified.

Antibiotic Therapy

Despite the clear role of empiric antibiotic therapy for acute diarrheal illnesses, particularly in travelers to areas with a high prevalence of infectious diarrhea or in hospitalized patients, there is no such set role in chronic diarrhea. In patients with chronic diarrhea, an empiric trial of antibiotics can be considered if the prevalence of infection is high in the community.

Anti-diarrheal Agents

The mechanism of action of most anti-diarrheal agents involves an interplay between an alteration in intestinal motility, increase of stool consistency, and mild absorptive or anti-secretory effects. These properties work together in aiding the absorption process by keeping fluid in the intestine and thus in contact with the mucosa for a longer period of time. In treating chronic diarrhea, it is of clinical importance to note that *after the fact dosing* is not appropriate. Instead, maximal benefit is achieved from scheduled dosing at bedtime or before meals.

Table 26.2 summarizes some of the agents that can be used as empiric or as a specific treatment of chronic diarrhea, which are reviewed in detail below.

Agents Used as Empiric or Specific Treatment of Chronic Diarrhea

Silicates are very safe medications, which function by binding bacterial enterotoxin. Kaolin and Attapulgite are the two drugs in this group.

Kaopectate: (kaolin + pectin) kaolin is a form of aluminum silicate and pectin is a carbohydrate, which is extracted from the rind of citrus fruit. In combination they bind bacterial toxins in the gastrointestinal (GI) tract and can change stool consistency. Kaopectate contained attapulgite until 2003 at which time its efficacy was questioned by the Food and Drug Administration (FDA). Kaopectate is still available in Canada but in the USA its formulation has been changed to contain bismuth subsalicylate.

Attapulgite: This binds to toxic substances in the GI tract. With limited efficacy, it can be used as an anti-diarrheal agent at a standard dose

Table 26.2
Treatment of Chronic Diarrhea

Drug class	Agent	Dose
Silicates	Kaopectate	30 ml every 30–60 min as needed. Max eight doses daily
Bulk-forming agents	Psyllium	10–20 g daily
	Polycarbophil	5–10 g daily
	Methylcellulose	5–20 g daily
Intraluminal agents	Bismuth	1 fluid ounce or two tablets every 30 min for up to eight doses in a 24-h period
Bile acid resins	Cholestyramine	4 g up to four times a day
	Colestipol	4 g up to four times a day
Opiates	Paregoric	5–10 ml, one to four times a day
	Loperamide	2–4 mg four times a day
	Codeine	15–60 mg four times a day
	Tincture of opium	2–20 drops or 0.6 ml four times a day
	Diphenoxylate	2.5–5 mg four times a day
	Morphine	2–20 mg four times a day
Enkephalinase inhibitor (δ-opiate receptor effects)	Racecadotril	1.5 mg/kg three times a day
Anticholinergics	Hyoscyamine	0.125–0.25 mg six times a day
	Dicyclomine	20 mg four times a day
	Methscopolamine	2.5 mg four times a day
	Glycopyrrolate	1–2 mg two to three times a day
Somatostatin analogue	Octreotide	50–250 μg three times a day
Ca channel blockers	Verapamil	
Alpha 2 adrenergic agonists	Clonidine	0.1–0.3 mg three times a day

of 600 mg up to seven times a day. These agents can be used in tube-fed patients to reduce the diarrhea associated with this type of feeding [8].

Bulk-forming agents are hydrophilic colloids that promote the retention of water by stool and lead to the formation of a gel. Stool fluidity is reduced by altering the texture and increasing the viscosity of the stool.

Chapter 26 / Empiric Treatment of Chronic Diarrhea 449

Bloating and abdominal pain are the most common side effects experienced. Patients suspected of having any type of stricture of their GI tract should not be treated with these agents. Also of note, even though these agents are not absorbed systemically, they may decrease the effect of other medications like warfarin, digoxin, and potassium-sparing diuretics [9].

Psyllium is a natural soluble fiber that is derived from the husks of the seeds of the plant, *Plantago ovata*. It is a bulk-forming agent that absorbs water in the colon and adds firmness to the stool. The change from watery to semi-formed stools will lead to improvement in patient symptomatology and will result in an increase in stool weight. Psyllium has been shown to improve fecal consistency and viscosity in subjects with experimentally induced secretory diarrhea using phenolphthalein [10]. It has become part of the treatment plan implemented in a variety of diseases including irritable bowel syndrome (IBS), chronic diarrhea of unknown etiology, fecal incontinence of loose stool [11], diarrhea associated with HIV infection [12], diarrhea associated with tube feeding [8] (without clogging the feeding tube at therapeutic doses) [13], and collagenous colitis [14].

In a pilot study, Murphy et al showed that psyllium effectively controlled radiation-induced diarrhea by decreasing stool frequency and symptom severity [15].

Methylcellulose is a semi-synthetic fiber derived from cellulose. It is non-digestible, non-toxic, and non-allergenic. It increases stool bulk and regulates its consistency by sequestering water from liquid stool giving it a role in the treatment of both diarrhea and constipation.

Polycarbophil is a semi-synthetic fiber with marked hydrophilic capacity in a dilute, alkaline environment. It has been used in the treatment of non-specific diarrhea and IBS. It appears to be safe with a high therapeutic index and usually does not interfere with digestion or absorption when used in its recommended dose. However, its beneficial effect may take several days to manifest [16]. Polycarbophil appears to increase colonic transit time in patients with IBS-diarrhea predominant thus decreasing bowel frequency. An improvement in the abdominal pain associated with this syndrome has also been observed [17].

It has also been shown to decrease nighttime soiling in patients who have undergone colectomy with ileal J-pouch anal anastomosis for ulcerative colitis [18].

Bismuth subsalicylate has been used for many decades to treat diarrheal illnesses. Although it is less effective than loperamide, it can decrease the number of unformed stools when compared to placebo [19]. Its mechanism of action is unknown, but it appears that the salicylate moiety may function via anti-secretory action. It also has bactericidal and anti-inflammatory properties. Its use in the treatment of microscopic colitis has been demonstrated, although with limited supporting data [20, 21].

Bismuth subsalicylate is a very safe option for treating mild diarrhea and has been used as an effective prophylactic/treatment agent for traveler's diarrhea in adults, but its use in children has been questioned secondary to the theoretical risk of developing Reye's syndrome, encephalopathy and salicylate intoxication with prolonged use [22, 23]. Therefore, it is not recommended in children less than 3 years of age and in those with viral illnesses. Other potential adverse effects that can be seen with its use include tinnitus and hyperpigmentation of the tongue and stool. It is recommended that the treatment period should not exceed 6–8 weeks and it should be followed by 8 weeks of bismuth-free intervals to decrease the rare incidence of bismuth toxicity [24].

Cholestyramine is a bile acid binder, which can be used for bile acid-induced diarrhea occurring after cholecystectomy or after small bowel resection [25–28]. It has also been used for treatment of pseudomembranous colitis [29–31], microscopic colitis [32–38], and chronic diarrhea associated with diabetes [39]. It has been shown to provide rapid and adequate relief of symptoms in diarrhea secondary to colitis not otherwise specified [34]. Case reports of patients with quinidine-induced diarrhea that have benefited from treatment with cholestyramine have been published [40]. In human immunodeficiency virus (HIV) patients with chronic diarrhea that is unresponsive to conventional anti-diarrheal treatment, a trial of bile acid sequestrating agents can sometimes be helpful, especially if they have bile acid malabsorption [41, 42].

Of note, bile acid-binding resins can bind other medications taken concurrently thus retarding their absorption. It is therefore important to dose these medications separately. High doses should be avoided given the risk of steatorrhea.

Budesonide is a glucocorticoid, which has a high affinity for the glucocorticoid receptor but undergoes extensive first-pass metabolism in the liver resulting in minimal systemic action. It has been used in several disease processes that respond to steroids with good outcomes, but with less systemic adverse effects.

Budesonide is approved by the FDA for use in patients with mild to moderate Crohn's disease of the ileum or ascending colon to maintain clinical remission for a 3-month period of time.

It has also proven beneficial in inducing disease remission in patients with microscopic colitis [43]. However, its benefit on a long-term basis has not been investigated well and disease relapse has been observed after its cessation [44].

Chapter 26 / Empiric Treatment of Chronic Diarrhea 451

Opiates and opiate-like medications are the most effective, non-specific anti-diarrheal treatment available. Whether the primary mechanism by which these agents exert their effect is via their anti-secretory properties versus their slowing of bowel transit is controversial [45–49]. Intestinal transit is mostly affected in the stomach and proximal intestine but in therapeutic doses, opiates also work in the proximal colon, rectum, and at the anal sphincter [50, 51].

Caution is advised when using anti-peristaltic agents in cases of infectious diarrhea as the resulting stasis may increase microorganism invasion and prolong the carrier state. This concern originated with a study showing prolonged fever in subjects with induced shigellosis who received lomotil [52]. The risk of toxic megacolon precludes the use of these agents in severe inflammatory bowel disease (IBD).

Another concern when using opiates and their derivatives is addiction. In most instances, physicians do not prescribe opiates at the dose and frequency that is needed to treat chronic diarrhea. Tolerance to the anti-diarrheal effect of these agents is rare and the effective dose remains the same for months to years [53]. With the exception of patients with a history of drug abuse, these medications are rarely abused when carefully monitored by a health-care practitioner. Loperamide and diphenoxylate should be prescribed first as they have the least addiction potential [54].

In addition to their risk of addiction, other side effects of these agents are respiratory depression, central nervous system (CNS) depression and delayed gastric emptying with resulting nausea and vomiting. Drugs in this category include paregoric, loperamide, codeine, tincture of opium, diphenoxylate with atropine, and racecadotril.

Paregoric: Also known as camphorated tincture of opium, paregoric has been used for many years for the treatment of diarrhea. It should not be confused with uncamphorated tincture of opium (usually referred to as "tincture of opium") as there is a difference between the two. Tincture of opium has 10 mg of morphine in each milliliter while paregoric has only 0.4 mg of morphine in each milliliter making it necessary to use larger quantities for the treatment of diarrhea.

Loperamide: Available over the counter, as imodium, loperamide is chemically related to narcotics, such as morphine. It does not, however, possess any of the narcotic analgesic properties or their euphoric effects even when used at high doses given its inability to cross the blood–brain barrier. Caution should be taken when it is used in patients with hepatic diseases as it undergoes extensive first-pass metabolism and can cause severe side effects including CNS depression.

The liquid form of loperamide can be used in treating tube feed-induced diarrhea. It has also been shown to be superior to placebo in treating chronic diarrhea caused by ileocolic disease or resection [55]. In a study comparing codeine phosphate, diphenoxylate, and loperamide, loperamide proved to be as effective as the other two with a better safety profile [56]. Although loperamide has been shown to reduce the duration of diarrhea in children, it should not be used in the management of acute diarrhea in this age group, given its potential life-threatening effects [7].

Codeine is an alkaloid found in opium. It is considered a prodrug as it is metabolized in vivo to the primary active compounds, morphine and codeine-6-glucuronide. Continuous use can induce physical dependence and addiction, however it is less addictive than other opiates with milder withdrawal symptoms.

Tincture of opium is an alcoholic herbal preparation of opium. It is a very potent narcotic secondary to its high concentration of morphine (10 mg/ml). Its clinical use is currently mostly limited to treating fulminant diarrhea that is unresponsive to other therapies. The typical dose of tincture of opium for the treatment of diarrhea is five drops by mouth four times a day, although refractory cases may require higher doses. When it is not available, liquid morphine (Roxanol) can be used but the dose needs to be cut in half as it is twice as concentrated as tincture of opium [51].

Diphenoxylate with atropine: Diphenoxylate is a synthetic phenylpiperidine derivative opiate agonist that is less potent than codeine. When used in high doses, it can cause euphoria and has analgesic effects. To limit the potential for abuse, atropine is added to diphenoxylate to produce anticholinergic side effects if more than 10 tablets are taken [51].

Racecadotril is an enkephalinase inhibitor with an anti-diarrheal effect. It has been proven effective and safe in hospitalized young children with acute watery diarrhea [57]. By inhibiting enkephalinase, the enkephalines can activate the opioid receptor and inhibit the secretion of chloride and fluid. This anti-secretory effect is independent of its effect on intestinal motility, which is a distinct property of this compound when compared to μ-opiate receptor agonists such as loperamide and diphenoxylate. The recommended dose is 100 mg three times a day for adults and 1.5 mg/kg three times a day for children. Racecadotril does not enter the CNS limiting its potential for neurotoxicity. Its use in young children, less than 2 years of age, in whom the blood–brain barrier is immature, can lead to CNS depression [58]. In addition, well-designed prospective studies of efficacy and safety should be carried out in children in the outpatient setting.

Anticholinergics function via an effect on bowel motility. Several side effects can result with their use including dry mouth, dizziness,

Chapter 26 / Empiric Treatment of Chronic Diarrhea   453

drowsiness, nausea, and blurred vision. Concurrent use of other medications with anticholinergic activity, such as tricyclic antidepressants, monoamine oxidase inhibitors, antihistamines, phenothiazines, antimuscarinics, and some of the antipsychotics can worsen these potential adverse effects.

Atropine is an anticholinergic drug, which competitively antagonizes the muscarinic receptor. Its use in the treatment of diarrhea is limited secondary to its possible side effects.

Hyoscyamine can be used as a sublingual preparation or extended release preparation. Its role in the treatment of diarrhea lies primarily in patients with diarrhea-predominant IBS.

Dicyclomine is similar to hyoscyamine, however there is no sublingual form available.

Methylscopolamine is also very similar to hyoscyamine but again there is no sublingual form available and it is more expensive than the other two.

Glycopyrrolate is once again similar to hyoscyamine but it has minimal CNS penetration, which results in less dizziness and drowsiness.

Octreotide is a somatostatin analogue, which is routinely used for treating more severe diarrhea resulting from carcinoid tumors and other neuroendocrine tumors [59]. It functions mainly by suppressing hormone secretion from tumor cells. In addition, it decreases gastrointestinal motility as well as fluid and electrolyte secretion. Octreotide can also be used in other types of refractory diarrhea such as that associated with acquired immunedeficiency syndrome (AIDS), chemotherapy, short gut syndrome, dumping syndrome, and graft versus host disease [60–63]. If there is no response to octreotide after two 2 weeks of use, it should be discontinued given its expense and the unlikelihood of a late response. Its role as a non-specific anti-diarrheal drug is limited [53].

Calcium channel blockers (CCBs): Calcium has an important role in the physiology and pathophysiology of gut smooth muscle cells and enteric neurons. CCBs have been used in the treatment of diarrhea resulting from microscopic colitis [64] and diarrhea-predominant IBS by their prolongation of colonic motility [65].

Clonidine is an α2-adrenergic agonist, which works mainly by an alteration of gut motility with an affect on intestinal transport. It stimulates sodium and chloride absorption and inhibits chloride secretion by interacting with its receptor on enterocytes [66–68]. It is mainly prescribed for patients with diabetic diarrhea [69], but it can also be used for secretory diarrhea of unknown etiology and diarrhea associated with opiate withdrawal [70]. Successful treatment of carcinoid-associated diarrhea with clonidine has been reported [71]. Secondary to its hypotensive effect, the use of clonidine is limited to cases of diarrhea refractory to opiates. Patients undergoing treatment with clonidine need to be hydrated well to decrease the risk of severe hypotension.

Phenothiazines are rarely used for the treatment of diarrhea. They function by altering bowel motility and cause a decrease in secretory action.

Proton pump inhibitors and histamine2 (H2) antagonists can be used to treat diarrhea associated with Zollinger–Ellison syndrome and systemic mastocytosis by decreasing gastric acid secretion.

Histamine1 (H1) antagonists can be used in the treatment of diarrhea associated with systemic mastocytosis via a decrease of intestinal secretions.

Serotonin antagonists can be used in patients with carcinoid syndrome. They can alter gut motility and decrease intestinal secretions.

Probiotics are live microorganisms, which confer a health benefit to the host if taken in adequate amounts. They can reduce the incidence and severity of antibiotic-associated diarrhea [72–76], which is dependent on the strain and dose of the probiotic used. Their use in immunocompromised patients and ones with a compromised intestinal barrier should be done cautiously. Probiotics can also be used in

Table 26.3
Probiotics used in gastrointestinal diseases

Product	Strain	Indication	Dose
Align	*Bifidobacterium infantis*	IBS	1 capsule daily
Florastor	*Saccharomyces boulardii*	AAD[a], CDAD[b]	1 capsule twice a day
Culturelle	*Lactobacillus rhamnosus GG*	Gas, bloating	1–2 capsules daily
VSL#3	*B. Bev, B. longum, B. infantis L. acidophilus, L. bulgaricus L. plantarum, L. casei, Streptococcus thermophilus*	IBS, UC, pouchitis	0.5–8 packets daily

[a] Antibiotic Associated Diarrhea
[b] C. Difficile Associated Diarrhea

Chapter 26 / Empiric Treatment of Chronic Diarrhea 455

travelers' diarrhea, diarrhea-predominant IBS, ulcerative colitis, and in the prevention of pouchitis. See Table 26.3 and the following chapter for a more detailed discussion on their use in diarrheal diseases.

REFERENCES

1. American Gastroenterological Association medical position statement: guidelines for the evaluation and management of chronic diarrhea. Gastroenterology 1999 Jun; 116 (6):1461–1463.
2. Alam NH, Majumder RN, Fuchs GJ, CHOICE Study Group. Efficacy and safety of oral rehydration solution with reduced osmolarity in adults with cholera: a randomized double-blind clinical trial. Lancet 1999; 354:296–299.
3. Atia AN, Buchman AL. Oral rehydration solutions in non-cholera diarrhea: a review. Am J Gastroenterol 2009; 104(10):2596–2604.
4. Fontaine O, Gore SM, Pierce NF. Rice-based oral rehydration solution for treating diarrhoea. Cochrane Database Syst Rev 2000; 30:CD001264.
5. Raghupathy P, et al. Amylase-resistant starch as adjunct to oral rehydration therapy in children with diarrhea. J Pediatr Gastroenterol Nutr 2006; 42(4):362–368.
6. Ramakrishna BS, Subramanian V, Mohan V, Sebastian BK, Young GP, Farthing MJ, Binder HJ. A randomized controlled trial of glucose versus amylase resistant starch hypo-osmolar oral rehydration solution for adult acute dehydrating diarrhea. PLoS One 2008; 3(2):e1587.
7. Guarino A, Albano F, Ashkenazi S, Gendrel D, Hoekstra JH, Shamir R, Szajewska H; European Society for Paediatric Gastroenterology, Hepatology, and Nutrition; European Society for Paediatric Infectious Diseases. ESPGHAN/ESPID evidence-based guidelines for the management of acute gastroenteritis in children in Europe. J Pediatr Gastroenterol Nutr 2008; 46 (Suppl 2):S81–S122.
8. Heather DJ, Howell L, Montana M, Howell M, Hill R. Effect of a bulk-forming cathartic on diarrhea in tube-fed patients. Heart Lung 1991; 20(4):409–413.
9. Lacy CF, Armstrong LL, Goldman MP, et al. eds. Drug information handbook, 11th edn. Hudson, OH: Lexi-Comp Inc., 2003.
10. Eherer AJ, Santa Ana CA, Porter J, Fordtran JS. Effect of psyllium, calcium polycarbophil, and wheat bran on secretory diarrhea induced by phenolphthalein. Gastroenterology 1993; 104(4):1007–1012.
11. Bliss DZ, Jung HJ, Savik K, Lowry A, LeMoine M, Jensen L, Werner C, Schaffer K. Supplementation with dietary fiber improves fecal incontinence. Nurs Res 2001; 50(4):203–213.
12. Sherman DS, Fish DN. Management of protease inhibitor-associated diarrhea. Clin Infect Dis 2000; 30(6):908–914.
13. Davidson LJ, Belknap DC, Flournoy DJ. Flow characteristics of enteral feeding with psyllium hydrophilic mucilloid added. Heart Lung 1991; 20(4):404–408.
14. Gubbins GP, Dekovich AA, Ma CK, Batra SK. Collagenous colitis: report of nine cases and review of the literature. South Med J 1991; 84(1):33–37.
15. Murphy J, Stacey D, Crook J, Thompson B, Panetta D. Testing control of radiation-induced diarrhea with a psyllium bulking agent: a pilot study. Can Oncol Nurs J 2000; 10(3):96–100.
16. Danhof IE. Pharmacology, toxicology, clinical efficacy, and adverse effects of calcium polycarbophil, an enteral hydrosorptive agent. Pharmacotherapy 1982; 2(1): 18–28.

17. Chiba T, Kudara N, Sato M, Chishima R, Abiko Y, Inomata M, Orii S, Suzuki K. Colonic transit, bowel movements, stool form, and abdominal pain in irritable bowel syndrome by treatments with calcium polycarbophil. Hepatogastroenterology 2005; 52(65):1416–1420.
18. Shibata C, Funayama Y, Fukushima K, Takahashi K, Ogawa H, Haneda S, Watanabe K, Kudoh K, Kohyama A, Hayashi K, Sasaki I. Effect of calcium polycarbophil on bowel function after restorative proctocolectomy for ulcerative colitis: a randomized controlled trial. Dig Dis Sci 2007; 52(6):1423–1426.
19. DuPont HL, Flores Sanchez J, Ericsson CD, Mendiola Gomez J, DuPont MW, Cruz Luna A, Mathewson JJ. Comparative efficacy of loperamide hydrochloride and bismuth subsalicylate in the management of acute diarrhea. Am J Med 1990; 88(6A):15S–19S.
20. Fine KD, Lee El. Efficacy of open-label bismuth subsalicylate for the treatment of microscopic colitis. Gastroenterology 1998; 114:29–36.
21. Amaro R, Poniecka A, Rogers A. Collagenous colitis treated successfully with bismuth subsalicylate. Dig Dis Sci 2000; 45(7):1447–1450.
22. Pickering LK, Feldman S, Ericsson CD, et al. Absorption of salicylate and bismuth from a bismuth subsalicylate-containing compound (Pepto-Bismol). J Pediatr 1981; 99:654–656.
23. Barrett MJ. Association of Reye's syndrome with use of Pepto-Bismol (bismuth subsalicylate). Pediatr Infect Dis 1986; 5:611.
24. Gorbach SL. Bismuth therapy in gastrointestinal diseases. Gastroenterology 1990; 99:863–875.
25. Eusufzai S. Bile acid malabsorption: mechanisms and treatment. Dig Dis 1995; 13(5):312–321.
26. Arlow FL, Dekovich AA, Priest RJ, Beher WT. Bile acid-mediated postcholecystectomy diarrhea. Arch Intern Med 1987; 147(7):1327–1329.
27. Hutcheon DF, Bayless TM, Gadacz TR. Postcholecystectomy diarrhea. JAMA 1979; 241(8):823–824.
28. Fromm H, Malavolti M. Bile acid-induced diarrhoea. Clin Gastroenterol 1986; 15(3):567–582.
29. Stroehlein JR. Treatment of Clostridium difficile Infection. Curr Treat Opt Gastroenterol 2004; 7(3):235–239.
30. Bartlett JG. Antibiotic-associated colitis. Dis Mon 1984; 30(15):1–54.
31. Moncino MD, Falletta JM. Multiple relapses of Clostridium difficile-associated diarrhea in a cancer patient. Successful control with long-term cholestyramine therapy. Am J Pediatr Hematol Oncol 1992; 14(4):361–364.
32. Abdo AA, Urbanski SJ, Beck PL. Lymphocytic and collagenous colitis: the emerging entity of microscopic colitis. An update on pathophysiology, diagnosis and management. Can J Gastroenterol 2003; 17(7):425–432.
33. Fernández-Bañares F, Salas A, Esteve M, Espinós J, Forné M, Viver JM. Collagenous and lymphocytic colitis. Evaluation of clinical and histological features, response to treatment, and long-term follow-up. Am J Gastroenterol 2003; 98(2):340–347.
34. Abdo AA, Beck P. Diagnosis and management of microscopic colitis. Can Fam Physician 2003; 49:1473–1478.
35. Baert D, Coppens M, Burvenich P, De Cock G, Lagae J, Rasquin K, Vanderstraeten E. Chronic diarrhoea in non collageneous microscopic colitis: therapeutic effect of cholestyramine. Acta Clin Belg 2004; 59(5):258–262.
36. Bohr J, Tysk C, Eriksson S, Abrahamsson H, Järnerot G. Collagenous colitis: a retrospective study of clinical presentation and treatment in 163 patients. Gut 1996; 39(6):846–851.

Chapter 26 / Empiric Treatment of Chronic Diarrhea   457

37. Mahmoud F, Khalife W, Elaprolu K, Khurana A. Microscopic colitis: a report of two cases. S D J Med 2005; 58(4):149–153.
38. Stroehlein JR. Microscopic colitis. Curr Opin Gastroenterol 2004; 20(1):27–31.
39. Valdovinos MA, Camilleri M, Zimmerman BR. Chronic diarrhea in diabetes mellitus: mechanisms and an approach to diagnosis and treatment. Mayo Clin Proc 1993; 68(7):691–702.
40. RuDusky BM. Cholestyramine therapy for quinidine-induced diarrhea. Case reports. Angiology 1997; 48(2):173–176.
41. Cramp ME, Hing MC, Marriott DJ, Freund J, Cooper DA. Bile acid malabsorption in HIV infected patients with chronic diarrhoea. Aust N Z J Med 1996; 26(3): 368–371.
42. Steuerwald M, Bucher HC, Müller-Brand J, Götze M, Roser HW, Gyr K. HIV-enteropathy and bile acid malabsorption: response to cholestyramine. Am J Gastroenterol 1995; 90(11):2051–2053.
43. Miehlke S, Heymer P, Bethke B, et al. Budesonide treatment for collagenous colitis: a randomized, double-blind, placebo-controlled, multicenter trial. Gastroenterology 2002; 123:978.
44. Miehlke, S, Madisch, A, Voss, C et al. Long-term follow-up of collagenous colitis after induction of clinical remission with budesonide. Aliment Pharmacol Ther 2005; 22:1115.
45. Coupar IM. Opioid action on the intestine: the importance of the intestinal mucosa. Life Sci 1987; 41:917–925.
46. McKay JS, Hughes S, Turnberg LA. The influence of opiates on intestinal transport. In: Csaky TZ, ed. Pharmacology of intestinal permeation 11. Berlin: Springer, 1984, pp. 381–390.
47. Awouters F, Megens A, Verlinden M, Schuurkes J, Niemegeers C, Janssen PAJ. Loperamide: survey of studies on mechanism of its anti-diarrheal activity. Dig Dis Sci 1993; 38: 977–995.
48. Kachel G, Ruppin H, Hagel J, Barina W, Meinhardt M, Domschke W. Human intestinal motor activity and transport: effects of a synthetic opiate. Gastroenterology 1986; 90:85–93.
49. Hughes S, Higgs NB, Turnberg LA. Loperamide has antisecretory activity in the human jejunum in vivo. Gut 1984; 25:931–935.
50. Read M, Read NW, Barber DC, Duthie HL. Effects of loperamide on anal sphincter function in patients complaining of chronic diarrhea with fecal incontinence and urgency. Dig Dis Sci 1982; 27:807–814.
51. Schiller LR. Review article: anti-diarrhoeal pharmacology and therapeutics. Aliment Pharmacol Ther 1995; 9(2):87–106.
52. DuPont HL. Adverse effect of lomotil therapy in shigellosis. JAMA 1973; 226(13):1525–1528.
53. Schiller LR. Chronic diarrhea. Curr Treat Opt Gastroenterol 2005; 8:259–266.
54. Jaffe JH, Kanzler M, Green J. Abuse potential of loperamide. Clin Pharm Ther 1980; 28:812–819.
55. Mainguet P, Fiasse R. Double-blind placebo-controlled study of loperamide (Imodium) in chronic diarrhoea caused by ileocolic disease or resection. Gut 1977; 18(7):575–579.
56. Palmer KR. Corbett CL, Holdsworth CD. Double-blind crossover study comparing loperamide, codeine and diphenoxylate in the treatment of chronic diarrhea. Gastroenterology 1980; 79:1272–1275.
57. Salazar-Lindo E, Santisteban-Ponce J, Chea-Woo E, Gutierrez M. Racecadotril in the treatment of acute watery diarrhea in children. N Engl J Med 2000; 343(7):463–467.

58. Lt Col Singh N, Lt Col Narayan S. Racecadotril: a novel antidiarrheal. MJAFI 2008; 64:361–362.
59. Degen L, Beglinger C. The role of octreotide in the treatment of gastroenteropancreatic endocrine tumors. Digestion 1999; 60 (Suppl 2):9–14.
60. Szilagyi A, Shrier I. Systematic review: the use of somatostatin or octreotide in refractory diarrhoea. Aliment Pharmacol Ther 2001; 15(12):1889–1897.
61. Fried M. Octreotide in the treatment of refractory diarrhea. Digestion 1999; 60 (Suppl 2):42–46.
62. Farthing MJ. The role of somatostatin analogues in the treatment of refractory diarrhoea. Digestion 1996; 57(Suppl 1):107.
63. Long RG, Adrian TE, Bloom SR. Somatostatin and the dumping syndrome. Br Med J 1985; 290:886–888.
64. Scheidler MD, Meiselman M. Use of verapamil for the symptomatic treatment of microscopic colitis. J Clin Gastroenterol 2001; 32(4):351–352.
65. Lu CL, Chen CY, Chang FY, Chang SS, Kang LJ, Lu RH, Lee SD. Effect of a calcium channel blocker and antispasmodic in diarrhoea-predominant irritable bowel syndrome. J Gastroenterol Hepatol 2000; 15(8):925–930.
66. Pamukcu R, Chang EB. Alpha-2-adrenergic agonists as antidiarrheal agents. A review of physiological and cellular mechanisms. In: Lebenthal E, Duffey M, eds. Textbook of secretory diarrhea. New York, NY: Raven Press, 1990, pp. 383–393.
67. Nakaki T, Nakadate T. Yamamoto S, Kato R. a-Adrenoceptors inhibit the cholera-toxin-induced intestinal fluid accumulation. Naunyn-Schmiedeberg's Arch Pharmacol 1982; 318:1814.
68. Morris AI, Turnberg LA. Influence of isoproterenol and propranolol on human intestinal transport *in* vivo. Gastroenterology 1981; 81:1076–1079.
69. Fedorak RN, Field M, Chang EB. Treatment of diabetic diarrhea with clonidine. Ann Intern Med 1985; 102:197.
70. DiStefano PS, Brown OM. Biochemical correlates of morphine withdrawal. 2. Effects of clonidine J Pharmacol Exp Ther 1985; 233(2):339–344.
71. Schwörer H, Münke H, Stöckmann F, Ramadori G. Treatment of diarrhea in carcinoid syndrome with ondansetron, tropisetron, and clonidine. Am J Gastroenterol 1995; 90(4):645–648.
72. D'Souza AL, Rajkumar C, Cooke J, Bulpitt CJ. Probiotics in prevention of antibiotic associated diarrhoea: meta-analysis. Br Med J 2002; 324(7350):1361.
73. Cremonini F, Di Caro S, Nista EC, et al. Meta-analysis: the effect of probiotic administration on antibiotic-associated diarrhoea. Aliment Pharmacol Ther 2002; 16(8):1461–1467.
74. Mcfarland LV. Meta-analysis of probiotics for the prevention of antibiotic associated diarrhea and the treatment of Clostridium difficile disease. Am J Gastroenterol 2006 Apr;101(4):812–822.
75. Szajewska H, Mrukowicz J. Meta-analysis: non-pathogenic yeast Saccharomyces boulardii in the prevention of antibiotic-associated diarrhoea. Aliment Pharmacol Ther 2005; 22(5):365–372.
76. Sazawal S, Hiremath G, Dhingra U, Malik P, Deb S, Black RE. Efficacy of probiotics in prevention of acute diarrhoea: a meta-analysis of masked, randomised, placebo-controlled trials. Lancet Infect Dis 2006; 6(6):374.

27 Probiotics for Diarrheal Diseases

Stefano Guandalini, MD

CONTENTS

INTRODUCTION
CLINICAL TRIALS IN THE PREVENTION
  AND/OR TREATMENT OF ACUTE DIARRHEA
PREVENTION OF DIARRHEA
PREVENTION OF
  ANTIBIOTIC-ASSOCIATED DIARRHEA
TREATMENT OF ACUTE DIARRHEA
TREATMENT OF PERSISTENT DIARRHEA
PREVENTION OF NECROTIZING
  ENTEROCOLITIS IN THE NEWBORN
USE OF PROBIOTICS IN INFLAMMATORY
  BOWEL DISEASES
CONCLUSIONS
REFERENCES

Summary

In recent years, a large body of literature has been generated on the use of probiotics. Regarded initially as alternative medicine, probiotics – mostly lactic acid bacteria – has gained their position in mainstream medicine, after a robust research activity covering both in vitro and in vivo studies, as well as randomized clinical trials. In terms of diarrheal diseases, the most promising applications

From: *Diarrhea, Clinical Gastroenterology*
Edited by: S. Guandalini, H. Vaziri, DOI 10.1007/978-1-60761-183-7_27
© Springer Science+Business Media, LLC 2011

appear in the prevention and/or the treatment of acute gastroenteritis, antibiotic-associated diarrhea, neonatal-necrotizing enterocolitis, and ulcerative colitis. It should be kept in mind that different strains of probiotics have different specificities, so no generalizations on the efficacy (or lack thereof) of "probiotics" should be made. This chapter will analyze the evidence for the use of probiotics in such diarrheal diseases; in some cases this is quite consolidated, in others still emerging.

Key Words: Probiotics, Diarrhea, IBD, IBS, NEC, VSL#3, *Lactobacillus GG*, *Saccharomyces boulardii*, *Bifidobacteria*

INTRODUCTION

Diarrheal diseases continue to represent a major threat to global health. The widespread use of oral rehydration solutions and the slowly improving hygienic standards in developing countries have resulted in a substantial decline in mortality from acute diarrhea, especially in young children. Mortality continues to be unacceptably high in these areas. It is currently estimated that approximately 1.6 million children below the age of 5 die each year from the immediate consequences of several billion episodes of diarrhea. In developed countries, on the other hand, while the burden of mortality from diarrheal diseases has largely regressed to now be considered marginal, these disorders still retain a high impact in terms of morbidity and of associated financial and social costs that range from hospitalizations to absenteeism from work and/or school, etc. The relatively recent introduction of an effective vaccination against rotavirus (that remains the single most common cause of acute-onset diarrhea worldwide) is expected to help reduce such a burden. It is nevertheless clear that even in developed countries there is currently a need for preventative and therapeutic strategies aimed at reducing the incidence, severity, and duration of acute diarrheal episodes. In the past several years a considerable amount of research has been done to verify if appropriate utilization of some probiotic strains may be the answer.

Most of the evidence currently available on the role of probiotics in treating or preventing acute diarrheal episodes originate from studies in infants and young children. This represents the age group in which diarrhea is more problematic, due do the higher risk of dehydration and electrolyte imbalances. It should also be noted that probiotics have been extensively evaluated in other gastrointestinal conditions associated with diarrhea such as necrotizing enterocolitis, antibiotic-associated diarrhea, and inflammatory bowel diseases (reviewed in [1]).

CLINICAL TRIALS IN THE PREVENTION AND/OR TREATMENT OF ACUTE DIARRHEA

As in many other inflammatory disorders, both gastrointestinal and extra-intestinal, the most studied probiotics for children and adults with acute diarrhea are bacteria of the genera *Lactobacillus* or *Bifidobacterium*, used either as single species or in mixed cultures with other bacteria (see Table 27.1). Other nonpathogenic genera, including *Escherichia, Enterococcus, Bacillus,* and nonbacterial organisms, such as the nonpathogenic yeast *Saccharomyces boulardii*, have also been extensively investigated. The yogurt-producing bacteria, *Lactobacillus bulgaricus* and *Streptococcus thermophilus* also have received some attention, especially in preventing diarrhea.

Table 27.1
Main probiotics in prevention and/or treatment
of diarrhea

Strain	Type
Lactobacillus	*acidophilus*[a]
	bulgaricus[a]
	casei[a]
	rhamnosus GG
	johnsonii
	paracasei
	plantarum[a]
	reuteri
	salivarius
Bifidobacteria	*animalis*
	bifidum
	breve[a]
	infantis[a]
	lactis
	longum[a]
Escherichia coli	Nissle 1917
Streptococcus	*salivarius* ssp. *thermophilus*[a]
Enterococcus	*fecium*
Yeasts	*Saccharomyces boulardii*

[a]Present in combination in the preparation "VSL#3".

PREVENTION OF DIARRHEA

Community Acquired

Only a few studies are available addressing the efficacy of probiotics in preventing the onset or mitigating the severity of community-acquired diarrhea. One of them is a prospective study by Oberhelman et al. [2] in a rural community in Peru. The study followed more than 200 infants and young children, mostly malnourished, receiving *Lactobacillus GG (LGG)* or placebo for 15 months. There were significantly fewer diarrheal episodes in children treated with *LGG* compared with placebo (5.2 vs. 6.0 episodes per child per year; $p = 0.028$). The benefit was particularly evident in non- breastfed children aged 18–29 months, as they experienced one fewer episode per child per year ($p = 0.005$).

Pereg et al. [3] followed 500 adults who were assigned to either yogurt-containing *L. casei* 10^{10} CFU/day or placebo. The incidence of diarrhea in the probiotic group and the control group was 12.2 and 16.1%, respectively, but the difference was not statistically significant.

Day-Care Acquired

Infants and young children attending day-care centers are notoriously at higher risk for common infectious diseases, including upper respiratory tract infections and diarrhea. Several randomized controlled trials (RCT) have been published on the efficacy of probiotics in decreasing the incidence and shortening the duration or severity of diarrheal episodes in this setting.

In a study published in 2000 [4], a yogurt-containing *L. casei* was administered to healthy children, 6–24 months of age, attending day-care centers for 12 weeks, followed by 6 weeks with no supplementation. A total of 779 children completed the study. The incidence of diarrhea between the treated and placebo groups was significantly different. Twenty-two percent of children in the control group had at least one attack of diarrhea compared to 15.8% of the children in the treatment group.

The efficacy of LGG was subsequently evaluated in a multicenter trial conducted in Finland in preschool children [5]. The probiotic was provided in milk with a concentration of 5×10^{10} CFU/ml and the reported intake was at least 200 ml/day for 30 weeks. No significant difference was observed between the study and the control groups in terms of frequency or severity of the episodes of diarrhea.

In an RCT, French investigators assessed the incidence of acute diarrhea in over 900 infants (4–6 months of age) who were fed a formula enriched by *Bifidobacterium breve* and *S. thermophilus* for a prolonged period of time [6]. Again, no significant difference was found in the

Chapter 27 / Probiotics for Diarrheal Diseases

incidence or duration of the diarrheal episodes or the number of hospital admissions. It must be noted, however, that the children in the probiotic-supplemented group experienced less severe episodes. They in fact had fewer instances of dehydration (2.5% vs. 6.1%, $p = 0.01$) and required fewer medical consultations (46% vs. 57%, $p = 0.003$), oral rehydration solution prescriptions (42% vs. 52%, $p = 0.003$), and formula changes (59% vs. 75%, $p = 0.0001$).

A multicenter RCT to evaluate the efficacy of a formula supplemented with *Bifidobacterium lactis* strain *Bb12* in the prevention of acute diarrhea in infants younger than 8 months living in residential nurseries or foster-care centers was conducted by another group of investigators also based in France [7]. Ninety healthy children received either the *Bb12* or a standard formula daily throughout their stay in the residential center for a total of almost 5 months. Also in this trial, the probiotic did not reduce the incidence of diarrhea when compared with placebo (28.3% vs. 38.7%). The only significant difference noticed was in the number of days with diarrhea; the *Bb12* group had 1.15 ± 2.5 days with diarrhea, with a daily probability of diarrhea of 0.84 vs. 2.3 ± 4.5 days and 1.55, respectively, in the control group ($p = 0.0002$ and 0.001).

Saavedra et al. [8] conducted a study in the United States comparing two different concentrations of *B. lactis Bb12* + *S. thermophilus* in formulas (either 1×10^7 or 1×10^6 CFU/g) in 118 children, 8–24 months of age. No significant differences were found between the two groups in growth, health-care attention seeking, day-care absenteeism, prevalence of diarrheal episodes, or other health variables.

In 2005, Weizman et al. [9] compared two different strains of probiotics: *B. lactis Bb12* vs. *L. reuteri* provided in formula as 1×10^7 CFU/g. The study was carried out for 3 months on almost 200 infants 4–10 months of age. In this case, both probiotics performed better than placebo for the number of diarrheal episodes (0.3 ± 0.1 vs. 0.1± 0.08 for *Bb12* and 0.02± 0.01 for *L. reuteri*, $p < 0.001$) and days with diarrhea (0.6 ± 0.2 vs. 0.4± 0.1 for *Bb12* and 0.15± 0.10 for *L. reuteri*, $p< 0.001$).

In 2007, Binns et al. [10] reported on the efficacy of a milk product containing probiotics and prebiotics on the incidence of diarrhea in almost 500 children attending 29 day-care centers in Perth, Australia. The probiotic employed was *B. lactis* (1.2×10^{10} CFU/day administered with a prebiotic blend) for 5 months. Even though the incidence of diarrhea was not significantly different between the study and the control group, the children in the study group had significantly fewer days with four or more stools, representing a reduction of about 20% in diarrheal rate.

The existing evidence suggests that the efficacy of probiotics in preventing diarrheal episodes in infants and children attending day-care centers or similar institutions, where the risk of acquiring infectious diarrhea is higher, is quite modest and of minimal clinical relevance.

Hospital Acquired

Patients in hospital wards are especially at risk of developing infectious diarrhea. In most instances, these episodes are due to a rapidly spreading *Rotavirus* infection and in fewer instances *Clostridium difficile*. Both agents can cause serious consequences, especially in ill infants and children that are already weakened by their underlying ailment, as well as in the elderly. Probiotics would therefore represent a welcome addition to the limited means available in preventing this disorder.

However, only a limited number of RCTs have evaluated the efficacy of probiotics for this purpose with conflicting results [11–13]. After careful analysis of these trials, it can be concluded that probiotics might have a role in protecting hospitalized patients from clinically significant diarrheal illness caused by rotavirus and possibly *C. difficile*. Further, adequately powered studies are needed to examine this possibility and compare different strains and doses of probiotics.

Traveler's Diarrhea

Diarrhea of acute onset, a common health problem, may affect from 5 to 50% of travelers, depending on the country being visited. The disorder is usually self-limited but up to 10% of the cases will develop persistent diarrhea of which, about 10% will eventually evolve into post-infectious irritable bowel syndrome. Many studies have therefore looked at the utilization of probiotics as a tool to prevent this bothersome event.

In a meta-analysis of 12 trials, McFarland [14] concluded that probiotics were able to prevent travelers' diarrhea significantly, based on the pooled relative risk (RR=0.85, 95% CI 0.79–0.91, $P < 0.001$). When analyzing the effect of single strains, it was evident that *S. boulardii* and a mixture of *L. acidophilus* and *B. bifidum* had significant efficacy. Importantly, no serious adverse reactions were reported in any of the 12 trials. Considering the possible reduction in the incidence of travelers' diarrhea and consequently the post-infectious irritable bowel syndrome, it appears that the preventive usage of either one of these probiotics could be helpful.

PREVENTION OF ANTIBIOTIC-ASSOCIATED DIARRHEA

Up to 40% of children and adults receiving oral antibiotics may develop diarrhea, which can be due to various causes, including *C. difficile*. In a recent meta-analysis published on the potential use of probiotics in preventing the incidence of antibiotic-associated diarrhea in children [15], 2000 children were evaluated. The most commonly investigated probiotics were Lactobacilli, *Bifidobacteria,* streptococci, and *S. boulardii*. The meta-analysis found that administration of either *LGG* or *S. boulardii*, but not other probiotic strains, reduced the incidence of antibiotic-associated diarrhea significantly.

TREATMENT OF ACUTE DIARRHEA

Arguably the most logical application for probiotics, the treatment of infectious diarrhea, has been the subject of extensive investigation. There are multiple publications since the mid-1990s with some excellent reviews addressing the role of probiotics in the treatment or prevention of diarrhea.

The probiotic strains most studied are LGG (17 clinical trials at the time of this writing [15–31], mostly randomized and placebo controlled), *S. boulardii* (six RCTs [17, 32–36]), and *L. reuteri* (four studies [37–40]), while other species such as *Escherichia coli* Nissle' 1917 [41–42], the heat-killed *L. acidophilus LB* [43–44] and the probiotic mixture *VSL#3* [45] have also been investigated, but received far less attention in this matter. Several meta-analyses are available that assess the efficacy of such probiotics.

In spite of some negative studies, it seems that the usage of *Lactobacillus GG* may cause a significant reduction in the duration of diarrhea. In a recent meta-analysis of 7 RCTs evaluating almost 1000 infants and young children [46] an average reduction of 1.1 days was seen with a 95% CI of 1.9–0.3. It also appears that *Lactobacillus GG* is most effective in rotavirus-induced diarrhea, where it may decrease the duration of diarrhea by 2.1 days. Furthermore, we evaluated the risk of running a protracted diarrheal illness (more than 7 days) in an RCT evaluating 287 patients [19] and found significant reduction in its incidence by using *Lactobacillus GG* (RR: 0.25; 95% CI: 0.09–0.75).

The effect of probiotics on the duration of hospitalization was evaluated in 535 patients in 3 RCTs and it was found that on average, there is a reduction by 1 day in the length of hospitalization. In two open label trials [20, 22] *LGG* administration could reduce the duration of rotavirus shedding which probably has epidemiologic significance.

Overall these data provide a rather robust evidence of efficacy for *Lactobacillus GG* in the treatment of acute diarrhea. One should, however, note that *Lactobacillus GG* appears to be less effective in bacterial diarrhea. It is also important to point out that correct dosage of this probiotic is crucial for its efficacy, with doses above 5 billion (5×10^9 CFU) per day being necessary.

Similar efficacy was shown for *S. boulardii*. In a recent re-assessment of a previously published meta-analysis [47, 48], Vandenplas et al. analyzed data from the pooled results of 6 RCTs involving 756 children. It was concluded that compared to placebo or no intervention, *S. boulardii* reduced the duration of diarrhea by almost 1 day.

This probiotic was comparable to LGG in preventing a protracted course of diarrhea.

L. reuteri was studied alone [30, 40] or in combination with *L. rhamnosus 19070-2* [38, 39] for its efficacy in reducing the duration of acute-onset diarrhea in children hospitalized or having diarrhea while in day care. In all circumstances the probiotic appeared to be able to reduce the duration of diarrhea, especially in cases caused by rotavirus, and shorten its shedding [39]. However, as only two groups of investigators have published results for this strain, general conclusions cannot be safely drawn at this time.

In a recent study in Nigeria [37], a combination of *L. reuteri* (strain *RC 14*) and *L. rhamnosus GR-1* was used in 24 adult female with HIV/AIDS, who were suffering from moderate diarrhea. Their CD4 counts were above 200 and none of them were receiving any anti-retroviral treatment or dietary supplements. Diarrhea resolved in 12/12 probiotic-treated subjects within 2 days, compared to 2/12 receiving yogurt for 15 days. While it would obviously be premature to apply these findings to clinical practice, it is exciting to see the appearance of potential applications for probiotics in these clinical settings.

As mentioned, *E. coli* Nissle' 1917 was also studied in two RCTs [41, 42]. Both investigations were multicenter trials which were conducted in Russia and Ukraine by the same group. Both studies showed a significant superiority of the probiotic compared to placebo in obtaining a faster recovery from acute-onset diarrhea in infants and toddlers [41]. A shorter duration of diarrhea lasting more than 4 days at study enrollment in young children was also seen [42].

VLS#3, a patented preparation containing seven different strains of probiotics, was used in an RCT conducted in India on 224 children with acute, rotavirus-induced diarrhea and proved to be significantly better than placebo in a preliminary report [45].

In summary, only a few probiotic strains have demonstrated efficacy in the treatment of diarrhea, especially acute-onset, infectious diarrhea

Chapter 27 / Probiotics for Diarrheal Diseases

in children and to a much lesser degree in adults. This is particularly true with rotavirus-induced diarrhea, especially if administered early in the course. It is important to know that the clinical relevance of such effect is moderate, as no more than 1-day reduction of disease duration should be expected. Only a few specific strains so far have evidence-based proof of efficacy, for which the dosage is crucial.

TREATMENT OF PERSISTENT DIARRHEA

Limited studies have been done addressing the application of probiotic therapy in treating children presenting with persistent diarrhea. One RCT was conducted in Argentina [50] with *S. boulardii* in which 89 children (6–24 months of age) received milk supplemented with *L. casei* and *L. acidophilus* strains *CERELA* 10^{10}–10^{12} CFU/g, or *S. boulardii* 10^{10}–10^{12} CFU/g twice a day for 5 days, while a third group received a placebo milk. Both *Lactobacillus* and *S. boulardii* significantly reduced the number of stools per day ($p<0.001$) and diarrheal duration ($p < 0.005$). Similarly, both probiotics significantly ($p < 0.002$) reduced vomiting as compared with placebo.

A second RCT [16] was performed with *LGG* in 235 Indian children, most of whom were malnourished, hospitalized for diarrhea lasting more than 14 days. The study showed the mean duration of diarrhea to be significantly lower in the cases than in controls (5.3 vs. 9.2 days, $p < 0.05$). Also, the duration of hospitalization was greatly reduced in children on *LGG* supplement (from 15.5 to 7.3 days, $p < 0.05$).

Clearly, no conclusions can be drawn based on only two trials. It is encouraging that probiotics may not only help in preventing diarrhea from running a prolonged course, as mentioned earlier, but can help in abbreviating the course of an already persistent diarrhea. This would be of particular importance in developing countries where malnutrition is still widespread.

PREVENTION OF NECROTIZING ENTEROCOLITIS IN THE NEWBORN

Necrotizing enterocolitis (NEC) is a very severe occurrence in premature infants, especially in those who are of very low birth weight (VLBW), with an incidence of around 3%. This complication occurs only in non-exclusively breastfed babies and has a multifactorial etiology including enteral feeding, pathogenic organisms, and altered enteric mucosal integrity. Predisposing factors include prematurity, low birth weight, mechanical ventilation, use of glucocorticoids and indomethacin, and low Apgar score at 5 min. NEC carries a substantial risk of complications, including intestinal failure owing to ischemia and/or subsequent resections, and carries a substantial mortality rate.

Probiotics containing *Bifidobacterium* and *Lactobacillus* are found in the stools of 5% of VLBW infants, and low colonization has been implicated as a predisposing factor for NEC.

Several investigations have been performed in at-risk premature infants to assess the potential of probiotics in preventing such ominous complications. A meta-analysis published in 2009, [51] assessed nine RCTs that enrolled preterm infants <37 weeks gestational age and/or <2500 g birth weight. A total of 1425 infants were included. The probiotics used were *LGG, L. acidophilus, Bifidobacterium infantis, B. breve, L. bifidus, S. thermophilus, B. infantis, S. boulardii.* The results showed that enteral probiotic supplementation significantly reduced the incidence of severe NEC and of mortality. A subsequent large multicenter study conducted on more than 400 preterm infants by Lin and colleagues also showed a highly significant protective effect of *L. acidophilus* and *B. bifidus* [52]. The patients receiving this supplementation were, in fact, much less likely to experience NEC of grade II or higher and even to die of unrelated causes. Given the hypothetical risk of administering live bacteria to such vulnerable, immunologically immature subjects, some caution must be exerted. The data available thus far are indeed very exciting and offer great hope for the prevention of NEC.

USE OF PROBIOTICS IN INFLAMMATORY BOWEL DISEASES

The potential for use of probiotics in these conditions appears great (reviewed in [53]), especially in light of the fact that the microflora plays an important role in inflammatory bowel disease (IBD). In spite of this, however, there is limited evidence available supporting the usefulness of probiotics in this condition [1].

Crohn's Disease

Only a few double-blind, placebo-controlled studies are available addressing the efficacy of probiotics in inducing and/or maintaining remission in patients with Crohn's disease. The majority of these studies are in adults, with invariably negative results [54].

Chapter 27 / Probiotics for Diarrheal Diseases 469

Table 27.2
Summary of possible uses of probiotics in diarrheal diseases

Indication	Probiotic	Dose	Notes
Prevention of day-care acquired diarrhea	Lactobacillus casei DN-114 001	100 ml of yogurt containing 10^8 CFU/ml	Present in a commercial yogurt
	Bifidobacterium lactis Bb12	1.5×10^8 CFU/l	Present in a proprietary milk formula
	Lactobacillus reuteri	1×10^7 CFU/g of formula	Present in a commercially available preparation
Prevention of traveler's diarrhea	Saccharomyces boulardii	250–500 mg/day	Present in a commercially available preparation
Prevention of antibiotic-induced diarrhea	Lactobacillus rhamnosus GG	$>5 \times 10^9$ CFU/day, better 10^{10}–10^{11}	Present in a commercially available preparation
	Saccharomyces boulardii	250–500 mg/day	Present in a commercially available preparation

Table 27.2
(continued)

Indication	Probiotic	Dose	Notes
Treatment of acute diarrhea	*Lactobacillus rhamnosus GG*	$>5 \times 10^9$ CFU/day, better 10^{10}–10^{11}	Present in a commercially available preparation, should be administered as early as possible. Can be administered in ORS
	Saccharomyces boulardii	5×10^9–10^{10} CFU (found in 250–500 mg)/day	Present in a commercially available preparation
Treatment of ulcerative colitis	*VSL#3*	450–3600 Billion lyophilized bacteria (one to eight sachets) per day	Present in a commercially available preparation
Prevention of community acquired or nosocomial diarrhea; treatment of persistent diarrhea; NEC; Crohn's disease			Data not yet adequate to provide recommendations

Ulcerative Colitis

More promising results have been produced by the use of probiotics in ulcerative colitis in adults (reviewed in [55]). Pediatric studies on the role of probiotics in IBD have been recently reviewed in [1].

A pediatric trial was published on 29 children who received *VSL#3* or placebo. Superior efficacy of this preparation when used along with prednisone and mesalamine was seen, when compared to these drugs alone [56]. Positive results of this probiotic mixture for adults with mild to moderate ulcerative colitis were also obtained recently by Sood and colleagues in a blinded, placebo-controlled study of 144 patients [57]. Although more evidence is needed, especially generated by large multicenter trials, it is fair to say that the prospective for a beneficial use of probiotics in patients with ulcerative colitis is good.

CONCLUSIONS

In the last few years, the status of probiotics has gone from alternative to main stream medicine, thanks to a remarkable body of investigations involving both basic science and a large number of well-conducted clinical trials. The role of probiotics in diarrheal diseases can be considered quite well documented in the treatment of acute diarrhea, prevention of antibiotic-associated diarrhea, and prevention of traveler's diarrhea. Additional areas of extreme interest, which will undoubtedly witness a vigorous research effort in the near future, are prevention of hospital-acquired diarrheas, prevention of NEC, treatment of ulcerative colitis, and the treatment of irritable bowel syndrome [58]. Table 27.2 lists possible uses of probiotics in diarrheal diseases based on current available evidence.

REFERENCES

1. Guandalini S. An update on the role of probiotics in the therapy of pediatric inflammatory bowel disease. Exp Rev Clin Immunol 2010;6:47–54.
2. Oberhelman RA, et al. A placebo-controlled trial of *Lactobacillus* GG to prevent diarrhea in undernourished Peruvian children. J Pediatr 1999;134(1):15–20.
3. Pereg D, et al. The effect of fermented yogurt on the prevention of diarrhea in a healthy adult population. Am J Infect Control 2005;33(2):122–125.
4. Pedone CA, et al. Multicentric study of the effect of milk fermented by *Lactobacillus casei* on the incidence of diarrhoea. Int J Clin Pract 2000;54(9): 568–571.
5. Hatakka K, et al. Effect of long term consumption of probiotic milk on infections in children attending day care centres: double blind, randomised trial. BMJ 2001:322(7298):1327.
6. Thibault H, Aubert-Jacquin C, Goulet O. Effects of long-term consumption of a fermented infant formula (with *Bifidobacterium breve c50* and *Streptococcus*

thermophilus 065) on acute diarrhea in healthy infants. J Pediatr Gastroenterol Nutr 2004;39(2):147–152.

7. Chouraqui JP, Van Egroo LD, Fichot MC. Acidified milk formula supplemented with *Bifidobacterium lactis*: impact on infant diarrhea in residential care settings. J Pediatr Gastroenterol Nutr 2004:38(3):288–292.

8. Saavedra JM, et al. Long-term consumption of infant formulas containing live probiotic bacteria: tolerance and safety. Am J Clin Nutr 2004;79(2):261–267.

9. Weizman Z, Asli G, Alsheikh A. Effect of a probiotic infant formula on infections in child care centers: comparison of two probiotic agents. Pediatrics 2005;115(1):5–9.

10. Binns CW, et al. The CUPDAY Study: prebiotic–probiotic milk product in 1–3-year-old children attending childcare centres. Acta Paediatr 2007:96(11): 1646–1650.

11. Mastretta E, et al. Effect of *Lactobacillus GG* and breast-feeding in the prevention of rotavirus nosocomial infection. J Pediatr Gastroenterol Nutr 2002;35(4): 527–531.

12. Saavedra JM, et al. Feeding of *Bifidobacterium bifidum* and *Streptococcus thermophilus* to infants in hospital for prevention of diarrhoea and shedding of rotavirus. Lancet 1994;344(8929):1046–1049.

13. Szajewska H, et al. Efficacy of *Lactobacillus GG* in prevention of nosocomial diarrhea in infants. J Pediatr 2001;138(3):361–365.

14. McFarland LV. Meta-analysis of probiotics for the prevention of traveler's diarrhea. Travel Med Infect Dis 2007;5(2):97–105.

15. Basu S, et al. Efficacy of high-dose *Lactobacillus rhamnosus* GG in controlling acute watery diarrhea in Indian children: a randomized controlled trial. J Clin Gastroenterol 2009;43(3):208–213.

16. Basu S, et al. Efficacy of *Lactobacillus rhamnosus* GG in acute watery diarrhoea of Indian children: a randomised controlled trial. J Paediatr Child Health 2007;43(12):837–842.

17. Canani RB, et al. Probiotics for treatment of acute diarrhoea in children: randomised clinical trial of five different preparations. BMJ 2007;335(7615):340.

18. Fang SB, et al. Dose-dependent effect of *Lactobacillus rhamnosus* on quantitative reduction of faecal rotavirus shedding in children. J Trop Pediatr 2009;55(5): 297–301.

19. Guandalini S, et al. *Lactobacillus* GG administered in oral rehydration solution to children with acute diarrhea: a multicenter European trial. J Pediatr Gastroenterol Nutr 2000;30(1):54–60.

20. Guarino A, et al. Oral bacterial therapy reduces the duration of symptoms and of viral excretion in children with mild diarrhea. J Pediatr Gastroenterol Nutr 1997;25(5):516–519.

21. Isolauri E, et al. A human *Lactobacillus* strain (*Lactobacillus casei* sp strain GG) promotes recovery from acute diarrhea in children. Pediatrics 1991;88(1):90–97.

22. Isolauri E, et al. Oral bacteriotherapy for viral gastroenteritis. Dig Dis Sci 1994;39(12):2595–2600.

23. Kaila M, et al. Viable versus inactivated lactobacillus strain GG in acute rotavirus diarrhoea. Arch Dis Child 1995;72(1):51–53.

24. Kaila M, et al. Enhancement of the circulating antibody secreting cell response in human diarrhea by a human *Lactobacillus* strain. Pediatr Res 1992;32(2): 141–144.

25. Majamaa H, et al. Lactic acid bacteria in the treatment of acute rotavirus gastroenteritis. J Pediatr Gastroenterol Nutr 1995;20(3):333–338.

Chapter 27 / Probiotics for Diarrheal Diseases

26. Pant AR, et al. *Lactobacillus* GG and acute diarrhoea in young children in the tropics. J Trop Pediatr 1996;42(3):162–165.
27. Rautanen T, et al. Management of acute diarrhoea with low osmolarity oral rehydration solutions and *Lactobacillus* strain GG. Arch Dis Child 1998;79(2): 157–160.
28. Raza S, et al. *Lactobacillus* GG in acute diarrhea. Indian Pediatr 1995;32(10):1140–1142.
29. Raza S, et al. *Lactobacillus* GG promotes recovery from acute nonbloody diarrhea in Pakistan. Pediatr Infect Dis J 1995;14(2):107–111.
30. Shornikova AV, et al. Bacteriotherapy with *Lactobacillus reuteri* in rotavirus gastroenteritis. Pediatr Infect Dis J 1997;16(12):1103–1107.
31. Misra S, Sabui TK, Pal NK. A randomized controlled trial to evaluate the efficacy of lactobacillus GG in infantile diarrhea. J Pediatr 2009;155(1): 129–132.
32. Billoo AG, et al. Role of a probiotic (*Saccharomyces boulardii*) in management and prevention of diarrhoea. World J Gastroenterol 2006;12(28):4557–4560.
33. Htwe K, et al. Effect of *Saccharomyces boulardii* in the treatment of acute watery diarrhea in Myanmar children: a randomized controlled study. Am J Trop Med Hyg 2008;78(2):214–216.
34. Kurugol Z, Koturoglu G. Effects of *Saccharomyces boulardii* in children with acute diarrhoea. Acta Paediatr 2005;94(1):44–47.
35. Ozkan TB, et al. Effect of *Saccharomyces boulardii* in children with acute gastroenteritis and its relationship to the immune response. J Int Med Res 2007;35(2):201–212.
36. Villarruel G, et al. *Saccharomyces boulardii* in acute childhood diarrhoea: a randomized, placebo-controlled study. Acta Paediatr 2007;96(4):538–541.
37. Anukam KC, et al. Yogurt containing probiotic *Lactobacillus rhamnosus* GR-1 and L. reuteri RC-14 helps resolve moderate diarrhea and increases CD4 count in HIV/AIDS patients. J Clin Gastroenterol 2008;42(3):239–243.
38. Rosenfeldt V, et al. Effect of probiotic *Lactobacillus* strains on acute diarrhea in a cohort of nonhospitalized children attending day-care centers. Pediatr Infect Dis J 2002;21(5):417–419.
39. Rosenfeldt V, et al. Effect of probiotic *Lactobacillus* strains in young children hospitalized with acute diarrhea. Pediatr Infect Dis J 2002;21(5):411–416.
40. Shornikova AV, et al. *Lactobacillus reuteri* as a therapeutic agent in acute diarrhea in young children. J Pediatr Gastroenterol Nutr 1997;24(4):399–404.
41. Henker J, et al. The probiotic *Escherichia coli* strain Nissle 1917 (EcN) stops acute diarrhoea in infants and toddlers. Eur J Pediatr 2007;166(4):311–318.
42. Henker J, et al. Probiotic *Escherichia coli* Nissle 1917 versus placebo for treating diarrhea of greater than 4 days duration in infants and toddlers. Pediatr Infect Dis J 2008;27(6):494–499.
43. Lievin-Le Moal V, Sarrazin-Davila LE, Servin AL. An experimental study and a randomized, double-blind, placebo-controlled clinical trial to evaluate the anti-secretory activity of *Lactobacillus acidophilus* strain LB against nonrotavirus diarrhea. Pediatrics 2007;120(4):e795–e803.
44. Salazar-Lindo E, et al. Effectiveness and safety of *Lactobacillus* LB in the treatment of mild acute diarrhea in children. J Pediatr Gastroenterol Nutr 2007;44(5):571–576.
45. Dubey AP, et al. Use of VSL[sharp]3 in the treatment of rotavirus diarrhea in children: preliminary results. J Clin Gastroenterol 2008;42(Suppl 3 Pt 1): S126–S129.

46. Szajewska H, et al. Meta-analysis: *Lactobacillus* GG for treating acute diarrhoea in children. Aliment Pharmacol Ther 2007;25(8):871–881.
47. Vandenplas Y, Brunser O, Szajewska H. *Saccharomyces boulardii* in childhood. Eur J Pediatr 2009;168(3):253–265.
48. Szajewska H, Skorka A, Dylag M. Meta-analysis: *Saccharomyces boulardii* for treating acute diarrhoea in children. Aliment Pharmacol Ther 2007;25(3): 257–264.
49. Hauck FH, et al. Imerslund-Grasbeck syndrome in a 15-year-old German girl caused by compound heterozygous mutations in CUBN. Eur J Pediatr 2008;167(6):671–675.
50. Gaon D, et al. Effect of *Lactobacillus* strains and *Saccharomyces boulardii* on persistent diarrhea in children. Medicina (B Aires) 2003;63(4):293–298.
51. Alfaleh K, Anabrees J, Bassler D. Probiotics reduce the risk of necrotizing enterocolitis in preterm infants: a meta-analysis. Neonatology 2009;97:93–99.
52. Lin H, et al. Oral probiotics prevent necrotizing enterocolitis in very low birth weight preterm infants: a multicenter, randomized, controlled trial. Pediatrics 2008;122:693–700.
53. Vanderpool C, Yan F, Polk DB. Mechanisms of probiotic action: implications for therapeutic applications in inflammatory bowel diseases. Inflamm Bowel Dis 2008;14(11):1585–1596.
54. Butterworth AD, Thomas AG, Akobeng AK. Probiotics for induction of remission in Crohn's disease. Cochrane Database Syst Rev 2008(3):CD006634.
55. Pastorelli L, et al. Emerging drugs for the treatment of ulcerative colitis. Expert Opin Emerg Drugs 2009;14(3):505–521.
56. Miele E, et al. Effect of a probiotic preparation (VSL#3) on induction and maintenance of remission in children with ulcerative colitis. Am J Gastroenterol 2009;104(2):437–443.
57. Sood A, et al. The probiotic preparation, VSL#3 induces remission in patients with mild-to-moderately active ulcerative colitis. Clin Gastroenterol Hepatol 2009;7(11):1202–1209.
58. Guandalini S, et al. VSL#3 improves symptoms in children with irritable bowel syndrome. A multicenter, randomized, placebo-controlled, double-blind, cross-over study. J Pediatr Gastroenterol Nutr 2010;51:24–30.

Subject Index

A

AA amyloidosis, 132

AAC, *see* Antibiotic-associated colitis (AAC)

AAHC, *see* Antibiotic-associated hemorrhagic colitis (AAHC)

Abdominal cramps, 7, 17, 21, 43, 45, 47, 228, 282, 301, 327, 417

Abdominal distension, 45, 83, 144, 215, 328, 344

Abdominal pain, 9, 17, 35, 40, 44, 46–53, 65, 67, 69, 77, 81, 83–84, 95, 109–110, 131, 142–144, 151, 160, 162, 166, 168, 194, 213, 215, 241–242, 244–245, 248, 253–257, 267, 276, 312, 318, 321, 325–326, 328–329, 333–336, 342–343, 345, 347, 350, 364, 371, 385, 434, 449

Abdominal X-rays, 87

Abetalipoproteinemia, 159, 169–171

Absorption, *see* Congenital disorders of digestion and absorption

Acanthocytosis, 170

Acetorphan, 398

Acetylcholine, 12, 178, 352, 403–404

Acetylcholinesterase inhibitors, 396, 404

Acetylsalicylic acid, 198

Achlorhydria, 192, 248, 259, 267, 272

Acid-tolerant aerobic organisms, 191

Acquired immunodeficiency syndrome (AIDS), 6, 51, 121, 368, 414, 453, 466

Acrodermatitis enteropathica (AE), 172–173

Actinobacter, 227

Acute diarrhea
  community-acquired, 4–6
  diagnosis, 20
  hospital-acquired, 6–7
  traveler's, 7–8

Acute gastroenteritis, 8, 290, 295, 349

Acute mesenteric ischemia (AMI), 251–253

Acute proctosigmoiditis, 416

Acute radiation injury, 143, 152

Adalimumab, 73, 76

ADAMTS-13, 44

Addison's disease (AD), 370–371
  causes and clinical features, 370
  gastrointestinal symptoms, 371
  treatment, 371

Adenosine triphosphate (ATP), 10

Adrenal gland, 370–373

Adult-type hypolactasia, 159, 163–164

Adverse reactions to food, 106–107

Aerobic organisms, 191

Aeromonas hydrophila, 47

AIDS, *see* Acquired immunodeficiency syndrome (AIDS)

Albendazole, 41, 49

Albumin, 68, 108, 118–120, 122–123, 125–126, 128, 130–134, 153, 345

Alcohol-related diarrhea, 379–387
  absorption and metabolism of alcohol in gut, 381
    "bacteriocolonic" pathway of ethanol oxidation, 381
    concentration of acetaldehyde, 381
    ethanol absorption, 381
    first-pass metabolism, 381
    gastrointestinal neuromuscular injury, 381
    mucosal permeability, 381
    non-oxidative metabolism, 381
  classification, 380–381
    alcohol hangover (*veisalgia*), 381
    alcohol-related organ dysfunction, 381
    alcohol withdrawal, 380
    concurrent dietary indiscretion, 380
  clinical presentation, 381–386
    alcohol hangover or *veisalgia*, 385
    alcohol-induced organ dysfunction, 385

From: *Diarrhea, Clinical Gastroenterology*
Edited by: S. Guandalini, H. Vaziri, DOI 10.1007/978-1-60761-183-7
© Springer Science+Business Media, LLC 2011

Alcohol-related diarrhea (*cont.*)
   alcohol withdrawal syndrome
      (AWS), 385
   binge drinking, 381–385
   chronic alcoholics, 385
   toxic alcohol-induced diarrhea, 385
   etiopathogenesis, 381–386
   pathophysiology of acute
      alcohol-induced diarrhea, 382–383
   pathophysiology of chronic
      alcohol-induced diarrhea, 383–384
   treatment, 386–387
   acute alcohol-related diarrhea, 386
   antibiotics, 387
   benzodiazepines, 387
   cholestyramine, 387
   chronic alcohol-related diarrhea,
      386–387
   clonidine, 387
   niacin and oral vitamin C, 387
   thiamine, 386
   ursodeoxycholic acid, 387
Allergic gastroenteropathy, 123
Allergy, 20, 87, 105–115, 220, 332, 394–395
Allopurinol, 416
Alopecia, 172, 218
Alpha 1-antitrypsin, 114, 128–130
Alpha 2-adrenergic agonist, 367, 443, 453
Alzheimer's disease, 404
Amebic colitis, 6, 21
American Academy of Microbiology report, 2
Amifostine, 149–150
Amino acids, 10, 118–120, 124, 165,
   167–169, 172, 274–275, 287, 382, 384
Aminoglycosides, 46, 231, 399
Aminosalicylates, 62, 65, 74, 76, 99, 247, 396
5-Aminosalicylic acid (5-ASA), 149
5-Aminosalicylate (5-ASA), 65, 149–150
Amitriptyline, 334
Amoxicillin, 74, 199, 412
Ampicillin, 39, 232, 412
Amyloidosis, 11, 16, 121, 132, 315, 435, 440
Anaerobic organisms, 191, 196, 364
Anemia, 23, 49, 67–68, 96, 110–111,
   122–123, 131, 145, 160, 169, 193,
   215–216, 226, 248, 251, 267, 274, 329,
   345, 360, 364–365, 371–373, 436
Anorectal dysfunction and incontinence, 364
   anal sphincter dysfunction, 364
   fecal incontinence, 364
   sphincter dysfunction, 364
Antacids, 19–20, 306, 330, 397, 402, 412
Anthraquinones, 300, 304–307, 403

Antibiotic-associated colitis (AAC), 48, 398
Antibiotic-associated hemorrhagic colitis
   (AAHC), 47
Antibiotics
   in bacterial overgrowth, 198–201
   drug-induced diarrhea, 412–413
   in IBD, 74
   in IBS, 336
   prevention of, associated diarrhea, 465
   in radiation enterocolitis, 151
Antibodies, 73, 75–76, 96, 108, 112, 129, 131,
   172, 219, 247, 249, 330, 345, 361–362,
   366, 372
Anticholinergics, 131, 333–334, 352–353,
   396, 404, 406, 443, 448, 452–453
Antidepressants, 334
   amitriptyline, 334
   desipramine, 334
   fluoxetine, 334
   imipramine, 334
   nortriptyline, 334
   paroxetine, 334
   serotonin reuptake inhibitors (SSRI), 334
   sertraline, 334
   tricyclic antidepressants (TCA), 334
Antidiarrheal agents, 53, 78, 151, 335,
   399, 417
Anti-endomysial IgA antibody
   (EMA-IgA), 219
Anti-endomysium antibodies, 219
Anti-inflammatory agents, 20, 114, 202, 255
Antimotility agents, 44, 53, 290, 364
Antiplasmin therapy, 132
Antiretroviral therapy, 50, 396, 398–399
Anti-social personality disorder, 300
Antispasmodic agents, 333
Anti-tissue transglutaminase IgA (TTG-IgA),
   96, 219, 222, 319
APOB gene, 161, 170
Apolipoprotein B, 161, 170–171
Appendectomy, 242–245
Appendicitis, 41, 46, 84, 111, 239,
   243–245, 293
APS, *see* Autoimmune polyglandular
   syndromes (APS)
Aquaporins (AQP), 283, 286, 289
Arf6 endocytic pathway, 286
Arthralgias, 38, 51, 95, 97, 216, 228–229
Arthritis, 41, 46–47, 67, 95, 190, 193, 216,
   225–226, 229–230, 416
Aspirin therapy, 348
Athletes' GI symptoms, 427–428
Atropine, 98, 410, 417, 451–453

Subject Index

Attapulgite, 447–448
Atypical celiac disease with extraintestinal
    manifestations
  arthritis and arthralgia, 216
  chronic hepatitis and
      hypertransaminasemia, 216
  dental enamel hypoplasia, 216
  dermatitis herpetiformis, 215–216
  iron deficiency anemia, 216
  neurological manifestation, 217
  osteopenia/osteoporosis, 217
  psychiatric disorders, 217
  short stature and delayed puberty, 216
Auranofin, 399, 416
Autoantibody testing, 129
Autoimmune disorders, 95–96, 210, 218
Autoimmune polyglandular syndromes
    (APS), 371–373
  type I, 371–372
    autoimmune hypoparathyroidism, 371
    autoimmune regulator (AIRE) gene, 371
    cholecystokinin deficiency, 372
    lymphangiectasia, 372
    muco-cutaneous candidiasis, 372
    superimposed Giardia infection, 372
  type II, 372–373
    myasthenia gravis, 372
    primary hypogonadism, 372
Autoimmune regulator (AIRE) gene, 371
Autonomic neuropathy, 11, 19, 315,
    362–364, 367
Azathioprine, 73, 75, 99, 124, 373
Azithromycin, 38, 42–44, 47, 54, 291–292
Azotorrhea, 182

B

Bacillus cereus, 282, 294
Bacterial overgrowth, 189–203, 363, 380
  clinical conditions
    gastroesophageal reflux, 195
    inflammatory bowel disease, 195
    irritable bowel syndrome, 194–195
    short bowel syndrome, 194
  14C xylose breath test, 364
  defined, 192
  diagnosis, 195–198
  mechanisms, 192–193
  symptoms, 193–194
  treatment
    antibiotics, 198–201
    dietary support, 201–202
    mechanical methods, 202
Bacteriotherapy, 46
Bacteroides, 191, 349

Balantidium coli, 49
Balsalazide, 149–150
Barium enema, 70, 94, 146–148, 239
Barium X-ray, 129
Benign conditions, 112, 125, 332, 345, 351
Benzodiazepines, 335, 386–387
Beta blockers, 370
Beta cells, 167
Beta-fructofuranoside fructohydrolase,
    165, 352
Bethanecol, 403
Bifidobacteria, 77, 191, 198, 461, 465
Bilateral retinal detachments, 122
Bile acid breath test, 360
Bile acid deficiency, 145, 171, 380, 386
Bile acid diarrhea, 13, 145, 152, 349, 383,
    386–387
Bile acid malabsorption, 97, 159, 171,
    311–312, 315, 348–349, 353, 360, 366,
    369–370, 380, 383, 386, 408–409,
    439–441, 450
Bile salt, 12–13, 15, 64, 66, 77, 169, 171, 246,
    347, 349, 353, 383, 387, 405–406
Bile salt-induced diarrhea, 12, 66, 246,
    347, 387
Biliary tract disease, 47
Biofeedback, 336, 366
Biomarkers, 85, 89, 272
Biopsy, 40, 47–49, 69, 71, 87, 95, 111, 124,
    142, 195, 198, 219, 230–232, 240, 249,
    255, 318–319, 321, 330, 345, 360–363,
    366, 439
Bisacodyl, 304, 306–308, 403
Bismuth subsalicylate, 53–54, 98, 398, 417,
    447, 449–450
Blastocystis hominis, 6, 49
Bloating, 23, 39, 64, 77, 83–84, 90, 151,
    193–194, 201, 215, 218, 228, 276, 327,
    333, 336–337, 426, 449, 454
Blood–brain barrier, 231, 451–452
Bloody diarrhea, 5, 17, 41, 45–47, 53–54, 65,
    144, 239–240, 242, 252, 301
Bone marrow
  biopsy, 240, 249
  transplantation, 125, 249, 373
Bowel dilation, 202
Bowel obstruction, 144, 151, 153–154,
    241, 249
Bowel perforation, 143
Brainerd diarrhea
  chronic secretory diarrhea, 321
  microscopic colitis, 321
  sporadic idiopathic secretory diarrhea, 321

478 Subject Index

Bristol Stool Chart, 437
Brush-border membrane, 118, 162, 164
Budesonide, 74–75, 98–99, 202, 366, 398, 447, 450
Bulk-forming agents, 443, 448–449

C

Ca^{2+}-activated Cl^- channel (CLCA), 282–283, 288
Caffeine, 77, 107, 337, 394, 396, 417, 427, 434
Calcitonin
  -secreting pancreatic endocrine tumors, 276
  thyroid-secreting, 12, 257, 408
Calcium channel blockers (CCB), 453
Calcium supplements, 167
Calprotectin, 21, 69, 198, 316–318, 347, 414, 436, 439
cAMP, *see* Cyclic adenosine monophosphate (cAMP)
Campylobacter, 4, 8, 14, 20–21, 35–36, 41, 51, 65–66, 68, 348
Cancer therapies, 125, 399–400
Capsule endoscopy, 126, 130, 147, 414
Carbamazepine, 98, 396, 404
Carbohydrate assimilation disorders, 162–167
  adult-type hypolactasia, 163–164
  congenital lactase deficiency, 162–163
  Fanconi–Bickel syndrome (FBS), 166–167
  fructose malabsorption, 166
  glucose–galactose malabsorption, 165–166
  sucrase–isomaltase deficiency, 164–165
Carbohydrate fermenters, *see* Small bowel bacterial overgrowth (SBBO)
Carbohydrate malabsorption, 19, 122, 163, 166–167, 312, 315, 319–320, 346, 350, 401, 436
Carcinoid syndrome, 12, 19, 121, 252, 257–258, 269–271, 315, 359, 368, 404, 454
CARD15, 64
Cardiac medications, 415–416
  digoxin, 415
  HMG-CoA reductase inhibitors, 416
  Na^+, K^+-ATPase pathway, 415
  ticlopidine, 415
Cardiomegaly, 129
Cardiovascular mortality, 184
CCK-A, 179–180
CCK-B, 179–180
CCK-mediated mechanisms, pancreatic secretion, 179

CD, *see* Celiac disease (CD)
CD4 T-helper cells, 6, 64, 211, 373, 466
$CD8^+$ lymphocytes, 106, 212
CDC, *see* Centers for Disease Control and Prevention (CDC)
Ceftriaxone, 42, 291–293
Celiac disease (CD), 14, 96, 119, 122, 146, 198, 210–212, 301, 312, 316, 330, 342, 344–345, 360–361, 365–366, 369–370, 435
  clinical presentation
    associated diseases, 217–218
    atypical, extraintestinal manifestations, 215–217
    typical, gastrointestinal manifestations, 214–215
  complications
    increased mortality rate, 222
    refractory celiac disease, 221–22
  diagnosis, role of serology, 219
  epidemiology, 210–211
  gluten free diet, 440
  pathophysiology
    immunology, 211–212
    pathology, 212
  serology, 360
  small bowel biopsy, 360
  treatment, 220–221
    ALV-003, 221
    American Dietetic Association guidelines, 220
    octapeptide (larazotide), 221
  in type 1 diabetes mellitus[a], 361
  type of screening test, 360
Celiac sprue, 94, 96, 99, 184
Cellulitis, 47, 132
Centers for Disease Control and Prevention (CDC), 2, 88, 322, 432
Central venous pressure, 127
Cephalexin, 201
Cephalosporins, 43, 47, 201, 256, 412
Certolizumab pegol, 73, 76
CFTR, *see* Cystic fibrosis transmembrane regulator (CFTR)
cGMP, 10–12, 283–284, 287, 290, 382
Charcot–Leyden crystals, 123, 129
Chemotherapy, 125, 248
  causing epithelial cell damage, 411
  and immunomodulators, 409–412
    EGF-receptor inhibitors, 411
    flavopiridol, 411–412
    fluorouracil, 410–411
    gradients from crypt to villus, 409

Subject Index

irinotecan, *see* Irinotecan-induced
  diarrhea
mycophenolic acid, 410
neutropenic enterocolitis, 411
oxaliplatin, 411
sorafenib-induced diarrhea, 411
transplant immunosuppressives, 410
tyrosine kinase inhibitor, 411
uracil–tegafur, 410
inducing diarrhea, 15, 23, 295, 396, 398,
  404, 409–412, 453
Cholecystectomy, 15, 274, 312, 450
Cholera, 5, 11–12, 38, 272, 282–285, 322,
  444–445
Cholestyramine, 77, 99, 145, 150, 152, 171,
  246, 349, 353, 360, 366, 386–387, 396,
  399, 407, 409, 412, 440, 448, 450
Cholinergic drugs, 403
  bethanecol, 403
  G protein-coupled muscarinic receptors,
    403
  G_q–PLC–IP3 pathway, 404
Chronic diarrhea, 3, 9, 15, 17–18, 22–23, 37,
  40, 93–94, 99, 111, 126, 215, 238, 245,
  257, 265–276, 288, 299–303, 311–312,
  314–315, 317–321, 342, 358, 362–365,
  371, 407, 409, 432–433, 435–436,
  443–455
Chronic diarrhea, empiric treatment, 443–455
  agents used, 447–455
    anticholinergics, 452
    atropine, 453
    attapulgite, 447
    bismuth subsalicylate, 449
    budesonide, 450
    bulk-forming agents, 448
    calcium channel blockers (CCB), 453
    cholestyramine, 450
    clonidine, 453
    codeine, 452
    dicyclomine, 453
    diphenoxylate with atropine, 452
    glycopyrrolate, 453
    H1 antagonists, 454
    hyoscyamine, 453
    kaopectate, 447
    loperamide, 451
    methylcellulose, 449
    methylscopolamine, 453
    octreotide, 453
    opiates, 451
    paregoric, 451
    phenothiazines, 454

polycarbophil, 449
probiotics, 454
proton pump inhibitors and H2
  antagonists, 454
psyllium, 449
racecadotril, 452
serotonin antagonists, 454
silicates, 447
tincture of opium, 452
antibiotic therapy, 447
anti-diarrheal agents, 447
dietary modifications, 446
oral rehydration solutions, 444–445
probiotics in GI diseases, 454
Chronic diarrheal disorders in adults
  carcinoid/carcinoid syndrome, 257–258
  chronic pancreatitis, 259
  gastrinomas/Zollinger–Ellison syndrome,
    258
  medullary thyroid cancer, 259
  somatostatinomas, 259
  tumors, 257
  vasoactive intestinal peptide tumor
    (VIPoma), 258–259
Chronic gastritis, 118
Chronic hepatitis and hypertransaminasemia,
  216
Chronic idiopathic diarrhea, 311–323
  Brainerd diarrhea, 321–322
  categories of, 312–313
  definition, 313–314
    fecal confusion/incontinence, 313
    loose stool consistency, 313
    pourable watery stools, 313
    soft or unformed stools, 313
    stool frequency/viscosity, 313
  differential diagnosis of, 314–317, 319–320
    bile acid malabsorption, 320
    causes, 312
    cholecystectomy, 312
    gastric surgery, 312
    intestinal resection, 312
    chronic idiopathic secretory diarrhea, 320
    Clostridium difficile toxin, 314
    colitis/Crohn's disease, 317
    gluten-sensitive enteropathy, 320
    malabsorption problems, 317
    negative microbiological studies, 319
    pancreatic exocrine insufficiency, 317
    protozoal stool antigen tests, 314
    quantitative stool collection, 317
    sugar malabsorption, 320
  duration, 314

Chronic idiopathic diarrhea (*cont.*)
etiologies, 322
Centers for Disease Control (CDC), 322
fluoroquinolones, 322
metronidazole, 322
sporadic/epidemic chronic idiopathic
secretory diarrhea, 322
evaluation of, 318–319
history and course of, 320–321
computerized tomography, 321
laxative screening, 321
opiate antidiarrheals, 321
quantitative culture of jejuna aspirate,
321
quantitative stool collection, 321
management of, 322–323
bile acid binders, 322
intravenous fluids, 322
oral rehydration solution, 322
tests, 317–319
Chronic idiopathic secretory diarrhea, 312,
320–323
Chronic infections, 9, 39
Chronic/intermittent watery diarrhea, 23, 41,
95, 320
Chronic mesenteric ischemia (CMI),
251–254
Chronic pancreatitis, 168, 178–179, 182, 184,
252, 259, 360, 380, 383, 446
Chronic peripheral lymphedema, 122
Chronic radiation injury, 143, 147–148, 150,
153–154
Churg–Strauss syndrome, 85
Chylomicron retention disease (CMRD),
161, 171
Chylous ascites, 122, 243
Ciprofloxacin, 41–42, 54, 74, 78, 199,
291–293, 387
Cirrhosis, 132–134, 169, 192, 251, 290, 380,
386, 406
Cisplatin, 142, 410–411
Citrobacter rodentium, 289
Citrulline, 169
Clavulanate, 74, 201
CLCA, *see* Ca^{2+}-activated Cl^- channel
(CLCA)
Clonidine, 358, 362–363, 386–387, 446, 448,
453–454
Clostridia, 191
Clostridium difficile, 7, 14, 20–21, 35–36,
44–45, 48, 51, 53–54, 66, 68, 121, 129,
193, 238, 252, 256–257, 314, 398,
412–413, 417, 464–465

colitis, 256–257
toxin, 314
Clostridium difficile infection (CDI), 3, 5–7,
44–46, 66, 71, 74, 78
complications, 44
treatment, 45
Clostridium perfringens, 21, 36, 48, 51, 53,
282, 294
Cl^- secretion, 282–288, 405, 413
CMRD, *see* Chylomicron retention disease
(CMRD)
CMV, *see* Cytomegalovirus (CMV)
Codeine, 77, 323, 365, 448, 451–452
Cognitive behavioral therapy, 336
Colchicine, 20, 396, 399, 416
Colectomy, 45, 66, 76, 99, 251, 254, 257, 449
Colicky abdominal pain, 48, 144
Colitis, *see* Gastroenteritis and colitis
Colocutaneous fistula, 240, 250
Colonic mucosa, 44, 46, 70, 94–96, 147, 347,
412, 427, 439
Colonic mucosal biopsy, 95
Colonoscopy, 47, 70, 94, 146, 317, 439–440
Community-acquired diarrhea
bacterial causes, 4–5
protozoal infections, 5–7
viral-induced, 4
Complex diarrheas, 399–400
"PINES" regulatory system in intestine, 400
Computerized tomography (CT), 70, 148–149
Congenital chloride diarrhea, 13, 288
Congenital disorders of digestion and
absorption
carbohydrate assimilation disorders,
162–167
classification, 160–161
lipid assimilation disorders, 169–171
malabsorption, 170–173
protein assimilation disorders, 167–169
Congenital lactase deficiency, 14, 160,
162–163
Congenital sucrase–isomaltase and trehalose
deficiencies, 14
Congenital syndromes
bile acid diarrhea, 13
chloridorrhea, 13, 315
sodium diarrhea, 13
Congenital zinc deficiency, 172–173
Congo red staining, 127
Constipation, 23, 48, 78, 185, 194, 213,
327–328, 333
Contamination, 4–7, 38–43, 46, 48, 197, 220,
248, 321, 428

Subject Index

Corticosteroids, 72, 74, 98, 124, 198, 202
Cortisol binding proteins, 122
Cow's milk protein allergy, 106
C-reactive protein, 68, 129, 330, 427
Crohn's disease (CD), 11–13, 15, 18, 23, 46,
  62–66, 67, 70–78, 85, 125, 131,
  146–147, 195, 239, 247, 257, 315–317,
  365, 414, 435, 450, 468, 471
Cromolyn, 88, 124
Cryptitis, 87, 97
Cryptosporidiosis, 40
Cryptosporidium, 6–7, 9, 12, 18, 20–21, 36,
  40, 69
CT angiography, 252–253
CT enterography, 70, 146, 148, 312
CT scan, 129, 146, 148, 230, 244, 252,
  255–256, 258
"Currant jelly stool", 239, 241
Cyclic adenosine monophosphate (cAMP),
  10–12, 15, 38, 180, 283–284, 287–288,
  290, 369–370, 382
Cyclophosphamide, 124
Cyclospora, 6, 20, 36, 40, 51, 318–319
Cyclospora cayetanensis, 40
Cyclosporine, 72, 75, 373
Cystic fibrosis, 119, 168, 171–172, 180, 185,
  282–283, 344–345
Cystic fibrosis transmembrane regulator
  (CFTR), 11, 180, 281–283, 287
Cytokines, 12–15, 89, 133, 152, 193, 212,
  383, 385, 427
Cytomegalovirus (CMV), 18, 20, 36, 49–50,
  65–66, 69, 71, 121, 131, 316, 318–319,
  398, 411
Cytotoxic chemotherapy, 269, 273
Cytotoxins, 14, 36, 44, 47, 252, 256, 412

D

DBE, *see* Double balloon enteroscopy (DBE)
3DCRT, *see* Three-dimensional conformal
  radiotherapy (3DCRT)
Deamidated gliadin peptides, 210
Dehydration, 17, 35, 37, 43, 95, 145, 154,
  160, 165–166, 172, 215, 273, 301, 318,
  320, 322, 344, 385, 398, 426, 428,
  432–433, 435, 443, 445, 460, 463
Dental enamel hypoplasia, 216
Dermatitis herpetiformis, 215–216, 435
Desipramine, 334
Diabetes medications, 407–408
  acarbose and tolbutamide, 408
  exenatide, GLP 1 inhibitors, 408
  metformin, 407

Diabetes mellitus, causes of diarrhea in
  autonomic neuropathy, 362
    anorectal dysfunction and incontinence,
      364
    bacterial overgrowth, 364
    intestinal fluid and electrolyte transport
      abnormalities, 362
    intestinal motility abnormalities,
      363–364
  bile acid malabsorption, 360
  CD, 360–361
  diabetic microangiopathy, 362
  drug/diet induced, 359
  lymphocytic colitis, 360
  pancreatic insufficiency, 360–362
Diabetic diarrhea, 358–359
  chronic diarrhea, 364
    biochemical examination, 365
    blood count, 365
    celiac serology, 365
    electrolyte/fluid deficits, 365
    leukocytosis, 365
    malabsorption, 365
    qualitative stool fat test, 365
    quantitative stool fat excretion, 365
  clonidine, 446
  definition, 359
  diabetes mellitus, *see* Diabetes mellitus,
    causes of diarrhea in
  GI symptoms, 358
  osmotic diarrhea, 359
  treatment of, 365–368
    alpha-2 adrenergic receptors, 367
    carcinoid syndrome, 368
    clonidine, 446
    codeine, 365
    endogenous gastrointestinal hormone,
      368
    gastric antrum, 368
    loperamide, 366
    mechanisms, criteria for diagnosis,
      and, 366
    orthostatic symptoms, 368
    quality of life (QOL), 365
    synthetic octapeptide analog, 368
    VIPomas, 368
    water and electrolyte transport in small
      bowel, 367
  type I diabetes mellitus (T$_1$DM), 358
  type II diabetes mellitus (T$_2$DM), 358
Diabetic microangiopathy, 362
  monoclonal antibodies, 362
  type IV collagen, 362

Diarrhea, 122, 226, 381
  associated with irritable bowel syndrome
    (IBS), 16
  associated with radiation enterocolitis, 142,
    144, 148
  classification and diagnosis, 18–19
  definition, 3
  drugs causing, 15–16, 394–395
  epidemiology
    acute diarrhea, 4–8
    chronic diarrhea, 9
    persistent diarrhea, 9
  etiologies, 17–19
  functional/motility-related, 19
  iatrogenic-/drug-induced, 15
  inflammatory, 14–15
  management, 433
  osmotic, 13
  pathophysiology
    disturbances, 11
    physiology, 10–11
  secretory, 11
  syndromes, 10, 14, 321
  therapy, 432
  in thyrotoxicosis, 11
Dicyclomine, 77, 333, 453
Diffusely adherent *E. coli* (DAEC), 8, 36, 37
Diffuse wall fibrosis, 145
Dilutional diarrhea, 308
  hypertonic solutions (high stool
    osmolality), 308
  hypotonic solutions (low osmolality), 308
Di-peptides, 119, 167
Diphenoxylate, 77, 98, 323, 398, 417, 448,
  451–452
Disaccharidase deficiency, 344–345
Disease states associated with protein-losing
  gastroenteropathy, 121
Distal venous thrombosis, 132
Diversion colitis, 66
D-lactate, 193, 197
Donepezil, 404
Double balloon endoscopy, 130
Double balloon enteroscopy (DBE),
  147–148, 414
Downregulated in adenoma (DRA),
  282–284, 288
Down syndrome, 217–218
Doxorubicin, 269, 274–275
Doxycycline, 46, 199, 231, 291
Drug/diet induced, diabetes mellitus, 359
  laxative, 360
  medication elixirs, 360

    metformin administration,
     359
Drug-induced diarrhea, 15, 393–417
  antibiotics, 412–413
  cardiac medications, 415–416
  chemotherapy and immunomodulators,
    409–412
  cholinergics/seritonergics/neuromodulators,
    403–405
  complex diarrheas, 399–400
  diabetes medications, 407–408
  diet, 400–402
    carbohydrate-induced diarrhea, 401
  endocrine medicines, 408–409
  fatty diarrhea, 398–399
  gastroenterology medications, 405–407
  HIV medications, 414–415
  inflammatory diarrhea, 398
  laxatives, 402–403
  mechanisms, 395
  NSAID, 413–414
  smoking-induced laxation, 404
  watery diarrhea, 397
    osmotic diarrhea, 397
    secretory diarrhea, 397–398
Drug-induced microscopic colitis, 98
Drugs used in the treatment of EE
  anti-IL-5, 89
  cromolyn, 88
  eotaxin-3, 89
  IL-4, 89
  IL-13, 89
  mepolizumab, 89
  montelukast, 88
  omalizumab, 88
  reslizumab, 89
Drugs used in treatment of gastroenteritis
  and colitis
  albendazole, 41
  aminoglycosides, 46
  Ampicillin, 39
  azithromycin, 38
  bismuth subsalicylate, 53
  ceftriaxone, 42
  cephalosporins, 43
  ciprofloxacin, 41
  doxycycline, 46
  fluoroquinolones (FQ), 37
  foscarnet, 50
  fosfomycin, 44
  fumagillin, 41
  ganciclovir, 50
  iodoquinol, 49

Subject Index

loperamide, 53
macrolides, 41
mebendazole, 49
metronidazole, 39
nitazoxanide, 39
paromomycin, 48
penicillin G, 39
pyrimethamine, 40
rifaximin, 38
tetracycline, 47, 49
tinidazole, 40
TMP–SMX, 38, 40
vancomycin, 45
4-D syndrome, *see* Glucagonomas
Duodenal eosinophilia, 88
Duodenotomy, 268
D-xylose, 128, 147–148, 196–197, 366, 384
Dynamic psychotherapy, 336
Dysentery, 6, 8, 42–44, 47–50, 65, 291, 293

E

E. coli, 5, 8, 12, 18, 20, 35–37, 43, 66, 69,
        240, 248–249, 282, 287–288, 348, 466
    O157:H7, 43–44, 69
EAEC heat-stable enterotoxin 1 (EAST1), 287
EATL, *see* Enteropathy-associated T-cell
        lymphoma (EATL)
EBRT, *see* External beam radiotherapy
        (EBRT)
Echocardiography, 129
Edema, 41, 48, 96, 111, 121–124, 126–127,
        131–133, 143, 147, 160, 228, 249,
        276, 364
Egg protein intolerance, 106
EGID, *see* Eosinophil-associated
        gastrointestinal disorder (EGID)
EKG, 129
Elective surgery, 131
Electrogastrography (EEG), 346
Electrolyte absorption/secretion, 9, 97, 317,
        362, 367, 400, 403–406, 453
Electron microscopy, 41, 133, 165, 172,
        226–227, 230, 232, 384
Enamel hypoplasia, 216
Encephalitozoon intestinalis, 41
Endocrine/hormonal diarrhea, 358
Endocrine medicines
    calcitonin, 408
    levothyroxine therapy, 408
    SeHCAT testing, 409
Endocrine neoplasia syndrome type 2a/2b
        (MEN-2a/MEN-2b), 259
Endocrine neoplasms, 266
    Carcinoid

diagnosis, 267
symptoms, 266–267
treatment, 268–269
gastrinomas
    diagnosis, 266
    symptoms, 266
    treatment, 268
glucagonomas, 275
neuroendocrine tumors, causes of, 275–276
somatostinomas, 273–274
systemic mastocytosis (SM), 275–276
vipomas
    diagnosis, 272
    symptoms, 272
    treatment, 273
Endocrine tumors, 11, 248, 266, 272–273, 275
Endocytosis, 106, 286
Endophthalmitis, 47
Endoplasmic reticulum (ER), 287
Endoscopic biopsies in protein-losing
        enteropathies, 130
Endoscopy, 70–71, 87, 94
Endotoxin, 380, 387
Enkephalinase inhibitor, racecadotril, 448, 452
Entameba histolytica, 6, 8, 14, 36, 48
Enteric anendocrinosis, 159, 172
Enteric-coated enzymes, 183
Enteroaggregative *E. coli* (EAEC), 5, 287
Enterochromaffin cells, 287, 413
Enteroclysis, 70, 146
Enterocolitis, 42
Enterocytozoon bieneusi, 41
Entero-enteric fistulas, 145, 154
Enterohemorrhagic *E. coli* (EHEC), 4–5, 8,
        14, 20, 36, 43, 65–66, 69, 289
Enteroinvasive *E. coli* (EIEC), 5–6, 20, 36, 43
Enterokinase deficiency, 107, 159, 168
Enteropathogenic *E. coli* (EPEC), 5, 8, 36–37,
        281–282, 284–286, 288–289, 292
Enteropathy, 119
    protein-losing, 117–134
Enteropathy-associated T-cell lymphoma
        (EATL), 221
Enterotoxigenic *E. coli* (ETEC), 5, 8, 12, 18,
        20, 35–37, 52, 282–283, 287, 292
Enterotoxins, 282–283
    Cl^- absorption, 288
    Cl^- secretion, 284–288
    impairment of water absorption, 289
    mechanisms in, causing diarrhea, 282
    Na^+ absorption, 288–289
    pathogens causing diarrhea, 291–294
    treatment, 289–295

Enzyme immunoassay (EIA), 39, 44–45, 293
Enzyme replacement therapy, 168
Eosinophil-associated gastrointestinal
    disorder (EGID), 82–85, 87–89
Eosinophilia, 40, 49, 85, 87–88, 110,
    123, 129
Eosinophilic ascites, 83, 88
Eosinophilic colitis (EC), 82
Eosinophilic enteritis, 81–82
    complications, 83
    diagnosis, 84–87
    etiology, 81
    evaluation, 87
    levels in GI tract of children, 86
    perspectives, 89
    six-food/antigen elimination diet, 88
    symptoms, 82–84
    treatment, 88–89
Eosinophilic esophagitis (EE), 82, 107,
    110, 114
Eosinophilic gastritis (EG), 82
Eosinophilic gastroenteritis, 82–83, 89, 107,
    110–111, 114, 121
Eosinophilic gastroenteropathies, 109, 114
Eosinophilic inflammation, 83, 85, 88–89
Eosinophilic myocarditis/thrombosis, 85
EPEC, *see* Enteropathogenic *E. coli* (EPEC)
Epithelial damage, 97
Epstein–Barr virus (EBV), 249
ER-associated degradation (ERAD), 287
Erbitux® (cetuximab), 411
Erythema, 96
Erythema nodosum, 46, 67–68, 435
Erythrocyte sedimentation rate (ESR), 68
Esophagogastroduodenoscopy (EGD),
    71, 440
EspF, 285–286, 289
EspG, 284, 286, 288–289
EspG2, 284, 288
ESPGHAN, *see* European Society for
    Pediatric Gastroenterology, Hepatology
    and Nutrition (ESPGHAN)
ETEC, *see* Enterotoxigenic *E. coli* (ETEC)
Ethanol, 381–382, 387
European Society for Pediatric
    Gastroenterology, Hepatology and
    Nutrition (ESPGHAN), 219, 290
Exocrine pancreatic insufficiency, 177–186
Exopolysaccharides, 149
External beam radiotherapy (EBRT), 149
Extraintestinal manifestations of IBD,
    65, 67
Exudative enteropathy, 119–120, 122, 125

F
Facial edema, 122
Factitious diarrhea, 299–309
    causes, 306
    clinical presentation, 301
    colonoscopy, 305
        biopsies, 305
        melanosis coli, 305
    diagnostic evaluation, 301–302
        biochemical findings, 301
        chronic volume depletion, 301
        hypocalcemia, 302
        potassium depletion, 302
        suspicion and easily obtainable
            stool/urine tests, 301
    epidemiology, 301
    laxative screens, 304–305
        ipecac, 304
        "laxative panel", 304
        magnesium-containing laxatives, 304
        negative, 304
        urine and stool test, 304
    management, 308–309
    room searches, 305–306
    stool characteristics, 306–308
        dilutional diarrhea, 308
        non-gap diarrhea, 307–308
        osmotic diarrhea, 306–307
    stool studies, 302–304
        in chronic diarrhea, 303
        fecal fat, 302
        negative, 302
        stool osmolality, measurement, 304
        stool osmolar gap, 302
        stool volume, 302
Factitious disorder (Munchausen syndrome),
    300
Fanconi–Bickel syndrome (FBS), 166–167
Fatigue, 38, 85, 225, 273, 385
Fat malabsorption, 13, 15, 64–65, 144, 148,
    171, 182, 201, 317, 371
Fat restriction, 132
Fat-soluble vitamin deficiencies, 193, 384
Fatty diarrhea, 398–399
    drugs inducing steatorrhea, 399
FDA, *see* Food and drug administration (FDA)
Febrile gastroenteritis, 38
Fecal calprotectin, 198, 414, 436, 439
Fecal elastase test, 182
Fecal fat, 22, 148, 181, 302, 330, 386,
    436, 438
Fecal incontinence, 66, 145, 313, 318, 320,
    327, 363–365, 434, 449

Subject Index

485

Fecal lactoferrin, 52, 69, 316, 436
Fecal lactoferrin assay (FLA), 69
Fecal leukocytes, 20–21, 44, 52, 69, 95, 147,
316–317, 436, 438–439
Fecal occult blood, 17, 23, 69, 129, 316,
318, 436
Fecal osmotic gap (FOG), 316
Fever, 7, 17, 20–21, 37–38, 41–47, 49–54, 67,
69, 78, 85, 95, 226, 228–230, 244–245,
249, 256, 282, 293–294, 301, 385,
433–435, 451
Fibroblast growth factor 19 (FGF19), 349
Fibrosing colonopathy, 185
Fine needle aspiration, 276
Fistulae, 143, 152, 247
Fluoroquinolones (FQ), 37–38
5-Fluorouracil, 142, 269, 274
Fluoxetine, 334
Flutamide, 416
Folic acid deficiency, 185
Fontan procedure, 127
Food
  intolerance, 66–67, 105–106, 351
  patch test, 87
  poisoning, 4, 17, 20, 39, 48, 282
  protein-induced enteropathy, 111, 114
  protein-induced proctocolitis, 112, 115
  proteins causing food allergies, 108
Food allergy, 107–109
  diagnosis
    eosinophilic gastroenteropathies, 114
    food protein-induced enterocolitis
      syndrome (FPIES), 114
    non-IgE mediated, 114
    oral allergy syndrome and immediate GI
      hypersensitivity, 112
    protein-induced enteropathy, 114
    protein-induced proctocolitis, 115
  in infancy, 111
  pathophysiology, 106–108
    antigens, 106–107
    glycoproteins, 106
    IgE, 107
    T lymphocytes, 108
  skin lesions in, 106
  symptoms
    IgE mediated, 109–111, 113
    non-IgE mediated, 111–112
Food and drug administration (FDA), 40,
75–76, 185–186, 335, 352, 401, 447, 450
Foodborne diarrheal illnesses, 34
Food protein-induced enterocolitis syndrome
(FPIES), 111, 114

Foscarnet, 50
Fosfomycin, 44
Frank anasarca, 122
Fructose, 401
  malabsorption, 160, 163, 166
Fumagillin, 41
Functional diarrhea (FD), 341–353
  bacterial overgrowth, 348
    diarrhea in irritable bowel syndrome
      (D-IBS), 348
    small bowel bacterial overgrowth
      (SBBO), 348
  bile acid malabsorption, 348–349
    cholestyramine, 349
    FGF19 feedback inhibition, 349
    SehCAT, 349
  clinical evaluation, 343–344
    defecation frequency, 344
    enteric infections, 344
    family diseases, 344
    "four F's", 344
    laxative/antibiotic use, 344
    stool consistency, 344
  differential diagnosis, 344–345
    antro-duodenal/colonic manometric
      studies, 345
    blood test, 345
    breath test, 345
    causes of diarrhea, 345
    pancreatic insufficiency, 345
    secondary disaccharidase deficiency, 344
    stool test, 345
    sweat test, 345
  epidemiology, 343
    functional gastrointestinal disorder
      (FGID), 343
    Italian National Health Service, 343
  fecal microbiota, 349–351
    psychosocial and parental factors,
      350–351
    role of nutrition, 350
  infection, 347–348
    bacterial gastroenteritis, 347–348
    colonic mucosal abnormalities, 347
    gastrointestinal infectious processes, 347
    parasitic, 347
    post-infectious irritable bowel syndrome
      (PI-IBS), 347
  motility, 346–347
    gastric motility, 346
    small bowel motility, 347
  non-specific chronic diarrhea (NSCD), 342
  pathophysiology, 345–346

486 Subject Index

Functional diarrhea (FD) (*cont.*)
   microbiota, 346
   parental factors, 346
   pharmacological treatment, 352–353
      anticholinergic agents, 352–353
      binding resins, 353
      enzymes, 352
      probiotics, 352–353
   prostaglandins, 348
   "Rome III criteria", definition, 343
   terminology, 342–343
      diarrhea-predominant irritable bowel
         syndrome D-(IBS), 343
      irritable bowel syndrome of infancy, 343
      toddlers diarrhea, 343
   therapy, 351
      dietary intervention, 351
      ominous malnutrition, 351

G

Gallbladder disease, 274
Gamma aminobutyric acid (GABA), 335
Ganciclovir, 50
Ganglioside (GM1), 285
Gastrectomy, 131
Gastric acid secretion, 192, 246, 267, 454
Gastrinomas, 258, 266–269
Gastrocolic reflex, 66–67
Gastroenteritis and colitis, 33
   classification, 35–36
   colectomy in severe, 45
   epidemiologic features, 51
   etiology, 34–35
   evaluation, 50–53
      fecal leukocytes and lactoferrin, 52–53
      stool culture, 53
   indications for diagnostic testing, 52
   infections, 36–50
   mimicking appendicitis, 48
   recommended diet in, 54
   symptoms, 37–40
   treatment, 53–54
      antidiarrheals, 53
      antimicrobials, 53–54
      rehydration, 53
Gastroenterology medications, 405–407
   chenodeoxycholic acid, 405–406
   cholestyramine, 407
   5-HT$_4$-receptor agonists, 406
      cisapride and tegaserod, 406
   mesalamine, 405
   misoprostol, 405
   octreotide, 407

olsalazine, 405
   proton pump inhibitor, omeprazole, 406
Gastroesophageal reflux, 195
Gastrointestinal bleeding, 143–144, 228,
   251, 382
Gastrointestinal (GI) symptoms, 84, 89, 110,
   213, 275, 358, 365, 368, 371, 427–428
Gastrointestinal (GI) tract, 82, 85–87, 89, 106,
   190–191, 194, 202, 276, 359, 413,
   426–427, 447
Genetic testing, 166–167
Gentamicin, 199, 201
GERD, 266–267
GI, *see* Gastrointestinal (GI) tract
Giant hypertrophic gastropathy, *see*
   Menetrier's disease
Giardia intestinalis, 39
Giardia lamblia, 6, 23, 35, 39, 348
Giardiasis, 20, 23, 184
GI bleeding, 153
Gliadin, 221
Glomerulonephritis, 160, 169
Glucagonomas, 275
Glucocorticoids, 74–75
Glucose breath hydrogen test, 194
Glucose–galactose malabsorption (GGM),
   165–166
GLUT2, 160, 166–167
GLUT5, 160, 166
GLUT7, 166
Gluten, 108, 115, 210–222, 382, 440
Gluten-free diet (GFD), 215–222, 366,
   370, 440
Glycoproteins, 106, 287
Glycopyrrolate, 448, 453
Golgi apparatus, 164, 171, 287
Gram-positive/gram-negative organisms, 191
Granulomatous disease, 129
Guillain–Barré syndrome, 41

H

H. pylori, 123, 131, 267, 351
HAART therapy, 415
Hamartomatous polyps, 251
H1 antagonists, 454
Hartmann pouch, 255
Headache, 38, 51, 385
Heart failure, 251, 254
Heat-labile enterotoxin (LT), 287
Hematochezia, 64–65, 67, 95, 238–239,
   242, 429
Hemolytic uremic syndrome (HUS), 43,
   248–249

Subject Index

Hemorrhagic colitis, 43, 47, 69, 249
Heparin sulfate proteins, 133
Hepatic artery embolization (HAI), 271
Hepatic cirrhosis, 192
Hepatic protein synthesis, 120–122
Hepatocytes, 167
Hepatomegaly, 160, 167, 228–229
Hepatosplenomegaly, 169
Herpes simplex virus, 69, 316
Hindgut carcinoids, 269
Hippel–Lindau syndromes, 274
HIV, 3, 5–6, 9, 37–38, 47, 49–51, 129
   medications, 414–415
      abacavir, 415
      didanosine, 415
      HAART therapy, 415
      lopinavir, 415
      ritonavir, 415
HIV-1, 283, 285, 288–289
HLA DQ2, 211–213, 218, 371
HLA DQ8, 211–213, 218
HLA DR3, 210, 371–372
HLA DR4, 210
HLA haplotypes, 211, 218
Homovanillic acid (HVA), 248
Hospital-acquired diarrhea, defined, 6
Hospitalization, 2–3, 5–7, 39, 42, 50, 54, 432, 460, 465–467
Hyalinized fibrotic lamina propria, 147
Hydrogen breath testing, 165–166, 382, 441
Hydrolysis, 165, 167, 384
5-Hydroxyindoleacetic acid (5-HIAA), 252, 258, 270, 272, 318
5-Hydroxytryptamine, 270, 335
   (serotonin) 3 receptor antagonists, 335
Hyoscyamine, 77, 333, 448, 453
Hyperammonemia, 168–169
Hyper and hypo-function of thyroid gland
   in hypothyroidism, 370
   thyroid gland-related diarrhea, treatment of, 370
      broad-spectrum antibiotics, 370
      carbimazole, 370
      propylthiouracil, 370
   in thyrotoxicosis, 368–370
      hyperphagia, 368
      hyperthyroidism, 368
Hyperchlorhydria, 268
Hypercholesterolemia, 124
Hypereosinophilic syndrome (HES), 85, 88–89
Hypergastrinemia, 267–269
Hyperglycemia, 167, 272

Hyperparathyroidism, 259, 269
Hypertransaminasemia and chronic hepatitis, 216
Hyperuricemia, 185
Hyperviscosity syndrome, 127
Hypnosis, 336
Hypnotherapy, 336
Hypoalbuminemia, 111, 120, 123, 125, 127, 132–133, 228–230
Hypobetalipoproteinemia, 161, 170–171
Hypocalcemia, 230, 302
Hypochloremia metabolic alkalosis, 302
Hypogammaglobulinemia, 39
Hypoglobulinemia, 120
Hypoglycemia, 167, 360
Hypokalemia, 215, 230, 248, 259, 267, 272–273, 301, 384
Hypoproteinemia, 118, 120, 122–123, 125–127, 365
Hypotension, 215, 242, 256, 270, 301, 367, 454
Hypothyroidism, 359, 369–370, 373

I

Iatrogenic-/drug-induced diarrhea, 15
IBD, *see* Inflammatory bowel disease (IBD)
IBS, *see* Irritable bowel syndrome (IBS)
Idiopathic bile acid malabsorption (IBAM), 440–441
   defective intestinal fibroblast growth factor 23, 441
   diagnosis, 440
      bile acid-binding resin, 440
      cholestyramine therapeutic trial, 440
      SeHCAT test, 440
Idiopathic diarrhea, *see* Chronic idiopathic diarrhea
IgA, 39, 106, 120, 122–123, 219, 330, 435
IgE, 87–89, 106–107, 109–110, 112–114, 120, 122, 134
   mediated food allergy
      eosinophilic esophagitis (EE), 110
      eosinophilic gastritis, 110
      eosinophilic gastroenteritis, 110–111
      immediate gastrointestinal hypersensitivity, 109
      oral allergy syndrome, 109
IgG, 45, 108, 120, 122–123
IgM, 120, 122–123, 127
Ileal resection, 12–13, 15, 22, 144–145, 245, 440, 444
Ileal sodium-dependent/bile salt transporter (ISBT), 171

Ileocolonic pathogens
  bacteria, 41–49
    Aeromonas hydrophila, 47
    Campylobacter, 41
    Clostridium difficile, 44–46
    Clostridium perfringens, 48
    Escherichia coli, 43–44
    Klebsiella oxytoca, 47–48
    non-cholera Vibrios, 46–47
    Plesiomonas shigelloides, 47
    Salmonella, 41
    Shigella, 42–43
    Tuberculosis, 47
    Yersinia, 46
  parasites, 48–49
    Balantidium coli, 49
    Blastocystis hominis, 49
    Entameba histolytica, 48–49
    trichuriasis (whipworm), 49
  viruses, 49–50
    cytomegalovirus (CMV), 49–50
Imipramine, 334
Immune dysfunction, polyendocrinopathy, enteropathy, X-linked syndrome (IPEX), 373
  azathioprine, 373
  CD4+CD25+ T cells (regulatory T cells), 373
  eczema/atopy, 373
  hypothyroidism, 373
  lymphadenopathy, 373
  "scurfin.", 373
  thrombocytopenia, 373
Immunodeficiency, 18, 40, 121, 160, 169, 345, 435
Immunoglobulin A (IgA), 106
Immunoglobulin deficiency, 127
Immunomodulating therapy, 227
Immunomodulators, 62, 69, 72–73, 75–76, 132, 152, 247, 409–412
Immunosuppressants, 124
IMRT, *see* Intensity-modulated radiation therapy (IMRT)
Incontinence, fecal, 66, 95, 145, 313, 318, 320, 327, 358, 363, 434, 449
Indium 111-labeled transferrin, 130, 414
Infant food allergy, 105–106, 109, 111
Infections in colitis
  ileocolonic pathogens
    bacteria, 41–49
    parasites, 48–49
    viruses, 49–50
  small intestinal pathogens

bacteria, 37–39
parasites, 39–41
viruses, 36–37
Inflammatory bowel disease (IBD), 62–63, 147, 184, 195, 344, 434
  diagnosis, 65–67
  diarrhea in, 64–65
  diet in, 77
  etiology, 63
  evaluation, 67–71
  pathophysiology, 63–65
  side effects causing diarrhea in, 65
  symptoms, 67
  treatment, 71–78
Inflammatory diarrhea, 14–15, 69, 398
  causes
    IBD, 14
    intestinal blood flow, reduction in, 15
    Clostridium difficile colitis, 398
  diagnosis, 18
  vs. noninflammatory diarrhea, characteristics, 18, 21
Infliximab, 73, 76, 247
Intensity-modulated radiation therapy (IMRT), 149–150
Interferon-γ, 133, 212, 227, 232
Intestinal failure, 153–154, 246, 468
Intestinal fluid and electrolyte transport abnormalities, 362–363
  alpha adrenergic receptors, 362
  characteristics of true diabetic diarrhea, 363
  chemical sympathectomy, 362
  octreotide/clonidine, 362
  pathophysiologic syndrome, 362
  streptozotocin, 362
Intestinal ion secretion, 11, 288
Intestinal ischemia, 124, 143, 238, 251–252, 254
Intestinal lymphangiectasia, 121–122, 126–128, 130, 132
Intestinal motility abnormalities, 363–364
  14C xylose, 364
  diagnostic approach to chronic diarrhea, 363
  manometry, 364
  orocecal transit time, 364
  prokinetic/antimotility agents, 364
  radioisotopic methods, 364
Intestinal mucosa, 14, 53, 111, 118–119, 121, 127, 162, 191, 210, 213, 221, 227, 230–232, 258, 382, 387, 413, 426, 444
Intestinal obstruction, 66, 83–84, 110, 131, 257, 269

Subject Index

Intestinal perforation, 43
Intestinal permeability, 124, 126, 129, 133, 221, 387, 413
Intestinal protozoa, 6, 9
Intestinal resection, 202, 312
Intestinal serotonins, 180
Intestinal sucrase–isomaltase (SIMD), 352
Intestinal transport, 289, 382, 399–400, 453
Intra-abdominal lymphoma, 231
Intra-abdominal sepsis, 153
Intraepithelial CD8+ TCRαβ T lymphocytes (IEL), 212
Intraepithelial lymphocytes, 16, 94, 97, 114, 212, 347, 414
Intussusception, 44, 84, 239, 241–242, 249, 251, 257
Inulins, 401
Invasive infections, 11, 14, 35, 38–39, 41–44, 48–49, 78, 251, 301, 309, 316, 411
Iodine deficiency, 369
Iodoquinol, 48–49
Ipecac, 304
Iressa® (geftinib), 411
Irinotecan-induced diarrhea, 410–411
  Hange-Shashito (TJ-14), natural inhibitor, 410
  neomycin, 410
  oral cyclosporin, 410
  probenecid, 410
  SN38 glucuronide deconjugation, 410
Iron deficiency anemia, 96, 145, 216
Irritable bowel syndrome (IBS), 95, 194–195, 314, 325–337, 435
  clinical manifestations, 326–327
    altered bowel habits, 327
    chronic abdominal pain, 326–327
    constipation, 327
    diarrhea, 327
    gastrointestinal symptoms, 327
  diagnoses, 22
  diagnostic approach/criteria, 329–331
    American College of Gastroenterology (ACG), 329
    Rome and Manning criteria, 329
    rules, 330
    symptoms of, 329–330
  dietary modification, 332–333
    bloating and gaseousness, 333
    bulking of stool, 333
    dairy and gas-producing foods, 332
    effect of fiber's mechanisms, 333
    formation of gels, 333
    intake of fiber, 332

  serum immunoglobulins, 332
  visceral hyperalgesia, 332
  medications, 333–336
    alternative therapies, 336
    antibiotics, 336
    antidepressants, 334
    antidiarrheal agents, 335
    antispasmodic agents, 333
    benzodiazepines, 335
    5-hydroxytryptamine (serotonin) 3 receptor antagonists, 335
    psychosocial therapies, 336
  Rome III criteria, 328
  subtypes of, 328
  symptoms, 320
  treatment, 331–333
    dietary modification, 332–333
    general principles, 331
    patient education, 332
    therapeutic relationship, 331–332
Irritable pouch syndrome (IPS), 66
Ischemic colitis, 18, 44, 47, 66, 71, 78, 146, 251–252, 254–255, 316, 335, 439
Isospora, 6, 9, 35–36, 40, 69
Isospora belli, 40
Isotretinoin, 396, 416

J

Jejunal aspirates, 194, 197, 364, 366
Jugular venous pressure, 129
Juvenile polyposis coli, 240, 251

K

Kaopectate, 447–448
145-kDa enzyme, 162
KDEL, 287
Keratitis, 47
KIT tyrosine kinase inhibitors, 276
Klebsiella oxytoca, 47–48

L

Lactase deficiency, 13–14, 17, 107, 159, 162–163, 202, 220
Lactase-phlorhizin hydrolase (LPH), 160
Lacteal exudates, 130
Lactobacilli, 149, 191, 198, 465
Lactobacillus bulgaricus, 164, 461
Lactobacillus GG (LGG), 294, 460, 465
Lactoferrin, 8, 21, 52, 316–318, 436, 439
Lactose breath hydrogen test, 195
Lactose intolerance, 66–67, 151, 162–163, 166, 314, 332, 337, 389, 446
Lactulase, 402
Lactulose

breath hydrogen test, 194
breath testing, 336
Ladd's procedure, 243
Lamina propria, 86, 94, 97, 119, 123, 127, 133, 147, 211, 227, 228, 230, 382
Laparotomy, 130, 241–245, 253–254, 276
Laxatives, 402–403
   abuse, 134, 272, 307, 308, 311, 435
   magnesium-containing salts, 402
   Miralax, 306–307
   sodium phosphates, 402
   stimulant laxatives, 403
Laxative screen, 307–308, 307–309, 321, 436
L-Dopa, 397, 416
Lethargy, 215, 228, 241, 301
Leukotoxins, 39
Lipid assimilation disorders, 169–171
   abetalipoproteinemia, 170
   chylomicron retention disease, 171
   hypobetalipoproteinemia, 170
   primary bile acid malabsorption, 171
Listeria monocytogenes, 38
Liver diseases, 75, 128
Longitudinal intestinal lengthening and tailoring (LILT) procedure, 246
Loperamide, 53, 98, 150–152, 290, 323, 365–366, 397, 428, 448
LPH, *see* Lactase-phlorhizin hydrolase (LPH)
LPI, *see* Lysinuric protein intolerance (LPI)
Lubiprostone, 402
Lung cancer, 95, 411
Lymphangiectasia in protein-losing gastroenteropathy
   elevated central venous pressure, 127
   Fontan procedure causing, 127
   hyperviscosity syndrome, 127
   Waldenstrom macroglobulinemia, 127
Lymphangiography, 130
Lymphatic drainage, 126–127
Lymphatic hydrostatic pressure, 120
Lymphatic obstruction, 120–122, 125, 129, 134, 243
Lymphocytic colitis, 62, 93–96, 98–99, 315, 321, 358, 360, 366, 369, 415
Lymphocytopenia, 122, 125–126
Lymphoid follicle hyperplasia, 115
Lymphoma, 121, 127, 146–147, 154, 221, 231, 241, 315, 435
Lysinuric protein intolerance (LPI), 168–169

M
Maalox, 402
Macrolides, 42, 231

Macular edema, 123
Magnesium salt, 402
Magnetic resonance imaging (MRI), 70
Magnetic resonance (MR) enteroclysis, 146
Malabsorption
   bile acid, 97, 159, 171, 311–312, 315–316, 320, 346
   carbohydrate, 19, 122, 159, 162–163, 312, 315, 319–320, 342, 346, 350–351, 368, 436
   congenital disorders, 171–172
   fructose, 159, 160, 164
   glucose–galactose, 107, 159, 165–166
   syndromes, 10, 19, 197, 311
Maldigestion, 19, 148, 159, 317–319, 398, 438
   See also Malabsorption
Malignant conditions, 122, 125, 251, 267–268, 272, 276
Malingering, 300
Manning criteria, 328–329
Marsh, 212–213, 219
Mast cells, 16, 123–124, 275–276, 347
Mebendazole, 49
Medullary carcinoma of thyroid, 12, 19, 315, 357, 408
Medullary thyroid cancer, 259, 276
Megaloblastic anemia, 193
Melanosis coli, 300, 305
Menetrier's disease, 118, 122–123, 131–132
Meningitis, 42, 47
6-Mercaptopurine, 99
Mesalamine, 72, 74, 149, 202, 405, 471
Mesalazine, 152, 405
Mesenteric ischemia, 316, 429
Mesenteric venous thrombosis (MVT), 251, 254
Metabolic abnormalities, 95
Metastatic carcinoid, 271
Metastatic colorectal carcinoma, 411
Metastatic disease, 146, 258, 269, 273–274, 276
Methicillin-resistant *S. aureus* (MRSA), 39
Methotrexate (MTX), 71–73, 124, 247, 373, 410
Methylcellulose, 448–449
Methylscopolamine, 453
Metronidazole, 39–40, 45, 48–49, 72, 74, 78, 126, 200–201, 256, 322
Microabscesses, 41
Microscopic colitis
   characteristics, 143
      abdominal pain/weight loss, 95

Subject Index

arthralgias and autoimmune disorders, 95
autoimmune disorders, 95
celiac disease, 95
chronic/intermittent watery diarrhea, 95
dehydration, 95
erythema/edema, 96
fever, 95
IBS, 95
incontinence, 95
metabolic abnormalities, 95
weight loss/steatorrhea/iron deficiency
anemia, 96
colonoscopy, 94
defined, 94
epidemiology, 93–94
female predominance, 95
incidence with age, 95
lung cancer, 96
histologic features, 95
cryptitis, 95
epithelial damage, 96
intraepithelial lymphocytosis, 96
neutrophils, 96
pathophysiological mechanisms, 97
bile acid malabsorption, 96
drug-induced microscopic colitis, 97
steroid therapy, 97
sigmoidoscopy, 94
treatment, 98–99
aminosalicylates, 98–99
azathioprine/6-mercaptopurine, 99
bismuth subsalicylate, 99
budesonide, 99
cholestyramine, 98–99
corticosteroids, 98
diphenoxylate/atropine, 98
loperamide, 98
prednisone, 98
surgical, 999
Microsporidia, 6, 20, 40, 51, 318
Microsporidiosis, 40
Midgut volvulus malrotation, pediatric
surgical disorders, 242–243
Migrating motor complex (MMC), 347
Milk protein allergic enteropathy, 119
Milk protein allergy, 105, 209, 220
Mineral deficiencies, 77
Miralax, 306–307, 402
Mitogen-activated protein kinases
(MAPK), 64
Mixed secretory and osmotic diarrhea,
172–173
Montelukast, 88

Motilin, 15, 397, 413, 427
Motor functions in digestion, 10–11
MR angiography, 253–254
99mTc-labeled dextran scintigraphy, 130
99mTc-labeled human immunoglobulin, 130
MTP gene, 170
Mucosal bleeding, 41
Mucosal diseases, 19, 118, 121, 336
Mucosal erosions, 120, 122–125,
122–126, 414
Mucosal erosions/ulcerations
protein losing gastroenteropathy with
benign/malignant conditions, 125
cancer therapies causing, 125
Crohn's disease, 125
hypoalbuminemia, 125
hypoproteinemia, 125
nonsteroidal anti-inflammatories
(NSAID) causing, 125
protein losing gastroenteropathy without
allergic gastroenteropathy, 123
H. pylori infection, 123
histology, 123
hypercholesterolemia, 124
hypoproteinemia, 122
Menetrier's disease, 122
symptoms, 123
systemic lupus erythematosis, 123
treatment, 124–125
usage of immunosuppressants, 124
Mucosal injury, 120, 125, 193, 276, 345
Multiple endocrine neoplasia I (MEN I),
258–259, 266
Multiple endocrine neoplasia syndrome type 1
(MEN-1), 258
Munchausen by proxy (Polle syndrome),
300, 304
Munchausen syndrome, 300
Myalgia, 38, 40
Mycobacterium, 23, 69, 231
Mycobacterium avium complex (MAC), 231
Mycobacterium tuberculosis, 23
Mylanta, 402

N

Na^+/H^+ exchangers (NHE), 283, 285, 288
Na^+/K^+-ATPase, 165
Natalizumab, 73, 76
Necrotizing enterocolitis (NEC), 238–241,
245, 467–468, 470–471
Neostigmine, 404
Neovascularization, 147
Nephrotic proteinuria, 128

Subject Index

Nephrotic syndrome, 120, 134
Neuroendocrine tumors
  medullary thyroid cancers (MTC), 276
  systemic mastocytosis (SM), 275–276
Neurofibromatosis type 1, 274
Neurogenin-3, 161, 172
Neurological manifestation, 217
Neutrophils, 21, 69, 97
NHE, *see* Na$^+$/H$^+$ exchangers (NHE)
Nitazoxanide, 39–40, 49
Nocturnal diarrhea, 67, 301, 327, 435
NOD2, 64
Noncaseating granulomas, 71
Non-CCK-dependent factors and pancreatic
    secretion, 180
Non-cholera Vibrios, 36, 46–47, 51
Non-correctible surgically strictures, 153
Non-enteric-coated enzymes, 183–184
Non-gap diarrhea, 307–308
  anthraquinones and bisacodyl, 307
    cascara, 307
    Danthron, 307
    rhein, 307
    senna, 307
  bisacodyl and sodium picosulfate, 308
  castor oil (*Ricinus communis*), 308
  oxyphenisatin and phenolphthalein,
      308
  rhubarb, ingestion of, 308
  thin layer chromatography, 307–308
Non-IgE mediated food allergy
  food protein-induced enterocolitis
      syndrome (FPIES), 111
  protein-induced enteropathy, 111
  protein-induced proctocolitis, 112
Non-inflammatory diarrhea, 12
  diagnosis, 23
  vs. inflammatory diarrhea, 18, 21
Non-neoplastic endocrine diseases, 357
  adrenal gland
    Addison's disease, 370–371
    APS, 371–373
  diabetic, 358–359
    chronic diarrhea, 364–365
    definition, 359
    diabetes mellitus, 359–364
    treatment of, 365–368
  hyper and hypo-function of thyroid gland
    in hypothyroidism, 370
    thyroid gland-related diarrhea, treatment
        of, 370
    in thyrotoxicosis, *see* Thyrotoxicosis
  IPEX, 373

Non-occlusive mesenteric ischemia (NOMI),
    253
Non-specific diarrhea, *see* Functional diarrhea
    (FD)
Nonsteroidal anti-inflammatories (NSAID),
    67, 97–98, 125–126, 276, 386, 398,
    413–414, 428
  acute proctocolitis, 414
  diclofenac, 414
  meclofenamate, 413
  non-invasive methods, 414
Non-structural protein 4 (NSP4), 283, 285,
    288–289
Noroviruses (Norwalk virus), 4, 7–8, 12, 18,
    20–21, 35–37, 51
North American Society for Pediatric
    Gastroenterology, Hepatology and
    Nutrition (NASPGHAN), 219
Nortriptyline, 334
NSAID, *see* Nonsteroidal anti-inflammatories
    (NSAID)
NSAID-induced injuries, 126
  treatment, 126
NSP4, *see* Non-structural protein 4 (NSP4)
Nuclear imaging, 125, 130, 134
Nutritional deficiencies, 153, 202, 228,
    274, 385

O

Obliterative endarteritis, 143
Occult blood, *see* Fecal occult blood
Octreoscans, 270
Octreotide, 131–132, 150, 152, 246, 258, 268,
    270–276, 362, 366, 397, 398, 407, 412,
    446–448, 453
Octreotide scan, 268, 274, 276
Ogilvie's syndrome, 404
Olestra, 402
Olsalazine, 65, 396, 405
Omeprazole, 268, 406
OMIM #182380, 165
OMIM #200100, 169
OMIM #201100, 172
OMIM 222700, 168
OMIM #223000, 162
OMIM 226200, 168
OMIM #227810, 166
OMIM #246700, 171
OMIM 276000, 168
OMIM #601295, 171
OMIM #610370, 172
Opiates, 276, 321, 323, 365, 417, 443,
    451–452, 452–454

Subject Index

Oral allergy syndrome and immediate GI hypersensitivity, 112
  associated with fresh fruits and vegetables, 109
  other food antigens, 109
  skin/lungs, 109
  symptoms, 109
Oral rehydration solution (ORS), 53, 289–290, 425, 444–445
  cereal-based ORS, 445
  hyponatremia, 445
  ingredient concentrations in reduced osmolarity ORS, 444
Oral rehydration therapy (ORT), 34, 38, 43, 53, 289, 433
Oral vaccines, 38
Orlistat, 396, 399, 402, 417
ORS, *see* Oral rehydration solution (ORS)
ORT, *see* Oral rehydration therapy (ORT)
Orthorexia, 401, 434
Osmotic diarrhea, 13, 162, 172–173, 306–307, 315, 317, 319, 397
  magnesium compounds with other agents, 306
    oral magnesium, 306
    polyethylene glycol 3350 (Miralax®), 306
    sodium sulfate (Glauber's salt), 307
Osteopenia/osteoporosis, 216–217
Osteoprotegerin, 8

P

Pancreatic calcification, 362
  hypoglycemic episodes, 362
  insulin sensitivity, 362
  secretin–cholecystokinin stimulation test, 362
Pancreatic endocrine tumors, 248, 273, 275–276
Pancreatic enzyme
  formulations and lipase content, 183
  supplement, 178, 181, 185, 446
Pancreatic enzyme supplementation, 185, 446
Pancreatic exocrine insufficiency, 181, 216
  CCK-mediated mechanisms in animals and humans, 179–180
  complications, pancreatic enzyme therapy, 185
  non-CCK-dependent factors affecting, 180
  physiology and definition, 181
  role of secretin, 180
  treatment, 181–183
Pancreatic insufficiency, 19, 178, 180–182, 184–186, 344–345, 360–362, 372, 380, 383, 386, 386, 438

Pancreatic islet
  cell tumors, 248
  tumors, 12
Pantoprazole, *see* Omeprazole
Paracrine-immuno-neuroendocrine system (PINES) regulatory system, 10, 400
Paradoxical diarrhea, 406
Paralytic ileum, 290, 404
Paraneoplastic syndromes, 247
Paregoric, 448, 451
Parenteral nutrition, 145, 153–154, 172, 195, 238, 245–246
Paromomycin, 48–49
Paroxetine, 334, 404
PAS-positive macrophages, 227–228, 230–232
Patch test, 87–88
Pathophysiological mechanisms, 97
Patients referral and evaluation, 431–441
  for bile acid malabsorption, 440
    SeHCAT test, 440
  classification of diarrhea, 432
  by gastroenterologists, 439
  history, 433–435
  IBAM, *see* Idiopathic bile acid malabsorption (IBAM)
  indications for children with acute diarrhea, 433
  physical examination, 435
    dermatitis herpetiformis, 435
    hyperthyroidism, 435
  by primary care physicians, 435–439
    Bristol stool chart, 437
    fecal calprotectin, 439
    Schilling's test, 436
    steatorrhea, 436
    stool analysis, 436
    stool osmotic gap, 438
    TSH and hemoglobin A1C, 436
    types of diarrhea, 438
  role of endoscopy, 439–44
    inflammatory bowel disease, 439
    microscopic colitis, 439
    positive celiac serology, 440
  for SIBO, 441
  treatment of dehydration, 434
PCR, 45, 48, 179, 226, 230–232, 292
Peanut allergy, 106, 108–109
Pediatric surgical disorders
  intussusception, 239–240
  midgut volvulus malrotation, 242–243
  necrotizing enterocolitis (NEC), 238–241
Penicillamine, 397, 416

Subject Index

Penicillin, 47, 231, 276
Penicillin G, 39, 231
Pentoxifylline, 150, 152
Peptide receptor radionuclide therapy (PRRT), 272
Pept-1 transporter, 118–119
Percutaneous endoscopic gastrostomy (PEG), 240, 250–251, 307
Period dominant power (PDP), 346
Periodic acid Schiff (PAS), 227–228, 230–232, 362
Peritonitis, 47–48, 131, 192, 241–242, 244, 249, 254–255
Persistent diarrhea, 3, 5, 8–9, 47, 49, 53–54, 162, 238, 247, 255, 287, 290, 314, 330, 343, 405, 446, 464, 467, 470
Phenothiazines, 453–454
Physician–patient relationship, 325, 326, 330–331, 337
Placebo response, 74, 88–89, 97–99, 149, 331–335, 404, 406–408, 449, 451, 462–463, 465–468
Plesiomonas shigelloides, 47
Pleural and pericardial effusions, 122
Polle syndrome, *see* Munchausen by proxy (Polle syndrome)
Polycarbophil, 448–449
Polycythemia, 429
Polyethylene glycol, 202, 304, 306–307, 402
Polylactosaminoglycan-containing receptors, 287
Polymorphisms, 8
Polypectomy, 251
Positron emission tomography (PET), 240, 249–250
Post-infectious irritable bowel syndrome (PI-IBS), 8, 41, 347, 464
Post-transplant lymphoproliferative disease (PTLD), 240, 249–250
Pre-albumin, 122
Prednisone, 72, 88, 99, 152, 471
Primary bile acid malabsorption (PBAM), 161, 171
Primary biliary cirrhosis, 406
Probiotics for diarrheal diseases, 459–471
acute diarrhea, treatment, 465–467
clinical trials in prevention of acute diarrhea, 461
Saccharomyces boulardii, 461
Clostridium difficile, 464
inflammatory bowel diseases, 468
Crohn's disease, 468
ulcerative colitis, 471

Lactobacillus GG (LGG), 468
NEC in newborn, prevention, 467–468
VLBW infants, 467–468
persistent diarrhea, treatment, 467
prevention of diarrhea, 461–464
antibiotic-associated diarrhea, 465
community acquired, 462
day-care acquired, 462–464
hospital acquired, 464
traveler's diarrhea, 464
Rotavirus, 464
VSL#3, 465
Probiotic therapy, 77, 145, 149–151, 201, 294, 336, 349, 399, 417, 454, 459–471
Proctopathy, 143, 145, 152
Proctosigmoidoscopy, 115
Propylthiouracil, 370
Prostaglandin analogues, 404–405
Protean manifestations, 87
Protein absorption, 118–119
amino acids, di- and tripeptides, 118–119
bacteria and cellular debris, 119
dietary requirement, 118
hydrolysis, 118
Pept-1 transporter, 118
Protein assimilation disorders, 167–169
enterokinase and trypsinogen deficiency, 168
lysinuric protein intolerance, 168–169
Protein kinase A (PKA), 180, 287
Protein-losing enteropathies, 132
clinical features
altered lymphatic drainage, 126–127
chylous ascites, 122
diarrhea, 122
edema, 122
frank anasarca, 122
intestinal lymphangiectasia, 122
malabsorption, 122
with mucosal erosions/ulcerations, 125–126
pleural and pericardial effusions, 122
without mucosal erosions/ulcerations, 122–125
yellow nail syndrome, 122
diagnosis, 127–130
protein absorption, 118–119
protein malabsorption and loss, 119–122
treatment, 131–133
antiplasmin therapy, 132
elective surgery, 131
fat restriction, 132
gastrectomy, 131

Subject Index

octreotide, 132
steroids, 132
Protein-losing gastrointestinal disorders, *see*
    Protein-losing enteropathies
Protein malabsorption and loss, 119–122, 182
  albumin, 119–120
  celiac disease, 119
  cystic fibrosis, 119
  diseases causing, 120
  hypoalbuminemia and hypoglobulinemia,
      120
  hypoproteinemia in, 120
  lymphatic obstruction/lymphatic
      hydrostatic pressure, 120
  lymphocytopenia, 122
  milk protein allergic enteropathy, 119
  mucosal erosions, 120
  mucosal injury, 120
  nephrotic syndrome, 120
  reduced concentrations of serum
      components, 122
  serum proteins, 119
  short bowel syndromes, 119
Protein malnutrition, 128
Proton pump inhibitors (PPI), 20, 98, 129,
    183–184, 192, 195, 202, 246, 267–268,
    397, 454
  and H2 antagonists, 454
Protozoal stool antigen tests, 314
PRSS1, 160, 168
Pseudomembranous colitis, 18, 121, 125, 256,
    316, 412, 414, 450
Psoriasis, 95, 435
Psychiatric disorders, 216–217
Psychotherapy, 336–337
Psyllium, 332, 448–449
Pulmonary proteinosis, 160, 169
Pyoderma gangrenosum, 67–68, 75, 435
Pyrimethamine, 40

Q

3q25-q26, 164

R

Racecadotril, 290, 294, 448, 451–452
Radiation enterocolitis
  classification, 142–143
  defined, 142
  diagnosis, 146
  endoscopy, caution in, 147
  medical therapy, 150–152
    antibiotics and probiotics, 151
    antidiarrheals, 150–151
    cholestyramine, 152

diet, 150–151
  hyperbaric oxygen (HBO), 152
  octreotide, 152
  prednisone and 5-ASA drugs, 152
  supplements, 151
  parenteral nutrition (PN), 153
  prevention, 148–150
  radiologic tests, 146
  risk factors, 144
  surgery, 153–154
  symptoms, 142–144
Radiation-induced diarrhea, 146, 150–152,
    154, 449
Radiation-related injuries, 125, 147
Radio Allergo Sorbent Test (RAST), 107,
    110, 112
Rectum, 10, 16, 35, 43, 62, 70, 72, 86, 110,
    143–144, 247, 269, 305, 327, 384, 451
Re-fistulization, 153
Refractory celiac disease, 221–222
Refractory diarrhea, 142–143, 153, 301, 453
Refractory sprue, *see* Refractory celiac disease
Rehydration, 34, 37–38, 50, 53–54, 289, 322,
    428, 434, 444–445, 460, 463
Reiter's syndrome, 41
Renal failure, 44, 248–249, 256
Respiratory disease, 47
Retinal-binding protein, 122
Reye's syndrome, 450
Rheumatologic disorder (HES), 88
Rifaximin, 38, 43–44, 54, 78, 151,
    200–201, 292
Rome criteria, 328–329
Ross Carbohydrate-Free formula, 166
Rotavirus(es), 4, 7–8, 12, 18, 20–21, 35–37,
    51, 211, 283, 285, 288–290, 294–295,
    460, 464–467
  affecting pediatric population, 37, 290
  cause of community-aquired diarrhea, 4–6
  -induced diarrhea, 290–291, 465–466
  in persistent diarrhea, 8–9
  responsible for hospital-acquired diarrhea,
      6–7, 471
  responsible for traveler's diarrhea, 8
  in secretory diarrhea, 11
  treatment in, induced
    racecadotril, 290
    with serum human immunoglobulins,
        295
  villous ischemia caused by, 37
Runner's diarrhea, 425–429
  clinical management, 427–428
    loperamide, 428

Runner's diarrhea (*cont.*)
    oral rehydration solutions, 428
    exercise effects, 426–427
    GI symptoms, 427–428
    incidence, 426
    race management, 428
    training implications, 428–429
        hematochezia, 429
        mesenteric ischemia, 429
        polycythemia, 429

S

Saccharomyces cerevisae, 165
Salmonella, 4, 7–8, 11, 14, 20–21, 35–36, 41–43, 51, 54, 65–66, 68, 348
SAR1B gene, 171
SBBO, *see* Small bowel bacterial overgrowth (SBBO)
Schilling test, 198, 386, 436
Schistosoma, 6
Secretin, 172, 179–180, 252, 258–259, 320, 362, 386, 427
Secretory diarrhea, 11–13, 16, 311, 315, 317–318, 320–323, 394, 397–398, 436
    chenodeoxycholic acid therapy, 405
    infectious, 12
    noninfectious causes, 13–13
    ursodiol, 405
    See also Chronic idiopathic secretory diarrhea; Non-inflammatory diarrhea
Selective serotonin reuptake inhibitors (SSRI), 404
    paroxetine and sertraline, 404
Selenium-75-homocholic acid taurine (SeHCAT), 440
    indicator of bile acid malabsorption, 440
75-Seleno-homocholic acidtaurine test (SehCAT), 348
Senna, 292, 298–299
Sepsis, 43, 46, 48, 77, 153, 238, 245, 247, 253
Septic arthritis, 47
Serial transverse enteroplasty procedure (STEP), 246
Serine protease-7 gene PRSS7, 168
Seronegative arthritis, 225, 230
Serotonin, 12, 16, 98, 180, 257, 259, 270–271, 276, 287, 334–335, 396, 404, 454
Serotonin 3 receptor antagonists, *see* 5-Hydroxytryptamine, (serotonin) 3 receptor antagonists
Serotonin reuptake inhibitors (SSRI), 98, 334, 396, 404
Sertraline, 334, 404

Serum chromogranin A, 270
Serum human immunoglobulins, 295
Serum proteins, 118, 120, 123, 134
SGLT1, *see* Sodium glucose transporter 1 (SGLT1)
Shigella, 4, 7–8, 11, 14, 20–21, 35–36, 42–43, 51, 65–66, 68–69, 348
Shock syndrome toxin 1, 39
Short bowel syndrome (SBS), 19, 22, 119, 171, 193, 194, 202, 239, 241, 245–246, 257, 316
Short-chain fatty acid (SCFA), 10, 164, 166, 194
Short stature, 160, 167, 216
    and delayed puberty, 215
SI gene, 164
Sigmoid, 10, 70, 87, 305
Sigmoidoscopy, 70, 94, 255–256, 330, 365, 439
Silicates, 443–444, 447
Sjögren syndrome, 217
Skin lesions in food allergy, 109
Skin prick test, 87, 107, 113
SLC7A7, 160, 168
SLC10A2, 161, 171
SLC39A4, 161, 172
Small bowel bacterial overgrowth (SBBO), 13, 19, 22, 65–66, 144–144, 148, 151, 189, 192–196, 311, 348, 380, 384, 386, 406, 436
Small bowel biopsies, 40, 111, 127, 198, 219, 318, 360, 366, 440
Small bowel disorders, 122
Small bowel enteroclysis, 146
Small intestinal and ileocolonic disease, 33
Small intestinal bacterial overgrowth (SIBO), 441
    hydrogen breath tests, 441
    test sugars, glucose and lactulose, 441
Small intestinal mucosal biopsy, 230–231
Small intestinal pathogens, 35
    bacteria
        Escherichia coli, 35
        Listeria monocytogenes, 36
        Staphylococcus aureus, 38–39
        Vibrio cholera, 35–36
    parasites
        Cryptosporidiosis, 40
        Cyclospora cayetanensis, 40
        Giardia intestinalis, 39
        Isospora belli, 40
        Microsporidiosis, 40
    viruses

Subject Index

norovirus, 37
rotavirus, 37
Sodium glucose transporter 1 (SGLT1), 160, 165, 282, 285, 289
Sodium picosulfate, 300, 308, 403
Solute carrier family 5, member 1(SLC5A1), 160, 165
Somatostatin, 152, 180, 252, 258–259, 267, 270–274, 315, 359, 363–364, 443, 453
Somatostatin analogue, octreotide, 152, 258, 453
Somatostatin-like immunoreactivity (SLI), 274
Somatostatinomas, 259, 267, 273–274
Somatostatin receptor SST2RA, 132
Sorbitol, 13, 19, 69, 330, 342, 344, 346, 350, 359, 364, 366, 382, 401
Sorbitol–MacConkey agar, 69
Soybean protein intolerance, 106
SPECT, 270
Sporadic/epidemic chronic idiopathic secretory diarrhea, 315
Squamous cell carcinoma, 411
16S ribosomal RNA, 226
SSRI, *see* Serotonin reuptake inhibitors (SSRI)
Staphylococcus aureus, 21, 35, 39, 282, 293
"Starbucks® diarrhea", 401
Stasis, 144–145, 202, 254, 363, 451
Steatorrhea, 95–96, 129, 181, 184–186, 193, 226, 363, 360–362, 386–387, 438
definition, 438
Steroids, 88, 96, 114, 132, 371, 450
Steroid therapy, 98–99
Stool
analysis, 133, 312, 436
antigen detection, *see* PCR
electrolytes, 303, 318, 362, 402, 436
osmolality, 22, 300, 302–304, 307–308, 317, 437
osmotic gap, 22, 437–438
pH, 163, 165–166, 307, 316, 438
tests, 21, 45, 256, 307, 318–319, 345
fat assessment, Sudan stain, 21, 316–318, 438
weight, 3, 22, 301, 312–313, 326, 413, 417, 428, 449
Streptococci, 191, 465
Streptococcus thermophilus, 164, 454, 461
Streptozotocin, 269, 274, 362
Strictures, 13, 62, 66, 70–71, 110, 129, 131, 143–147, 151–153, 185, 194

Strongyloides, 6, 88, 316, 411
Strongyloides stercoralis, 88
Sucrase–isomaltase deficiency, 107, 159, 164–165
Sudan stain, stool fat assessment, 21, 316–317, 438
Sulfamethoxazole, 38, 74, 78, 199, 201, 226, 293
Sulfasalazine, 72, 77, 149, 152
Superior mesenteric artery (SMA), 253
Surgical disorders presenting with diarrhea
in adults
acute mesenteric ischemia (AMI), 253–255
chronic mesenteric ischemia (CMI), 253–24
Clostridium difficile colitis, 256–258
intestinal ischemia, 251
ischemic colitis, 254–255
mesenteric venous thrombosis (MVT), 251
chronic diarrheal disorders in adults
carcinoid/carcinoid syndrome, 257–258
chronic pancreatitis, 259
gastrinomas/Zollinger–Ellison syndrome, 258
medullary thyroid cancer, 259
somatostatinomas, 259
tumors, 257
vasoactive intestinal peptide tumor (VIPoma), 258
pediatric chronic diarrheal disorders
inflammatory bowel diseases (IBD), Crohn's disease and ulcerative colitis, 247
juvenile polyposis coli, 251
percutaneous endoscopic gastrostomy (PEG), 250
post-transplant lymphoproliferative disease (PTLD), 249–250
short bowel syndrome, 245–246
tumors, 247–248
verotoxigenic *E. coli* infection and hemolytic uremic syndrome (HUS), 248–249
pediatric surgical disorders
appendicitis, 243–245
intussusception, 241–242
midgut volvulus malrotation, 242–243
necrotizing enterocolitis (NEC), 238–241
Surgical management in IBD, 76
Syndecans, 133

Systemic lupus erythematosus (SLE), 85, 124, 132, 254
Systemic mastocytosis (SM), 12, 275–276, 454

T
Tacrolimus, 373
T-cell receptor (TCR), 211
TDH, *see* Thermostable direct hemolysin (TDH)
Technetium 99m-labeled human serum albumin, 130
Technetium 99m scintigraphy, 130
Telangiectasias, 147
Tenesmus, 7, 17, 21, 35, 42–43, 64, 67, 143, 144, 435
Terminal ileum, 62, 68, 70, 87, 142, 144–145, 171, 191, 241, 245, 347
Tetracycline, 47, 49, 74, 78, 200, 291, 399, 416
Th1 cytokines, 64, 212
Th2 cytokines, 64, 84, 89
Theophylline, 15, 20, 395–397, 416
Thermostable direct hemolysin (TDH), 283, 288
Thin layer chromatography (TLC), 300, 304, 307–308
Three-dimensional conformal radiotherapy (3DCRT), 149–150
Thrombocytopenia, 44, 169
Thrombotic thrombocytopenic purpura (TTP), 43–44, 54
Thyroid binding proteins, 122
Thyroid disease, 360, 369–370, 370–372
Thyroidectomy, 276
Thyroiditis, 217–218
Thyroid-secreting calcitonin, 12
Thyrotoxicosis, 368–369, 408
  barium examination, 368
  cAMP signaling, 369
  COFA, 369
  gluten-free diet, 370
  pulmonary hydrogen excretion, 368
  T3 hyperthyroidism, 369
  thyroid disorders, 359
Tincture of opium, 397–398, 448, 451–452
Tinidazole, 40
Tissue infections, 47
Tissue transglutaminase, 96, 210, 219, 319, 330
Tissue transglutaminase 2 (TG2), 210
T lymphocytes, 108, 212, 250, 347
TMP–SMX, *see* Trimethoprim–sulfamethoxazole (TMP–SMX)

TNF-α (alpha), 62, 73, 75–76, 133
Tocopherol, 150–152
Toddlers diarrhea, *see* Functional diarrhea (FD)
Toxic alcohol-induced diarrhea
  diethylene glycol, 385
  isopropanol, 385
Toxocara, 88
Trace metal deficiencies, 122
Transactivator factor peptide (Tat), 283, 285, 288–289
Transforming growth factor-β (TGF-β), 15
Traveler's diarrhea, 4, 7, 16, 37, 38, 53, 292, 352, 450, 464, 469, 471
Treatment of microscopic colitis, 98–99, 450
Treatment of protein-losing enteropathies, 131–133
  antiplasmin therapy, 132
  elective surgery, 131
  fat restriction, 132
  gastrectomy, 131
  octreotide, 131
  steroids, 132
Trehalose deficiency, 14
Trichuriasis (whipworm), 49
Tricyclic agents, 334
Tricyclic antidepressants (TCA), 334, 337, 453
Triglycerides, 132, 169–170, 201, 387
Trimethoprim, 38, 74, 78, 199, 201, 226, 293
Trimethoprim–sulfamethoxazole (TMP–SMX), 38, 40, 43, 46–47, 231
Tripeptides, 118–119, 167–168
Tropheryma whipplei, 225
Tropical sprue, 14, 19, 121–122, 192
Trypsinogen deficiency, 159, 168
Tuberculosis, 18, 23, 36, 47, 76, 121, 130, 146–147, 316, 318, 411
Tumors, 11–12, 19, 247–248, 257–260, 265–269, 275–276, 307, 320–321, 453
  associated diarrhea, octreotide, 443
  chronic diarrheal disorders, 257
Tumor necrosis factor alpha (TNF-α), 64, 73, 75–76, 133, 427
Turner syndrome, 217
Type 1 (insulin-dependent) diabetes, CD associated with, 218
Type III secretion system (T3ss), 288
Typhoid fever, 41–42

U
Ulceration, 36, 41, 49, 70, 96, 120–121, 122–125, 143, 146–147, 249–250, 255, 258, 413

Subject Index

499

Ulcerative colitis (UC), 11, 18, 23, 61–64, 67, 70–74, 76, 85, 121, 125, 146, 239, 247–248, 257, 315–316, 369, 405, 439, 443, 449, 460, 470

Ulcerative jejunitis, 146

Ulcerative proctitis, *see* Ulcerative colitis (UC)

UNICEF, *see* United Nations Children's Fund (UNICEF)

Unilateral edema, 122

United Nations Children's Fund (UNICEF), 53, 290

United States Pharmacopeia (USP), 182–183

Upper extremity edema, 122

Urgent bowel movements, 312

UV epifluorescence microscopy, 40

V

Vancomycin, 45, 200, 256

Vandetanib, 276

Vanillylmandelic acid (VMA), 240, 248, 252

Vascular endothelial injury, 44

Vasoactive intestinal peptide tumor (VIPoma), 19, 240, 248, 252, 258, 267, 272–273, 315, 357, 363–364

Vasoactive intestinal peptide (VIP), 12, 240, 248, 252, 258, 272–273, 282, 318

Verotoxigenic *E. coli* infection, 248–249

and hemolytic uremic syndrome (HUS), 248–249

Vibrio cholerae, 5, 12, 18, 20–21, 35, 38, 282, 284, 289, 291

Vibrio parahaemolyticus, 5, 46, 281, 287–288

Video capsule endoscopy (VCE), 70, 147–148

Villous atrophy, 111, 212, 383, 416

Vipomas, 272–273, 368

Viral enteritis, 66–67

Virotoxin, 288–289

Virulent bacterial colonization, 238

Vitamin B_{12}, 148, 193, 198, 202, 232, 245, 384, 436

Vitamin C, 149, 380, 386–387

Vitamin deficiencies, 145, 154, 193, 380, 384

Vitamin D supplements, 164

Vitamin E, 149, 152, 170–171

Vitamin malabsorption, 122

Vomiting, 7, 20–21, 37–40, 47–48, 51, 83–84, 109–111, 123, 143–144, 160–161, 165, 168, 213, 241–242, 244, 248, 254, 276, 282, 293–294, 304, 321, 371, 384–385, 434, 451, 467

VSL#3, 149, 454, 460, 465, 470–471

W

Waldenstrom macroglobulinemia, 127

Water absorption impairment, 145, 259, 286, 427

Watery diarrhea/stools, 6, 8, 12, 17, 21–23, 37–38, 40–41, 43, 47–48, 95, 215, 240, 248, 252, 256, 259, 267, 272, 290–294, 315–316, 320–321, 387, 398, 452

Watery diarrhea, hypokalemia, and achlorhydria (WHDA) syndrome, 248, 259

Weight loss, 23, 40–41, 48–49, 67, 83, 95–96, 110–111, 123, 142, 144–145, 151, 189, 215, 225–226, 242, 249, 253, 267, 274, 301, 312, 318, 320, 364, 368, 398, 402, 435

Werner's syndrome, *see* Multiple endocrine neoplasia I (MEN I)

Whipple's disease, 184, 440

Central nervous system (CNS) involvement in, 231–232

clinical features, 228–230

diagnosis, 230–231

epidemiology and etiology, 226

erythrocyte sedimentation, 230

extraintestinal manifestations, 225, 226

treatment, 231–232

WHO, *see* World Health Organization (WHO)

Williams syndrome, 217–218

World Health Organization (WHO), 2, 34, 53, 289–290, 444

WR-1065, 149

X

X-rays, 87, 129–130

Y

Yeast overgrowth, 194

Yellow nail syndrome, 122

Yersinia, 14, 18, 20–21, 36, 46, 51, 69, 287, 293

Yersinia enterocolitica, 20, 43, 62, 287, 293

Z

ZES, *see* Zollinger–Ellison syndrome (ZES)

Zinc, 53, 159, 172–173, 275, 290, 380, 384, 386–387

Zinc deficiency, 172–173

ZIP4, 161, 172–173

Zollinger–Ellison syndrome (ZES), 12, 258, 266, 273, 454